THE ENCYCLOPEDIA OF

THE BRAIN AND BRAIN DISORDERS

CONTENTS

Foreword vii

Acknowledgments ix

Introduction xi

Entries A to Z 1

Appendixes

Appendix I: Self-Help Organizations 378

Appendix II: Professional Organizations 389

Appendix III: Governmental Organizations 391

Appendix IV: Helpful Web Sites 393

Appendix V: Read More About It 397

Appendix VI: Research Periodicals 399

Glossary 405

References 408

Index 412

1387

FOREWORD

This book represents an exciting revision of *The Encyclopedia of the Brain and Brain Disorders, Second Edition*. In addition to updating the previous edition, Facts On File asked Carol Turkington and me to update and incorporate the content from our *The Encyclopedia of Memory and Memory Disorders* into this book. The rapid pace at which researchers are advancing our understanding of these subjects makes staying current on the state of that knowledge quite challenging. We trust you will find the resulting text even more informative, entertaining, and understandable than the previous editions of both books.

We have kept the user-friendly features of the previous editions of *The Encyclopedia of the Brain and Brain Disorders* and *The Encyclopedia of Memory and Memory Disorders* that made them popular with readers. We have received feedback from school librarians, who tell us that high school students consult this and other books in the Facts On File Library of Health and Living series for information for term papers and school reports. College students (including my son and his friends at Clemson University) tell me the books in this series have been helpful in preparing more complex reports, research papers, and theses.

My physician and psychologist colleagues tell me that they appreciate the availability of such concise, thorough sources of information on sometimes esoteric concepts. I certainly intend to keep a copy next to my desk for quick reference. We have gone to great lengths to provide explanations that are simple but not simplistic, while thoroughly covering topics. Carol and I have attempted to make the information contained in each entry as thorough as possible, while making them understandable to a wide audience. Toward that end, I have shared drafts of this edition with many colleagues as well as with my wife, who is probably the most knowledgeable psychologist in the field of school psychology and early childhood neuropsychology that I know. I appreciate their ongoing feedback.

As you read through the entries in this book, note that terms in small capital letters have their own entries or a variant of the entry. We have moved references to organizations and Internet Web sites to appendixes at the back of the book and have included many additional online sources in the reference section. I am a child and adolescent psychologist and member of the American Psychological Association and, as such, I am also a subscriber to an increasing number of professional publications that have both paper and online editions. I find that downloading online versions of publications enables me to take the information with me anywhere and keeps my bookshelves free of old journals that I hesitate to toss. Six years ago, I never thought that I would have my entire music library and all 20,000 photographs in my collection on an iPod, along with all my home movies and the PowerPoint presentations for all the courses I teach.

Thank you for using this text. I hope you find it a valuable resource. I am already beginning to think about the next edition, which will probably come out about the same time as the next edition of the *Diagnostic and Statistical Manual on Mental*

Disorders. Already, there are rumblings about new and revised psychiatric diagnoses. Please feel free to forward any comments or suggestions to me in care of Facts On File if there is something you would like to see added to the next edition, or if you found particular entries especially helpful or confusing, or just to say hello. I look forward to hearing from you.

—Joseph R. Harris, Ph.D.

ACKNOWLEDGMENTS

As the coauthor of *The Encyclopedia of the Brain and Brain Disorders, Third Edition*, I find myself in the same position as the evening news anchor who parades in front of the cameras while the production team goes unnoticed. It is without false modesty, and with great pride and gratitude, that I have the privilege of thanking the following individuals.

Carol Turkington has always spoiled me with the works we wrote together, in some of which our names will never appear, over the past 15 years. She always worked directly with the publishers and editors, which left me more time for research and relieved me of having to deal with publishers' editorial staffs. When James Chambers, Facts On File executive editor, asked me to complete this revision myself due to Carol Turkington's illness, I had some trepidation about working with the Facts On File editorial team, whom I did not know. I knew Carol always loved working with FOF, but I feared their staff might not be patient with someone with a full-time job (two, in fact) and who was recovering from major surgery after a nearly fatal accident. Mr. Chambers has been a dream of an executive editor: He has invariably been generous, accessible, and open. He has given me everything I have requested, and I know from our time working together these past several months that he would go the extra mile to give me anything I need to complete this edition. Jane Hickok, project editor, with whom I have worked the most directly, has been incredibly patient with my fumbling through completion of this book in the midst of the most impossible six months of my life: It has been as if every force of the universe has worked against completion of this book, yet Jane has always told me to breathe and make sure I do not put too much on my plate. She has that rare talent of editing my copy that forces me to slam my increasingly warped Chinese serenity balls against my head and shout, "Why didn't I write it that way to begin with?" Mr. Chambers and Ms. Hickok have made the editorial process a pleasure. I look forward to a long relationship with Facts On File and with them in particular.

My family, friends, and coworkers have invariably given me suggestions, criticisms, and emotional support to help keep me moving. My wife, Elaine, the most gifted school psychologist and preschool neuropsychologist I know, has been tireless in giving me suggestions and criticisms to improve this book (and myself!). Carol and I have repeatedly tried to get her to work with us on our books, but she has left that to me, probably to avoid showing me up. My son, Ross, and my (hopefully) daughter-in-law-to-be, Heather Boling, have kept me in touch with the undergraduate set, helping me recall that group's need for quick, to-the-point references for term papers and class projects. My graduate students at Converse College, never shy about giving me criticisms, have kept me on my toes: They have given me invaluable feedback on my handouts and PowerPoint presentations, many of which found their way into this book. My pal Dr. Stephanie Thomas, child and adolescent psychiatrist extraordinaire, who helps me care for the young people in my charge, has always made the time for me to buttonhole her about psychiatric issues, new psychiatric drugs, and medical issues outside psychiatry. She has also been my friend during some very rough times. I seem to be drawn to brilliant women.

Finally, I have procrastinated in saying goodbye to my writing partner and mentor, my best friend, Carol Ann Turkington. Carol died on December 22, 2007, after a heroic battle with breast cancer. Carol, never the kind of person to want attention or sympathy, managed to keep from me how ill she was until the very end—and then I had to learn how grave her health had become from our agent, Gene Brissie. My first conversation with Carol 15 years ago began as a discussion about writing but ended as mutual bragging about her then three-year-old daughter, Kara (who still calls me "Uncle Joe"), and my then seven-year-old son, Ross (who still calls Carol "Aunt Carol"). She was such a proud mom: She kept me current on Kara for the past 15 years and always followed Ross's life closely. I will never forget how proud she was to accompany Kara to Kara's first formal tea, with elbow-length gloves and the works. In addition to my sweet Kara, who is now a beautiful and brilliant young woman, Carol leaves behind her adoring husband, Michael. I always worked so well with Carol, I think, because not only was she the premier medical writer of our time, but she was also such a warm and loving mom and wife, someone who became the little sister I always wanted. My people, the Cherokee, have a phrase *oginali ulv* (ᎣᎩᎾᎵ ᎤᎸ) that roughly means "sister friend"—a sister you chose and who chooses you rather than one related to you by birth. Carol was certainly that. Put your finger anywhere in this book, and you will see Carol Turkington.

If Carol were still here, she would join me in thanking you for allowing us to share the information in this book with you.

Joe Harris

INTRODUCTION

This book has been designed as a guide and reference to a wide range of terms related to the brain and brain disorders, to memory and memory disorders, and to additional information and addresses of organizations that deal with the brain and brain disorders. It is not a substitute for prompt assessment and treatment by experts trained in the diagnosis of neurological problems.

In this revised edition, we have combined the *Encyclopedia of the Brain* and the *Encyclopedia of Memory and Memory Disorders,* updating, streamlining, and adding new terms where appropriate. New topics include such topics as

- infantile neuroaxonal dystrophy (INAD)
- neuronal migration disorders (NMDs)
- meningococcal vaccines
- pneumococcal meningitis
- rivastigmine (Exelon)
- Pervasive Developmental Disorders (PDDs)
- TORCH Disorders

In addition, almost every entry has been revised, many with extensive updates, with the newest information on autism and autism spectrum disorders (ASDs), atherosclerosis, learning disabilities and psychological testing, neurofibromatosis, polio, prions, rabies, antidepressants (including the updated FDA warnings), tacrine (Cognex), dysautonomia, echoencephalography, donepezil (Aricept), the brain, aphasia, acalculia, acoustic neuroma, acoustic reflex, AIDS dementia complex (ADC), Alzheimer's disease, estrogen and the brain, ADHD and new treatments, ergoloid mesylates (Hydergine), chronic fatigue and immune dysfunction syndrome (CFIDS), and corticobasal degeneration.

The appendixes in the back of the book have been updated, with the latest addresses, phone numbers, and Internet Web sites for all self-help, professional, and governmental organizations

Information in this book comes from the most up-to-date sources available and includes some of the most recent research in the fields of neurology and neuropsychology. Readers should keep in mind, however, that changes occur very rapidly in this field. References have been provided for readers who seek additional sources of information.

Carol Turkington
Cumru, Pennsylvania

ENTRIES A TO Z

abaissement du niveau mental A term meaning "lowering of the level of consciousness" invented by French psychiatrist PIERRE JANET to describe the weakening control of consciousness prior to DISSOCIATION. Today this term usually refers to ALTERED STATES OF CONSCIOUSNESS.

Janet believed this altered state of consciousness was found not just in dissociation but also in multiple personality, trances and automatic writing. He used the term to describe the weakening of willful control of consciousness and the subsequent dissociation into autonomous parts that might not be aware of each other.

Swiss psychoanalyst Carl Jung picked up Janet's term to describe schizophrenia; Jung believed this lowering of consciousness was the root of the mental disorder. In 1902 in Paris Jung became a student of Janet and was influenced by Janet throughout his life.

While Janet wrote widely in French, very few of his works have been translated into English.

abducens nerve Also known as the sixth cranial nerve, this nerve (together with the third and fourth cranial nerves) is responsible for eye movements. It supplies just one muscle of each eye, which is responsible for moving the eye outward. This nerve originates from the abducens nucleus in the PONS (part of the BRAIN STEM) and emerges from the brain right below it. It then extends through the skull, entering the back of the eye socket through a gap between the skull bones.

Because it has such a long way to travel through the skull, this nerve is often injured in fractures along the base of the skull or by a disorder (such as a tumor) that distorts the brain. Damage to this nerve can cause double vision or an eye disorder called strabismus.

abscess, brain A collection of pus surrounded and caused by inflamed tissue in or on the brain. Abscesses cause symptoms because of the increase in local pressure and/or local nerve tract damage. They are most often found in the frontal and temporal lobes of the CEREBRUM in the FOREBRAIN.

Except for head injuries, brain abscesses are almost always caused by infection from other areas of the body. About 40 percent of these abscesses are caused by sinus or middle-ear infections; the rest are caused by infection following penetrating brain injury or blood-borne infection. There may be multiple abscesses from blood-borne infections such as endocarditis and some of the immunodeficiency disorders.

Brain abscesses are relatively rare today because the widespread use of antibiotics controls many inflections in the early stages.

Symptoms and Diagnostic Path
The most common symptoms are headache, memory problems, drowsiness and vomiting, visual problems, fever, and epileptic seizures.

Treatment Options and Outlook
Abscesses are treated with high doses of intravenous antibiotics, but because antibiotics alone may not cure the problem, surgery may be needed to drain or remove the abscess. After the operation, antibiotics are usually given for up to two months. During surgery, a section of the skull is opened to provide access to the abscess and to facilitate drainage. If the abscess has penetrated any area of the skull, some of the affected area may be removed.

It is sometimes difficult to locate and remove all traces of the infection, and recovery may be complicated by reinfection. Because many patients experience epilepsy after brain abscesses, anticonvulsant drugs are often administered after removal or drainage of the abscess. (See also CRANIOTOMY.) They are fatal in about 10 percent of cases; many of the remaining 90 percent suffer brain dysfunction (such as EPILEPSY).

abstract memory A person's general store of knowledge. This type of memory has a huge capacity for storing meanings of events and objects. Its center is believed to be located in the CORTEX, the brain's outer gray layer. Damage to the temporal, parietal, and occipital cortex affects abstract memory in different ways.

acalculia Generalized difficulty in dealing with mathematical concepts. Brain lesions are often associated with difficulty in solving arithmetic problems.

Symptoms and Diagnostic Path

People with acalculia often substitute one operation for another; for example, a person may add when asked to subtract, or combine numbers instead of calculating correctly (such as adding 2 plus 3 and getting 23). Lesions in the left parietal lobe often result in acalculia.

Acalculia can be diagnosed by asking the patient to perform arithmetic problems requiring simple operations, such as addition and subtraction. If the patient can perform these operations, then standardized achievement tests may be used to assess the person's ability to complete more complex arithmetic questions such as word problems or algebra problems.

Treatment Options and Outlook

Successful treatment of acalculia varies depending on the cause. The loss of mathematical ability due to dementia secondary to a stroke, neurological disease (such as ALZHEIMER'S DISEASE or Huntington's chorea), or exposure to neurotoxins requires treatment of the underlying cause to the extent pos-

sible. Many elderly, for example, suffer reversible dementia due to medication mismanagement but experience an alleviation of symptoms when they receive assistance in managing their medications. Elderly individuals experiencing severe depression after the death of a spouse may see a general improvement in cognitive ability after they begin taking antidepressant medications. Individuals who have experienced stroke may respond favorably to occupational therapy or medications to help them regain at least some of their former cognitive abilities. Many elderly who fear technology benefit from learning how to use electronic calculators instead of relying on their ability to perform mathematical calculations in their heads. One of the authors (Dr. Harris) has worked as an expert examiner in Social Security disability cases in which former bookkeepers and accountants, who formerly engaged in amazing feats of calculation (such as running their fingers down a lengthy grocery store list and having the sum by the end of the tape) could no longer engage in their former employment following strokes, development of Alzheimer's disease, or, as in several cases, AIDS-related complex.

Children who suffer from acalculia frequently improve their mathematical abilities when they receive special education services. For example, a child with visual processing deficits may learn mathematical operations and principles when his or her special education program relies on tactile stimuli such as abaci, counting beads they can manipulate, or containers full of marbles or buttons they can count out, subtract, etc.

The treatment outlook for acalculia varies according to the cause and severity of the disorder. Cultural-familial deficits caused by lack of exposure to educational stimulation in the home before the child begins attending school, whether due to parents' lack of education or their own acalculia, frequently show quick improvement once children begin attending school and receiving special or remedial education. Acalculia due to delays in brain maturation or damage, such as due to the mother's exposure to teratogens during pregnancy, may lend themselves more to management than to remediation. For example, IEP teams may allow students with acalculia to use calculators in classroom activities in which classroom rules ordinarily prohibit calculators. IEP teams also have the option, depending on the severity of a mathematics-based learning disability, to have the student's entire mathematical instruction take place in a special education classroom or provide a shadow to accompany them to their science and mathematics classes to assist them in understanding and performing required mathematical calculations.

acetylcholine   A common chemical NEUROTRANS-MITTER found at all nerve-muscle junctions, as well as many sites in the central nervous system. Acetylcholine was the first neurotransmitter discovered by scientists; it was isolated in the 1920s from one of the nerves that regulate heart function.

The actions of acetylcholine are called cholinergic actions; those actions are blocked by anticholinergic drugs. Acetylcholine is stored in tiny vessels called synaptic vesicles at the tips of cholinergic axon terminals. After acetylcholine is released and acts on nerve or muscle fibers, it is broken down into choline and acetate by an enzyme called acetylcholinesterase. This breakdown of acetylcholine by acetylcholinesterase helps reabsorb choline and acetate back into the releasing neuron.

Acetylcholine is a common neurotransmitter in humans, in animals, and in insects. Because of this, many insecticides contain substances that interfere with the activity of acetylcholinesterase (the enzyme that destroys acetylcholine). While these insecticides kill pests, they can also poison humans.

Acetylcholine operates as a primary neurotransmitter in brain areas that handle processing of learning and memory, of states of vigilance and awareness. As such, it was no surprise that ALZHEIMER'S DISEASE would be related to acetylcholine dysfunction. In this disease, the region of the brain chiefly responsible for the synthesis of acetylcholine undergoes degeneration.

acetyl-L-carnitine (ALC)   A molecule found naturally in the body responsible for carrying fats into the mitochondria (the energy-producing part of the cells) and regarded by some scientists as one of the most promising chemicals for the treatment of ALZHEIMER'S DISEASE.

Long-term administration of ALC, which is found in many common foods (including milk), has preserved spatial memory in aged rats. Some studies suggest that ALC also may play an important part in protecting the brain from the effects of aging. One study has found that ALC helps nourish certain receptors in the brain that are important for learning. In addition, other animal research suggests that ALC interferes with the formation of lipofuscin, a substance that is associated with a reduction of cognitive ability in the aged.

In human studies, ALC has been found to increase short-term memory, attention span, and alertness of those with Alzheimer's disease and other forms of senility. It also is said to increase the brain levels of choline acetyltransferase and to increase dopamine activity. (Dopamine deficiencies in the brains of Alzheimer's patients are believed to be the primary reason behind low levels of ACETYLCHOLINE, which can lead to muddy thinking, confused memory, slow reflexes and depression.)

ALC has been available in Italy since 1986, where it is classified as a NOOTROPIC DRUG and is used to treat Alzheimer's disease and age-associated memory impairment.

acoustic nerve   Also known as the auditory nerve, this is part of the VESTIBULOCOCHLEAR NERVE (eighth cranial nerve). This nerve carries sensory impulses from the cochlea (the part of the inner ear that detects sounds) to the hearing center in the brain, where the impulses are translated as sounds.

acoustic neuroma   A benign tumor of the cells that surround the auditory nerve, a branch of the VESTIBULOCOCHLEAR NERVE (eighth cranial nerve) responsible for balance and hearing. This type of tumor is also known as an eighth-nerve tumor, a schwannoma, neurolemmoma, or an auditory nerve tumor.

Acoustic neuromas can cause hearing loss on the affected side. Usually slow growing and benign; several types of tumors can grow on the auditory nerve, but the most common is an acoustic neuroma.

The cause is unknown, except for the few tumors associated with NEUROFIBROMATOSIS, a hereditary neurological disorder.

Symptoms and Diagnostic Path

The most common symptom is hearing loss in the affected ear. Most people with this type of tumor have balance problems, headache, ringing in the ears, facial numbness, and hearing loss in one or both ears.

Auditory, balance, and hearing tests (including a brain stem auditory-evoked response test and a CAT SCAN) can reveal these tumors.

Treatment Options and Outlook

There are three treatment options: observation, surgical removal, or radiation. Since acoustic neuromas are benign and produce symptoms by pressure on surrounding nerves, careful observation over a period of time may be all that is necessary.

When a small tumor is discovered in an older patient, observation to determine the growth rate of the tumor may be acceptable if there are no serious symptoms. In this case, MRI scans are performed from time to time, and if the tumor does not grow significantly, observation is continued. However, if the tumor gets progressively bigger, treatment may become necessary.

If diagnosed early, the tumor can be removed without damaging the person's hearing. If detected too late, these tumors can be life threatening.

Although the surgical removal of such tumors is complex and delicate, few patients die from the surgery because of modern technology and early detection.

Long-term eye problems affect at least half of those who have had an acoustic neuroma removed, in addition to possible taste disturbances, problems with voice or swallowing, and (if the facial nerve has been injured or removed during surgery) some degree of facial paralysis.

With small tumors, it may be possible to save what is left of the patient's hearing, but medium or large tumors have usually destroyed enough of the nerve that the ability to hear cannot be restored by surgery. The particular hearing problems common to people who have had acoustic neuromas include difficulty locating the direction of sound, problems hearing persons who are speaking softly, and understanding speech in a noisy environment.

Radiation therapy is a third technique used to treat these tumors, based on the principle that radiation delivered precisely to the tumor will stop its growth while minimizing injury to surrounding nerves and tissue. This noninvasive procedure can be performed either as a one-dose treatment on an outpatient basis, or with several doses ranging from several days to several weeks.

In single-dose treatments, hundreds of high-dose small beams of radiation are aimed at the tumor. This treatment has been very successful, with only a few side effects, such as facial weakness or numbness.

In multidose treatment, called fractionated stereotactic radiosurgery (FSR), smaller doses of radiation are given over a longer period of time, requiring the patient to return to the treatment location each day for several weeks. Each visit only takes a few minutes and most patients can go back to their normal routine before and after each treatment. This type of noninvasive treatment involves a shorter recovery with preservation of hearing in many cases. However, radiation treatment is limited to small or medium tumors, and the long-term results are not yet known. Radiation treatment is a way of controlling the tumor's growth without removing it.

Untreated, the tumor first distorts the eighth cranial nerve; as it grows larger, it can press on the seventh, fifth, and ninth cranial nerves. Eventually it can grow so large that it protrudes from the canal into the brain behind the mastoid bone and, if untreated, can eventually lead to death.

acoustic reflex A reflex contraction of a small muscle in the middle ear that stiffens the chain of hammer, anvil, and stirrup to protect the inner ear. This important reflex serves a protective role in the brain. Because of links between the cochlear nerve and the RETICULAR FORMATION (the network of cells in the BRAIN STEM that plays an important role in sleep and arousal), a person will wake up when hearing a loud, unexpected noise.

acquisition The process of encoding or recording information in the first stage of the memory process (followed by storage and retrieval/recall). If a person can't remember something, it may be because the information was never recorded in the first place (a failure of acquisition), although it is most likely a problem of retrieval.

ACTH   See ADRENOCORTICOTROPIC HORMONE.

acute idiopathic polyneuritis   The medical name for GUILLAIN-BARRÉ SYNDROME.

addiction   The physiological and psychological dependence on a particular chemical substance produced by the habitual use of a certain drug. Addiction is typically an interaction among personality, environment, biology, and social acceptability. Denied the required dose of a drug, an addicted user goes through a period of agonizing withdrawal. Experts are still debating whether the motivation for continual drug abuse springs from a wish to avoid withdrawal or to achieve the drug-related pleasure.

Many types of drugs are abused, including MARIJUANA, AMPHETAMINES, HALLUCINOGENS (such as LSD), TRANQUILIZERS, and ANTIDEPRESSANT DRUGS. Alcohol and tobacco are probably the substances that have addicted the largest number of people. Most drugs, when abused, carry the risk of dependency.

Currently, the most rapidly addictive substance is COCAINE, especially when it is smoked in the form of crack; the cocaine high is swift, a sudden euphoria that explodes in a rush within 15 seconds of the first puff. Unfortunately, this euphoria is short lived, evaporating within 5 to 15 minutes. The sensation of confidence and clarity can suddenly vanish, leaving the user with an over-powering urge to retain that state again with another "hit."

Not all drugs are physically addicting; marijuana and hashish seem to be psychologically addictive. In addition, the psychedelic drugs LSD and mescaline, which interfere with transmitters like SEROTONIN and NORADRENALINE, appear to set off neither a physical nor psychological dependency. Even cocaine, which may create a strong psychological

dependency, seems to create only a mild physical dependency.

Surprisingly, even the "hard" drugs such as heroin do not always result in addiction. On average, only about 10 percent of the people who snort cocaine or shoot heroin will go on to become full-fledged addicts, but the reason why some people become addicted and others do not has never been fully understood. Experts believe that environment and heredity play a part. Because human beings appear to crave stimulation, satisfaction, and pleasure, they are capable of turning to chemicals if a healthy path to these goals is not found.

There is a wide range of addictive drugs. Rapid-acting opiates (including heroin, MORPHINE, and meperidine) provide pain relief, contentment, and emotional detachment; long-term effects include weight loss, reduced sex-hormone levels, and physical and psychological dependence. Withdrawal can cause cramps, gooseflesh, and diarrhea.

The NICOTINE in tobacco increases the pulse rate and blood pressure, reduces appetite, and relaxes regular users; long-term use can cause physical and psychological dependence, respiratory disease, and a number of cancer risks.

Tranquilizers such as the BENZODIAZEPINES reduce emotional responses and alertness and relax muscles; long-term use causes physical and psychological dependence. Withdrawal may cause anxiety and sleep problems.

Amphetamines can cause appetite and sleep loss and increase heart rate and blood pressure; long-term use can lead to malnutrition and psychological dependence. Withdrawal can cause protracted sleep, depression, and increased appetite.

BARBITURATES can reduce tension, enhance sleep, and cause intoxication in high doses; long-term use can cause physical and psychological dependence and lead to sleep disturbances. Withdrawal can cause anxiety, possible DELIRIUM TREMENS, and convulsions.

Alcohol can cause poor coordination, suppressed inhibitions, and slow mental processes. It can produce physical and psychological dependence, the risk of brain, nerve, and heart damage, cirrhosis, and certain cancers. Withdrawal can lead to delirium tremens and convulsions.

Marijuana and hashish can cause euphoria and, after long-term use, can lead to loss of drive and impaired learning ability. There are no withdrawal symptoms. Both, however, can cause teratogenic effects (developmental malformations), even when the father consumes them before conception.

Hallucinogens (LSD, mescaline, and MDMA) cause perceptual distortions and arousal; long-term use can lead to flashbacks and possible brain damage.

adrenaline   Secreted by the adrenal glands, this neurotransmitter and hormone readies the body for action. Adrenaline is also known as EPINEPHRINE. The release of adrenaline increases heart rate and blood pressure, and diverts blood flow from the skin and gastrointestinal area to parts of the body where it is needed in times of survival-oriented action.

adrenocorticotropic hormone (ACTH)   Also called corticotropin, this hormone is produced by the PITUITARY GLAND and stimulates the outer layer of the adrenal gland to release various corticosteroid hormones. ACTH is also needed to maintain the adrenal cortex cells. ACTH production is partly controlled by the HYPOTHALAMUS (an area in the center of the brain) and partly by the level of hydrocortisone in the blood.

When ACTH levels rise too high, hydrocortisone production is increased, which suppresses the release of ACTH from the pituitary gland. If ACTH levels are too low, the hypothalamus releases its hormones, stimulating the pituitary gland to increase ACTH production.

ACTH levels increase in response to stress, emotion, injury, infection, burns, surgery, and low blood pressure.

Disorders of ACTH include Cushing's syndrome, a pituitary-gland tumor that causes excess ACTH production, which in turn results in an excess of hydrocortisone produced by the adrenal cortex.

age-associated memory impairment (AAMI)   See MILD COGNITIVE IMPAIRMENT.

aging and memory   As a person ages, the functioning of the memory process begins to slow down, affecting different types of memory in different ways. There are many reasons why this memory deterioration occurs: malnutrition, depression, medications, as well as a range of organic problems in the aging brain itself.

Researchers believe there are several possible reasons for this age-related memory deterioration, although none has been demonstrated conclusively. First of all, there are a range of reversible reasons for an age-related loss: depression, medications (especially the BENZODIAZEPINES used to treat anxiety), dietary irregularities, thyroid deficiency, alcohol, and marijuana.

There is also a wide range of organic reasons that underlie this type of memory loss. While scientists once thought that age brought an irreversible loss of cells in the cerebral cortex, they have now completely changed their minds. Today researchers believe that major cell loss appears to occur in a tiny region toward the front of the brain called the basal forebrain and in the HIPPOCAMPUS and AMYGDALA, which control memory and learning. Loss of these cells causes a drop in the production of the neurotransmitter ACETYLCHOLINE, vital to memory and learning. Patients with ALZHEIMER'S DISEASE for example, have marked decreases in this vital neurotransmitter.

Unfortunately, the hippocampus—probably one of the most important brain structures involved in memory—is highly vulnerable to aging. Studies have found that up to 5 percent of the nerve cells in the hippocampus evaporate with each decade past middle age. This could mean a loss of up to 20 percent of total hippocampal nerve cells by the time people enter their 80s.

Damage to this area of the brain may be a result of stress hormones such as cortisol, made in the adrenal glands.

It may be that as the brain ages, the speed with which information is processed decreases so that retrieving stored material takes longer. Or memory problems may occur because of dying neurons or decreased production of neurotransmitters (chemicals like acetylcholine that allow brain cells to communicate with each other).

Memory problems also may be linked to the fact that as a person ages, the brain shrinks and the cells become less efficient. In addition, things can happen to the brain to accelerate its decline—a person can be genetically unlucky, be exposed to toxins such as lead, or make bad choices in life, as by smoking and drinking to excess. All those things will accelerate memory decline.

Or it could be that an aging person's ability to retrieve memories may be impaired directly. Studies have shown that older people may have problems recalling a list of words but have no problem picking out those previously seen words from a longer list. Because they can recognize these previously seen words, it is obvious that the memory of the words has been stored somewhere in the brain—it is just harder to retrieve them (remember) than recognize them (picking from a list). In this case, a list may serve as a visual cue to help a person retrieve the memory.

Age-related memory problems also may be due to differences in ENCODING (storing information). Those people with the best ability to remember at any age tend to cloak new information with details, images and "cues." When they are introduced to a new acquaintance, for example, they notice the physical appearance of the person and link it in some way to the person's name, fitting the introduction into a context they already understand. Researchers have discovered that with age, a person is less able to organize this information effectively, perceiving less and noticing fewer details. In fact, researchers have documented a drop in effective encoding strategies during the 20s and traced a further, more gradual decrease over the life span. For these reasons, older people have the most difficulty when attempting unfamiliar tasks that require rapid processing—such as learning how to program a videocassette recorder or operating a computer.

About half of elderly men and women with severe intellectual impairment have Alzheimer's disease; another fourth suffer from vascular disorders (especially multiple strokes) and the rest have a variety of problems, including BRAIN TUMOR, abnormal thyroid function, infections, pernicious anemia, adverse drug reactions and abnormalities in the spinal fluid. (See STROKE.) A good diagnosis is important because all of these other disorders can be treated.

Decline in Mental Ability

The chief decline in mental ability among healthy older people is in "executive function"—the ability to perform several tasks at once or to switch back and forth rapidly between tasks, which the frontal lobe, specifically the prefrontal lobe, controls.

And while semantic memory (general vocabulary and knowledge about the world) often stays sharp through the 70s, memory for names (especially those not used frequently) begins to decline after age 35. While short-term memory does not decline as a person ages, long-term and episodic memory (remembering the time and place something occurred) does deteriorate.

The elderly also suffer from SOURCE AMNESIA (forgetting where something was learned). Spatial visualization skills (the ability to recognize faces and find one's car) already have begun to wane by the time a person enters the 20s.

An older person's ability to recall memories from long ago does not necessarily have anything to do with memory; the memories are not being remembered from long ago, but merely from the last time the story was told. This is why memories that have been retrieved many times may be distorted.

While some specific abilities do decline with age, overall memory remains strong through the 70s; research studies have shown that the average 70-year-old performs as well on such a test as do 25 to 30 percent of 20-year-olds. In fact, many older people in their 60s and 70s score significantly better in verbal intelligence than young people.

There is significant evidence that memory loss is not an inevitable part of aging, according to experts at Harvard University. Studies of nursing home populations controlled for age bias and excess anxiety showed that patients were able to make significant improvements in memory through rewards and cognitive challenges.

While some memory loss is common, it is usually benign and memory function diminishes only slightly with the years. Physical exercise and mental stimulation improve mental function in some people. Animal studies in California reveal that rats living stimulating lives, with plenty of toys in their cages, have larger brain cells and longer dendrites.

So while it is true that the brain does become less effective as a person ages, it is generally because of disuse rather than disease. And just as it's possible to strengthen a muscle by lifting weights, it's also possible to challenge the brain to become more efficient.

"The use-it-or-lose-it principle applies not only to maintaining muscular flexibility, but to high levels of intellectual performance as well," says psychologist K. Warner Schaie, Ph.D., director of the Gerontology Center at Pennsylvania State University. Dr. Schaie, who's been tracing the mental meanderings of 4,000 people for more than 30 years, is an international authority on mental stimulation and the aging brain. He believes that by running through some daily mental drills—sort of like practicing scales on a piano—a person can prevent intellectual breakdown. In fact, he's discovered that you can reverse a downward mental slide through a combination of mental gymnastics and problem-solving skills.

Only recently have scientists figured out that a person's brain doesn't gradually self-destruct during aging—that there is some choice over when, and how much, mental ability is lost, says gerontologist Robert Butler, M.D., director of the National Institute on Aging and winner of the Pulitzer Prize for his book *Why Survive? Being Old in America* (1985). "There is no overall decline with age," Butler says. "In fact, judgment, accuracy and general knowledge may increase."

Researchers once thought that by age 13 a person's brainpower began a slow downward spiral until—by about age 70 or 80—there would be barely enough brain cell wattage to power a penlight. More recent studies have exploded that myth.

Schaie's long-term study has looked at how older people handle skills ranging from identification of a rotated object to finding the square root of 243. He found that after about age 30, most people reach a plateau that is usually maintained until about age 60; after that, there are small declines depending on ability and sex. It's not until the 80s that any sort of serious mental slowdown occurs.

The capacity to focus on a task or follow an argument remains strong throughout life. The bad news, according to some neuropsychologists, is that memory may decline by 50 percent between ages 25 and 75. But the good news is that wisdom and critical thinking do not decline.

Slowing Mental Decline

It is possible to slow down a mental decline, some experts say. Evidence from animal research suggests that stimulating the brain can not only stop cells from shrinking, it can actually increase brain size. Studies show that rats living in an enriched environment had larger outer brain layers, with larger, healthier neurons. The rats also had brains with more cells responsible for providing food for the neurons. Those rats kept in a barren cage with nothing to play with were listless and had smaller brains.

Some scientists now believe that humans can also improve their brain function and even reverse a decline by challenging themselves with active learning or by living in an "enriched" environment. In fact, stimulating environments can even counteract the brain shrinkage due to old age.

In addition, research has found that exercised brain cells have more dendrites (the branchlike projections that allow the cells to communicate with each other). With age, a stimulating environment encourages the growth of these dendrites, and a dull environment lowers their number. That's why scientists believe that a person's socioeconomic status often predicts mental decline, since people who don't have a lot of disposable income often can't afford very stimulating environments. Researchers conclude that fewer, smaller brain cells is the price a person pays for failing to stimulate the brain.

There are probably as many memory aids as there are things to be remembered. As far back as the late 19th century, psychologist William James was busy coming up with ways to put some pizzazz into his brain cells. He came to the conclusion that it's possible to improve memory by improving the way facts are memorized . . . which is why every music teacher since has translated the notes of the scale (E, G, B, D, F) into "Every Good Boy Does Fine."

But no matter what method is used to remember the name of the new neighbor, a zip code, or the third law of quantum mechanics, the amount of time spent trying to remember is crucial. Researchers have found it's always better to sit down once or twice a day to try to remember things than to try to cram 10 hours of study in at one time. People pay attention to what interests them. If older people must read and remember something, they should try to find a room where they can read without too many distractions. Also, it helps to be an active reader, reading a sentence as a critic would, ready to locate an inconsistency, checking against what is already known.

If a memory problem is caused by any sort of brain disease, memory strategies aren't going to help. But if the brain is structurally healthy, odds are these strategies will provide some improvement in memory and problem-solving skills.

Normal memory changes with age. Among these changes are

- reduced attention span
- slowed thinking process (particularly apparent when dealing with new problems or a problem that needs an immediate reaction)
- fewer memory strategies (older people use fewer cues than younger people)
- longer learning time

Some features of memory that do not normally change with age include

- short-term memory
- semantic memory
- retention of well-known information
- searching technique (Searching may take longer, but the technique does not change.)
- interference (New information in one area competes with original information, which makes it hard to break old habits.)

aging and the brain Aging does not necessarily cause an irreversible loss of cells in the cerebral cortex; major cell loss appears to be in the basal forebrain, in the HIPPOCAMPUS and AMYGDALA (site of memory and learning). The loss of these cells, in turn, causes a drop in the production of the neurotransmitter ACETYLCHOLINE, a chemical that is vital to memory and learning. Not surprisingly, ALZHEIMER'S DISEASE patients have markedly low levels of this vital neurotransmitter.

Unfortunately, the hippocampus—probably one of the most important brain structures involved in memory and learning—is highly vulnerable to aging, and up to 5 percent of the nerve cells in the hippocampus evaporate with each decade past middle age. This could add up to a loss of up to 20 percent of total hippocampal nerve cells by the time a person enters the eighth decade of life.

Damage to this area of the brain may be caused by stress hormones such as cortisol. Rat studies have found that stress-induced increases in cortisol prematurely age the hippocampus. In addition, excessive amounts of FREE RADICALS (toxic form of oxygen) can also build up as a person ages, damaging the hippocampus.

However, the aging brain can also be negatively affected by a whole host of other factors, such as MALNUTRITION, alcohol, DEPRESSION, and medications (especially the BENZODIAZEPINES used to treat anxiety). In addition, there are a range of organic problems that can occur in the brain itself. Functional brain problems may also be caused by dying neurons or decreased production of neurotransmitters (chemicals like ACETYLCHOLINE that allow brain cells to communicate with each other).

In addition, there are physical changes in the aging brain—tissue actually shrinks and the cells become less efficient, according to researchers at the Neuroscience Laboratory of the National Institute of Aging in Bethesda, Maryland. In addition, hereditary problems, environmental toxins, or poor lifestyle choices (smoking, substance abuse, and the like) can accelerate the decline in brain function.

About half of the elderly men and women with severe intellectual impairment have Alzheimer's disease; another fourth suffer from vascular disorders (especially multiple STROKES), and the rest have a variety of problems, including a BRAIN TUMOR, abnormal thyroid function, infections, pernicious anemia, adverse drug reactions, and abnormalities in the cerebrospinal fluid (HYDROCEPHALUS). A good diagnosis is important because most of these other disorders can be treated.

The chief problem among healthy older people is a decline in their ability to perform several tasks at once or to switch back and forth rapidly between them. While general vocabulary and knowledge about the world often stays sharp through the seventies, memory for names begins to decline as early as age 35. Moreover, the ability to recognize faces and find one's car (spatial ability) has already begun to wane by the time a person enters the twenties. While long-term memory does not usually decline as a person ages, short-term and episodic memory (remembering the time and place something occurred) does deteriorate with age.

While some specific abilities do decline with age, overall brain function remains strong through the 70s. In fact, many people in their 60s and 70s score significantly better in verbal skills than young people.

However, brain deterioration may not be inevitable. Studies of nursing home populations showed that patients were able to make significant improvements in cognitive ability when given rewards and challenges. Furthermore, physical exercise and mental stimulation can even improve mental function in some people as they age. A stimulating environment strengthens the brain and a dull environment weakens it.

The brain often becomes less effective as a person ages because of disuse rather than disease. Just as it is possible to strengthen a muscle by lifting weights, it is also possible to challenge the brain to become more efficient. Some scientists believe that by mentally challenging the brain, such as practicing daily mental drills and problem-solving challenges, a person can prevent intellectual breakdown and reverse a decline. Engaging in mental activity such as Sudoku is also related to a lower incidence of Alzheimer's disease.

Researchers believe that after about age 30, most people reach an intellectual plateau that is usually maintained until about age 60; after that, there are small declines, depending on ability, gender, and health. For many people, it is not until the 80s that any sort of serious mental slow-down occurs. The capacity to focus on a task or follow an argument remains strong throughout life.

Evidence from animal research suggests that brain stimulation stops cells from shrinking and can also increase brain cell and dendrite branching. Studies show that rats living in an enriched environment had larger outer brain layers with healthier neurons and more cells responsible for providing food for the neurons. Rats kept in a barren cage had smaller brains and apathetic behavior.

Some scientists now believe that humans can also improve their brain function or reverse a decline by challenging themselves with active learning or by living in an "enriched" environment. Scientists suggest that a person's socioeconomic status can predict mental decline because poverty often goes hand-in-hand with an unstimulating environment. Fewer, smaller brain cells is the price a person pays for failing to stimulate the brain.

agnosia A neurological condition in which patients fail to recognize objects even though they show no signs of sensory impairment. The problem in recognizing objects is often restricted to particular types of stimuli, such as colors or objects, and may take quite subtle forms.

Symptoms and Diagnostic Path

For example, in facial agnosia (PROSOPAGNOSIA) patients cannot recognize a familiar face, but they can recognize the person's voice. Even odder, some facial agnosics can't recognize their own faces in a mirror, although their concept of self is intact; it is just that the face in the mirror and the connection to the self has vanished. There are indications that patients with facial agnosia also may have problems recognizing other classes of stimuli (such as makes of cars or species of birds).

Because an object can be recognized only if the sensory information about it can be interpreted, a person must be able to recall memorized information about similar objects. Agnosia is caused by damage to those parts of the brain responsible for this necessary interpretative and memory recall. The most common causes of this type of brain damage are stroke and head injury. In addition, tumors of the parietal lobe of the cerebral hemispheres also frequently cause agnosia.

Sigmund Freud invented the term *agnosia,* meaning "state of not knowing." It can be contrasted with APHASIA (inability to recall words and construct speech).

In addition to facial agnosia, there are other types: In *visual agnosia,* the patient is unable to verbally identify visual material, even though he or she may be able to indicate recognition of it by other means (such as gestures). In *color agnosia,* a patient can't recognize colors; if asked to pick out a blue sweater, he or she cannot do so. There is nothing wrong with a color agnosic's eyesight and he or she is not color blind; it is just that colors are devoid of meaning.

There is a wide variety of agnosias for sound (sensory agnosia): These can include *pure word deafness,* the inability to recognize spoken words although the patient can read, write and speak, and react to other sounds. In *cortical deafness,* the patient has problems discriminating all kinds of sounds.

Somatosensory agnosia is the inability to recognize objects by shape or size. ANOSOGNOSIA is the inability to recognize the fact that you are ill; a patient may feel sick but cannot make the connection between the symptoms and the perception "I'm sick."

Reduplicative paramnesia, or CAPGRAS SYNDROME, is a rare disorder in which patients fail to recognize other people and places they know well. The effect can be induced by showing a patient a picture and then, a few minutes later, producing the same picture again. A patient with reduplicative paramnesia may say she has seen a similar picture but insist that it is definitely not the one she is now looking at. This disorder is believed to have a psychological origin, although more recent research suggests there may be an organic cause. It is typically associated with CONFABULATION, speech problems, and a denial of illness.

Treatment Options and Outlook

The primary cause of agnosia must first be determined and treated if possible. Treatment for the particular form of agnosia is limited to support for the sufferer.

agraphia The loss or lessened ability to write, although the patient has normal hand- and arm-muscle function. A form of APHASIA, agraphia is caused by brain damage (usually within the parietal-temporal-occipital association cortex), such as from a BRAIN TUMOR or HEAD INJURY.

Symptoms and Diagnostic Path

Writing requires a complex sequence of mental processes, including word selection, spelling recall, execution of hand movements, and visual agreement that written words match their mental representation. These varied processes apparently take place in a number of connected brain areas; damage to any of them can cause different types and severity of agraphia. Agraphia rarely occurs alone; it often appears with loss of the ability to read (ALEXIA) or a general disturbance in speaking.

Treatment Options and Outlook

While there is no specific treatment for agraphia, some of the lost writing skills may eventually return.

See also APRAXIA; DYSPHASIA.

AIDS and the brain Neurological complications occur in at least 70 percent of patients who are diagnosed with acquired immunodeficiency syndrome (AIDS); at autopsy, 80 to 90 percent of patients are found to have neurological abnormalities.

Some of these complications occur in early stages of the disease, while others do not show up until late in the course of the condition. Complications include MENINGITIS, ENCEPHALOPATHY, AIDS DEMENTIA COMPLEX, CYTOMEGALOVIRUS, ENCEPHALITIS, TOXOPLASMOSIS, STROKE, MYELOPATHY, and PERIPHERAL NEUROPATHIES.

AIDS dementia complex (ADC) One of the most frequent and serious neurological complications of AIDS, this marked mental deterioration has been reported in up to 30 percent of AIDS patients in advanced stages of the disease. The symptoms are due to the direct infection of the brain by the human immunodeficiency virus (HIV).

Human immunodeficiency virus was established as the cause of AIDS in 1983; by 1985, it was understood that it was a type of virus that primarily infects macrophages and leads to chronic disease such as ENCEPHALITIS. Researchers believe that infection of the nervous system occurs in most cases and that it takes place very early—perhaps at the time when the blood first tests positive for the HIV virus—although the infected person may not show symptoms for quite some time. About one-fourth of all AIDS patients first seek help when they experience symptoms of AIDS dementia complex.

The disease was first described in 1983, but the diagnostic criteria for AIDS devised by the U.S. Centers for Disease Control was modified to allow a diagnosis of AIDS solely on the basis of dementia in a person who is HIV-positive, without any evidence of other opportunistic infection.

Dementia is found at increasing rates throughout the course of an AIDS infection—from about 3 percent at the time AIDS is first diagnosed to 8 to 16 percent of HIV positive outpatients to more than 60 percent in AIDS patients who die; some estimates place the occurrence closer to 90 percent at time of death.

Many neuroscientists believe that the N-methyl-D-aspartate (NMDA) receptor on nerve cells plays a role in AIDS dementia; the receptor triggers nerve-cell death when over-excited by NMDA or by glutamate (see TOXIC ENCEPHALOPATHY). Some experts suspect that HIV may destroy nerve cells indirectly by prompting the overproduction of a brain chemical called quinolinic acid, which can cause toxic effects at high levels.

Still, experts point out that most AIDS patients develop dementia despite pentamidine treatment, although they admit that the inhaled form of the drug that is usually given may not reach the brain as efficiently as an injection would. On the other hand, injected pentamidine can cause seizures in some people.

Diagnostic studies have revealed that the brains of people with ADC typically show cortical atrophy and enlarged ventricles.

The cause of ADC is not fully known at present. Since the amount of virus in the brain does not correlate well with the degree of dementia, most investigators believe that secondary mechanisms are also important in the development of ADC.

Symptoms and Diagnostic Path

Early symptoms of AIDS dementia include forgetfulness, poor concentration and confusion, movement problems (unsteady gait, leg weakness), apathy, depression, agitation, and behavioral changes. Patients become apathetic and lose interest in the environment, becoming socially withdrawn. Some patients may become overtly psychotic.

Most studies suggest that even if the brain is infected early, cognitive ability remains relatively unimpaired until the later stages of the disease. Although dementia is fairly common in advanced stages of AIDS, scientists are not sure whether people who test positive for HIV but who have no symptoms are already mentally impaired; it is clear that otherwise asymptomatic HIV carriers do not generally exhibit signs of AIDS dementia. Studies have shown that less than one percent of those who are HIV carriers but have no symptoms have AIDS dementia.

Children with AIDS experience a much higher percentage of AIDS dementia. About 60 percent go on to develop the disorder, probably because children better resist opportunistic infections and live long enough to develop dementia. It occurs primarily in more advanced HIV infection when the CD4 cell counts are relatively low. While the progression of dysfunction is variable, it is regarded as a serious complication, historically predicting death in less than one year.

Neurologists can diagnose ADC by ruling out alternative conditions. This routinely requires a careful neurological examination, brain scan (MR or CT), and a lumbar puncture to evaluate the cerebrospinal fluid. No single test is available to confirm the diagnosis, but the constellation of history, laboratory findings, and examination reliably establish the diagnosis when performed by experienced clinicians.

Treatment Options and Outlook

The drug zidovudine (AZT) is the best treatment so far for ADC since it is able to cross the BLOOD-BRAIN BARRIER. Other antiviral drugs, including D4T, nevirapine, and abacavir, are also effective.

alcohol and the brain   Alcohol is a central nervous system depressant that, in higher concentrations, is a NEUROTOXIN. It acts on the brain's RETICULAR FORMATION and spinal cord, depressing brain activity and thus reducing anxiety, tension, and inhibitions. In moderate amounts, alcohol can impart feelings of relaxation and confidence because the alcohol loosens the control exercised by higher brain centers. However, tests show that alcohol also interferes with the brain's activities, slowing reactions; even a few drinks four times a week can affect the brain.

Whether moderate social drinking (no more than one or two drinks per day) damages the brain is not clear, but most physicians agree that limited quantities of alcohol do not usually produce nerve-cell damage (unless the person is already an alcoholic).

Chronic drinking and alcoholism can cause a variety of neurological problems, including mental deterioration and muscle damage; alcohol withdrawal can cause minor tremors to DELIRIUM TREMENS (DTs), a potentially fatal syndrome characterized by extreme agitation, hallucinations, and a very high fever. Alcoholism is one of the most serious and prevalent medical problems in the United States; at least 12 to 15 percent of the population may be alcoholics. As many as 70 percent of known alcoholics display neurological abnormalities, according to the National Council on Alcoholism and Drug Dependence, Inc., a nonprofit educational organization.

The more alcohol in the bloodstream, the more it impairs concentration and judgment and the more the drinker's false confidence is increased. Excess amounts of alcohol are toxic to the brain, causing possible unconsciousness and even death.

Blood alcohol level is determined by the amount of alcohol consumed, whether or not there is food in the stomach, and how physically large the drinker is. A drinker begins to feel less inhibited when the level of alcohol reaches 0.05 percent. When the blood concentration reaches 0.1 percent, the drinker becomes clumsy; in most states, this is considered the legal limit of sobriety. As blood-level content increases, more and more brain control centers are affected. At a blood level above 0.2 percent, the motor area of the brain is significantly depressed and the drinker begins to stagger and

become uncoordinated. Emotional centers including the LIMBIC SYSTEM are also affected, leading to unpredictable outbursts.

As the blood level increases, effects become more serious: at 0.3 percent, the drinker is completely confused and may fall into a stupor; anything above 0.4 percent induces coma; and a level of 0.5 percent depresses activity in the MEDULLA OBLONGATA, the part of the BRAIN STEM that controls breathing. This will lead to death from respiratory failure in two to three hours (lower blood alcohol levels of about 0.4 percent can be fatal if they rise suddenly, such as when a drinker drinks an entire bottle of alcohol in a few minutes).

Exactly how alcohol affects individual brain cells is not completely understood. Alcohol works on the reticular formation, the part of the brain that plays a major role in attention and awareness, and coordinates information from the sensory systems to the brain's higher centers. It also can impair function of the CEREBELLUM, producing many of the symptoms of cerebellar disease such as slurred speech, jerky gait, and posture and movement problems.

Habitual drinkers experience a tolerance for alcohol so that nerve cells in the brain become less and less responsive to a given amount of alcohol. Paradoxically, however, after years of drinking, many alcoholics experience a reduced tolerance.

EFFECTS OF BLOOD ALCOHOL LEVELS	
Percent Concentration	**Observable Effects**
.05	Flushed face, euphoria, false confidence
0.1	Disturbed thinking, coordination, irritability, reduced self-control, irresponsible behavior
0.2	Marked confusion, unsteady gait, slurred speech, unpredictable behavior
0.3–0.4	Extreme confusion and disorientation, drowsiness, delayed or incoherent reaction to questions progressing to coma
0.5	Risk of death due to breathing arrest (although habitual drinkers may survive such high levels)

One theory is that long-term alcohol abuse damages the right frontal lobe of the CEREBRAL CORTEX, which is responsible for spatial skills and perception. This could be the reason why verbal skills (controlled mainly by the left side of the cortex) are relatively unharmed.

Research suggests that some individuals seem predisposed to become alcoholics; the inherited trait appears to be a decreased reaction to the effects of drinking during the first three to five drinks. Because the person's brain does not quickly indicate drunkenness, the drinker consumes more alcohol. Asians and Native Americans are genetically inclined to experience drunkenness earlier and more powerfully than drinkers of other races; it is unclear whether this puts them at higher risk for alcoholism, although, statistically, alcoholism is rampant among Native Americans.

Prolonged alcohol abuse can permanently impair brain function, causing visible changes in the brain. For example, the brain actually shrinks in size because the brain cells begin to waste away. CAT SCANS can measure the shrinkage by detecting an increase in the size of VENTRICLES, the fluid-filled cavities in the central part of the brain lying beneath the cerebral cortex. The ventricles enlarge because alcoholics have less brain and more empty space. Another measure of brain shrinkage is the size of the sulci—the valleys in the folds of the cortex. As the brain atrophies, the valleys widen.

This wasting of the brain can cause loss of some mental capabilities in nonverbal skills, such as the ability to solve problems involving shapes and space, to reason abstractly, and to perform physical tasks that require eye-hand coordination. On the other hand, often-repeated verbal skills such as vocabulary and word comprehension tend to be retained.

Short-term memory loss is a classic problem among alcohol abusers who have problems remembering new information. People over age 40 experience the most short-term memory problems after drinking—but even people age 21 to 30 experience some short-term memory loss. Women in particular appear to be more susceptible to the toxic effects of alcohol; women alcoholics seem to experience both verbal and spatial cognitive problems, whereas men only seem to have spatial cognitive problems.

Even social drinkers have memory problems of the same kind, albeit milder, related to the amount of alcohol they drink. Occasional drinkers are less affected than those who drink often.

Not all the damage experienced by alcoholics is caused directly by alcohol, however. The most severe brain condition found in chronic alcoholism is related to vitamin deficiency; in this way, chronic alcohol abuse may lead to WERNICKE'S ENCEPHALOPATHY, a condition characterized by sudden confusion as well as impaired coordination, sensory perception, and REFLEXES. Untreated, this syndrome may lead to coma and death. Administration with large doses of thiamine, a vitamin, can reverse some of these symptoms. If treatment is not begun early enough, Wernicke's encephalopathy can escalate into KORSAKOFF SYNDROME, a syndrome characterized by severe amnesia, apathy, and disorientation.

While most alcohol-induced memory problems seem to disappear when the person stops drinking, chronic abuse may cause irreversible damage. Most Korsakoff patients must be institutionalized for life.

Drinking alcohol during pregnancy can be especially harmful to a woman's unborn baby because alcohol readily crosses the placenta, where it can affect the vulnerable developing nervous system of the fetus. Heavy or chronic alcohol abuse by pregnant women can lead to FETAL ALCOHOL SYNDROME, a condition found in infants when alcohol interferes with normal brain development. These infants have abnormally small heads, with a smaller-than-normal brain size, usually with some degree of MENTAL RETARDATION.

However, even light to moderate drinking probably affects the developing fetus. Many authorities advise pregnant women not to drink at all because only a few glasses of alcohol can be harmful if taken during a critical period of fetal brain development, causing slight but measurable mental deficits. The most critical time for such fetal damage occurs from weeks two to eight after conception, during organogenesis, when cells are differentiating into organs, before many women even know that they are pregnant.

In addition to the administration of thiamine, the central nervous system effects of alcohol abuse can be reversed in most cases except for the most severe. As soon as an alcoholic stops drinking, brain size begins to increase; both the ventricles and SULCI grow smaller, causing the brain to grow larger. At the same time, performance tests begin to improve. Verbal abilities, if impaired, appear to improve fastest, followed by sensory and motor function. The more complex abilities of short-term memory, visuo-spatial learning, and abstract thinking improve at slower rates. Still, even years after giving up drinking, alcoholics may have some cognitive deficits.

alcohol idiosyncratic intoxication A marked behavioral change (usually aggressive) caused by drinking an amount of alcohol insufficient to induce intoxication in most people. This behavior change, which is usually atypical for the person, is usually followed by AMNESIA for the period of intoxication.

Some experts believe the phenomenon is really a dissociative disorder in which aggressive and destructive behaviors are likely to be prominent.

See also KORSAKOFF SYNDROME.

alexia The inability to recognize and name written words by a person who had been literate, severely disrupting the ability to read. The disability is caused by brain damage from stroke or head injury to a part of the cerebrum. It is considered to be a much more serious reading disability than dyslexia.

See also AGRAPHIA; APHASIA; APRAXIA; DYSLEXIA AND MEMORY; DYSPHASIA.

Alpers' disease A rare, progressive genetic neurodegenerative disease of the cerebrum. First signs of the disease, which include intractable seizures and failure to reach developmental milestones, usually occur in infancy. While some researchers believe that Alpers' disease is caused by an underlying metabolic defect, no consistent defect has been identified.

Symptoms and Diagnostic Path
Symptoms include developmental delay, progressive MENTAL RETARDATION, poor muscle tone, spasticity, DEMENTIA, and a type of seizure that consists of repeated muscle jerks. Optic atrophy may also occur, often leading to blindness. Although there may not be any physical signs of chronic liver dysfunction, many patients suffer liver impairment and failure.

The only way to diagnose the disease is at autopsy.

Treatment Options and Outlook
There is no way to slow down its progression. Treatment is symptomatic and supportive. Anticonvulsants may be used to treat the seizures, but the anticonvulsant valproate may increase the risk of liver failure. Physical therapy may help to relieve spasticity and maintain or increase muscle tone.

Those with the disease usually die within the first 10 years of life, usually from liver failure, although cardiorespiratory failure also may occur.

alphabetical searching A type of verbal method for improving memory in which the subject works through the alphabet in the hope that a particular letter will act as a retrieval cue for a forgotten word or name. Alphabetical searching is believed to be effective only when the person already has a great deal of information about the word (its length, whether it is common, the number of syllables, and so on).

alpha waves A type of brain wave that occurs when the brain is "at rest" and not receiving sensory input. One of the four main types of brain waves, alpha (together with beta) rhythms are the most often found in healthy waking adults, usually with eyes closed; slower rhythms are found during sleep, in early childhood, and during serious illness.

Brain waves are recorded by ELECTROENCEPHALOGRAPHY; the alpha waves are in the 8–13 hertz range. According to British researchers in the 1940s, alpha waves may reveal a person's personality based on the type of activity of this wave. Type R (for "responsive") people have alpha rhythms that predominate when their eyes are closed and their minds are relaxed. The waves are blocked when the eyes are open or during mental effort. About two-thirds of all people tested were Type R.

Type P ("persistent") subjects exhibited alpha rhythms with eyes open or closed or when struggling with mental problems. About one-sixth of subjects were type Ps, who seem to perceive by sound or touch much better than by forming visual images.

Type M ("minus") subjects showed no noticeable alpha rhythms at any time, whether or not their minds were busy or at rest or whether their eyes were open or shut. About one-sixth of all adults are type M, who always think in visual images.

altered states of consciousness Qualitative alterations in the overall pattern of mental functioning, so that the person feels consciousness is radically different from the way it normally functions.

Alzheimer, Alois (1864–1915) German neuropathologist who first diagnosed Alzheimer's disease in 1906 during the autopsy of a 51-year-old patient who had died with severe dementia. Alzheimer's, a disease characterized by progressive loss of memory, had never before been isolated as a brain disorder.

During the autopsy, Alzheimer noted two abnormalities in the woman's brain—neuritic plaques and NEUROFIBRILLARY TANGLES.

Alzheimer worked with colleagues Emil Kraepelin and Franz Nissl in the research lab at the psychological clinic of the University of Munich, where they conducted research on the underlying disease processes in the nervous system that caused DEMENTIA PRAECOX. While Nissl invented new staining techniques to better study nerve cells, Alzheimer discovered the disease process for Alzheimer's disease. Alzheimer also served as a professor at Breslau University from 1913 until he died in 1915.

Alzheimer's disease The most common cause of dementia, this chronic condition is characterized by irreversible memory loss, disorientation, speech and balance problems, and decline of the intellect. This fatal disorder affects the cells of the brain, producing intellectual impairment in up to 4.5 mil-

lion Americans who are usually in the sixth decade of life; about 60,000 patients are between 40 and 60. The disease kills about 120,000 Americans each year and is the fourth leading cause of death among the elderly (behind heart disease, cancer, and stroke).

The number of Americans with Alzheimer's has more than doubled since 1980, and that number is expected to continue to grow. By 2050, the number of individuals with Alzheimer's could range from 11.3 million to 16 million.

About half of the elderly men and women with severe intellectual impairment have Alzheimer's disease; another fourth suffer from vascular disorders (especially multiple STROKES), and the rest have a variety of problems, including BRAIN TUMOR, abnormal thyroid function, infections, pernicious anemia, adverse drug reactions, and abnormalities in the cerebrospinal fluid. An early diagnosis is important because most of these other disorders can be treated.

Alzheimer's disease, which is the most common of the more than 70 forms of dementia, is characterized by abnormal fibers in the brain that appear under the microscope as a tangle of filaments (neurofibrillary tangles). These tangles were first described in 1906 by German neurologist Alois Alzheimer, M.D., who discovered them after performing an autopsy on the brain of a 51-year-old woman afflicted with dementia. Newer diagnostic techniques indicate there are other brain cell changes common in Alzheimer's disease, including groups of degenerated nerve endings (called plaques) that disrupt the passage of electrochemical signals in the brain. The larger the number of plaques and tangles, the greater the disturbance in intellectual functioning and memory.

The early onset form of the disease has been linked to genes on chromosomes 21 and 14; a cholesterol-processing gene pair called apolipoprotein E-type IV (apoE-IV) has been identified as the carrier of a 90-percent risk of the disease by age 80. This gene is located on chromosome 19; a person may have up to two copies of the gene pair—and the more copies, the higher the risk of contracting Alzheimer's, according to researchers, and the earlier in life individuals are affected. The gene is fairly common; 15 percent of the overall population has one of this gene pair, and one percent has two. But not everyone with apoE-IV will develop the disease.

In recent research, scientists have discovered that apoE promotes the formation of amyloid plaques in the brain. ApoE-IV is the most aggressive stimulator of this plaque formation; apoE-III causes fewer plaques and apoE-II can even slow plaque formation.

But while researchers have made great strides in untangling the mystery, scientists still do not know how to prevent or cure Alzheimer's disease. However, some scientists suspect that an imbalance between different kinds of apoE proteins may cause plaque formation. If Alzheimer's is related to a specific protein imbalance, it may be possible to alter diet or lower the protein that is too high. Researchers believe they will be able to develop a diagnostic tool that could screen for the gene pair, enabling counselors to make judgments about whether a person's likelihood of contracting the disease is high or low, early or late. Researchers cautioned that their conclusions about the gene can be applied only to families where members have late-onset Alzheimer's, the most common form of the disease.

In addition to the apoE-4 cholesterol-processing gene found on chromosome 19 (which must be inherited from both parents in order to produce the disease), British researchers have identified a genetic defect associated with an inherited form of Alzheimer's disease that occurs in only a fraction of Alzheimer's patients.

The defective gene, located on chromosome 21, causes cells to insert a single incorrect amino acid while manufacturing a substance called amyloid precursor protein (APP). Family members not affected by the disease and 100 unrelated, normal individuals from the local population lacked the genetic error. DNA analysis of 18 individuals with early-onset Alzheimer's in 16 other families revealed two members of one family bearing the same mutation. The finding adds fuel to the assumption that there are many underlying causes of Alzheimer's disease.

The link between chromosome 21 and Alzheimer's disease was discovered because nearly all Down syndrome people (with a defect on the same chro-

mosome) who live to their late 30s develop brain degeneration similar to that seen in Alzheimer's disease.

Other studies suggest that the gene for amyloid precursor protein is on chromosome 21, and a few cases of Alzheimer's disease are linked to a defective APP gene.

However, there are also a large number of Alzheimer's disease patients with no family history of the disease; these sporadic cases suggest there must be other factors influencing the development of the disease. In addition to the Alzheimer's gene, there is some evidence that some forms of the disease may be due to a "slow virus"; it is also possible that the disorder is caused by an accumulation of toxic metals in the brain or by the absence of certain kinds of endogenous brain chemicals.

Research has found accumulated amounts of aluminum within the affected nerve cells of subjects having the classic neurofibrillary tangles of Alzheimer's disease. Other studies have shown high amounts of aluminum, iron, and calcium in the brains of Chamorro natives of Guam, who had died of AMYOTROPHIC LATERAL SCLEROSIS or PARKINSONISM-dementia. This population is adversely affected by these two chronic disorders, both of which were previously suspected to be transmitted by a slow-acting virus. But now scientists suspect that there is a link between their environmental deficiency in calcium and magnesium and the excess of aluminum and other metals. The studies are important because of the similarity between parkinsonism-dementia and Alzheimer's disease.

Mercury, selenium, zinc, and other elements have also been studied to see whether there is a link with Alzheimer's disease, but so far no evidence has been found.

Other investigations are looking at excitotoxins, chemicals that overstimulate nerve cells to the point of killing them. Some excitotoxins are found in certain food, such as the cycad seed eaten on the island of Guam; others occur naturally within the body. Under certain conditions, the neurotransmitters glutamate and aspartate (contained in the artificial sweetener aspartame) can become toxic to nerve cells.

Most brain function depends on messages transmitted from cell to cell by a chemical carrier (or neurotransmitter). Scientists have identified in Alzheimer's patients a striking reduction of up to 90 percent in a brain enzyme called choline acetyltransferase. This enzyme is critical in the biosynthesis of ACETYLCHOLINE. In addition, scientists have found low levels of the neurotransmitter acetylcholine important in the formation of memories in the same areas of the brain where plaques and tangles occur.

Some scientists focused on proteins such as beta-amyloid, a major component of neuritic plaques, but more recent research has found these proteins in the brains of healthy subjects—not just those with Alzheimer's disease. Beta-amyloid is a fragment of a normal protein, amyloid precursor protein. Researchers showed that beta-amyloid is used in the cells' ordinary activities and that the levels of the protein in the cerebrospinal fluid of healthy subjects were no different than in the fluid of those with Alzheimer's disease. Before this, scientists thought the protein was present only in the brains of people with Alzheimer's, and they thought the protein caused the massive slaughter of brain cells that characterize the condition. Now scientists wonder if Alzheimer's might be caused by a dangerous mutation of beta-amyloid or an abnormal reaction to normal P-amyloid.

Some researchers believe that the disease could be caused by a slow-acting virus that produces symptoms years after a person is exposed. Unlike most viral diseases, however, Alzheimer's disease is not transmissible, and it is not similar to other viral disease patterns. If it is caused by a virus, then it is not a conventionally-recognized one.

There are other rare dementias that are caused by unusual viruses, including CREUTZFELDT-JAKOB DISEASE, KURU, and Gerstmann-Sträussler-Scheinker syndrome. Because these dementias have similar brain changes to Alzheimer's disease, scientists hope that studying them may reveal clues about how a slow-acting virus may play a role in brain disease.

Symptoms and Diagnostic Path

Symptoms vary from patient to patient. In the early stages, the patient notices increasing memory loss that may be selective, often accompanied by some loss of previously well-established memory and a worsening short-term memory. The forgetfulness soon becomes a far more profound memory loss than simply misplacing keys or forgetting a name. If a patient misplaces eyeglasses, that is normal forgetfulness; if he or she cannot remember that he or she *wears* glasses, it could be a sign of Alzheimer's. The person may compensate by writing lists or asking others for help. Patients may feel anxious and depressed because of the memory problems, but these symptoms are often unnoticed.

The patient may have a problem with remembering recent events; the patient may neglect to turn off the oven, may recheck to see if jobs are done, and may repeat already-answered questions.

As the disease worsens, the signs become more pronounced. This early forgetfulness gradually evolves into a second stage of severe memory loss (especially for recent events). Patients may remember things that happened long ago, but they cannot remember yesterday's dinner menu or what they heard on television. They may become disoriented in time or place and begin to lose their way even in familiar territory. Their concentration and ability to calculate numbers worsens, and they may begin to have trouble finding the right word (dysphasia). The patient's conversation becomes more and more senseless, and judgment begins to be affected.

As their problems deepen, patients begin to experience sudden unpredictable mood changes; personality changes begin to appear as well. As mental ability declines, daily activities become more difficult—and then impossible. Patients cannot concentrate, and they begin to forget about bathing, dressing, brushing their teeth, and shaving.

In the third stage, the patient becomes seriously disoriented and confused and may suffer from psychosis, HALLUCINATIONS, and paranoid delusions. Symptoms are usually worse at night. Some people become demanding, unpleasant, and even violent, forgetting everything they ever knew about social behavior. Other patients become docile and helpless; many wander from home and may not be able to find the way back. Others get lost inside their own house.

Patients forget to eat and cannot remember where they are or even who they are. They no longer recognize friends or members of their own family.

Eventually, even the most dedicated family members can no longer care for the person, and hospitalization is necessary.

While the symptoms are progressive, there is a great deal of variation in the rate of change from person to person. In some patients, there may be a rapid decline, but more commonly many months pass with little change. In later stages, the patient's immobility may result in pneumonia, bedsores, and feeding problems, shortening the remaining life expectancy by as much as one-half. The disease may last between three to 15 years before the patient dies.

There is a difference between age-associated memory impairment (AAMI) and Alzheimer's disease. AAMI may remain unchanged for years, but Alzheimer's disease is progressive, interfering with the normal activities of daily life. In addition, Alzheimer's disease affects more than memory; it affects the ability to use words, compute figures, solve problems, and reason. It results in changes in mood and personality.

Doctors at specialized centers can correctly diagnose "probable Alzheimer's" 80 percent to 90 percent of the time.

Short of autopsy, the only way a physician can diagnose Alzheimer's is to rule out other diseases. It must be clear that the memory problems are not the result of mild, occasional forgetfulness caused by normal aging. Depression, which can affect memory, must also be ruled out.

If other diseases have been ruled out, a diagnosis of Alzheimer's disease can usually be made based on medical history, mental status, and consistent symptoms. In addition, the doctor may order a MINI-MENTAL STATE EXAMINATION (MMSE), a common test of mental function. In the MMSE, a health professional asks a patient a series of questions about everyday mental skills. Another popular mental status test is the "mini-cog," in which a patient must complete two tasks: to remember and repeat the names of three common objects and to draw a clock face showing all 12 numbers in the right places and indicating a time specified by the examiner.

An electroencephalogram may show a general slowing of certain brain waves or patterns that may help confirm the presence of Alzheimer's. Tests of blood and urine may be done to help the doctor eliminate other possible diseases. In some cases, testing a small amount of spinal fluid also may help. Tests of memory, problem solving, attention, counting, and language can help a doctor pinpoint specific problems.

The doctor may want to do a brain scan, including a computerized tomography (CT) scan, a magnetic resonance imaging (MRI) scan, or a positron emission tomography (PET) scan.

Information from the medical history and any test results help the doctor rule out other possible causes of the person's symptoms. For example, thyroid gland problems, drug reactions, depression, brain tumors, and blood vessel disease in the brain can cause symptoms similar to Alzheimer's disease. Periodic neurological exams and psychological testing help evaluate the progress of the disease.

Treatment Options and Outlook

It is imperative that patients be under the care of a physician who can consult with a neurologist. As yet, doctors can neither prevent nor cure Alzheimer's disease, although it is possible to ease some of the symptoms with drugs.

The first drugs to be approved for the treatment of Alzheimer's are the CHOLINESTERASE INHIBITORS, which include DONEPEZIL (Aricept), approved for all stages of Alzheimer's; RIVASTIGMINE (Exelon), approved for mild to moderate Alzheimer's disease; and GALANTAMINE (Razadyne), also approved for mild to moderate stages. TACRINE (Cognex) was the first cholinesterase inhibitor approved, but today it is rarely prescribed because of associated side effects, including possible liver damage.

These drugs are designed to prevent the breakdown of a chemical messenger in the brain called acetylcholine, which is important for memory and thinking. About half of the people who take cholinesterase inhibitors experience a modest improvement in cognitive symptoms.

MEMANTINE (Namenda) was approved to treat moderate to severe Alzheimer's disease. Classified as an "uncompetitive low-to-moderate affinity N-methyl-D-aspartate (NMDA) receptor antagonist," it is the first Alzheimer drug of this type approved in the United States. It appears to work by regulating the activity of glutamate, one of the brain's specialized messenger chemicals involved in information processing, storage, and retrieval.

Vitamin E supplements also are often prescribed to treat Alzheimer's disease because they may help protect brain cells, although recent research casts doubt on their effectiveness. Normal cell functions create a harmful byproduct called a FREE RADICAL, a kind of oxygen molecule that can damage cell structures and genetic material. This damage, called oxidative stress, may play a role in Alzheimer's disease. Cells have natural defenses against this damage, including the antioxidants vitamins C and E, but with age some of these natural defenses decline.

Because problem behaviors are also a part of Alzheimer's disease, there are several effective treatments designed to help control behavior. Experts recommend nondrug treatment of behavioral symptoms as a first option. (Indeed, some medications can worsen dementia symptoms.)

Changes in lighting, color, and noise can greatly affect behavior. Dim lighting may make some people with Alzheimer's uneasy, and loud or erratic noise can lead to confusion and frustration. This is particularly apparent as evening approaches—the so-called sundowning effect, in which patients become more confused, restless, and agitated with the transition from day to night.

Patients should stay active for as long as possible, and may enjoy singing, playing music, painting, walking, playing with a pet, or reading. They benefit from established routines for bathing, dressing, cooking, cleaning, and laundry.

Severe behavioral symptoms are treated with medication. In some cases, drugs like donepezil or tacrine, used to improve thinking and memory, may also improve behavior. Several other drugs can treat problem behaviors, including antipsychotics such as haloperidol (Haldol); antianxiety drugs such as alprazolam (Xanax), buspirone (Buspar), or diazepam (Valium); or many of the antidepressants such as fluvoxamine (Luvox), nefazodone (Serzone), or paroxetine (Paxil).

Anti-inflammatory drugs may delay or slow down the development of Alzheimer's.

People with arthritis are less likely to develop Alzheimer's, which may be due to their use of anti-inflammatory drugs, since doctors think brain inflammation occurs as one stage in the development of Alzheimer's. These drugs may limit brain scarring and also reduce the inflammation caused by a type of gene (Interleukin-1) that worsens inflammation.

Of all the common nonsteroidal anti-inflammatory drugs (NSAIDs), ibuprofen may be the most effective. In studies of these drugs, scientists found they seemed to lower the incidence of Alzheimer's by between 30 and 75 percent. This research reinforces an earlier study that compared NSAID use in twins, finding that a twin who used NSAIDs regularly was 10 times less likely to develop Alzheimer's than the twin who was not taking an NSAID.

Investigators are uncertain why some other drugs had no effect; the drugs that do not seem to prevent Alzheimer's include aspirin, which is also an anti-inflammatory drug, and acetaminophen (for example, Tylenol), which is not.

Most drugs being tested today attempt not to cure but to treat the cognitive symptoms, including memory loss, confusion, and problems in learning, speech, and reasoning.

Other drug researchers are excited about a substance called hyperzine A, a chemical found in a type of tea brewed with club moss (*Huperzia serrata*) that the Chinese have insisted for hundreds of years improves memory. Chemists at the Mayo Clinic in Jacksonville, Florida, have been studying hyperzine A, a potent and selective acetylcholinesterase inhibitor. Acetylcholinesterase is an enzyme that breaks down acetylcholine, a key chemical messenger in the brain involved in awareness and memory; an acetylcholinesterase inhibitor like hyperzine A blocks acetylcholinesterase. Like the drug tacrine, hyperzine A prevents acetylcholinesterase from breaking down acetylcholine, thus raising synaptic levels of acetylcholine in the brain and possibly improving memory. Researchers say hyperzine A is a more effective, more specific agent than tacrine, but the drug has not been approved by the FDA.

HYDERGINE, an extract of a type of fungus that grows on rye, has been approved by the FDA as another treatment. Hydergine has been used in the United States for all forms of dementia.

Recent trends in behavioral management are moving away from the use of drugs and focusing on nondrug management, including better environmental design, patient monitoring systems, organized activities, and programs tailored to individual needs. Proper nutrition is very important, although special diets are not usually needed.

Other experimental strategies include the use of certain substances such as an infusion of the protein NERVE GROWTH FACTOR directly into the brain; this protein is found in healthy brains but is deficient in Alzheimer's patients. In animal studies, a catheter is surgically implanted under the skin and scalp, leading into a hole drilled in the skull to allow a catheter tip to enter the brain. The catheter infuses the drug directly into the brain at a set rate from a refillable pump implanted under the skin in the abdomen. The pump is powered by a battery that lasts about two years.

While it is helpful if the patient can continue a daily routine and be encouraged to do a little more than the patient feels can be done, when the condition becomes severe, a special setting with professional staff and full-time care may be required.

Risk Factors and Preventive Measures

Age is the most clearly established risk factor; most victims of Alzheimer's disease are over 65. Family history is another risk factor; many studies show that those with relatives with Alzheimer's disease are more likely to develop the disease than someone with no such family history. Other potential risk factors include toxins, head injury, and gender.

One of the hottest areas of research in the early 21st century is centered around the prevention of Alzheimer's disease. While there are no sure preventives at the moment, there are several interesting possibilities.

Vaccines Researchers at Elan Pharmaceuticals of South San Francisco vaccinated mice that were genetically engineered to develop plaques with a fragment of beta amyloid in 1999. A year later, seven of nine mice remained plaque free. Then the scientists vaccinated year-old mice whose brains were riddled with plaques, and discovered that the plaques started to melt away.

Since that discovery, the first tests of the vaccine have shown that it is safe in humans, but experts say it is far too soon to tell if the vaccine will actually work to prevent the development of Alzheimer's. Experts theorize that the vaccine, which is made from beta-amyloid protein, would stimulate a person's immune system to recognize and attack the protein.

Despite the vaccine's promise, there are a number of reasons the method that worked in mice may not prevent or halt Alzheimer's in humans. First, the plaques may be a symptom of the disease, rather than the cause. In addition, Alzheimer's patients have other changes in the brain that the mice do not fully exhibit, such as tangles of protein inside nerve cells.

A second vaccine—this one a simple nasal spray—developed by researchers at Brigham and Women's Hospital in Boston prevents the plaque buildup in the brain.

Vitamin E Some researchers believe this antioxidant vitamin may protect memory from the effects of disease and prevent its onset. In one study of Alzheimer's patients at the University of California, San Diego, very high doses of the vitamin did slow down the progression of symptoms. However, vitamin E is not recommended specifically for the treatment of Alzheimer's because there is no direct evidence that it prevents the disease.

Vitamin E is an antioxidant and may prevent nerve cell damage by destroying toxic free radicals (by-products of normal cell metabolism). Some scientists think free radicals are discharged by immune cells that are in the brain responding to chronic brain inflammation from Alzheimer's. The free radicals may attach to molecules in the nerve cell membrane and disrupt function.

Because vitamin E has other health benefits, researchers say there is no reason not to take it whether or not it has been shown to help memory. However, vitamin E has been associated with increased bleeding in vulnerable patients, so patients should discuss taking vitamin E with a doctor.

Estrogen replacement Estrogens have strong effects on the brain. Some experts suspect that Alzheimer's disease in older women may be related to estrogen deficiency, because estrogen may interact with nerve growth factors and delay the degeneration of neurotransmitters that facilitate memory and learning.

Studies have shown that hormone replacement therapy (which includes estrogen) can boost a woman's performance on memory tests, and may reduce the chance of getting Alzheimer's. On the other hand, estrogen may increase the risk of breast cancer, gall bladder disease, high blood pressure, and stroke, so it is often not recommended for women with a history of any of these conditions.

Studies show that estrogen replacement therapy (ERT) after menopause can reduce a woman's risk of developing Alzheimer's by 30 percent to 50 percent. In June 1997, the report of a long-term study from the National Institute on Aging (NIA) documented that estrogen replacement therapy in postmenopausal women was associated with a 50 percent reduction in the risk of developing Alzheimer's disease. In all, 472 women were studied for 16 years. Another NIA study documented the effects of estrogen in slowing the decline of visual memory in 288 women. The study showed that women who received ERT during the memory testing period performed better than women who had never taken estrogen.

Scientists still do not understand how estrogen lowers the risk of Alzheimer's disease or delays the onset of symptoms. It may help brain cells survive, slowing the onset of the disease, or it may help prevent the formation of beta-amyloid fibers (a protein associated with neuron damage) in the brain. Another theory is that estrogen works as an antioxidant to protect nerve cells.

While research suggests that taking estrogen may help women prevent the onset of Alzheimer's, it does not work for women who already have been diagnosed with the condition. Once a woman has been diagnosed with Alzheimer's disease, estrogen will not reverse the situation.

Nondrug prevention   Some experts think that maintaining mental fitness may delay onset of dementia. One study of a large order of nuns found that the sisters had significantly lower rates of Alzheimer's disease than others, even though their average age was 85. Interestingly, most other factors affecting the nuns (such as diet and environment) are no different than among the lay population. What was different is that many of the nuns have advanced academic degrees and lead an intellectually challenging life into old age.

Lifelong mental exercise and learning may promote the growth of additional synapses (the connections between neurons) and delay the onset of dementia. Other researchers argue that advanced education gives a person more experience with the types of memory and thinking tests used to measure dementia. This advanced level of education simply may help some people "cover" their condition until later.

Alzheimer's disease, early onset   Although Alzheimer's disease is generally thought of as an older person's problem, it also can affect those in their 30s, 40s, or 50s. The behavioral symptoms are the same no matter when the disease strikes, but the younger patient with AD *is* different.

Younger patients may have more problems expressing thoughts and feel even more frustration at the situation. In addition, while the symptoms may be noticed, they will often be confused with psychiatric disorders or some sort of "midlife crisis." This preconceived idea that AD is an "old person's disease" may lead even the physician to disregard AD as a possible diagnosis. In this event, a second opinion should be obtained from a physician who is familiar with the diagnosis of dementia-type illnesses.

Families are encouraged to seek legal advice as soon as possible after receiving a diagnosis; this is even more important for the family of younger patients.

While a person with AD finds that friendships often fade away as the disease progresses, younger patients may find friends breaking away even sooner because they are faced with the reality that AD can strike someone so young.

amblyopia   A permanent loss of visual acuity caused by a failure in the link of nerve connections in the visual pathway between the retina and the brain commonly called "lazy eye." The eye is functionally sound. If normal vision is to develop during infancy and childhood, it is important that clear, corresponding visual images are formed on both retinas so that compatible nerve impulses pass from the eyes to the brain. If no such images are received, normal vision cannot develop. If images from the two eyes are very different, one will be suppressed to avoid double vision, and normal vision may not develop in one of the eyes.

The primary cause of the failure to develop a normal visual pathway is a squint in very young children, in which only one eye focuses on a selected object while the brain suppresses a different image from the other eye. The problem could also develop as a result of congenital cataracts or severe focusing errors in a young child (such as when one eye is normal and the other has a severe astigmatism that causes a blurry image).

Symptoms and Diagnostic Pathway
Symptoms are reduced vision in one eye that did not receive adequate use.

Treatment Options and Outlook
Amblyopia must be treated as soon as possible; after age eight, it is physiologically too late for the brain to make proper connections in the visual pathway. For amblyopia caused by squinting, the patient must cover the good eye to force the poor eye to function normally. Glasses or surgery to place the deviant eye in the correct position also may be required. Glasses may also help correct severe focusing errors, and congenital cataracts may be removed surgically.

With early diagnosis and treatment, sight can be restored to the lazy eye.

amino acids The fundamental building blocks of protein. "Amino acids" refers to any of a number of organic compounds containing an amine and a carboxyl group. The body uses amino acids as the basic substance from which to construct not only proteins, but NEUROTRANSMITTERS as well.

Individual amino acid molecules are linked together by chemical bonds (called peptide bonds) to form short chains of peptides called polypeptides. In turn, hundreds of these polypeptides are linked together to form a protein molecule. One protein differs from another in the way their amino acids are arranged.

A total of 20 different amino acids make up all the proteins found in the human body; 12 can be made within the body (known as nonessential amino acids). The other eight (called the essential amino acids) must be obtained from the diet and cannot be produced by the body. In addition, there are about 200 other amino acids not found in proteins but which play an important part in chemical reactions within cells.

Animal sources usually provide a wider range of amino acids than do plant sources, so people on a vegetarian diet must be especially careful that their selection of food includes all of the essential amino acids.

Because the amino acids are responsible for producing neurotransmitters, some researchers believe that boosting the brain's supply of certain amino acids should also increase the production of neurotransmitters, affecting both mood and cognition. Two amino acids have been singled out for particular study: TRYPTOPHAN and TYROSINE.

Some studies have suggested that tryptophan may ease depression and boost effectiveness of antidepressants. In addition, several controlled trials have suggested that tyrosine appears to improve alertness and cognitive performance in the face of stress.

On the other hand, increasing the pool of amino acids does not necessarily mean more neurotransmitters will be made.

amnesia Loss of the ability to memorize or recall stored information. In most cases of amnesia, the patient has problems storing information in long-term memory and recalling this information.

There are many theories that explain the underlying mechanism of amnesia and many different causes, including brain damage from injury or disease. *Anterograde amnesia* is the loss of memory for events following trauma; *retrograde amnesia* is a loss of memory for events preceding the trauma. Some patients experience both types of amnesia.

Amnesia following an injury (such as a concussion) in areas of the brain concerned with memory function is known as *traumatic amnesia*. Degenerative disorders such as ALZHEIMER'S DISEASE or other types of DEMENTIA may also cause amnesia, as can infections such as ENCEPHALITIS or a thiamine deficiency in alcoholics. Amnesia could also be caused by a BRAIN TUMOR, a STROKE or a SUBARACHNOID HEMORRHAGE, or certain types of mental illness for which there is no apparent physical damage.

Transient Global Amnesia

This type of uncommon amnesia refers to an abrupt loss of memory for a few seconds to a few hours without loss of consciousness or other impairment. During the amnesia period, the patient cannot store new experiences and suffers a permanent memory gap for the period of time during the amnesic episode. There may also be loss of memory encompassing many years prior to the amnesia attack; this retrograde amnesia gradually disappears, although it leaves a permanent gap in memory that does not usually extend backward more than an hour before onset of the attack. These attacks, which may occur more than once, are believed to be caused by a temporary reduction in blood supply in certain brain areas. Sometimes, they act as a warning sign of an impending stroke.

The attacks, which usually strike healthy, middle-aged patients, may be set off by many things, including sudden temperature changes, stress, overeating, or sexual intercourse. While several toxic substances have been associated with transient global amnesia, it is believed that the attacks are usually caused by a transient cerebral ischemia to regions of the brain involved in memory.

Posthypnotic Amnesia

Amnesia may also occur after HYPNOSIS, either spontaneously or by instruction, making the memory of an hypnotic trance vague and unclear, much the way a person has trouble recalling a dream. If a hypnotized subject is told that he or she will remember nothing after awakening, the subject will experience a much more profound posthypnotic amnesia. However, if the patient is rehypnotized and given a countersuggestion, he or she will awaken and remember everything; therefore, experts believe this phenomenon is clearly psychogenic.

The amnesia may include all the events of the trance state or only selected items—or it may occur in matters unrelated to the trance. Memory for experiences during the hypnotic state may also

return (even after a suggestion to forget) if the subject is persistently questioned after awakening. It was this observation that led Sigmund Freud to search for repressed memories in his patients without the use of hypnosis.

Psychogenic Amnesia

Several types of amnesia belong to a different class of amnesia than those types caused by injury or disease; called psychogenic amnesia, they are induced by hypnotic suggestion or occur spontaneously in reaction to acute conflict or stress (usually called hysterical). This type of amnesia may also extend to basic knowledge learned in school (such as mathematics), which is never seen in organic amnesia unless there is an accompanying APHASIA or dementia. These types of amnesia are completely reversible, although they have never been fully explained.

In one type of mixed amnesia, organic factors may also be involved in the development of psychogenic amnesia, and an accurate diagnosis may be difficult. This complex intermingling of true organic memory problems with psychogenic factors can prolong or reinforce the memory loss.

It is quite common for a brain-damaged person to experience a hysterical reaction in addition to brain problems. For example, one patient who developed a severe amnesia that impaired the formation of new memories after carbon-monoxide poisoning went on to develop hysterical amnesia that continued to sustain the memory loss.

In psychogenic amnesia, there is no fundamental impairment in the memory process or in the consolidation or retention of information. Instead, the problem lies in accessing stored or repressed (usually painful) memories. This inability to recall painful memories is a protection against bringing into consciousness ideas associated with profound loss or fear, rage, or shame.

This type of amnesia usually can be treated successfully by procedures such as hypnosis. A normal mentally healthy person is assumed to be integrated within a unified personality. But under traumatic conditions, memories can become detached from personal identity, making recall impossible. Modern accounts of hysterical amnesia have been heavily influenced by SIGMUND FREUD, who attributed the problem to a need to repress information injurious to the ego.

With this theory, the memory produces a defense reaction for the individual's own good. This explains why psychogenic amnesia occurs only in the wake of trauma and is consistent with the high incidence of depression and other psychiatric disorders in those who go on to develop psychogenic memory problems.

There are four types of psychogenic amnesia: localized, selective, generalized, and continuous. *Localized amnesia* is the failure to recall all the events during a certain period of time, usually the first few hours after a disturbing event. *Selective amnesia* is the failure to recall some but not all of the events during a certain time period. *Generalized amnesia* is the inability to recall any events from a person's entire life, and *continuous amnesia* is the failure to recall events subsequent to a specific time up to and including the present.

amnesia and crime   A great deal of amnesia for crime has a psychogenic origin; that is, the crimes are so horrific that the criminal must not remember in order to remain sane. For example, between 23 and 65 percent of murderers claim to have amnesia related to their crimes.

But not all criminal amnesia is of a self-protective nature; some criminals do not remember their crimes because they have SCHIZOPHRENIA or DEPRESSION. In these cases, their amnesia may be an intrinsic part of their illness. In addition, many violent crimes are committed by alcoholics during "blackouts." During such a blackout, the person is not unconscious or stuporous—just drunk.

If a defendant claims amnesia for the crime with which he is charged, it could be argued that he is unfit for trial or that he can plead "automatism." This means that the behavior was carried out involuntarily and without conscious intent. Crimes committed during an alcoholic blackout are not included in this plea, since it is assumed that people are aware of the effects of alcohol and are therefore responsible for their actions while drunk.

Amnesia for a crime may be a form of emotional defense that arises after the crime has been committed; this does not therefore imply a lack of conscious involvement during the amnesic period itself.

No cases have been found in which a defendant was acquitted due to an organic amnesic state.

amnesic syndrome   A permanent, global disorder of memory following brain damage from accident or illness that does not result in a general deterioration of memory function, but selectively impairs some aspects of memory while leaving others normal.

For example, patients with this syndrome score very badly on clinical memory tests but perform normally on intelligence tests, such as the Wechsler Adult Intelligence Scale. Therefore, a person with amnesic syndrome will have a memory quotient (MQ) between 20 to 40 points below the IQ. In particular, these patients score very poorly on tests of the retention of novel information (such as paired-associate learning or free recall), but they have no problem understanding a normal-length sentence— they just cannot remember it for any length of time. Skills learned before the onset of the syndrome, such as riding a bike or driving, are unaffected.

The amnesic syndrome can be caused by lesions in two distinct parts of the brain: the DIENCEPHALON and the MEDIAL TEMPORAL LOBE of the CORTEX. Damage can be caused by a wide range of problems, including disease, neurosurgery, BRAIN TUMOR or HEAD INJURY, STROKE and deprivation of oxygen (anoxia). It also may be caused by a TRANSIENT ISCHEMIC ATTACK (TIA) that briefly blocks blood flow to the HIPPOCAMPUS.

amphetamines   Also known as uppers or "pep pills," this group of stimulant drugs facilitate the release of certain NEUROTRANSMITTERS, in particular norepinephrine and dopamine. Amphetamine also blocks the reuptake mechanisms for neurons using these neurotransmitters. Consequently, higher levels of transmitter that remain available longer tend to overactivate neurons. This is the cause of the amphetamine "high." Because of this ability, amphetamines are often abused for their stimulant effects. Their manufacture and distribution are governed by the Controlled Substances Act.

The short-term effects of amphetamine use include reduced appetite and increased heart rate and blood pressure. Long-term effects include malnutrition and psychological dependence and psychosis. Withdrawal symptoms range from excessive sleep to large appetite and depression.

amusia   The loss of the ability to comprehend or reproduce musical tone.

amygdala   A group of related nuclei located at the base of the temporal lobe that connects the impulses from the olfactory system and the CORTEX, and provides emotional content to memory. Sensory information from certain cortical areas enters the LIMBIC SYSTEM directly through the amygdala.

Because the amygdala connects to the HIPPOCAMPUS, it has been believed for a long time to play a role in memory. While most now believe the amygdala does not itself process memory, it is believed to be a source of emotions that imbue memory with meaning. For example, the remembrance of a memory or a whole stream of recollection often brings with it a burst of emotion—evidence that the amygdala is most likely involved.

amyloid precursor protein (APP)   A protein molecule found in the brain, heart, kidneys, lungs, spleen, and intestines. The normal function of APP in the body is unknown. In ALZHEIMER'S DISEASE, plaques are made when an enzyme snips APP apart at a specific place and then leaves the fragments—BETA-AMYLOID—in brain tissue where they come together in abnormal deposits.

amyotrophic lateral sclerosis (ALS)   Also known as Lou Gehrig's disease, this is a progressive, degenerative brain disease that attacks nerves in the brain and spinal cord that control muscular activity. As brain cells die, they can no longer control movement.

Symptoms and Diagnostic Path
Weakness begins in the hands and arms (and more rarely, legs), together with wasting and quivering of muscles, stiffness, and cramping. Eventually, all limbs are affected equally. However, there is no loss of sensation, and bladder function remains normal. Eventually the patient becomes totally paralyzed.

Weakness usually spreads to include the muscles involved in breathing and swallowing, leading to death within four years. However, a few people have lived more than 20 years after the diagnosis. The final stages of the disease leave the patient unable to speak, swallow, or move, but the intellect and awareness remain untouched by disease.

The body has many kinds of nerves. Some are involved in the process of thinking, memory, and detecting sensations, and others handle vision, hearing, and other body functions. The nerves that die in ALS are the motor neurons that provide voluntary movements and muscle power. The heart and the digestive system are made of a different kind of muscle, and their movements are not under voluntary control. Therefore, the heart and digestive system are not involved in ALS. Breathing also may seem to be involuntary, but although a person cannot stop the heart, it is possible to hold the breath.

No single test can diagnose ALS; instead, it is primarily diagnosed based on symptoms, a full medical history, and neurologic exams at regular intervals that can assess whether symptoms are worsening. In addition, a series of tests to rule out other diseases may be performed, including

- electromyography (EMG), a special technique that detects electrical activity in muscles
- nerve conduction velocity (NCV)
- magnetic resonance imaging (MRI)

Based on the symptoms and results, the physician may order tests on blood and urine samples to eliminate the possibility of other diseases.

Treatment Options and Outlook
There is no cure for ALS, although riluzole (Rilutek), the first drug treatment, has been approved. Riluzole may lessen motor neuron damage by decreasing the release of glutamate. Clinical trials with ALS patients showed that riluzole prolongs survival by several months, mainly in those patients who have trouble

swallowing, and lengthens the time before a patient needs ventilation. However, riluzole cannot treat damaged motor neurons, and there are possible risks: patients taking the drug must be monitored for liver damage and other possible side effects.

Other treatments are aimed at easing symptoms and improving the quality of life and use medications to treat fatigue and muscle cramps, control spasticity, and reduce excess saliva and phlegm. Drugs also are available to help patients with pain, depression, sleep disturbances, and constipation. Pharmacists can give advice on the proper use of medications and monitor a patient's prescriptions to avoid risks of drug interactions.

Gentle, low-impact aerobic exercise such as walking, swimming, and stationary bicycling can strengthen unaffected muscles, improve cardiovascular health, and help patients fight fatigue and depression; stretching exercises can help prevent painful spasticity and shortened muscles.

ALS patients who cannot speak may work with a speech therapist to learn ways to speak louder and more clearly or, later on, to use nonverbal means and aids, such as speech synthesizers and computer-based communication systems. These methods and devices help patients communicate when they can no longer produce sounds.

When the muscles weaken, use of nocturnal ventilatory assistance (intermittent positive pressure ventilation [IPPV]) or bilevel positive airway pressure (BIPAP) may be used to aid breathing during sleep. Eventually, patients may need respirators (a machine that inflates and deflates the lungs).

anencephaly The absence of the brain, top of the skull, and spinal cord at birth; this is an extreme form of SPINA BIFIDA.

Anencephaly occurs in about five out of every 1,000 pregnancies, but only in about one-third of cases does the pregnancy continue to term.

The lack of brain development is caused by a failure in the development of the neural tube, the nerve tissue in the embryo that eventually develops into the spinal cord and brain. While doctors do not know why this occurs, cases have been linked to low levels of folic acid in the mother's diet. There also may be a genetic component to the problem.

Maldevelopment of the neural tube also may cause HYDROCEPHALUS. Collectively, these birth defects are known as NEURAL TUBE DEFECTS and are assumed to have similar causes.

Symptoms and Diagnostic Path
This birth defect is detectable early in pregnancy by measuring alpha-fetoprotein, by ultrasound scanning, and by amniocentesis. If anencephaly is detected, the parents may want to consider termination of the pregnancy since there is no chance the child can survive after birth.

Treatment Options and Outlook
Most infants born with this condition are stillborn or live only a few hours after birth.

aneurysm, brain Ballooning of an artery leading to the brain due to pressure of blood flowing through a weakened area. The weakening may be caused by disease, injury, or a defective artery wall. A cerebral aneurysm often occurs as a swelling where the arteries branch at the brain's base, which is usually caused by a congenital weakness.

There are several reasons why an aneurysm would form in a blood vessel. The muscular middle layer of an artery might have a congenital weakness, and normal blood pressure can cause a ballooning at the weak point. Aneurysms of smaller vessels may occur with blood poisoning as a result of local infection on the artery wall.

Symptoms and Diagnostic Path
Cerebral aneurysms may last for many years without causing any symptoms, but because they are located in the brain, they are extremely dangerous. Sudden enlargement or bursting of an aneurysm in the brain will produce immediate signs much like those of a stroke—dilated pupils, drooping eyelid, rigid neck, severe headache, and unconsciousness.

CAT or MRI SCANS can provide critical information about this type of aneurysm.

Treatment Options and Outlook
Unruptured brain aneurysms are sometimes treated to prevent rupture, and surgery or minimally invasive endovascular coiling techniques can be used to

treat brain aneurysms. However, not all aneurysms are treated right away.

Surgery The main goals of treatment once an aneurysm has ruptured are to stop the bleeding and potential permanent damage to the brain and reduce the risk of recurrence. During surgery, a surgeon must first remove a section of the skull (CRANIOTOMY), spread the brain tissue apart, and place a metal clip across the neck to stop blood flow into the aneurysm. After clipping the aneurysm, the bone is secured in its original place, and the wound is closed.

Coil embolization or endovascular coiling Endovascular therapy is a minimally invasive procedure that treats the aneurysm from within the blood vessel, in a process known as coil embolization, or "coiling." Unlike surgery, endovascular coiling does not require open surgery. Instead, physicians use X-rays called fluoroscopic imaging to treat the disease from inside the blood vessel, threading a catheter into the patient's brain via the leg artery. Tiny platinum coils are threaded through the catheter, blocking blood flow into the aneurysm and preventing rupture.

Studies suggest that endovascular coiling produces substantially better patient outcomes than surgery, and the relative risk of death or significant disability at one year for patients treated with coils was 22.6 percent lower than in surgically treated patients.

angiography A type of diagnostic technique that enables blood vessels to be seen on X-ray film after a deep artery has been injected with a dye.

The procedure can detect brain tumors and help the surgeon see the pattern of blood vessels and the amount of blood that is feeding a tumor. By detecting a cerebral blood vessel with an unnatural appearance, an angiogram can help detect diseases that affect cerebral blood flow. *Carotid angiography* sometimes is performed on patients suffering from TRANSIENT ISCHEMIC ATTACKS (brief symptoms of stroke lasting less than 24 hours) to see whether there is a block or a narrowing in one of the carotid arteries in the neck supplying blood to the brain. *Cerebral angiography* can demonstrate the presence

of an aneurysm within the brain or reveal a brain tumor before surgery.

Procedure

First, contrast dye is injected through a fine catheter inserted into the carotid artery deep in the neck. Then, skin and tissues around the artery are numbed with local anesthetic, followed by a needle inserted through the skin into the artery; a long thin wire with a soft tip is inserted through the needle, the needle is removed, and the catheter is then threaded over the wire into the blood vessel. An X-ray is used to guide the tip of the catheter into the vessel to be examined; the contrast dye allows a rapid sequence of X-rays to be taken to study the flow of dye along the vessels.

Risks and Complications

There are some risks involved with this procedure. While it is possible to experience an allergic reaction to the dye, new contrast agents have lowered the risk of a severe reaction to less than one in 80,000 exams. Blood vessels may be damaged at the puncture site, anywhere along the vessel during passage of the catheter, or at the dye injection site.

Techniques have been modified recently to allow for treatment in addition to diagnosis; in *balloon angioplasty,* small balloons can be inflated at the tip of a catheter to expand a narrowed or blocked segment of artery. Other material can be injected to reduce or shunt blood supply away from a tumor, and medication to control bleeding or treat tumors can be infused directly into the local blood supply targeted at individual organs.

animal memory Not all animals possess a memory in a human sense. Animals farther down on the evolutionary ladder possess a rudimentary perceptive memory, genetically programmed to help them survive, but a productive memory that depends on recall developed later in animal evolution.

Ants, for example, live a deceptively complex life of rigid job descriptions and interrelated socialization patterns, but they are unable to recognize each other based on a memory of past experience. Instead, they detect chemical signals to identify each other; they live their busy little lives based entirely on the way they interpret smells. By extracting a chemical that would normally identify larvae and attaching the chemical to fake larvae, scientists were able to show that ants could not distinguish fakes from real larvae. To an ant, if it smells like larvae, it is larvae, and ants have no ability to adapt to any other circumstance or possibility. Animals without such memory cannot adapt their behavior to changing circumstances; their adaptation relies only on natural selection.

Birds are farther along, evolutionarily speaking. While they are still largely guided by inborn instincts, they also are able to adapt to their circumstances using recognition based on memory. If a scientist moves eggs from one nest to another, birds can recognize their own eggs and reclaim them: The bird's past experience molds its present behavior. This is the difference between recognition based on memory and identification based on genetically programmed instinct.

Higher animals, such as dogs, cats, and wild animals, rely on the adaptive value of the memory to a much greater degree. An elephant stuck in quicksand will, once freed, always remember the danger of quicksand and avoid it. This type of memory based on recognition is memory of the highest order; many domestic animals are capable of it.

aniracetam   One of a class of NOOTROPIC drugs that some studies suggest may be capable of improving cognitive performance on a number of intelligence and memory tests. Its chemical structure is similar to PIRACETAM, a drug being investigated in the treatment of ALZHEIMER'S DISEASE.

Studies suggest it stimulates the function of certain brain receptors. Both long- and short-term memory improvement has been shown in research. It appears to be a general enhancer of transmitter release for a number of transmitter systems.

Aniracetam is not approved for distribution in any country. Other names for aniracetam include Draganon, RO 13-5057, and Sarpul.

Anna O   was a young Viennese woman and "hysteria" patient in the late 19th century whose real name was Bertha Pappenheim. She was called "Anna O" by JOSEF BREUER and SIGMUND FREUD, who described her treatment in their book *Studies on Hysteria.*

Anna O was treated by Breuer from 1880 to 1882 for a range of psychosomatic problems and dissociative absences. Freud learned about her case after her treatment by Breuer, but her case led him to the technique of letting patients talk about their problems.

Breuer and Freud did not agree on the fundamental cause of dissociative absences. Breuer insisted they were a form of autohypnosis, while Freud believed they served as a defense mechanism, a protection against harmful thoughts.

Anna O was quite hypnotizable and excellent at self-hypnosis, and Breuer hypnotized her almost daily for hours at a time. Before the onset of her hysteria, she had often hallucinated an alternate world she called her private theater, a fairy-tale world in which she lived her life. If her father had not contracted a fatal case of tuberculosis, she might have spent the rest of her life in her dream world, but she was called upon to stay alert and nurse her father.

Although a bright, energetic woman, her culture expected her to live a life of quiet self-denial. She spent her time tending her dying father, never revealing any emotion and never earning a respite from her duties. Yet despite her resentment, she did not rebel openly. Her father's illness brought about a crisis in her life; she could no longer retreat into her private world, but she could not bear her new life, either. First, she experienced a hysterical cough while hearing an orchestra playing as she tended her father. She wished she could be at the party, and then immediately felt guilty for wanting to dance while her father lay dying. She coughed instead and continued to cough whenever she heard music. She had altered her emotional memory; she associated music with happiness, but then remembered her father and despised her wish for fun, changing the association with music.

After six months, she retreated to her bed, where she alternated between consciousness and DISSOCIATION. During conscious periods, she seemed normal except that she stayed in bed and exhibited a variety of odd behaviors—speaking only English, coughing when hearing music, and hating water. When she retreated into her dream world, she lost the abilities of recognition and perception. She did not see or hear people, although Breuer could break through to her and maintain contact by steady speech. Anna did not, however, perceive strangers.

When Breuer brought a colleague to see her, she did not perceive him, and recognized that there was another person in the room only when he blew cigar smoke at her. She looked for the source of smoke, saw the stranger and ran.

Eventually Anna O recovered apparently on her own, although her changed circumstances helped. (Her father died and she entered a sanitarium where she had no responsibilities.) While Breuer's intensive therapy relieved some of her symptoms, she developed others, and when he stopped her treatment she was no better than when she had begun two years before. Many more years passed before she was healthy, but eventually she became an important figure in Austria's feminist movement.

Anna O's case shows that emotional memory failures don't need to have an objective cause—they can be related to a patient's own perceptions. While Breuer could attempt to treat her symptoms, he couldn't address the inequities of Viennese society.

anomia A type of APHASIA involving the inability to verbalize the names of people, objects, and places. It appears to relate to speech output, since patients usually have no problem understanding when the object is named for them.

anosognosia A type of AGNOSIA in which people do not recognize that they are ill because they cannot make the connection between the fact of symptoms and the perception "I'm ill."

anoxia The complete disruption of oxygen supply to a given cell. This loss of oxygen causes a disruption of cell metabolism and can be fatal to the cell unless it is corrected within a few minutes. Anoxia

refers to oxygen deprivation, as opposed to ischemia, which produces a loss of oxygen and other blood constituents.

See also HYPOXIA.

anterior commissure A collection of nerve cells that connects the brain's two hemispheres. It is smaller and appeared earlier in evolution than the CORPUS CALLOSUM. Recent research has suggested that in men, this part of the brain is smaller than in women, even though men's brains are generally larger than women's brains. The larger commissure in women may help explain, at least in part, why the two hemispheres of the female brain seem to work together on activities ranging from language to emotional responses.

See also CEREBRAL COMMISSURE.

anterior communicating artery A short artery located in the FOREBRAIN that connects the two arteries in the front of each hemisphere. Aneurysms often occur along this artery, which can cause a type of AMNESIA when the aneurysm bursts, damaging the forebrain.

See also ANEURYSM, BRAIN.

anterograde amnesia See AMNESIA.

anticholinergics Anticholinergics are a group of ACETYLCHOLINE-blocking drugs that are used to treat irritable bowel syndrome and certain types of urinary incontinence, Parkinson's disease, asthma, and other diseases. They also have a reputation as amnesic drugs.

These drugs act as antagonists to the actions of cholinergic nerve fibers (or cells), usually of the parasympathetic nervous system. These cholinergic nerve cells are those that use acetylcholine as their neurotransmitter. Drugs that have anticholinergic effects block the transmission of this neurotransmitter, preventing the communication between nerve cells and altering behavior. Most psychoactive drugs have anticholinergic effects in both the central and the peripheral nervous systems.

Depending on the dose, the anticholinergics SCOPOLAMINE, atropine, and glycopyrrolate all can produce sedation and lack of vigilance. The most famous of the memory-clouding anticholinergics is scopolamine, a belladonna alkaloid that is a particularly potent amnesic agent. Other anticholinergics include heterocyclic antidepressants, antipsychotics, antihistamines, antiparkinsonian drugs, and some hypnotics.

Research studies suggest that after a patient has received an anticholinergic drug, memory retention remains intact but effortful retrieval is impaired. It is believed that the neurochemical processes disrupted by these drugs are not involved in maintaining information in memory; rather they control the encoding process, which leads to a deficiency of retrieval.

If a patient takes several of these drugs together—or takes too many of any one kind—the combination can cause a crisis called the anticholinergic syndrome. Symptoms of this include dry mouth, constipation, urinary retention, decreased sweating, fever, flushing, discoordination, tachycardia, confusion, delirium, disorientation, agitation, visual and auditory hallucinations, anxiety, restlessness, pseudoseizures, and delusions. Treatment for anticholinergic syndrome is anticholinesterase therapy.

anticoagulant drugs This group of drugs prevents abnormal blood clotting and is used to prevent and treat STROKE or TRANSIENT ISCHEMIC ATTACKS. If the drugs are given by injection, they begin to work within a few hours; those given by mouth work within a day. They increase the effect of an enzyme that blocks the activity of coagulation factors that are needed for blood to clot.

By interfering with the blood-clotting mechanism, these drugs can prevent an abnormal blood clot from forming; if a clot already exists, the drugs can stop it from growing larger and reduce the risk of a piece of it breaking off and blocking another blood vessel. Unlike thrombolytic drugs, these drugs do not dissolve clots that already exist.

anticonvulsant drugs A group of drugs used to prevent SEIZURES or to interrupt a seizure taking place by inhibiting the excess electrical activity in the brain and blocking its spread. Anticonvulsants include carbamazepine, clonazepam, diazepam, ethosuximide, phenobarbital, phenytoin, primidone, and valproic acid.

The choice of drug is determined by the type of seizure; in long-term seizure prevention, more than one type of drug may be needed.

Adverse effects include reduced concentration, memory problems, poor coordination, and fatigue.

See also EPILEPSY.

antidepressant drugs Drugs that appear to correct a chemical imbalance or dysfunction in the brains of depressed people by boosting the level of NEUROTRANSMITTERS. Each of the major classes of antidepressants, which includes MONOAMINE OXIDASE (MAO) INHIBITORS, CYCLICS, and SEROTONIN inhibitors—affect different neurotransmitter systems in different ways.

Most of these drugs usually take at least 10 days before they begin to work and up to two months before they are fully effective; they all carry some type of side effects of varying intensity.

The complex array of various brain chemicals and processes that influence depression tend to differ from one patient to the next; because there is no foolproof way to identify which neurotransmitters may be causing depression, prescribing antidepressants may be a trial-and-error process until the right one is found.

For many people, the first antidepressant is often not the right antidepressant. In fact, only a little more than half of all patients who are given antidepressants find relief with their first prescription. No one is quite sure how or why antidepressants work, and no one can predict who will respond to which drug. The best a physician can do is to look at a person's symptoms and try to match those symptoms with an antidepressant.

There is no one miracle antidepressant that works better than any other, all the time, for everybody. Because depression itself is a complex disease with many causes, doctors must choose among a wide range of antidepressants that work on different brain systems and affect different processes.

Cyclic antidepressants are a class of traditional drugs that treat depression by boosting the level of several different neurotransmitters (NOREPI-NEPHRINE, EPINEPHRINE, serotonin, and DOPAMINE) by blocking their reabsorption. MAO inhibitors destroy enzymes responsible for breaking down monoamine neurotransmitters, boosting the neurotransmitter levels. In general, MAOIs are used to treat those who do not respond to tricyclics. Some of the newer antidepressants (selective serotonin reuptake inhibitors) interfere with the reuptake of a specific neurotransmitter (serotonin).

Antidepressants include the tricyclics amitriptyline, amoxapine, clomipramine, desipramine, doxepin, imipramine, nortriptyline, and protriptyline; the tetracyclic maprotiline (Ludiomil); monoamine oxidase inhibitors (MAOIs) isocarboxazid (Marplan), phenelzine (Nardil), and tranylcypromine; the selective serotonin reuptake inhibitors (SSRIs) fluoxetine, paroxetine, citalopram, fluvoxamine, and sertraline; and the structurally unrelated compounds bupropion, nefazodone, mirtazapine, venlafaxine, and trazodone. LITHIUM is another antidepressant used to treat bipolar disorder (manic depression).

FDA Warnings

Due to the well-documented side effects of antidepressant medications in individuals ages 18 to 24, in 2004 the FDA proposed that antidepressant manufacturers update their black box warnings on their products' labeling. Those warnings should, according to the FDA, alert consumers to the possibility of suicidality, especially during the first month of treatment. The medications identified thus far as having increased suicidality in adolescents and young adults include the following:

Anafranil (clomipramine)
Asendin (amoxapine)
Aventyl (nortriptyline)
Celexa (citalopram hydrobromide)
Cymbalta (duloxetine)
Desyrel (trazodone HCl)
Elavil (amitriptyline)
Effexor (venlafaxine HCl)
Emsam (selegiline)
Etrafon (perphenazine/amitriptyline)
fluvoxamine maleate

Lexapro (escitalopram oxalate)
Limbitrol (chlordiazepoxide/amitriptyline)
Ludiomil (maprotiline)
Marplan (isocarboxazid)
Nardil (phenelzine sulfate)
nefazodone HCl
Norpramin (desipramine HCl)
Pamelor (nortriptyline)
Parnate (tranylcypromine sulfate)
Paxil (paroxetine HCl)
Pexeva (paroxetine mesylate)
Prozac (fluoxetine HCl)
Remeron (mirtazapine)
Sarafem (fluoxetine HCl)
Seroquel (quetiapine)
Sinequan (doxepin)
Surmontil (trimipramine)
Symbyax (olanzapine/fluoxetine)
Tofranil (imipramine)
Tofranil-PM (imipramine pamoate)
Triavil (perphenazine/amitriptyline)
Vivactil (protriptyline)
Wellbutrin (bupropion HCl)
Zoloft (sertraline HCl)
Zyban (bupropion HCl)

Side Effects

Side effects from antidepressants generally fall into three categories: Sedation; dry mouth, blurry vision, constipation, urinary problems, increased heart rate, and memory problems; and dizziness on standing up (orthostatic hypotension). Many antidepressants can produce rapid heartbeat, tremor, and sexual problems (loss of interest or inability to reach orgasm). Those that interfere with dopamine (such as Wellbutrin and Asendin) may produce movement disorders and endocrine system changes. Blocking serotonin may create stomach problems, insomnia, and anxiety.

Those that work on the other side of the synapse, blocking receptors that pick up neurotransmitters, have other side effects, depending on which receptors are affected. Blocking histamine H1 receptors produces weight gain and sedation; muscarinic receptor blockade causes dry mouth, constipation, blurry vision, and memory problems.

This is why a tricyclic such as amitriptyline (Elavil) causes so many side effects—it blocks the absorption of both norepinephrine and serotonin, plus four different receptors (Alpha$_1$, Dopamine D$_2$, Histamine H$_1$, and muscarinic).

Each drug has a profile of its own particular side effects. Tricyclics often cause dry mouth, constipation, sedation, nervousness, weight gain, and diminished sex drive. MAOIs interact with certain foods and other medications to produce potentially fatal high blood pressure. Such antidepressants as the SSRIs (including Prozac, Paxil, and Zoloft) produce fewer side effects than MAOIs or tricyclics because they affect fewer brain pathways, but nausea, headache, and sexual problems may occur.

Still, even though a drug is characterized by certain side effects, it does not mean a patient will experience any of them. In addition, many antidepressants can be taken before bed so that the side effects will occur during sleep. If a bedtime dose makes a patient too sleepy the next morning, a dose at dinner may be a better idea. A physician can work with a person's schedule to find the dosage timetable that works best.

If antidepressants lower sex drive, cause impotence, or interfere in orgasm, these side effects can be eliminated by adding another drug or changing the antidepressant.

antiemetic drugs A group of drugs used to treat nausea and vomiting; many work by reducing nerve activity at the base of the brain, suppressing the vomiting reflex. Antihistamine drugs and anticholinergic drugs also reduce the vomiting associated with vertigo by suppressing nerve activity in the balance center in the inner ear. Some antiemetics cause drowsiness, and some should not be taken during pregnancy because they may cause birth defects.

antioxidant A substance that chemically neutralizes FREE RADICALS (potentially harmful, highly-charged atoms on molecules). The most common free radical is a species of oxygen. In the brain, it can chemically interact with lipids (the main component of a cell wall), harming the neuron. New research suggests that antioxidants can neutral-

ize free radicals before they begin to damage the brain's cells.

While a certain amount of free radicals are necessary to maintain proper body function, high levels are toxic to brain (and body) cells. Each day, the body generates thousands upon thousands of these free radicals in response to ultraviolet (UV) light, smoke, or pollution. Once activated, they destroy the cells in the brain and elsewhere in the body.

Some of the most common of the antioxidants include vitamins C (found in citrus fruits) and E (found in eggs, butter, and vegetable oil).

antipsychotic drugs A group of drugs used to treat psychoses (mental disorders involving loss of contact with reality) that block the action of certain NEUROTRANSMITTERS in the brain. These drugs are especially helpful in the treatment of SCHIZOPHRENIA and MANIC-DEPRESSION and are also used to calm or sedate patients with other mental disorders (such as DEMENTIA). The antipsychotic drugs include the phenothiazines (such as chlorpromazine, fluphenazine, perphenazine, thioridazine, and trifluoperazine) and various other medications including haloperidol, thiothixene, or LITHIUM, which is used specifically to treat the symptoms of mania.

Most antipsychotics block the action of DOPAMINE, a neurotransmitter found in the brain. Excess dopamine activity has been associated with many forms of psychoses. Lithium may control symptoms of mania by reducing activity in certain nerve impulse transmitters (SEROTONIN and NOREPINEPHRINE) that influence emotional status and behavior.

Adverse Effects

While these drugs have been helpful in controlling irrational thinking, aggressive behavior, and HYPERACTIVITY, serious side effects have appeared with increasing prominence. Especially troublesome is TARDIVE DYSKINESIA, which began to appear in large numbers of people during the 1970s. This movement disorder is caused by high doses of neuroleptic drugs for more than six months and appears primarily in adults and the elderly, although children can also be affected. Certain areas of the body are especially affected, including lips, eyes, jaw, arms, legs, and trunk; movements are usually involuntary and irregular and may be confused with PARKINSONISM (a disorder with symptoms similar to those of PARKINSON'S DISEASE). Protruding tongue, lip and facial contortions with eye blinks, and unplanned opening of the jaw are common. Slow, writhing movements and rapid, jerky expressions are also found, together with a rocking movement of the trunk. In some adults, the condition is irreversible.

Most of the antipsychotics also can cause drowsiness or lethargy; other possible side effects include dry mouth, blurry vision, and urinary problems.

anxiety An unpleasant emotional state ranging from mild discomfort to intense fear that some scientists believe may be the result of an elevated level of arousal in the CENTRAL NERVOUS SYSTEM. This excess arousal would lead a person to react more excitedly and adapt more slowly to events surrounding him or her.

While a certain amount of anxiety is normal, it can become a symptom when the anxious feelings interfere with normal daily activities.

Symptoms and Diagnostic Path
The most common symptoms of anxiety center around the chest, including palpitations (more forceful, irregular heartbeat), throbbing or stabbing pains, air hunger (inability to take in enough air), feelings of tightness in the chest, and a tendency to hyperventilate (sigh or overbreathe).

Other symptoms include headaches, neck spasms, back pain, and an inability to relax, together with restlessness, tremors, and sense of tiredness. The symptoms of anxiety may include a feeling of impending doom in the absence of any particular threat.

Stomach symptoms include dry mouth, feelings of distention, diarrhea, nausea, appetite changes, swallowing problems, and constant belching.

Treatment Options and Outlook
Effective treatment may include reassurance, counseling, and therapy, together with antianxiety drugs (such as the BENZODIAZEPINES).

aphasia A neurological condition in which language comprehension or expression is disturbed due to brain dysfunction, affecting the ability to speak and write and/or the ability to comprehend and read the written word. *Aphasia* is a complete absence of these skills, while *dysphasia* refers to a disturbance in these abilities. A STROKE or a HEAD INJURY are the most common causes of brain damage leading to aphasia.

Symptoms and Diagnostic Path
The speech problems caused by brain damage are different from speech problems caused by dysfunction in other parts of the body. Related disabilities with aphasia include word blindness (ALEXIA) or writing problems (AGRAPHIA).

Language functions within the brain are situated in the dominant cerebral hemisphere, especially in the Broca's and Wernicke's areas, and in the pathways that connect the two. Damage in this area is the most common cause of aphasia. A patient with damage to BROCA'S AREA will experience problems in expressing language; speech is labored, slow, and dysrhythmic. However, the few words that are uttered are meaningful. A patient with a damaged WERNICKE'S AREA will experience problems in comprehending language; speech is fluent, but because of the comprehension problems, the meaning is disturbed. The patient will have problems choosing the right word or the correct grammatical form; writing is affected, and spoken or written commands may not be understood. Irrelevant words intrude.

In *global aphasia*, the patient has an almost or complete inability to speak, write, or understand spoken or written words, usually with widespread damage to the dominant cerebral hemisphere. This is the most severe type of aphasia. Patients with *nominal aphasia* have problems naming objects or finding words, although the person may be able to choose the correct name from several offered. This condition may be caused by general cerebral dysfunction or damage to a specific language area. In *mixed nonfluent aphasia*, patients have sparse and effortful speech which resembles that seen in patients with severe Broca's aphasia. However, unlike people with Broca's aphasia, they only have limited comprehension of speech and cannot read or write beyond an elementary level. People with *anomic aphasia* have a persistent inability to supply the words for the things they want to talk about (especially significant nouns and verbs), referred to as word-finding difficulty. As a result, their speech is grammatically fluent but their speech is full of vague circumlocutions and expressions of frustration. They understand speech well, and in most cases, read adequately. Their problem in finding words is as evident in writing as in speech. In *developmental aphasia,* the problem is caused by delayed development of the central nervous system.

Treatment Options and Outlook

Treatment strives to improve communication by helping the person use remaining abilities, restore language abilities as much as possible, compensate for language problems, and learn other methods of communicating. Treatment may be offered in individual or group settings.

Individual therapy focuses on the specific needs of the person, whereas group therapy offers the chance to use new communication skills in a comfortable setting. Family involvement is often a crucial component of aphasia treatment so that family members can learn the best way to communicate.

While aphasia may improve after a stroke or head injury, the more severe the aphasia, the less chance for improvement. Speech therapy is the primary treatment. The most effective treatment begins early in the recovery process. How much a patient will improve depends on the cause of the brain damage, the area of the brain that was damaged, the extent of the brain injury, and the age and health of the individual. Additional factors include motivation and handedness. Educational level may also be important.

apnea   A prolonged cessation of breathing that can be caused by a brain stem damage from STROKE, TRANSIENT ISCHEMIC ATTACK, or HEAD INJURY.

Breathing is an automatic process that is controlled by the respiratory center in the brain stem; these breathing centers send nerve impulses to the muscles of the chest and diaphragm that regulate lung expansion and deflation.

apolipoprotein E (ApoE)   A protein whose main function is to transport cholesterol; one form of this protein has been linked to late-onset ALZHEIMER'S DISEASE. The gene for this protein is found on chromosome 19.

There are three forms of ApoE: e2, e3, and e4; ApoE-4 is associated with about 60 percent of late-onset Alzheimer's cases and is considered a risk factor for the disease. A person can have two ApoE-4 genes (one inherited from each parent), one ApoE-4 gene (inherited from one parent, but not the other), or no ApoE-4 variants at all. It seems that the ApoE-4 gene doesn't guarantee who will get Alzheimer's disease, but is an indication of who is more vulnerable.

It appears that the more ApoE-4 variants a person has, the quicker he or she will get Alzheimer's (if the person gets it at all). Research suggests that those with two E-4 varieties experience onset by age 80 to 85; those with one experience onset by age 90 to 95; those with none of the E-4 varieties don't get the disease until age 95 to 100—if at all.

But not everyone with the gene goes on to develop Alzheimer's. Experts think that other factors, such as diseases like diabetes or atherosclerosis, boost the chance that the gene carrier will develop Alzheimer's. In one study of 6,000 healthy people over age 65, those who carried the ApoE-4 gene and who also had diabetes, atherosclerosis, or a circulation problem in hands, feet, or legs, had a much higher risk of memory and thinking problems than those without the gene or the illnesses. Those with both atherosclerosis and ApoE-4 had more than an eightfold increased risk for problems in learning and memory. (And atherosclerosis alone also increased the risk for memory problems.)

Experts believe that people who have the gene should modify their lifestyle in order to prevent diabetes or heart disease. By watching diet and getting plenty of exercise, it is still possible to head off possible causes of dementia.

It is possible to be tested for the ApoE gene variant, but the test is a strong predictor of risk only for those younger than age 70.

apoplexy   An outdated term for STROKE. Symptoms include sudden loss of consciousness, paralysis, or loss of sensation. The usual cause of apoplexy is the rupture of a brain artery or blockage by a clot.

appestat   Outdated term referring to the region of the brain within the HYPOTHALAMUS that controls food intake. It is believed that appetite suppressants probably decrease the sense of hunger by altering the chemical characteristics in this area. Stimulating the appestat with electrodes provokes overeating in satiated lab animals.

appetite   The desire for food that can be a pleasant sensation in anticipation of eating (as compared to HUNGER, an unpleasant feeling triggered by a physiological need for food). A person's appetite is regulated by two parts of the brain—the HYPOTHALAMUS and the CEREBRAL CORTEX—and is a sensation learned by enjoying a variety of food that smells and tastes good. When combined with hunger, it can provide the body with enough foods to maintain health.

How hungry a person feels at any one time is dependent on the amount of glucose circulating in the blood, which is monitored in the brain. Temporary appetite loss (known medically as anorexia) can be caused by a range of illnesses or minor emotional upsets. A more chronic loss of appetite may be the sign of a more serious illness or mental disorder. Physical causes of loss of appetite could include STROKE, BRAIN TUMOR, or BRAIN INJURY causing damage to the hypothalamus or cerebral cortex. Other possible physical problems linked to appetite loss include stomach problems, gastric ulcers, or liver disorders (such as hepatitis).

In addition, some youngsters between ages two and four may refuse food; this is usually considered to be a normal phase of child development (if there are no other symptoms).

Under normal conditions, healthy people can go hungry for a day or two without causing harm to the brain, as long as plenty of fluids are consumed.

appetite stimulants   Although a variety of drugs have been prescribed (including alcohol and iron-containing elixirs), there are no known drugs that safely and effectively stimulate the APPETITE.

See also APPETITE SUPPRESSANTS; HUNGER.

appetite suppressants   A group of drugs that suppress the APPETITE, probably by affecting the HYPOTHALAMUS, the part of the brain that controls the desire to eat. Common appetite suppressants include diethylpropion, fenfluramine, mazindol, phenmetrazine, phentermine, and phenylpropanolamine.

Side Effects
Common side effects include dry mouth, insomnia, dizziness, palpitations, and restlessness. Taking an appetite suppressant for more than six weeks may lead to dependence; however, newer drugs are less addictive than the amphetamines that used to be prescribed for appetite control.

Taking appetite suppressants with alcohol may cause increased sedation; taking them with CAFFEINE may cause excessive stimulation. Taken with food or drinks containing tyramine (such as Chianti, robust red wines, vermouth, ale, or beer) can cause an increase in blood pressure.

See also APPETITE STIMULANTS; HUNGER.

apraxia   The inability to make purposeful movements despite normal muscles and coordination because of nerve tract damage within the CORTEX (the main mass of the brain) that translates the *idea* for movement *into* the movement. People with apraxia usually know what they want to do, but they seem to be unable to remember the sequence of actions necessary to make the movement. The brain damage may be caused by HEAD INJURY, infection, STROKE, or BRAIN TUMOR.

Symptoms and Diagnostic Path
There are several different types of apraxia, depending on the part of the brain that has been damaged. A person who cannot carry out a spoken command to make a particular movement but who can unconsciously make that movement has *ideomotor apraxia*. AGRAPHIA (writing problems) and EXPRES-

SIVE APHASIA (severe speaking problems) are both special forms of apraxia.

Treatment Options and Outlook

Recovery from head injury or stroke varies widely from one patient to the next; degree of recovery often depends on severity of the initial injury. Even in the best of situations, however, there is usually some deficit that remains, and it may require considerable effort for the patient to relearn the lost skill.

See also ALEXIA; DYSPHASIA.

aprosodia A condition caused by damage to certain sections of the right brain hemisphere in which speech can become flat and emotionless, or in which the emotional qualities of speech and gestures are not completely comprehended or executed. The speech of a person with this condition lacks cadence, stress, different tones, and emotional gestures.

arachnoiditis A fairly rare condition characterized by chronic inflammation and thickening of the brain's ARACHNOID MEMBRANE that may develop several years after MENINGITIS, or after bleeding beneath the arachnoid membrane. It also may be caused by a variety of diseases, such as SYPHILIS; from head injury; or from errors in diagnostic procedures such as MYELOGRAPHY or lumbar puncture. Usually, however, no cause is ever found.

Symptoms and Diagnostic Path

Although symptoms vary with the severity of the disorder, they can include epileptic seizures, headache, blindness, numbness, tingling, stinging leg pain, or spastic paralysis.

Arachnoiditis is a disabling disease causing intractable pain and brain deficits. As the disease progresses, some symptoms may worsen and become permanent.

· Treatment Options and Outlook

There is no cure. The goal of treatment should be to return the patient to a normal life. Conservative therapy such as pain management is generally rec-

ommended. In those patients whose arachnoiditis is progressive, surgery to remove adhesions is only mildly effective because scar tissue continues to develop. Surgery also exposes the already-irritated spinal cord to more trauma.

Few people with this disorder are able to continue working. In some cases, progressive paralysis may occur.

arachnoid membrane The middle of the three layers (MENINGES) of connective tissue surrounding and protecting the brain and the spinal cord.

archicortex Older region of the CEREBRAL CORTEX that includes the LIMBIC SYSTEM, although usually refers to the HIPPOCAMPUS only.

Aretaeus of Cappadocia (A.D. 81?–138) This Greek physician from Cappadocia made the distinction between mental and nervous diseases and described the characteristics of EPILEPSY. He led a revival of the teachings of HIPPOCRATES and is believed to be second only to Hippocrates in his keen observational abilities. He adhered to the pneumatic school of medicine, believing that health was maintained by "vital air." Pneumatists felt that an imbalance of the *humors* (blood, phlegm, choler, and melancholy) disturbed the *pneuma* (breathing), which is characterized by an abnormal pulse. Actually, however, Aretaeus practiced the methods of several different schools of medical thought.

His contributions were forgotten until the discovery of two of his manuscripts in 1554 that described pleurisy, diphtheria, tetanus, pneumonia, asthma, and epilepsy. He also gave diabetes its name and gave the earliest clear description of that disease.

See also BRAIN IN HISTORY.

Arnold-Chiari malformation A congenital disorder characterized by a distortion of the base of the skull; the lower BRAIN STEM and parts of the CEREBELLUM are longer than normal and protrude through the opening for the spinal cord at the base of the skull. This condition is commonly associated with NEURAL TUBE DEFECTS and HYDROCEPHALUS.

Symptoms and Diagnostic Path

In most cases, symptoms begin during infancy; however, the onset of symptoms may be delayed until adolescence or adulthood. Symptoms usually include vomiting, muscle weakness in the head and face, difficulty swallowing, and varying degrees of mental impairment. Paralysis of the arms and legs also may occur.

Adults and adolescents with Chiari malformation who previously had no symptoms may show signs of progressive brain impairment as they grow older, such as involuntary, rapid, downward eye movements. Other symptoms include dizziness, headache, double vision, deafness, an impaired ability to coordinate movement, and episodes of acute pain in and around the eyes.

Treatment Options and Outlook

Surgery to repair the meningeal sac's protrusion into the spinal cord helps stabilize the Arnold-Chiari malformation's effects. In combination with the implantation of shunts to relieve pressure on the brain, this usually results in periods of significant alleviation of symptoms. However, symptoms usually return as the hydrocephalus redevelops.

arteriogram   Another term for angiogram.
See also ANGIOGRAPHY.

arteriography, cerebral   Also known as coronary angiography, this is an X-RAY examination of an artery that has been outlined by the injection of a contrast dye. The technique is used to detect diseases of the vascular system, such as carotid artery disease or brain aneurysms.

Procedure

Cerebral arteriography is used to show the extent and location of arteriosclerosis in the brain's major arteries. It is an important tool that helps doctors diagnose patients with cerebrovascular disease that can lead to stroke.

Risks and Complications

While arteriography is key in evaluating many people who are at high risk of stroke, occasionally it can lead to complications. Patients with cerebrovascular disease are at special risk for such complications. For example, STROKE can occur during the procedure or in the first few hours after it is over.

See also MAGNETIC RESONANCE IMAGING.

ascending reticular activating system   A complex net of cells in the BRAIN STEM concerned with attention, sleep, and wakefulness. It is called "ascending" because of the widespread flow of information it sends into the neocortex.

Asperger's syndrome   A condition characterized by sustained problems with social interactions and social relatedness and the development of restricted, repetitive patterns of interests, activities, and behaviors. Asperger's syndrome is usually considered a subtype of high-functioning autism (see AUTISTIC DISORDER). Although the correct modern term is *Asperger's disorder,* according to the *Diagnostic and Statistical Manual, Fourth Edition—Text Revision (DSM-IV-TR);* (the manual used to diagnose mental conditions), it is also sometimes called Asperger syndrome or Asperger's syndrome.

The disorder is named for Hans Asperger, a Viennese pediatrician who first documented the cluster of characteristics of the syndrome in the 1940s.

Asperger's disorder is one of five conditions grouped under the umbrella category of PERVASIVE DEVELOPMENTAL DISORDERS (PDD) because all five share a number of characteristics: impairments in social interaction, imaginative activity, verbal and nonverbal communication skills, and a limited number of interests and activities that tend to be repetitive. The other four disorders in the PDD group include autism, RETT SYNDROME, childhood disintegrative disorder, and PDD–Not Otherwise Specified (PDD-NOS). The umbrella term *pervasive developmental disorders* was first used in the 1980s to describe this class of disorders having similar symptoms or characteristics.

Asperger's was believed to be a milder variant of autism, but without the delays in cognitive or language development. In 1994 Asperger's was first classified as a pervasive developmental disorder.

The validity of this condition, as opposed to high-functioning autism, remains controversial. Inconsistencies in the way the term has been used and the lack, until quite recently, of recognized official definitions has made it difficult to interpret the research available on this condition. Even now, some clinicians will use the term to refer to persons with autism who have IQs in the normal range, or to adults with autism, or to PDD-NOS. Recent official definitions emphasize differences from autism, e.g., in terms of better communication (particularly verbal) skills. It also seems likely that the condition overlaps, at least in part, with some forms of learning disability.

Many children with pervasive developmental disorders, such as Asperger's disorder, also meet the diagnostic criteria for ATTENTION DEFICIT HYPERACTIVITY DISORDER (ADHD). However, ADHD should not be diagnosed when there is Asperger's, since all the ADHD symptoms can be attributed to the other condition. Clinicians who overlook other symptoms of Asperger's tend to diagnose these children as ADHD.

Like many learning disorders, Asperger's is believed to be more common in males, although more research needs to be done to understand its genetic origins. According to the National Institutes of Health, Asperger's disorder occurs in one out of every 500 Americans—more often than multiple sclerosis, Down syndrome, or cystic fibrosis. It is estimated that more than 400,000 families are affected by this condition.

While biological factors are of crucial importance in the etiology of autism, so far brain imaging studies with Asperger's cases have found no consistent pattern or evidence of any type of lesion, and no single location of any lesion.

Associated medical conditions such as fragile X syndrome, tuberous sclerosis, neurofibromatosis, and hypothyroidism (sluggish thyroid) are less common in Asperger's disorder than in classical autism. Therefore, scientists suspect there may be fewer major physical brain problems associated with Asperger's than with autism.

Symptoms and Diagnostic Path

Often there are no obvious delays in language or cognitive development, or in age-appropriate self-help skills. While these individuals possess attention deficits, problems with organization, and an uneven profile of skills, they usually have average and sometimes gifted intelligence.

Individuals with Asperger's syndrome may have problems with social situations and in developing peer relationships. They may have noticeable difficulty with nonverbal communication, impaired use of social gestures, facial expressions, and eye contact. There may be certain repetitive behaviors or rituals. Though grammatical, speech is peculiar due to abnormal inflection and repetition. Clumsiness is prominent both in speech and physical movements. Individuals with this disorder usually have a limited area of interest that excludes more age-appropriate common interests, such as single-minded obsessions about cars, trains, doorknobs, hinges, astronomy, or history.

When compared to autism, Asperger's disorder usually appears later in life, with less severe social and communication problems. Clumsiness and single-minded interests are more common, and verbal IQ is usually higher than performance IQ (in autism, the reverse is usually true). The outcome is usually more positive than for autism. Children with Asperger's disorder have impaired social interactions similar to those of children with autism, as well as stereotyped or repetitive behaviors and mannerisms and nonfunctional rituals. However, language skills are normal and sometimes superior to those of an average child, although their speech is usually described as peculiar, such as being stilted and focusing on unusual topics. Children with Asperger's usually have normal IQ.

Most of the individuals with Asperger's syndrome are interested in having friends, but lack the social skills to begin or maintain a friendship. While high-functioning autistic individuals also may be social but awkward, they are typically less interested in having friends. In addition, high-functioning autistic individuals are often delayed in developing speech/language.

Treatment Options and Outlook

While there is no cure, early intervention has been shown to be effective. The need for academic and social supports increases through the school years, and by adolescence many children develop symptoms of depression and anxiety. One recent focus of therapy has been the use of therapy animals, especially dogs. It is important to continue supports into adulthood to ensure affected adults can lead productive lives.

Symptoms can be managed using individual psychotherapy to help the individual to process the feelings aroused by being socially handicapped. Other treatments may include parent education and training, behavioral modification, social skills training, educational interventions, and medication. Symptoms and appropriate medications include

- hyperactivity, inattention, and impulsivity: stimulants (methylphenidate, dextroamphetamine, methamphetamine, pemoline), clonidine, and tricyclic antidepressants (desipramine, nortriptyline)
- irritability and aggression: mood stabilizers (valproate, carbamazepine, lithium), beta blockers (nadolol, propranolol), neuroleptics (risperidone, haloperidol)
- preoccupations, rituals, and compulsions: antidepressants (fluvoxamine, fluoxetine, clomipramine)
- anxiety: antidepressants (sertraline, fluoxetine, imipramine, clomipramine, nortriptyline)

association The connection of one item to be remembered with others a person already knows. For example, the easiest way to tell the difference between *stationery* and *stationary* is that you use stationery to write a letter; to remember how to spell *believe*, never believe a lie. Association can be used consciously to remember information; but it also can occur unconsciously. The experience of hearing or seeing something that reminds one of something else occurs because such sounds or sights somehow were linked together in the past, so that remembering one bit of information automatically drew the other bit of information with it.

association areas Areas in the NEOCORTEX that are not concerned with primary sensory processing but that have a secondary role in integrating sensory information with other brain systems. Many scientists suspect that these areas play a large role in thinking and memory.

astrocytoma A usually malignant brain tumor, the most common type of GLIOMA (arising from supportive brain cells called GLIAL CELLS). This type of tumor most often occurs in the CORTEX.

Although all types of this tumor are serious, they are divided into grades according to their growth rate and malignancy, with grade I the slowest tumor that may spread throughout the brain without causing symptoms for many years. The so-called benign astrocytoma is slow growing, but it may spread to large areas of the brain and may be encapsulated in a cyst.

The astrocytoma may occur in the cerebral hemispheres of adults or in the cerebellum, brain stem, or the optic nerve of children.

Symptoms are similar to other types of tumors and depend on the area affected. There are three types of astrocytomas: low-grade, anaplastic, and glioblastoma multiforme. A *low-grade astrocytoma* may occur in either the cerebrum of adults and children, or in the cerebellum of children. An *anaplastic astrocytoma* is moderately malignant and commonly spreads to surrounding brain tissue. The most malignant type of astrocytoma is a grade 4 *glioblastoma multiforme*, which spreads rapidly throughout the brain and is resistant to treatment.

The usual treatment is surgery, but very few astrocytomas can be completely surgically removed. Usually, radiation therapy follows surgery, and radiation retreatment may be required.

asymmetry in the brain Many parallel areas (especially in the CORTEX) are larger in one hemisphere than in the other. For example, the PLANUM TEMPORALE, an important component in the understanding of speech, is larger in the left hemisphere in most healthy people.

The normal asymmetry of the brain appears to be reversed in the brains of those with SCHIZOPHRENIA. In these patients, for example, the planum temporale is much larger in the right hemisphere, which may help to explain their garbled speech.

ataxia Shaky movements and unsteady gait caused by the brain's failure to regulate the body's posture and the strength and direction of limb movements. Ataxia is usually the result of brain damage in the CEREBELLUM or spinal cord, caused by infection, HEAD INJURY, BRAIN TUMOR, toxins, MULTIPLE SCLEROSIS, and so on.

Cerebellar ataxia causes clumsiness in intentional movements, including walking, speaking, and eye movements. *Sensory ataxia* (unsteady movements that are exaggerated when the patient closes the eyes) occurs from a lack of sensory feedback.

Friedreich's ataxia is a fatal genetic disease characterized by the degeneration of nerve tissue in the spinal cord and of nerves that control muscle movement in the arms and legs. It may be inherited as a recessive or dominant trait and may strike anyone from a very early age up to and beyond age 50. While it is similar to multiple sclerosis, MS is not inherited and is believed to have a different origin.

atherosclerosis A disease of the arteries characterized by buildup of fat deposits on the inner walls, eventually obstructing blood flow. Atherosclerosis is one of the primary causes of STROKE, the third most common cause of death (after cancer), which occurs when blood flow to the brain is reduced or cut off.

The probability that this condition will occur is increased with certain risk factors, such as cigarette smoking, high blood pressure, obesity, physical inactivity, high cholesterol level, family history, and male gender. The risk also increases as patients age, since more plaques develop with each passing year.

Moderating or eliminating the risk factors (especially early in adult life) can significantly reduce the probability that a person will develop atherosclerosis—or at least delay its onset. For example, diet should be low in saturated fat and salt; patients should stop smoking, treat high blood pressure, get regular exercise, control cholesterol, and maintain control of diabetes.

Symptoms and Diagnostic Path
Atherosclerosis produces no symptoms until the arteries are so clogged that blood flow begins to slow down. Narrowing of the arteries supplying blood to the brain may cause TRANSIENT ISCHEMIC ATTACKS (TIAs), which temporarily mimic the signs and symptoms of a stroke.

Medical history, ANGIOGRAPHY (X-rays after injection of radiopaque dye), ultrasound, or plethysmography (pulse pattern tracing) can reveal atherosclerosis.

Treatment Options and Outlook
Once the damage has been done, medication alone cannot unclog the arteries. However, various medications can slow or sometimes even reverse the effects of atherosclerosis. Cholesterol medications can lower a person's low-density lipoprotein (LDL) cholesterol (the "bad" cholesterol), slowing, stopping, or even reversing the buildup of fatty deposits in the arteries. Boosting high-density lipoprotein (HDL) cholesterol ("good" cholesterol) also can help. These types of drugs include statins and fibrates.

Antiplatelet medications (such as aspirin) can lessen the chance that platelets will stick and clump in narrowed arteries, forming a blood clot or more blockage. By thinning the blood with an anticoagulant, such as heparin or warfarin (Coumadin), clots can be prevented.

Medications to control blood pressure, such as beta blockers, angiotensin-converting enzyme (ACE) inhibitors, and calcium channel blockers, all can help slow the progression of atherosclerosis.

Finally, physicians sometimes recommend other medications to control specific risk factors for atherosclerosis, such as diabetes. Sometimes medications are not enough, and more aggressive treatment is needed. Patients with severe symptoms, failing organs, or a blockage that threatens muscle or skin tissue, may require surgery or a more invasive procedure, including angioplasty, endarterectomy, thrombolytic therapy, or bypass surgery.

During an angioplasty, a long, thin tube is inserted into a blocked or narrowed artery, and a wire with a deflated balloon is passed through the tube into the narrowed area. The balloon is then inflated, compressing the deposits against the artery walls. A mesh tube called a stent may be left in the artery to help keep the artery open. Angioplasty may be performed using lasers.

In some cases, fatty deposits must be surgically removed from the walls of a narrowed artery in a procedure called an endarterectomy. When the procedure is performed on arteries in the neck (the carotid arteries), it is called a carotid endarterectomy. An artery blocked by a blood clot can be treated by inserting a clot-breaking drug directly into the artery where the clot is located. Called thrombolytic therapy, this drug will break up the clot.

Failing all else, bypass surgery may be performed to create a graft bypass using a vessel from another part of the body, or a tube made of synthetic fabric. This allows blood to flow around the blocked or narrowed artery.

One day, researchers may use targeted gene therapy to treat atherosclerosis. Researchers have discovered many genes that play a role in the development and progression of atherosclerosis.

athetosis Slow writhing movements made involuntarily, often as a result of a dysfunction deep within the brain. When associated with the jerky movements of chorea, it is called choreoathetosis. This condition is often found in those with HUNTINGTON'S DISEASE, CEREBRAL PALSY, ENCEPHALITIS, or other brain disorders. It also may occur as a side effect to certain medications.

See also TARDIVE DYSKINESIA.

attention and the brain The brain is capable of paying attention to relatively few outside events at the same time. "Attention" is in fact a highly directed process that depends on a person's alertness, concentration, and interest.

Scientists have learned about attention by studying patients who have suffered BRAIN DAMAGE and experienced a subsequent inability to pay attention. For example, a patient who has injured one side of the brain may ignore anything that happens on the opposite side of the body. Another may wave only one hand when commanded to wave both hands.

Such problems are known as "neglect" and may result in bizarre behavior such as applying makeup on only one side of the face or ignoring food on one side of the plate. The problem does not involve paralysis, however; the person is physically capable of the required activity but has a neurological malfunction that affects selective attention.

According to research, focused attention is a process distributed throughout the brain that begins with a "red alert" in the reticular structures, progressing within an interlocking system involving sensation, movement, and emotion. The degree of our attention is mediated by a variety of factors, including interest, internal state (hunger, and so on), and emotional significance. Brain damage anywhere along this system can result in attention disorder.

Although some parts of the brain—especially the right hemisphere—are more important in the process than others, there is no one "attention center" in the brain.

attention deficit disorder (ADD) with or without hyperactivity The former term used to define ATTENTION DEFICIT HYPERACTIVITY DISORDER (ADHD), used in the *Diagnostic and Statistical Manual of Mental Disorders, III-Revised (DSM-III-R)*. It was replaced by the term *ADHD* used in the current *DSM-IV-TR.*

attention deficit hyperactivity disorder (ADHD) A group of behavioral problems marked by inattention, hyperactivity, and impulsiveness, formerly called attention deficit disorder (ADD), hyperactivity, hyperkinetic syndrome, and/or minimal brain dysfunction.

ADHD's wide variety of names and definitions occurs primarily because the symptoms of this syndrome are complex and varied; many times, all these behaviors do not appear in one child at any one time.

ADHD is presumed to be a brain condition that affects between 3 percent and 7 percent of the population. Since the early 1990s, scientists have worked to pinpoint the differences found in brain scans between the normal brain and the ADHD brain. Recently, scientists have been able to localize the brain areas involved in ADHD, finding that areas in the FRONTAL LOBE and BASAL GANGLIA are reduced by about 10 percent in size and activity in children with ADHD. Still other research has implicated dysfunction of the reticular activation system in many cases of ADHD.

Studies in the past few years have shown that boys with ADHD tend to have brains that are more symmetrical than those of non-ADHD boys. Three structures in the brains of boys with ADHD were smaller than in non-ADHD boys of the same age: prefrontal cortex, CAUDATE NUCLEUS, and the globus pallidus. The prefrontal cortex is thought to be the brain's "command center"; the other two parts translate the commands into action.

There is also evidence that not only are some of the structures slightly varied, but the brain may use these areas differently. Watching brain scans, researchers discovered that boys with ADHD have an abnormal increase of activity in the frontal lobe and certain areas below it. These areas work in part to control voluntary action. This meant that the ADHD boys were working harder to control their impulses than non-ADHD boys. When the ADHD boys were given Ritalin, this abnormal activity quieted down. This effect was not seen in the non-ADHD boys. This means that Ritalin may act differently on ADHD brains compared to "normal" brains.

Although brain scans (called functional magnetic resonance imaging or fMRI) are expensive and may not be covered by insurance, they may provide a more accurate way to diagnose ADHD. As scientists explore more of the brain, ADHD may be thought of more as a disorder than a behavioral problem.

Dopamine levels in the brain also appear to play a major role in ADHD. The National Institute of Mental Health released the results of a major clinical trial focusing on ADHD that found that medication that boosts the level of dopamine in the brain is the most successful type of treatment.

Experts believe that at least some cases of ADHD may be inherited, and that it may involve both brain structures in the frontal lobe related to attention, impulse control, and executive function, as well as neurotransmitters and subtle imbalances in brain chemistry. Other children may experience abnormal fetal development that affects the areas of the brain controlling attention and movement.

Symptoms and Diagnostic Path

Both children and adults with ADHD consistently display inattention, hyperactivity, and impulsivity. People who are inattentive may have trouble establishing and maintaining attention and concentration, and may get bored with a task after just a few minutes. Those who are hyperactive seem to feel restless and are constantly in motion, finding it hard to sit still. People who are impulsive have a problem with curbing their immediate reactions and tend to act before they think. Other symptoms may include problems in school, with friends, and with behavior.

ADHD and learning disabilities frequently occur together, but they are not the same condition. Learning disabilities include difficulty with receiving, organizing, understanding, remembering, and offering information. ADHD involves difficulty with paying attention to information. Between 10 percent and 20 percent of all school-age children have learning disabilities. Of those with learning disabilities, between 4 percent and 12 percent of all school-age children will also have ADHD, making it the most common childhood neurobehavioral disorder.

In addition, ADHD behaviors are often found in children with other problems, such as TOURETTE SYNDROME, MENTAL RETARDATION, CEREBRAL PALSY, EPILEPSY, or SCHIZOPHRENIA.

Although ADHD is a common childhood behavioral disorder, it can be difficult to diagnose and even harder to understand. Once viewed as a disorder of childhood, primarily involving hyperactivity and the inability to pay attention, ADHD is now seen as a lifelong condition that may not include physical restlessness or hyperactive behavior at all. It may also be the source of unusual talents or giftedness in specific areas.

In recent years, there has been growing interest in ADHD as well as concerns about possible overdiagnosis. In surveys among pediatricians and family physicians across the country, wide variations were found in diagnostic criteria and treatment methods for ADHD. Indeed, the definition and treatments of ADHD continue to evolve; in the 1990s, there was an extraordinary surge in the level of focus on ADHD and in the incidence of diagnosis among children and adults. It is likely that the present level of understanding of the disorder, as well as current methods of diagnosis and treatment, will continue to develop rapidly in the coming years.

Once thought to be a disorder primarily affecting young hyperactive boys, ADHD is both more complicated and more pervasive. In particular, experts now know that children do not typically "outgrow" the condition, nor does it affect only males. The present gender ratio ranges from three to one to seven to one, males to females.

ADHD is primarily diagnosed through a combination of individual and family history, individual behavioral assessments, and information about behavior from parents, teachers, and others.

Tests for ADHD include measures to evaluate inattention, distractibility, and memory, along with tests to identify coexisting conditions such as learning and language problems, aggression, disruptive behavior, depression, or anxiety. This type of assessment should take at least one to two hours, or more if the picture is complicated or unclear. The interview should include input from several people, including at least one parent.

In addition, certain medical conditions such as hypothyroidism, juvenile diabetes, and seizure disorders must be ruled out as causes of the child's inability to pay attention. Increasingly, psychologists and physicians are reluctant to make the diagnosis alone, favoring a joint diagnosis after they have gathered all necessary medical, psychological, and behavioral information.

Formerly called attention deficit disorder, with or without hyperactivity, this disorder has been renamed attention deficit hyperactivity disorder (ADHD) and includes three subtypes:

- **inattentive subtype** (formerly known as attention deficit disorder, or ADD): with signs that include being easily distracted, an inability to pay attention to details, not following directions, losing or forgetting things like toys, notebooks, or homework

- **hyperactive-impulsive subtype** (formerly known as attention deficit hyperactivity disorder, or ADHD) include fidgeting, squirming, blurting out answers before hearing the full question, difficulty waiting, running or jumping out of a seat when quiet behavior is expected

- **combined subtype** (the most common of the subtypes) includes those signs from both of the subtypes above, and can be seen with or without hyperactivity

To be considered for a diagnosis of ADHD, a child must display these behaviors before age seven and the behaviors must last for at least six months, and they must be considered "maladaptive." For a diagnosis, the behavior must also negatively affect at least two areas of a child's life (such as school, home, or friendships).

ADHD is diagnosed using the criteria in the *Diagnostic and Statistical Manual of Mental Disorders, Fourth Edition (DSM-IV)*. Diagnostic criteria include

Inattention

- often fails to give close attention to details or makes careless mistakes in schoolwork, work, or other activities

- often has difficulty sustaining attention in tasks or play activities

- often does not seem to listen when spoken to directly

- often does not follow through on instructions and fails to finish schoolwork, chores, or duties in the workplace (not due to oppositional behavior or failure to understand instructions)

- often has difficulty organizing tasks and activities

- often avoids, dislikes, or is reluctant to engage in tasks that require sustained mental effort (such as schoolwork or homework)

- often loses things necessary for tasks or activities (such as toys, school assignments, pencils, books, or tools)

- is often easily distracted by extraneous stimuli

- is often forgetful in daily activities

Hyperactivity-Impulsivity

- often fidgets with hands or feet or squirms in seat
- often leaves seat in classroom or in other situations in which remaining seated is expected
- often runs about or climbs excessively in situations in which it is inappropriate (in adolescents or adults, may be limited to subjective feelings of restlessness)
- often has trouble playing or engaging in leisure activities quietly
- is often on the go
- talks excessively
- often blurts out answers before questions have been completed
- often has difficulty awaiting turn
- often interrupts or intrudes on others

The American Academy of Pediatrics recently developed new guidelines for the diagnosis of ADHD with input from a panel of medical, mental health, and educational experts. The new guidelines, designed for primary care physicians diagnosing ADHD in children aged six to 12 years, include the following recommendations:

- ADHD evaluations should be performed by the primary care clinician for children who show signs of school difficulties, academic underachievement, troublesome relationships with teachers, family members, and peers, and other behavioral problems.
- Questions to parents, either directly or through a previsit questionnaire about school and behavioral issues, may help alert physicians to possible ADHD.
- In diagnosing ADHD, physicians should use *DSM-IV* criteria, which requires that symptoms be present in two or more of a child's settings, and that the symptoms interfere with the child's academic or social functioning for at least six months.
- The assessment of ADHD should include information obtained directly from parents or caregivers, as well as a classroom teacher or other school professional, regarding the core symptoms of ADHD in various settings, the age of onset, duration of symptoms, and degree of functional impairment.
- Evaluation of a child with ADHD should also include assessment for coexisting conditions: learning and language problems, aggression, disruptive behavior, depression, or anxiety.
- Because as many as one-third of children diagnosed with ADHD also have a coexisting condition, other diagnostic tests (sometimes considered positive indicators for ADHD) have been reviewed and considered not effective. These tests include lead screening, tests for generalized resistance to thyroid hormone, and brain image studies.

Of course, all children sometimes have trouble paying attention, following directions, or being quiet, but for children with ADHD, these behaviors occur more frequently and are more disturbing.

Treatment Options and Outlook

There is no cure for ADHD, but a combined program of medication and behavioral therapy can help and is often prescribed to treat ADHD. In fact, researchers have demonstrated that a combination of medication and behavior management is superior to either alone. With the advice and cooperation of a child's pediatrician, teachers, counselors, and family members, the child can have a normal life in spite of this disorder.

Medication For most children and adults with ADHD, medication is an important part of treatment that is not used to control behavior but to ease the symptoms of ADHD. Stimulants appear to work by altering the levels of transmitters in the brain by which the different nerve cells communicate.

Between 70 and 80 percent of children with ADHD respond positively to these medications, with improvements in attention span, impulsivity, and behavior, especially in structured environments. Some children also demonstrate improvements in frustration tolerance, compliance, and even handwriting. Relationships with parents, peers, and teachers may also improve.

These medications may also be effective in adults who have ADHD. The reaction to these medications can be similar to that experienced by children with ADHD—a decrease in impulsivity and an increase in attention. Many ADHD adults treated with medication report that they are able to bring more control and organization to their lives. Other medications, such as antidepressants, can be helpful when depression, phobic, panic, anxiety and/or obsessive-compulsive disorders are present.

Drugs commonly prescribed include stimulants such as METHYLPHENIDATE (Ritalin), dextroamphetamine (Dexedrine or Dextrostat), and single-entity amphetamine (Adderall). While these drugs can be addictive in teenagers and adults, they do not seem to be addictive in children. Nine out of 10 children improve on one of these stimulants, so if one does not work, others are tried. It may seem strange to give stimulants to children with hyperactivity and attention deficit problems, but instead of making the child act out more, these drugs reduce the hyperactivity and increase the attention span. The drugs also help children with ADHD control their behavior. A child using these drugs may actually become quieter and more attentive.

Sometimes, however, none of these medications work. In this case, some children may respond well to antihistamines usually prescribed for allergies, or such antidepressants as Elavil, Prozac, Tofranil, or Norpramin. Clonidine, a drug normally used to treat high blood pressure, may ease some symptoms of ADHD. With any of these medications, adjusting the dosage for each child is vital for treating the symptoms of ADHD.

Side effects Stimulant drugs do cause side effects. Most doctors feel that the potential side effects should be carefully weighed against the benefits before prescribing drugs to children with ADHD. While taking these medications, some children may lose weight, have stomachaches or have less appetite, and temporarily grow more slowly. The rate of brain growth slows down in some children who take these drugs, although there is a marked rebound in brain growth when these drugs are discontinued. Others may have trouble falling asleep and become irritable. Some doctors worry that stimulants may worsen the symptoms of TOURETTE SYNDROME, although recent research

suggests this is not true. Many doctors believe if they carefully monitor a child's height, weight, and overall development, the benefits of medication far outweigh the potential side effects. Side effects that do occur can often be handled by reducing the dosage.

Drug controversy Still, the use of stimulants for children with ADHD—especially Ritalin—is not without controversy. Critics worry that Ritalin and other stimulant drugs are prescribed unnecessarily for too many children, since many things—including anxiety, depression, allergies, seizures, or problems at home or school—can make children seem overactive, impulsive, or inattentive. They argue that many children who do not have ADHD are drugged anyway as a way to control disruptive behaviors.

Critics also worry that so many of the nation's children are given these drugs without any real understanding of the future side effects. Ritalin is one of the most commonly prescribed drugs for children, yet there are concerns about its long-term effects.

There are no studies on children who have taken Ritalin for more than 14 months. Ritalin affects the brain in a way very similar to cocaine, one of the most addictive substances known. Critics worry that children who take Ritalin may be more likely to use illegal drugs in the future, or that they might be more likely to smoke as adults. These concerns are fueled by research showing that rats that were exposed to stimulants were more likely to choose cocaine, suggesting that early exposure to some drugs may make a person more likely to abuse drugs in the future. However, the data on whether there is a link between Ritalin and later substance abuse are controversial.

Some studies show that Ritalin makes people more prone to addiction to certain substances, but other researchers insist that children with ADHD are not more likely to use drugs of any type later in life.

Behavioral treatment Many experts believe that the best way to manage the symptoms of ADHD is to combine drug treatment with behavioral methods. Medication can help to control some of the behavior problems that may have led to family turmoil, but more often there are other aspects of a child's problem that medication will not affect.

Even though ADHD primarily affects a person's behavior, the simple fact of having ADHD can trigger serious emotional problems as well. Some of these children have very few experiences that build their sense of worth and competence. If they are hyperactive, they are often punished for being disruptive. If they are too disorganized and unfocused to complete tasks, they may be branded "lazy." If they are impulsive, shove classmates, and interrupt, they may lose friends. If they are unlucky enough to have a related conduct disorder, they may get in trouble at school or with the police.

The daily frustrations that are a part of having ADHD can make people feel abnormal or stupid. In many cases, the cycle of frustration and anger has persisted for so long it may take years to alleviate.

For this reason, parents and children may need special help to develop techniques to manage the behavior patterns that have become ingrained. In such cases, mental health professionals can help the child and family develop new attitudes and ways of relating to each other.

Behavior treatments include coaching, a process of individual support that focuses on understanding maladaptive patterns of behavior, identifying goals and strategies for change, and providing consistent reinforcement and feedback. For younger children, such an approach may involve behavioral rating scales, consistent feedback, and reinforcement for positive behavioral change. For adults, the approach may focus on identifying and describing goals and strategies. In either case, focusing on the role of individual responsibility and choice is a vital component, as is developing a consistent pattern of feedback and reinforcement.

In individual counseling, the therapist helps children or adults with ADHD learn to feel better about themselves. The therapist can also help people with ADHD identify and build on their strengths, cope with daily problems, and control their attention and aggression.

In group counseling, people learn that they are not alone in their frustration and that others want to help. Sometimes only the child with ADHD needs counseling, but often the entire family can benefit from support. If the child is young, parents can learn techniques for coping with and improving their child's behavior.

Several intervention approaches are available and different therapists tend to prefer one approach or another. Knowing something about the various types of interventions makes it easier for families to choose the best therapist for their own situation.

In psychotherapy, patients talk with the therapist about their thoughts and feelings, explore problem behaviors, and learn different ways to handle their emotions. If someone who has ADHD wants to gain control of symptoms more directly, more direct kinds of intervention are available.

Cognitive-behavioral therapy helps people directly change their behavior instead of only concentrating on understanding their feelings and actions. The therapist may help an individual learn to think through tasks and organize work, or encourage new behavior by giving praise each time the person acts in the desired way. A cognitive-behavioral therapist can use these techniques to help a child with ADHD learn to control his or her fighting, or an impulsive teenager to think before speaking.

Social skills training can help children learn new behaviors by watching the therapist model appropriate behavior like waiting for a turn, sharing toys, or responding to a bully.

Support groups can also be helpful, linking people who have common concerns. Many adults with ADHD and parents of children with ADHD find it useful to join a local or national support group. Many groups deal with issues of children's disorders. Members of support groups share frustrations and successes and provide referrals.

Because ADHD affects all aspects of a child's home and school life, experts recommend parent education and support groups to help family members learn how to help the child cope with frustrations, organize environments, and develop problem-solving skills. Special parenting skills are often needed because children with ADHD may not respond as well to typical parenting practices—especially punishment. Instead, children with ADHD should learn how to reinforce their positive behaviors themselves, and learn how to solve problems. Children who take medications and practice these behavior techniques do better than those who rely on medication alone.

Parenting skills training, offered by therapists or in special classes, gives parents tools and techniques for managing their child's behavior. One such technique is the use of "time out" when the child becomes too unruly or out of control. During time outs, the child is removed from the agitating situation and sits alone quietly for a short time to calm down. (Time-out should not be confused with isolation, which is a punishment technique.) Parents may also be taught to give the child quality time each day, in which they share a relaxed activity. During this time together, the parent looks for opportunities to point out what the child is doing right, and praises strengths and abilities. An effective way to modify a child's behavior is through a system of rewards and penalties. The parents (or teacher) identify a few desirable behaviors that they want to encourage in the child, such as asking for a toy politely. The child is told exactly what is expected in order to earn a small reward, which is awarded when he or she performs the desired behavior. The goal is to help children learn to control their own behavior and to choose the more desired behavior. The technique works well with all children, although children with ADHD may need more frequent rewards.

Parents also may learn to structure situations in ways that will allow their child to succeed. If a child is easily overstimulated, parents may try allowing only one or two playmates at a time. If the child has trouble completing tasks, parents may help the child divide a large task into small steps, then praise the child as each step is completed.

Stress management methods such as meditation, relaxation techniques, and exercise can increase the parents' tolerance for frustration, enabling them to respond more calmly to their child's behavior.

Other behavioral treatments that may be helpful in treating children with ADHD include play therapy and special physical exercise.

Play therapy may help a child who has fears and anxieties, but these are not the key problems among most ADHD children. Special physical exercises are usually designed to boost coordination and increase a child's ability to handle activities that can be overstimulating. Most ADHD children do have problems in these areas, but this is not the cause of ADHD. While these exercises may help, they seem to work mostly because they get parents to pay more attention to the child, which boosts self-esteem.

auditory agnosia A defect, loss, or failure in development of the ability to comprehend spoken words, caused by disease, injury, or malformation of the hearing centers of the brain. A person with auditory agnosia may or may not be able to reliably respond to an audiometric test or may give very different results at different times.

auditory brain stem response (ABR) test A diagnostic test that determines how well certain portions of the hearing system in the brain respond to sounds.

As nerve impulses pass through the lower levels of the brain from the auditory nerve on their way to higher brain centers, they make connections in the brain stem. The ABR measures this electrical activity in the brain stem. This test is useful for detecting hearing loss in newborns, to diagnose auditory disorders, and for confirming nonorganic hearing loss. This test can be performed on individuals of any age—even the youngest infant.

The test consists of a brief tone that causes a small variation in electrical potentials that can be recorded from the scalp. Clicks or tone pips are fed into the ear, and a computer analyzes the results to see if the brain activity changes. Rather than a true test of the entire process of hearing, the ABR determines whether hearing signals are reaching higher brain centers.

By repeating the sound up to 100 times and averaging the response by computer, the responses can be enhanced while eliminating random background electrical activity. Auditory thresholds can be established that are quite close to those that can be obtained in conventional hearing tests.

Development of new sound-delivery systems and recording electrodes now allow the use of ABR for monitoring people with head injuries.

auditory cortex An area of the brain situated in the TEMPORAL LOBE that is critical to HEARING. The auditory cortex connects to the cochlear nerve fibers that respond to a specific sound frequency.

auditory-evoked potentials   Slight electrical signals in the brain read from an electroencephalogram that have a characteristic pattern and occur in response to repetitions of identical sounds. The characteristic pattern (or wave form) indicates that the brain has responded to the test sound and that the sound must therefore have been heard by the client. Tests of auditory-evoked potentials are useful for those who cannot participate in hearing tests, such as the very young or mentally retarded patients.

See also AUDITORY BRAIN STEM RESPONSE TEST.

auditory memory   The memory for sound. This type of sense memory is particularly strong among great musicians; the great conductor Arturo Toscanini, for example, could remember a score after hearing it one or two times and could write it out from memory 40 years later.

auditory nerve   See ACOUSTIC NERVE.

auditory perception   The ability to receive, identify, discriminate, understand, and respond to sound.

autism, early onset   Children whose symptoms of autism appear during the first year of life. (Children whose symptoms appear between ages one and two are referred to as having *late-onset* or *regressive* autism. Although some researchers argue that the regression is not real or that congenital autism was simply unnoticed by the child's parents, many parents do report that their children had completely normal speech, behavior, and social skills until some time between one and two years of age.)

The cause of autism is unknown and extremely controversial. Many scientists believe autism may be related to some type of brain dysfunction.

Symptoms and Diagnostic Path

After a normal first month or two, autistic infants typically become increasingly unresponsive, screaming when cuddled and growing more aloof. Later on, the child will avoid eye contact and will be extremely resistant to change. Any attempt at altering the routine will cause severe tantrums; rituals develop in play, and often the child becomes attached to unusual objects or collections, or is obsessed with a particular idea. This hysterical need for "sameness" makes it very difficult to teach an autistic child new skills.

There are usually delays in speech; if the child does speak, it is usually immature, unimaginative and robotic, with frequent echoing of words or phrases. Behavioral abnormalities include rocking, self-injury, flicking or twiddling fingers, walking on tiptoe, hyperactivity or sudden screaming fits. Sometimes, the child may have one outstanding special skill (such as rote memory, artistic or musical talent).

While half of all children with autism are not diagnosed until age four to six, it is possible to diagnose a child as early as 18 months old. Since the earlier the condition is identified the earlier treatment can begin and the better the prognosis for the child, early diagnosis is critically important. A good diagnosis can identify if a child does not have autism; if autism does exist, the evaluation can determine the seriousness of the problem, and place the child "on the autism spectrum."

Because there are no medical tests for autism, a diagnosis must be based on observing the person's communication, behavior, and developmental levels. Even in very early childhood, parents can begin to observe their child to make sure certain developmental milestones are reached.

There appears to have been a rapid increase in the number of children diagnosed with AUTISTIC DISORDER, especially in California, which has an accurate and systematic centralized reporting system of all diagnoses of this disorder. Whereas autism once accounted for 3 percent of all developmental disabilities, in California it now accounts for 45 percent; other countries report similar increases. Experts disagree as to whether—and why—there has been a dramatic increase in autistic disorder over the past two decades; some insist the increase is simply due to better diagnosis, while others argue that the increase is an actual boost in numbers. Many experts say that the rise may not be due to more cases that occur, but rather that more cases are being diagnosed.

Treatment Options and Outlook

There is no known treatment that is reliably effective at all times for all children, although special schooling, behavioral therapy, support and counseling for parents and families may help. Medication may be useful to treat the accompanying epilepsy or hyperactivity. Still, children can learn skills, coping mechanisms, and strategies to ease various symptoms. Intensive, appropriate early intervention greatly improves the outcome for most young children. Most programs will build on the interests of the child, teach functional skills in a highly structured manner using behavioral techniques, follow a consistent schedule of activities, and include visual cues. Some symptoms may lessen as the child ages, and others may disappear altogether; with appropriate treatment, many problem behaviors can be changed so that the person may appear to no longer have autistic disorder. However, most patients continue to show some residual symptoms to some degree throughout their entire lives.

In addition to a preschool program, children with autism should be trained in functional living skills at the earliest possible age. Learning to cross a street, to buy something in a store, or ask for help are critical skills, and may be hard even for those with average intelligence. Training is aimed at boosting a person's independence and providing opportunities for personal choice and freedom.

Studies show that individuals with autistic disorder respond well to a highly structured, specialized education program tailored to the individual's needs, typically addressing functional communication, social interaction skills, preacademic skills, adaptive behavior, and play. Techniques from the field of applied behavior analysis are recommended by many experts. Initially, most young children with autistic disorder require a small ratio of children to adults to ensure effective intervention. Ideally, this should include some opportunities for one-to-one instruction.

Many schools today have an inclusion program in which the child is in a regular classroom for most of the day, with special instruction for a part of the day. This instruction should include such skills as learning how to act in social situations and in making friends. Although higher-functioning children may be able to handle academic work, they, too, need help to organize tasks and avoid distractions.

During middle and high school years, instruction should include practical matters such as work, community living, and recreational activities, and include work experience, using public transportation, and learning skills that will be important in community living. While some autistic behaviors improve during the teenage years, others may get worse. Increased autistic or aggressive behavior may be one way some teens express their newfound tension and confusion. At an age when most teenagers are concerned with popularity, grades, and social skills, teens with autism may realize they are different from their peers. Unlike their classmates, they do not have friends, they may not date, or they may not be planning a career. For some, the sadness that comes with such realization motivates them to learn new behaviors and acquire better social skills.

Treatment is most successful when geared toward the individual's particular needs. An experienced specialist or team should design the individualized program, which may include applied behavior analysis, occupational therapy, physical therapy, speech language therapy, and medication. More controversial treatments may include sensory integration, dietary interventions, vitamins and supplements, music therapy, vision therapy, or auditory integration training.

During the course of childhood and adolescence, children with this condition nevertheless usually make some developmental gains. Those who show improvement in language and intellectual ability have the best overall prognosis. Although some individuals with autistic disorder are able to live with some measure of partial independence in adulthood, very few are able to live entirely on their own.

autism spectrum disorders (ASDs)   A relatively new term that encompasses autism and similar disorders that is gradually replacing the term *pervasive developmental disorders*. This group of disorders is characterized by varying degrees of problems with communication skills, social interactions, and restricted, repetitive, and stereotyped patterns of behavior. The autism spectrum disorders include ASPERGER'S SYNDROME (tends to include milder symptoms), AUTISTIC DISORDER (autism), and pervasive developmental disorder-not otherwise specified (PDD-NOS), a condition with very minor symptoms or symptoms that do not meet specific criteria for other autism spectrum disorders.

While half of all children with one of the autism spectrum disorders are not diagnosed until age four to six, it is possible to diagnose a child as early as 18 months. Since the earlier the condition is identified the earlier treatment can begin and the better the prognosis for the child, early diagnosis is critically important. A diagnosis can identify whether a child does not have an autism spectrum disorder; if one of the spectrum disorders does exist, the evaluation can determine the seriousness of the problem, and place the child "on the autism spectrum."

Because there are no medical tests for the autism spectrum disorders, a diagnosis must be based on observing the person's communication, behavior, and developmental levels. Even in very early childhood, parents can begin to observe their child to make sure certain developmental milestones are reached. A three-year-old child should be able to imitate adults and playmates, play make-believe with dolls, and use pronouns or plural words. Parents might want to check with a pediatrician if their child has not mastered these skills.

autistic disorder   A severe developmental disorder known popularly as autism, which affects a person's ability to communicate, form relationships with others, and respond appropriately to the environment. Autistic disorder is a "spectrum disorder," which means that its symptoms can appear in a wide variety of combinations from mild to severe. It is one of a group of related disorders known collectively as the AUTISM SPECTRUM DISORDERS.

Left untreated, many children with autistic disorder will not develop effective social skills and may not learn to communicate or behave appropriately. Very few individuals recover completely without any intervention.

The result of a neurological disorder that affects the functioning of the brain, autistic disorder has been estimated to occur in as many as one in 500 people. Its prevalence rate makes it one of the most common developmental disabilities, four times more common in boys than in girls and not related to race, ethnic origin, family income, lifestyle, or education.

Although a single specific cause of the disorder is not known, current research links autistic disorder to biological or neurological differences in the brain. The disorder has been associated with maternal German measles infection, phenylketonuria (an inherited disorder of metabolism), tuberous sclerosis (an inherited disease of the nervous system and skin), lack of oxygen at birth, encephalitis, and infantile spasms. It is neither a mental illness nor a behavior problem, and it is not caused by bad parenting. No known psychological factors in the development of the child have been shown to cause autistic disorder.

Genetics appear to play an important role in the development of some cases of autistic disorder, and some studies have suggested that individuals with autistic disorder may have weakened immune systems. Some experts believe that in some children, the immune system is weakened either due to faulty genes or exposure to certain chemicals, which may predispose the child to autism. Exposure to additional environmental toxins may then trigger autistic disorder.

The possible role of vaccinations, many of which were added to the vaccination schedule in the 1980s and are typically administered to children between ages one and two, is a matter of considerable controversy. Prior to 1990, about two-thirds of children with autistic disorder displayed symptoms at an early age, and only one-third initially appeared to be developing appropriately, regressing some time after age one. Starting in the 1990s, the trend has reversed—fewer than one-third evidence early-onset symptoms, and two-thirds develop symptoms in their second year.

The concept of a link between autism and vaccines is controversial. Some experts believe that the measles-mumps-rubella (MMR) combination vaccine or thimerosal, a mercury-based preservative in childhood vaccines, is implicated in autistic disorder in some children. In response to these concerns, manufacturers of children's vaccines have removed thimerasol from almost all vaccines administered to children.

On the other hand, the National Institute of Child Health and Human Development (NICHD) argues there has been no conclusive, scientific evidence that any part of a vaccine, nor any combination of vaccines, causes autistic disorder. In 2001, the Institute of Medicine (IOM) and the American Academy of Pediatrics (AAP) released findings from their separate reviews of the available evidence on a possible link between vaccines and autism. Both groups independently found that existing evidence does not support such a connection. Still, research continues into the link between autistic disorder and vaccines, including research into the effects of thimerosal on the immune system.

See also AUTISM, EARLY ONSET.

autistic savants Individuals who lack normal intelligence but who possess one outstanding mental ability, such as a so-called photographic memory or the ability to do complex mathematical calculations in their heads. Autistic savants were formerly called idiot savants (meaning "wise idiot"), a term invented in 1887 by J. Langdon Down, a pioneer in the study of mental retardation. Autistic savants are usually incapable of activities of daily living other than their one ability and are often unable to reason or to comprehend meaning.

The savant syndrome is six times more likely to appear in males than females. Although it is considered rare, almost 10 percent of children diagnosed with autism may exhibit this syndrome.

No matter what their particular talent, all savants share a prodigious memory; their skills may appear in a range of areas, including calendar calculating, music, rapid calculating and mathematics, art or mechanical ability.

One of the more common patterns that can be found among savants is a triad of mental retardation, blindness, and musical ability.

In 1988 the movie *Rain Man* won an Academy Award for best picture for its portrayal of a prodigious autistic savant; the feats of this savant were based on actual clinical literature.

autobiographical memory A uniquely human function of early memories that begins at a certain point in childhood. It depends on a child's ability to speak, since it requires linguistic representations of events. The phenomenon of infantile amnesia was first identified by SIGMUND FREUD, but since Freud's time, scientists have learned that as children grow older they learn to share memories with others and acquire the narrative forms of memory recounting. Such recountings are effective in reinstating experienced memories only after the children can use another's representation of an experience in language as a reinstatement of their own experience. This requires an ability to understand language that appears in the mid- to late preschool years. (See also AMNESIA, CHILDHOOD; MEMORY IN INFANCY.)

automatic gestures Habitual routines (such as locking your front door) that, because they are performed without any conscious thinking or awareness, may not be recorded in memory and therefore may not be recalled at a later date.

automatic processing Memory functions are carried out with a minimum amount of conscious attention. While it is often argued that processing activities (such as ENCODING and RETRIEVAL) require different levels of attention, automatic processing tasks are disrupted only slightly by the simultaneous performance of other more demanding tasks regardless of their precise nature—and automatic processing disrupts only minimally the performance of these other tasks. In contrast, EFFORTFUL PROCESSING is disrupted by and disrupts other demanding tasks performed at the same time.

autonomic nervous system A system of nerves that controls involuntary functions such as heart rate, blood pressure, hormone flow, and so on. It consists of a network of nerves divided into two parts: the SYMPATHETIC NERVOUS SYSTEM and the PARASYMPATHETIC NERVOUS SYSTEM (PNS).

The sympathetic nervous system boosts activity in the body, increasing the heart and breathing rates as part of the body's "fight or flight" response. The parasympathetic nervous system includes nerves that branch off from both ends of the CENTRAL NERVOUS SYSTEM (from the head and base of the spine). The brain stem sends signals to the PNS, which acts as a sort of brake on the body's systems.

In normal conditions, these two systems balance each other, but during exercise or when facing stress, the sympathetic system takes over. During sleep, the parasympathetic system asserts more control.

Physicians can treat certain disorders by administering drugs that affect the autonomic nervous system; for example, anticholinergic drugs block the effect of ACETYLCHOLINE, reducing muscle spasms. Beta-blockers can slow the heart rate by blocking the action of EPINEPHRINE and NOREPINEPHRINE on the heart.

averaged evoked response   A recording of brain activity in response to a specific stimulus that is repeated and averaged over time. The averaged evoked response helps discriminate a specific response from other unrelated brain activity.

axon   A long unbranched fiber extending from a neuron that carries nerve impulses to other cells. In some exceptional cases, an axon also may receive input.

balance The ability to remain upright and not fall over when walking is a complex process that depends on a continuing flow of information to the brain about the position of the body. The body maintains its balance due to a complex integration of this information combined with a constant flow of instructions from the brain to various parts of the body, performing the necessary changes to keep the body in balance.

The brain receives information about body position from many sources: eyes, sensory nerves in skin, muscles, and joints, and the three semicircular canals of the labyrinth in the inner ear that detect placement and speed of head movements. The CEREBELLUM is the part of the brain mainly responsible for collecting and integrating this information and conveying data to other motor centers to coordinate body movement.

Anything that affects the cerebellum, such as a tumor or a STROKE, may cause clumsiness, speech disorders, and other features of impaired muscular coordination.

See also VESTIBULAR SYSTEM.

barbiturates A group of sedative drugs also known as tranquilizers that work by mimicking brain chemicals related to sedation, depressing activity in the brain. Barbiturates slow down the activity of nerves that control many mental and physical functions, such as emotions or heart rate.

Barbital was the first of the barbiturates that appeared in 1903; it was originally widely prescribed for anxiety, insomnia, and seizures. More than a dozen different barbiturates are currently on the market, although their use has rapidly declined in the past 10 years and is strictly controlled because they are habit forming and widely abused. Overdoses can be fatal.

Common barbiturates include amobarbital, pentobarbital, phenobarbital, secobarbital, and thiopental. Phenobarbital is still used to treat EPILEPSY, and thiopental is used to induce anesthesia. Barbiturates are sometimes used to reduce cerebral blood pressure. However, BENZODIAZEPINES and other drugs have replaced barbiturates in treating insomnia and anxiety.

Side Effects

If used longer than four weeks, barbiturates can produce dependence. Withdrawal effects (insomnia, twitching, nightmares, convulsions) may occur if treatment is stopped abruptly. Gradually, higher and higher doses of the drug are needed to produce the same effect. Other adverse effects include drowsiness, staggering, and excitability. *Taking alcohol with barbiturates will dangerously depress brain activity,* which can slow down breathing. Like all other central nervous system depressants, barbiturates can lead to coma when taken in overdose. They are especially dangerous when combined; most drug-related hospital emergency admissions involve overdoses of these depressants.

See also CENTRAL NERVOUS SYSTEM DEPRESSANTS.

Bartlett, Sir Frederic C. (1896–1969) An English psychologist who believed that the brain stores information by using what it already knows and placing a new pattern over a similar old one.

Bartlett's work was a departure from the popular theories and style of psychologist Hermann Ebbinghaus, who tested his own ability to memorize nonsense syllables. This memorization could be called rote learning, but modern researchers understand that what Ebbinghaus was really studying was rote learning without arousal—in other words, factual memory for events that have no emotional importance. And because rote learning without arousal is a poor way to construct memory, it is not surprising that Ebbinghaus and his colleagues concluded that memory doesn't work very well or endure for a very long time.

While Bartlett developed his technique as a way of sidestepping problems in memory study, it limited his ability to understand memory. He believed that memory was simply a storage bin for objective items that were either retained or not—a point of view that eventually was challenged by psychologists who believed that subjective factors also are vital to memory systems.

Bartlett did not believe that only objective factors should be studied; his work during the 1930s was designed to test the way people usually use their memories. As he described in his book *Remembering: A Study in Experimental and Social Psychology* (1967), Bartlett believed that remembering is active; it is not the reactivation of memory traces that have been filed away but an imaginative reconstruction built out of the relationship of the attitude toward a mass of organized past reactions and to little details. Therefore, he noted, memory is hardly ever exact, and he agreed with Sigmund FREUD that personal view greatly affects memory.

In one of his most famous studies, he told an American Indian war story filled with unusual details; when it was over, subjects were asked to repeat the story after 15 minutes and then after four and six months. As time passed, the story grew shorter and shorter, and its Indian point of view disappeared. What Bartlett's study revealed was that memory alters information, omitting and distorting facts depending on personal prejudices and turning a puzzling but emotionally rich story into something that is dull but understandable.

Bartlett believed that what was going on was the operation of something he called a schema—an underlying subjective organizing principle. A person's memory of the Indian tale changed over time to conform with that person's underlying personal schema.

basal forebrain Nuclei in the deep regions of the forebrain containing neurons that release the NEUROTRANSMITTER called ACETYLCHOLINE. The basal forebrain includes the medial septum, which projects to the HIPPOCAMPUS; the band of Broca, which projects to the hippocampus and AMYGDALA; and the NUCLEUS BASALIS OF MEYNERT, which projects to the NEOCORTEX and amygdala. Damage to these structures of the brain is believed to contribute to organic AMNESIA. It is also a primary focus of ALZHEIMER'S DISEASE.

basal ganglia Clusters of paired nuclei deep within the CEREBRUM and the upper parts of the BRAIN STEM that play an important part in producing smooth, continuous muscular actions and in stopping and starting movement. They may also affect the development of skills and habits, and—according to recent research—may help coordinate thinking.

Fibers pass from almost every region of the cerebral CORTEX (especially the motor cortex) to the basal ganglia. After processing in the basal ganglia, nerve signals are then transmitted back to the supplementary motor area and premotor cortex of the frontal lobe.

The three major nuclei of the basal ganglia are the CAUDATE, the putamen, and the globus pallidus. The SUBSTANTIA NIGRA and the AMYGDALA are also considered as part of the basal ganglia.

Diseases or degeneration of the basal ganglia and their connections may lead to the appearance of involuntary movements, trembling, and weakness such as those found in PARKINSON'S DISEASE. In fact, much of what scientists know about this part of the brain was learned during the study of Parkinson's disease.

PARKINSONISM, a disorder characterized by a masklike face, rigidity, and slowed movements, is caused by neuron damage in the substantia nigra of the basal ganglia. These neurons normally release the neurotransmitter DOPAMINE. As these dopaminergic neurons die, brain levels of dopamine decrease. The drug LEVODOPA (which is transformed into dopamine in the brain) is used to treat Parkinson's disease.

Malfunctions in this area may also be associated with SCHIZOPHRENIA.

See also BRAIN DAMAGE; CARBON MONOXIDE POI-
SONING; CAUDATE NUCLEUS; HUNTINGTON'S DISEASE.

basilar membrane   A flexible membrane in the
cochlea of the ear that is attached to the bony shelf
and divides the coil of the cochlea lengthwise into
two compartments. On one side of the membrane
is the perilymph fluid of the scala tympani; on the
other side is the organ of Corti. As sound vibrations
disturb the perilymph fluid, they are transferred
through the basilar membrane to the organ of Corti
and on, to the hair cells inside.

The movement of the hair cells is translated into
electrical activity, which eventually reaches the
auditory cortex in the brain to interpret sound.

See also HEARING.

Batten disease   A degenerative neurological disease affecting children, characterized by progressive seizures, dementia, intellectual failure, loss of
motor skills, and blindness. The condition is usually
fatal by age 20. Also known as neuronal ceroid
lipofuscinoses, this condition is subtyped by age of
onset into *infantile* (Santavouri-Haltia), *late infantile*
(Jansky-Bielschowsky), *juvenile* (Spielmeyer-Vogt),
or *adult* (Kufs') disease.

Afflicting about two to four of every 100,000
newborns, it is the most common neurodegenerative disorder of childhood. In the past, the only
way physicians were able to distinguish Batten
disease from other conditions was by noting the
accumulation of certain pigments and proteins
within neurons and many other cell types, which
either caused the illness or was a byproduct of the
true problem.

The mutant gene responsible for the devastating
brain disorder is located on chromosome 16. Most
Batten patients have an identical chunk of this
chromosome missing. Identification of this gene
could help physicians diagnose the disease quickly,
and scientists hope that a treatment may be found
if they can determine how the protein encoded by
the gene works in healthy people.

Batten disease is an autosomal recessive disorder, which means that a child must inherit two
copies of the defective gene, one from each parent. When both parents carry one defective gene,
each of their children faces a one-in-four chance of
developing the condition. At the same time, each
child also faces a 50 percent chance of inheriting
just one copy of the defective gene. Individuals
with one defective gene are known as carriers,
meaning they do not develop the disease but they
can pass the gene on to their own children. Adult
Batten disease may be inherited as an autosomal
recessive disorder or, less often, as an autosomal
dominant disorder. In autosomal dominant inheritance, all people who inherit a single copy of the
disease gene develop the disease. As a result, there
are no unaffected carriers of the gene.

Symptoms and Diagnostic Path
Affected children suffer mental impairment, worsening seizures, and progressive loss of sight and
motor skills as years pass. Eventually, children
with Batten disease become blind, bedridden, and
unable to communicate. At present, the disease is
always fatal.

Because vision loss is often an early sign, Batten disease may be first suspected during an eye
exam when an eye doctor can detect a loss of cells
within the eye that occurs in the three childhood
types of the disease. However, because the same
cell loss also occurs in other eye problems, the
disorder cannot be diagnosed just by this sign by
itself. Typically, an eye specialist or physician who
suspects Batten disease may refer the child to a
neurologist, who can diagnose Batten disease on
the basis of medical history and skin tests, electroencephalogram (EEG), and electrical studies
of the eyes (VISUAL-EVOKED RESPONSES and elec-
tro-retinagrams [ERG], brain scans, and enzyme
assays).

Treatment Options and Outlook
No specific treatment can stop or reverse the symptoms. However, seizures can sometimes be reduced
or controlled with anticonvulsant drugs.

Physical and occupational therapy may help
patients retain some function.

Adding vitamins C and E, and limiting vitamin
A in the diet appeared to help slow the disease in
some cases. However, vitamin therapy ultimately
did not change the fatal outcome of this disease.

B-complex vitamins   See VITAMINS, B-COMPLEX.

behavioral treatments of memory disorders   Techniques to improve memory that include chaining (breaking up a task into smaller units taught one at a time), flooding, or modeling. Behavioral treatments of memory problems work well because they are adaptable to a wide range of patients, the goals are small and specific, and treatment can be tested continually and easily.

The theoretical approaches underlying behavioral therapy draw upon a number of fields within psychology. While behavioral treatments have been used in rehabilitation for years, only recently have they been tried to ease acquired cognitive impairments.

A behavior program for patients with memory problems should specify the behavior to be changed, state the goals of treatment, measure deficit to obtain a baseline, plan/begin treatment, monitor progress, and change the procedure if needed.

Bell's palsy   The most common type of facial paralysis, this temporary problem is caused by damage or injury to one of the two facial nerves. Bell's palsy typically affects only one of the paired facial nerves and one side of the face, although in some rare cases it can affect both sides. Bell's palsy is most common between ages 30 and 60; each year about 40,000 Americans develop the problem.

Most scientists believe that a viral infection, such as viral meningitis or the common cold sore virus (*herpes simplex*), causes the disorder as the facial nerve swells and becomes inflamed in reaction to the infection.

Symptoms and Diagnostic Path
Symptoms of Bell's palsy usually begin suddenly and peak within 48 hours, and may include twitching, weakness, or paralysis, drooping eyelid or corner of the mouth, drooling, dry eye or mouth, impaired taste, and excessive tearing; the palsy often causes significant facial distortion.

Treatment Options and Outlook
There is no cure or standard accepted course of treatment. Some cases are mild, and the symptoms usually fade away by themselves within two weeks. For more lasting symptoms, treatment may include the antiviral drug acyclovir combined with an anti-inflammatory drug such as the steroid prednisone. Painkillers such as aspirin, acetaminophen, or ibuprofen may ease pain. Some physicians believe that no treatment is necessary, although the eyes must be protected if they do not close. A temporary patch or ointment may be recommended for sleeping; eyedrops may also help.

Usually a temporary problem, recovery begins within a few weeks and may be complete within a few months. If the paralysis partially improves by the end of the first week, there will probably be a good outcome.

Recovery from total paralysis may not be complete; if the damage to the facial nerve is quite severe, the fibers may be irreversibly damaged.

Bender-Gestalt test   One of the most widely used components of the typical psychological examination of adults and children. Dr. Lauretta Bender developed the test in 1938 to help tell the difference between ENDOGENOUS BRAIN DAMAGE and EXOGENOUS BRAIN DAMAGE.

The test requires subjects to copy nine geometric figures. There are several scoring systems for children and adults; the results provide an estimate of the person's ability to draw what they see. The test also provides a way of gauging the ability to transfer an image from SENSORY MEMORY to SHORT-TERM MEMORY.

benzodiazepines   A class of tranquilizers that are among the best known and most widely prescribed drugs in the world, used primarily to control symptoms caused by anxiety or stress. They work by depressing brain function, relieving anxiety, and promoting sleep. The drugs slow down the activity of nerves that control many mental and physical functions, such as emotions or heart rate.

The first benzodiazepine was marketed as an antianxiety drug in 1960 under the trade name Librium; three years later, its relative, Valium (DIAZEPAM), was introduced. By the mid-1970s, one of every seven Americans was taking Librium or Valium and more than 100 million prescriptions a year were being written. While in terms of sales they were among the most successful drugs in history, they were beginning to be overprescribed for a range of emotional problems that might have been better treated without drugs. By the mid-1980s fewer prescriptions for these two drugs were written after repeated warnings of overdose.

The benzodiazepines are still widely used because they can relieve anxiety while being much less sedating and dangerous than BARBITURATES. They are also fairly safe drugs; while it is possible to commit suicide by overdosing on either Valium or Librium, it is not easy.

Benzodiazepines can strengthen the sedating effects of alcohol or barbiturates and can also increase their depressant effects on important brain centers (especially the areas that control breathing).

Scientists believe that benzodiazepines, barbiturates, and alcohol all act on the same synapses in the brain, although benzodiazepines act in a slightly different site than the others.

Side Effects

Daytime drowsiness, dizziness and forgetfulness, unsteadiness, slowed reactions. Drowsiness usually wears off after a few weeks. Chronic users may become dependent when taken for more than three or four weeks, and tolerance can develop in time. Stopping benzodiazepines abruptly may lead to withdrawal symptoms (anxiety, nightmares, restlessness), but these are less severe than with other addictive drugs.

besipirdine An acetylcholine-boosting drug currently being studied as a possible treatment for ALZHEIMER'S DISEASE. The drug mimics acetylcholine, a chemical necessary for brain cell communication, which is severely depleted in Alzheimer's.

beta-amyloid protein A normally harmless protein found in the brain that, in ALZHEIMER'S DISEASE, is triggered by an unknown stimulus to fold and twist into a different shape. As it changes, the protein begins forming abnormal strands that build up on brain cells, forming plaques and killing them.

These plaques appear to be made, in part, from protein molecules called AMYLOID PRECURSOR PROTEIN (APP)—that normally are essential components of the brain. Plaques occur when an enzyme snips APP apart at a specific place and then leaves the fragments (beta-amyloid) in brain tissue, where they come together in abnormal plaque deposits.

It appears that beta-amyloid also induces another harmless brain protein, tau, to become a killer as well. (See TAU PROTEIN.) Together, the two destroy the brain cells of people with Alzheimer's, forming the plaques and tangles that have been the hallmarks of the disease since it was first described in 1907 by Alois Alzheimer. Scientists disagree about whether it's the sticky plaques of beta-amyloid in the brain or the tangles of tau protein inside brain nerve fibers that play a more central role in the destruction of brain cells. Most Alzheimer's researchers have focused attention on amyloid as the substance that kills brain cells. They believe excessive amounts of beta-amyloid are toxic to neurons in the same way that too much cholesterol is toxic to the cells in blood vessel walls.

What is known is that increases of beta-amyloid in brain tissue are associated with increasing severity of mental decline, with the highest levels of beta-amyloid found in the brains of patients with the greatest degree of dementia. See also DEMENTIA; PRESENILINS.

beta-endorphins See ENDORPHINS.

beta wave A type of BRAIN WAVE. Beta I waves, like alpha waves, show the brain's readiness for action; beta II waves show intense mental activity.

Binet, Alfred (1857–1911) French psychologist known as the father of modern intelligence testing, who played a major role in the development of experimental psychology.

Alfred Binet was born in Nice, France, on July 11, 1857, the only child of an artist mother and a physician father. His parents divorced when he was young and he was reared by his mother, who went with him to Paris where he entered law school at the age of 15. After receiving his license to practice law in 1878, he decided instead to study medicine. Eventually, he dropped out of college without getting a medical degree when he became interested in psychology. He never completed a degree in psychology, but continued to read and study psychological topics.

French education changed profoundly at the end of the 19th century, when laws made it mandatory for children aged six to 14 to attend school. Suddenly, scientists began to focus on the mental development of children with a new intensity. Interested in individual differences in mental performance, Binet developed tests and puzzles that he tried out on his own daughters, Madeleine and Alice. It was through this study of his daughters that he began to discover the importance of attention span on the development of adult intelligence, and in 1890 he published three papers describing his observations of his daughters. Using these observations, Binet argued against the prevailing view that lack of intellect in certain fields was an illness.

His discovery of different kinds of memory led to a government appointment to develop tests intended to identify areas of mental weakness in schoolchildren. He began to study the effect of suggestibility in experiments with children, and discovered that age played a major role in the development of children's mental faculties.

In 1891 he joined the Laboratory of Physiological Psychology at the Sorbonne; three years later he became its director. At the lab, he studied memory, thinking, hypnosis, handwriting, and perception.

Theodore Simon applied for a research position under Binet's supervision just at the time when French officials were becoming particularly concerned with mental subnormality in light of the new education laws. As a result, Binet and Simon tried to develop a test that would estimate intelligence. The two came up with a test consisting of 30 items, standardized on groups of about 50 "normal" children of different ages and 45 "subnormals." This constituted the first major test of intelligence, published by Binet and Simon in 1905.

The tests were revised in 1908, and again in 1911 right before Binet's death. Binet's death, only six years after the first use of his test meant that necessary revisions and refinements were left largely to others.

Binswanger's disease An extremely rare form of dementia characterized by lesions in the white matter deep inside the brain, resulting in loss of memory, thinking, and learning. The disease is a slowly progressive condition for which there is no cure, often marked by strokes and partial recovery. Patients with this disorder usually die within five years after its onset.

Symptoms and Diagnostic Path

In addition to memory and learning problems, patients usually show signs of abnormal blood pressure, stroke, blood problems, mood disorders, disease of the large blood vessels in the neck, and disease of the heart valves. Other prominent features of the disease include urinary incontinence, difficulty walking, Parkinson-like tremors, and depression. These symptoms, which tend to begin after the age of 60, are not always present in all patients and may sometimes appear only as a passing phase. Seizures may also be present.

Treatment Options and Outlook

There is no specific treatment for Binswanger's disease. Medications can be used to control high blood pressure, depression, abnormal heart rhythms, and low blood pressure.

biofeedback A technique in which a person uses information about a normally unconscious body function such as blood pressure, to gain conscious control over that function. Biofeedback may help in the treatment of stress-related conditions such as hypertension or migraine.

The subject is connected to a recording instrument that can measure one of the unconscious body activities—blood pressure, pulse rate, body temperature, muscle tensions, sweat on the skin, brain waves, or stomach acidity. The subject receives the information (feedback) on the changing levels of the body activities from alterations in the instrument's signals (flashing lights, fluctuating needle, changing sounds).

With practice, the person starts to become aware of how he or she is feeling whenever there is a change in the recording instrument's signal. Relaxation techniques also may be used to bring about a change in the signal; the instrument's response may indicate which methods of relaxation work best.

Eventually the subject learns to change the signal by consciously controlling the body function being tested. Once learned, control can be exerted without the equipment.

biological clocks   See CIRCADIAN RHYTHM; JET LAG; MELATONIN.

bipolar disorder   A form of mental illness, previously referred to as manic-depressive disorder, in which the patient swings between extremes of mania and deep DEPRESSION. The problem seems to result from imbalance in the activity of certain NEUROTRANSMITTERS (SEROTONIN, DOPAMINE, and NOREPINEPHRINE) that influence emotion and behavior.

While bipolar disorder can be crippling in the acute phase, more than 80 percent of people who are afflicted recover. However, repeated episodes can seriously disrupt a person's life and may lead to suicide. Moreover, some experts believe that such recurrent, progressive depression is a result of structural changes in the brain as the disease worsens; some physicians recommend keeping some patients on LITHIUM for long periods of time to prevent the subsequent almost-impossible-to-reverse deterioration.

Symptoms and Diagnostic Path

A number of physical illnesses (especially brain disorders), some types of drug abuse, and a family history for the disorder are all established factors. Researchers have located at least one defective gene on chromosome 11 that appears to be linked to the disorder. One study found that in sets of identical twins, if one twin had bipolar disorder, there was a 50 percent chance that the other twin would develop the disorder. The concordance rate in fraternal twins is only 10 percent, the same as for other siblings. Moreover, adopted children have been found to suffer from bipolar disorder at a rate that matches their birth parents instead of their adoptive parents, although environment and upbringing do play a role in the development of the disease.

Treatment Options and Outlook

In severe cases, hospitalization may be required. Lithium is the drug of choice; it works best for people who have had no more than three episodes of mania. About 20 percent of patients will have a complete remission on lithium; the rest will respond in varying degrees. In about 30 percent of patients, lithium smooths out the periods of mania hut does not control the episodes of depression; in these cases physicians may prescribe a selective serotonin reuptake inhibitor (a type of antidepressant). Other patients respond to the anticonvulsants Tegretol or Depakote.

birth injury to the brain   Any problem that occurs during the birth process that carries the risk of ANOXIA (loss of oxygen) can have a potentially devastating effect on a newborn's brain. Damage to the brain may either be localized or diffuse (a much more serious problem); loss of oxygen during birth for longer than about five minutes will likely cause serious damage.

Brain problems linked to birth trauma can include CEREBRAL PALSY, MENTAL RETARDATION, EPILEPSY, AUTISM, ATAXIA, LEARNING DISABILITIES, SCHIZOPHRENIA, and MICROCEPHALY.

blackouts, alcoholic   A common phenomenon among alcoholics and normal drinkers who overindulge, involving a loss of memory during the drunken state. During a blackout, the individual is not unconscious or incapacitated, and usually possesses most of his or her faculties.

Symptoms and Diagnostic Path

Experts once believed that blackouts were a form of state-dependent forgetting, that is, a person can remember information learned in a state only when in that state. In other words, a person who commits a crime while drunk would only remember that crime while drunk. However, at least one research study did not support this theory. in a study of five convicted murderers who had committed their crimes while drunk and claimed amnesia for their activities, the murderers were allowed to become drunk. None recalled their crimes while drunk, and when they were sober again all had varying degrees of amnesia for the experiment.

In one form of alcoholic blackout, called en bloc, the person experiences AMNESIA that has a clear beginning and end; in this form, the patient knows there has been a "lost period." In a second form of blackout, the person is not aware of any amnesia and also may have exhibited memory problems while drinking without any recollection of them.

Researchers believe that alcoholic blackouts occur because the original level of alcohol intoxication was enough to disrupt the physiological processes involved in forming memories.

blood-brain barrier   A protective filtering mechanism of the blood vessels of the brain that keeps out (or slows down) many substances in the blood. The barrier utilizes a semipermeable membrane separating circulating blood from fluid surrounding brain cells. This barrier serves to protect the brain from some poisons and unwanted chemicals.

Blood vessels have small windows to allow for the passage of food and oxygen into all parts of the body and the return to the blood of cellular waste products. But the blood vessels of the brain are highly selective, which is helpful when it comes to keeping out harmful chemicals but not so beneficial when it also excludes substances such as chemotherapy drugs.

Fortunately, blood vessels near tumors are often damaged, which may allow drugs and lymphocytes into the tumor area. Research is currently looking at the possibility of further disrupting this blood-brain barrier by certain drugs or by hyperthermia (increased temperature of brain tissue). In addition, drugs may be injected directly into the cerebrospinal fluid or directly into an artery feeding into a brain tumor.

Some medications given first can temporarily allow passage of other drugs through the blood-brain barrier.

Boston remote memory battery   The most extensive test for RETROGRADE AMNESIA, devised by Marilyn Albert in 1979. Its three components each have easy and hard questions; the easy questions reflect information that might be answered on the basis of general knowledge, while the hard questions reflect information whose recollection relies much more on remembering a particular time period.

Unfortunately, the test is considered to be culture-specific and cannot be used with patients outside the United States. (See also ASSESSMENT OF MEMORY DISORDERS.)

botulism   A serious form of food poisoning that selectively affects the CENTRAL NERVOUS SYSTEM. The toxins are rapidly absorbed by the gastrointestinal tract and bind to brain tissue; in fatal cases, death is often caused by a failure of the cardiac and respiratory centers in the brain. Botulism is caused by contamination with the botulin toxin, produced by the bacterium *Clostridium botulinum,* which thrives in improperly preserved foods (especially canned meat).

Because the toxin is not stable when heated, it is generally destroyed when boiled at 100°C for one minute (or if the food is sterilized by pressure cooking at 250°F for 30 minutes).

C. botulinum occurs as harmless inactive spores in air, water, and food. When the spores are deprived of oxygen, however (such as inside a sealed can or jar), they begin to grow, producing one of the most deadly toxins known to humans—7 million times more deadly than cobra venom. Still, even inside a sealed jar, the spores will not grow if the food is very acidic, sweet, or salty (such as canned fruit juice, jams, and jellies, sauerkraut, tomatoes, and heavily salted hams). Canned foods that *are* susceptible to contamination include green beans, beets, peppers, corn, and meat.

Although the spores are invisible, it is possible to tell if food is spoiled by detecting a broken vacuum seal (when the spores grow, they give off gas that makes cans and jars lose their seal so that jars will burst or cans will swell). Any food that is spoiled or whose color or odor does not seem right inside a home-canned jar should be destroyed without tasting or even sniffing, because the spores can be fatal in small amounts.

Botulism is more common in the United States than anywhere else in the world, due to the popularity in this country of home canning. The name is derived from the Latin word for sausage (*botulus*), which was chosen after some people in the 1800s were poisoned with contaminated sausages. Cases of botulism from commercially canned food are rare because the U.S. Food and Drug Administration enforces strict health standards.

Botulism also can occur if the bacteria in the soil enters the body through an open wound.

Symptoms and Diagnostic Path

Onset of symptoms may vary from 12 to 36 hours, although they can appear as soon as three hours or as late as two weeks after ingestion of contaminated food. The earlier the symptoms, the more severe the reaction and the higher rate of fatality. Cranial nerve symptoms include double or blurred vision, drooping eyelid, difficulty or pain on swallowing, or slurred speech. This is followed by a descending paralysis that affects all the muscles. Throughout the course of the illness, the patient's mind remains clear, but almost all patients have breathing problems. Other symptoms include nausea and vomiting, diarrhea, stomach cramps, and headache.

Death usually occurs in untreated cases from suffocation as a result of the paralysis of breathing muscles.

Infant botulism may include constipation, facial muscle flaccidity, sucking problems, irritability, lethargy, and floppy limbs.

Treatment Options and Outlook

Prompt administration of the antitoxin (type ABE botulinus) lowers the risk of death to 25 percent. The Centers for Disease Control in Atlanta, Georgia, is the only agency with the antitoxin; this is the agency that makes the decision to treat the problem. Local health departments should be called first.

A patient should vomit immediately after eating food known to contain botulism toxin, but because vomiting may not be complete and the disease can be caused by only a small amount of toxin, botulism may still develop.

In infant botulism, once symptoms appear it is often too late to administer the antitoxin. Two-thirds of those who are poisoned will die; the rest face a long recovery period.

brain The brain is an organ of jellylike consistency that sits atop the spinal cord and controls all bodily processes, including thought and emotion, speech, and memory. It consists of two halves, or hemispheres, separated by a groove called the CORPUS CALLOSUM. Each side of the brain contains three areas: the BRAIN STEM, the CEREBELLUM, and the CEREBRUM. The brain stem controls basic bodily functions such as breathing and heart rate. The cerebellum controls coordination and balance. The cerebrum controls such complex and complicated functions as thinking, speaking, and reading.

At three pounds, the adult human brain weighs about as much as a sack of sugar. It is about 75 percent water and accounts for approximately 2 percent of an adult's body weight. If one could harness the electricity produced by the brain, it could power a 10-watt lightbulb. The brain consumes about 20 percent of the oxygen taken into the body. The number of brain pathways capable of producing thought is the number 1 followed by 10.5 million kilometers of zeroes printed in a standard 12-point font.

Although the above facts make the human brain fascinating, ancient anatomists were confused by the brain and considered it "stuffing." As educational television programs like to point out, the ancient Egyptians thought the brain served no function other than to maintain the shape of the skull. Ancient medical procedures involved extracting the brain through the nose with forceps. The EDWIN SMITH SURGICAL PAPYRUS, which archaeologists believe was written about 1,700 years before the common era, contains the earliest reference to the brain. The papyrus mentions the brain eight times and describes the symptoms of two patients with compound skull fractures.

In the fifth century B.C., Pythagorean Alcmaeon de Croton produced the oldest writings describing the brain as the location of mental functions. Before that time, anatomists believed the heart controlled mental functions and emotions. Hippocrates, writing in the fourth century B.C., stated that the brain was responsible for intelligence. Aristotle, who also wrote in the fourth century B.C.E., stated that the heart was responsible for intelligence and the brain served to cool the blood. Aristotle claimed humans are more intelligent than other animals because we have a larger brain to cool the blood.

In the 10th century A.D., Arab physician Najab ud-din Muhammad provided the earliest descriptions of neurological disorders in detail, such as agitated depression, priapism, impotence, schizophrenia, and mania. In the 11th century A.D., another Arabic physician, Alhazen, contributed to the field that ultimately became psychology by arguing in his *Book of Optics* that vision occurs in the brain rather than the eyes and that people's expectations affect their interpretations of what they see.

Medical historians point to the invention of the microscope in the 16th century C.E. as leading to many rapid advances in medicine because physicians could study tiny structures in detail. Camillo Golgi in the late 1800s developed staining procedures that allowed him to discern individual NEURONS. Santiago Ramón y Cajal, using Golgi's microscopic techniques, formulated the neuron doctrine, which states that the neuron is the functional unit of the brain. PIERRE-PAUL BROCA, also working in the late 1800s, suggested that certain regions of the brain controlled certain functions. He identified BROCA'S AREA as the site controlling expressive speech. CARL WERNICKE, working from the late 1800s until his death due to injuries he received in a bicycle accident in 1905, discovered WERNICKE'S AREA, which controls receptive language, or the understanding of speech.

Nerve Cells

Nerve cells are the building blocks of brain tissue. These cells receive signals from other cells by accepting NEUROTRANSMITTERS, which are chemicals manufactured by NEURONS and released by the axon terminals into fingerlike structures called DENDRITES. The neurons then send an electrical impulse down the nerve shaft, or AXON, where the axon terminals release neurotransmitters for intake by the next neurons in the chain. ACETYCHOLINE is a neurotransmitter that plays a role in SHORT-TERM MEMORY, THIRST, body temperature,

and motor function. EPINEPHRINE stimulates the FIGHT-OR-FLIGHT RESPONSE. NOREPINEPHRINE affects LONG-TERM MEMORY, HUNGER, and the sleep-wake cycle. SEROTONIN is another neurotransmitter that affects emotions, sleep, and the feeling of being full after meals. ENDORPHIN and ENKEPHALIN influence emotion, PAIN, pleasure, and appetite. The MYELIN SHEATH is a fatty membrane that covers the axon, providing insulation, thereby increasing the efficiency of the nerve impulse.

Cranial Nerves

There are 12 nerves in the brain, referred to as CRANIAL NERVES, FIRST through TWELFTH. The OLFACTORY NERVE (first) controls the sense of smell; the OPTIC NERVE (second) controls vision; the OCULOMOTOR NERVE (third) controls eye movements; the TROCHLEAR NERVE (fourth) controls lateral movement of the eyeball; the TRIGEMINAL NERVE (fifth) controls reception of sensation from the face and stimulation of facial/oral muscles involved in eating; the ABDUCENS NERVE (sixth) controls stimulation of the lateral rectus that supplies the eye; the FACIAL NERVE (seventh) controls the sensation of TASTE from the forward two-thirds of the tongue and also controls the movements involved in facial expression; the VESTIBULOCOCHLEAR NERVE (eighth) controls sensation of the stimuli necessary for balance and movement; the GLOSSOPHARYNGEAL NERVE (ninth) controls reception of taste from the rear one-third of the tongue; the VAGUS NERVE (tenth) controls reception of special sense of taste from the epiglottis and controls the muscles necessary for voice and resonance; the SPINAL ACCESSORY NERVE (eleventh) controls neck muscles; and the HYPOGLOSSAL NERVE (twelfth) controls swallowing and SPEECH articulation.

Hemispheres of the Brain

The brain is divided into the left and right hemispheres. We must not make overly broad generalizations, but researchers have identified specialization differences between the two sides. The left hemisphere exerts the most control over sequential, analytical, verbal, logical, linear, algorithmic processing, and present/past reasoning, and the right hemisphere mostly controls simultaneous, holistic, imagistic, intuitive holistic algorithmic processing, and present/future reasoning. However, contrary to the notion the media presents that only one side of the brain works at a time, imaging studies demonstrate that even when the brain is engaged in so-called left-brain or right-brain activities, the other side of the brain shows some activity.

Brain Stem

The brain stem, also known as the MESENCEPHA-LON, is the most primitive part of the brain. It is an extension of the spinal cord. It is part of the REPTILIAN BRAIN, sometimes called the snake brain. It regulates the same primitive functions as reptiles' brains, including waking, breathing, and heart rate. Notable structures within the brain stem include the MEDULLA, PONS, MIDBRAIN, and RETICULAR FORMATION. The latter structure is especially important in awareness, attention, and sleep. The 12 cranial nerves begin in the brain stem.

Cerebellum

The cerebellum (Latin for "little brain") is the second-largest part of the brain. It is an outgrowth of the HINDBRAIN. It sits beneath the cerebrum and is directly behind the brain stem. The cerebellum controls body movement and balance and helps maintain body posture and muscle coordination.

Limbic System

The LIMBIC SYSTEM lies on both sides of and underneath the THALAMUS, under the cerebrum. It is important in the regulation of emotions and the formation of memories. The limbic system helps maintain bodily homeostasis, the regulation of the body's "normal state." It also regulates the functioning of the PARASYMPATHETIC NERVOUS SYSTEM (PNS) and the SYMPATHETIC NERVOUS SYSTEM (SNS). It receives input from many sources, including the vagus nerve, reticulor formation and brain stem, optic nerve, neurons, olfactory nerve, and the HYPOTHALAMUS. The limbic system sends instructions to the rest of the body via the autonomic nervous system and the PITUITARY GLAND.

The HIPPOCAMPUS is a part of the limbic system located in the medial temporal lobe. It is important in general MEMORY, spatial memory, and navigation. Its effects on general memory include new memories for events, DECLARATIVE MEMORY, and episodic memory. The hippocampus affects our ability to recall how to get to where we are going as well as the ability to find shortcuts.

The AMYGDALA consists of two almond-shaped groups of neurons on either side of the thalamus, at the lower end of the hippocampus. When researchers stimulate the amygdala, laboratory animals become physically aggressive. If researchers remove the amygdala, animals become very tame and passive and no longer experience sexual arousal.

The septum lies in front of the thalamus. It is responsible for the sexual orgasm. The cingulate gyrus is part of the cerebrum that lies closest to the limbic system, just above the corpus callosum. The cingulate gyrus provides the pathway from the thalamus to the hippocampus. The cingulate gyrus is responsible for focusing attention on emotionally important events and associating memories for smells and pain.

The BASAL GANGLIA include the CAUDATE NUCLEUS, putamen, globus pallidus, and SUBSTANTIA NIGRA. The basal ganglia lie over and to the sides of the limbic system and are responsible for repetitive behaviors, reward experiences, and focusing attention.

Cerebral Cortex

The CEREBRAL CORTEX is the series of folded bulges (called *gyri*) we commonly refer to as GRAY MATTER. The folds allow the cerebral cortex to include much more surface area than would be possible with a smooth surface. Two-thirds of the surface of the cerebral cortex is contained within those folds. Gray matter is composed of neurons and unmyelinated nerve fibers. The oldest part of the cerebral cortex, from an evolutionary standpoint, is the hippocampus, also known as the *archicortex*. The most recently evolved part of the cerebral cortex is the six-layered neocortex. The cerebral cortex contains the FRONTAL LOBE, PARIETAL LOBE, TEMPORAL LOBE, and OCCIPITAL LOBE.

The frontal lobe is located at the front of the brain and includes the prefrontal cortex. The frontal lobe controls our motor functions, higher-order thinking (also called executive functions), planning, reasoning, judgment, impulse control, and memory.

The parietal lobe is behind the CENTRAL SULCUS and above the occipital lobe. It is important in cognition, information processing, pain and touch sensation, spatial orientation, speech, and visual perception.

The temporal lobe is in front of the occipital lobe and beside the FISSURE OF SYLVIUS. The temporal lobe is important in regulating emotional responses, hearing, memory, and speech. It contains two structures that are crucial in speech, Broca's area, which governs the expression of language, and Wernicke's area, which governs the understanding of speech.

Sympathetic Nervous System

The sympathetic nervous system (SNS) controls heartbeat and the secretion of HORMONES. It consists of two chains of nerves passing from the spinal cord and extending through the body. It regulates the release of norepinephrine, which triggers the release of glucose from energy stores and increases blood flow to the skeletal muscles during the fight-or-flight response.

Parasympathetic Nervous System

The PARASYMPATHETIC NERVOUS SYSTEM (PNS) works to counter the action of the sympathetic nervous system (SNS) by calming heart rate and respiration, normalizing the body after the need for the fight-or-flight response has passed. It works through the release of acetylcholine. It is made up of two chains of nerves, one passing from the brain and the other leaving the lower spinal cord.

The Future of Brain Research

Knowledge of the brain has advanced rapidly in recent years and science is quickly closing in on discovering more about the brain's role in our daily functioning. Medicine and psychology have long assumed that the brain serves an important role in disorders such as attention deficit hyperactivity disorder (ADHD), mental illness, and learning disabilities, but there is still much to learn about the precise role of brain processes in these disorders. Researchers are employing cutting-edge imaging, brain wave analysis, and understanding of brain chemistry to attempt to identify the mechanisms involved in these disorders and eventually improve our ways of preventing and treating them. Increased precision of imaging techniques helps us study the living brain without having to rely on autopsy studies, thereby allowing researchers to pose predictions regarding brain activity and narrow down possible explanations for disorders such as epilepsy. Increased sophistication in pairing of computers with imaging and other analytical techniques offers much promise for increasing our understanding of the brain and BRAIN DISORDERS.

brain cells There are two kinds of brain cells: NEURONS (nerve cells) and GLIA. While the majority of brain cells (85 percent) are glia, it is the remaining 15 percent—the neurons—that make the brain the most important organ in the body.

Glial cells play a supportive role in brain function, helping to remove waste products, supplying nutrients, maintaining electrical balance, and guiding the brain's development. The neurons, on the other hand, control the body's emotions, activities—and the ability to think.

Neurons in the brain are structurally the same as nerve cells throughout the body, with a main cell body composed of a nucleus and cytoplasm. The nucleus contains the genetic material that allows a cell to reproduce; the cytoplasm provides energy for the cell. Neurons have very long extensions called AXONS that allow neurons to communicate with each other. At the end of each axon are many branches that touch a neighboring neuron. One neuron has more than 10,000 "antennae," called DENDRITES, that receive impulses from the axons of other neurons. The human brain has more than 15 billion neurons.

brain damage Degeneration or death of nerve cells and tracts within the brain, which may be localized in particular areas (causing specific defects) or more diffuse, causing mental problems or severe physical handicap. Memory is very sensitive to brain damage, since it is dependent on such a wide range of interacting processes; even limited brain damage may affect some of these processes. Many brain structures seem to be involved in the process of memory, including the HIPPOCAMPUS, hypothalamus, THALAMUS, and TEMPORAL LOBE. Damage to any of them can cause memory problems.

Most people with organic amnesia will have experienced one of the following: HEAD INJURY, cerebral vascular accident, progressive DEMENTIA, BRAIN TUMOR, toxic disorder, brain surgery or nutritional disorder. (See CEREBROVASCULAR ACCIDENT [CVA].)

Memory deficits may be a lifelong handicap for brain-damaged patients and their families. Such patients are liable to a greater risk of personal danger (by forgetting a lighted cigarette or a pot on the stove), increased annoyance from others by repeatedly failing to remember, and social isolation.

Localized brain damage can occur as a result of a head injury (especially those that penetrate the skull) or from a STROKE, brain tumor or BRAIN ABSCESS. It also may be caused by damage to the brain at birth from jaundice (excess bilirubin levels). The BASAL GANGLIA also may be damaged by CARBON MONOXIDE POISONING.

Diffuse brain damage may result from hypoxia (lack of oxygen in the brain) that may occur during birth; from cardiac or respiratory arrest; or from poisoning, drowning, electric shock or prolonged convulsions. It also may be caused by the accumulation of toxic substances in the brain, as occurs in phenylketonuria or galactosemia, or of environmental poisons (such as lead or mercury). Other possible causes include brain infections (such as encephalitis) or, rarely, a reaction after immunization. In addition, there is some evidence that the tips and undersurface of the temporal lobes may be more susceptible to traumatic damage than other parts of the brain; if so, then memory problems following diffuse brain damage may in fact indicate hippocampal damage. Encephalitic patients, too, may suffer extensive temporal lobe lesions (although the virus does not always attack this area).

Patients who have suffered head injury or stroke are likely to experience memory problems in addition to other symptoms. Unlike nerves in the limbs or trunk, nerve cells and tracts in the brain and spinal cord do not recover their function if they have been destroyed. However, patients may improve somewhat after brain damage as they learn to use other parts of the brain to compensate for the loss.

The ability to store and recall memories following brain injury may be affected in quite different ways from one patient to the next. This is because there is not just one kind of memory, but many—verbal and nonverbal memory, visual and auditory memory, short-term and long-term memory, episodic and semantic memory. Moreover, even in the same patient, some memory functions may work fine while others show more disruption.

There are three main ways to improve memory performance for brain-damaged patients—physical treatment (such as medication) and internal and external aids.

Internal aids include mnemonics, rehearsal strategies, or anything a patient does mentally to the information to be remembered. External aids include diaries, notebooks and calendars, alarm clocks, gadgets and computers. Environmental aids also may be used to help mold behavior in patients with severe memory problems, for example, lines may be painted on the ground to help them find their way around. One hospital geriatric unit reduced its incontinency problem among patients by painting all the lavatory doors a different color from other doors.

The effectiveness of external aids is related to the attitude toward their use; in some cases patients need counseling before they will accept the aids. One of the most effective aids is the combination of a digital alarm watch and a notebook with the day's activities; whenever the alarm goes off, the patient consults the notebook.

The ability of a brain-damaged patient to recover memory depends on the cause and site of the damage, the individual's personality, and how motivated he or she is to recover. Indeed, researchers agree there is little evidence that practice by itself will significantly improve a brain-damaged person's memory. (See also MEMORY FOR FACES; VISUAL IMAGERY METHOD.)

brain death Complete and irreversible cessation of all brain function, usually measured by lack of electrical signals on ELECTROENCEPHALOGRAMS taken over a period of at least 12 to 24 hours, even if the heart and lungs continue to function with help from a machine. This time period is important because brain activity may be temporarily depressed by some forms of drug reactions or poisons. If there is a suspicion of intoxication with CENTRAL NERVOUS SYSTEM DEPRESSANTS, the diagnosis of brain death cannot be made.

Brain dead means the patient cannot breathe spontaneously, has no memory, consciousness, knowledge, thought, touch, sight, or any other sense. The brain is irreparably destroyed and begins to deteriorate.

The concept of brain death does not apply to patients who exist in a persistent vegetative state or to other severe degrees of brain damage. Decisions concerning these patients must be made based on other criteria.

While the legal definition of brain death (also called irreversible coma) may vary from state to state, it is usually taken to mean the absence of REFLEXES, movements, and independent breathing.

This legal definition may become important when considering whether the patient's organs should be donated and in determining whether or not to turn off a ventilator. Because blood supply to organs is important if they are to be transplanted with the best chance for success, they should be taken after the brain is dead but while the heart and lungs are still functioning.

The American Bar Association, the American Medical Association, the National Conference of Commissioners on Uniform State Laws and the President's Commission for the Study of Ethical Problems in Medicine have proposed a model statute to come up with a more standard definition of death. This proposed statute (called the "uniform determination of death act") says:

> An individual who has sustained either (1) irreversible cessation of circulation and respiratory functions or (2) irreversible cessation of all functions of the entire brain, including the brain stem, is dead. A determination of death must be made in accordance with acceptable medical standards.

The concept of brain death has been accepted by the Roman Catholic Church and by those attending the First World Meeting on Transplantation of Organs. In 1972, the American Neurological Association accepted brain death as a definition of death.

brain development in children Research has revealed that the first three years of life are critical in the development of the brain and that there is far more to brain development than luck or heredity. Not only does environment affect how large and how fast a child's brain grows, but it helps direct the actual wiring of the brain's circuitry.

Every baby is born with about 100 billion brain cells—no more will develop during the child's lifetime. Brain cells connect with each other across tiny spaces called SYNAPSES, joining together to form systems that perform different functions.

During the first eight months after birth, neurons join together quickly, so that after eight months, a baby may have as many as 1 quadrillion synapses. In order to become permanent, however, these connections must be reinforced through everyday experience and stimulation by caregivers and other people. Many of those early connections are never reinforced, so that by age 10, a child has only about half as many (500 trillion) synapses—about the same number as an adult.

The child's brain develops from the least complex part, the BRAIN STEM, which controls basic involuntary life functions like heart rate and body temperature, to the most complex (the top layer of the brain called the CORTEX), which controls reasoning and abstract thought.

The brain systems that control vision and language begin forming quite early. What a baby sees and hears at a very young age has a profound and long-term impact on vision and language skills.

Simple interactions may be the most important factors in the development of connections in a child's brain. Through this contact, the child is stimulated to develop important sensory functions while absorbing the sensation of love that is critical to healthy emotional development.

Because different systems in the brain develop at different times, specific parts of a child's brain must be stimulated within a specific time span in order to develop normally. If the crucial environmental cues do not occur during these periods, the parts of the brain that regulate those functions may not develop appropriately. For example, the window of opportunity for the development of vision occurs from birth to about six months of age. Children who get little visual stimulation during this time will not develop the necessary brain cell connections and vision problems may result.

The critical window for the development of speech and vocabulary is between birth and three years of age, and is so important that the sounds children hear in those years will largely determine the size of their adult vocabulary. Children who do not hear language regularly early in life do not learn to think as well as those who are exposed to a lot of spoken language.

Between the ages of one and four, children develop the capacity to understand logic and mathematical concepts. There is also a great deal of evidence suggesting that experience with music at an early age may improve a child's mathematical ability. Children who have little experience with math and logic during this stage may have more trouble learning those skills later in life.

Just as healthy emotional development is important during the early years, the negative impact of stress, trauma, and neglect can have a terrible impact on the developing brain. Research clearly shows that abuse and trauma early in life can raise the levels of the stress hormone called cortisol. High levels of cortisol washing over the brain can cause certain areas that regulate emotional response and attachment to be 20 percent to 30 percent smaller than normal. Children who have been traumatized develop ineffective response patterns, such as hyperarousal (hyperactivity, anxiety, impulsivity, and sleep difficulties) or dissociation (daydreaming and fantasy), more commonly seen in girls.

Children need nurturing human interaction to help develop the cortex and limbic system (the top layers of the brain that control higher levels of thought and help regulate impulsive emotional response). Neglect and trauma can create a brain that is very good at primitive emotional behavior but not so good at developing mature, reasoned responses. Serious neglect and abuse can affect the actual physical development of the brain. Successful intervention must start early and be intensive and ongoing.

See also DEVELOPMENT OF THE BRAIN.

brain disorders Impairments in the structure or function of BRAIN tissues that result in functional impairment or decreased quality of life. Brain dis-

orders reveal themselves through behavioral, cognitive, consciousness, medical, motor, and sensory symptoms. Procedures to diagnose brain disorders consist of medical and nonmedical procedures. Brain disorders come from many sources. Some of the more common sources include BRAIN TUMORS, infectious diseases, genetic disorders, BRAIN INJURY, lifestyle factors, mixed causes, and unknown causes.

Symptoms and Diagnostic Path

People who suffer from brain disorders and the family members of such people frequently first see signs of those disorders in behavioral symptoms. Psychologists and medical personnel assess people suspected of having brain disorders for *activities of daily living* (ADLs). At the most basic level, ADLs refer to self-care skills, such as bathing, dressing and undressing, eating, moving between bed and a chair, voluntary control of toileting, and walking. For example, members of a Marine squad may notice that one of their fellow Marines has stopped caring for his normal hygienic needs following a head injury after he was struck by shrapnel from the explosion of an improvised explosive device. Or perhaps an elderly grandmother, who has always been fastidious in her cleanliness and her appearance, abruptly begins to dress in a slovenly fashion and wet or soil herself. Family members frequently notice elderly relatives begin to walk in a shuffling manner for no obvious reason. The examining professional will, in such cases, conduct diagnostic procedures to determine the source of the changes in behavior. Thorough behavioral assessment can point the physician to the area of the brain that is likely causing the behavioral difficulties. For example, difficulties expressing coherent thoughts might suggest to the physician to perform an MRI of BROCA'S AREA, or abrupt deterioration in vision may suggest studies of the OCCIPITAL LOBE.

Many cognitive symptoms of brain disorders reveal themselves first in academic settings. ACAL- CULIA (a dysfunction in mathematics reasoning), AGRAPHIA (written expression dysfunction), ALEXIA (the inability to read words), AMUSIA (the inability to recognize musical tones), CUE-DEPENDENT FOR- GETTING, and LANGUAGE DELAY may only become evident in school, where educators detect children whose abilities seem deficient in comparison with other children's. Other disorders, such as AGNOSIA, ANOMIA, ANOSOGNOSIA, APROSODIA, AUDITORY AGNOSIA, AMNESIA, DYSPHASIA, HALLUCINATION, and MEMORY DISTORTIONS may occur at any phase of life.

Some symptoms of brain disorders relate to our ability to maintain an appropriate level of CONSCIOUSNESS. UNCONSCIOUSNESS, DELIRIUM, GRAND MAL SEIZURES, and PETIT MAL SEIZURES cause individuals or their caregivers to seek immediate medical attention. Others, such as perceptual aberrations, result from traumatic brain injury and should prompt individuals to seek medical attention, although many people initially ignore these symptoms and only seek help after their symptoms begin to worsen.

Some medical symptoms such as HYPERBILIRUBIMIA, HYPOGLYCEMIA, OCCIPITAL NEURALGIA, PERIPHERAL NEUROPATHY, and TRIGEMINAL NEURALGIA may require extensive diagnostic examinations to determine their cause and identify the underlying condition.

Motor symptoms of brain disorders can be especially disturbing to individuals who experience them. For example, PARKINSONISM, postural rigidity, TREMOR, and exaggerated movements may occur because of PARKINSON'S DISEASE, CONCUSSION, side effects of medication, or other underlying causes. APNEA, APRAXIA, ATAXIA, ATHETOSIS, CATAPLEXY, CHOREA, DYSARTHRIA, DYSAUTONOMIA, DYSKINESIA, and DYSTONIA are frequently part of a group of other symptoms that lead to diagnosis of a brain disorder.

Sometimes brain disorders reveal themselves through sensory disturbances such as OLFACTORY FATIGUE or VERTIGO.

Medical diagnostic procedures for brain disorders and imaging techniques in particular have shown remarkable advances in accuracy and availability in recent years. The medical fields of NEUROLOGY and NEUROPSYCHIATRY have long relied on X-RAYS to obtain diagnoses. More recent advances in imaging provide additional tools for determining the health of the living brain, including cerebral arteriography, the COMPUTERIZED AXIAL TOMOGRAPHY (CAT) SCAN, MAGNETIC RESONANCE IMAGING (MRI) and FUNCTIONAL MAGNETIC RESONANCE IMAGING (fMRI) scans, POSITRON EMISSION TRANSAXIAL TOMOGRAPHY (PETT) scans, ULTRASOUND SCANS, and SPECT (SINGLE-PHOTON EMISSION COMPUTERIZED TOMOGRAPHY) scans render images of varying degrees of accuracy, allowing examination of the brain noninvasively.

Additional components of the NEUROLOGICAL EXAM include the AUDITORY BRAIN STEM RESPONSE (ABR) TEST, AUDITORY-EVOKED POTENTIALS, AVERAGED EVOKED RESPONSE, CEREBRAL BLOOD-FLOW STUDIES, ECHOENCEPHALOGRAPHY, the GLUCOSE UTILIZATION SCAN, LUMBAR PUNCTURE (LP), MYELOGRAPHY, nerve conduction studies, the SPINAL TAP, and VISUAL-EVOKED RESPONSES.

NEUROPSYCHOLOGY is the psychological specialty that deals with cognitive and behavioral aspects of neurological disorders. The NEUROPSYCHOLOGIST conducts a NEUROPSYCHOLOGICAL ASSESSMENT of varying degrees of complexity according to the needs of the patient and medical specialists with whom the neuropsychologist is consulting. At the initial stage, this assessment may consist of a brief MENTAL STATUS EXAMINATION, such as the MINI-MENTAL STATE EXAMINATION (MMSE). This level of evaluation provides brief screening of executive functioning—the ability to perform simple calculations, demonstrate an awareness of the world or current events (such as the name of the current president), and follow one-step instructions—and memory—recalling several objects after certain times have passed and following instructions with several steps.

Once the neuropsychologist has made a preliminary determination of the subject's assessment needs, the next step is to include additional instruments. Intelligence tests, such as the STANFORD-BINET INTELLIGENCE SCALE, FIFTH EDITION, or one of the Wechsler series, including WECHSLER ADULT INTELLIGENCE SCALE—FOURTH EDITION (WAIS-IV); WECHSLER INTELLIGENCE SCALE FOR CHILDREN, FOURTH EDITION (WISC-IV); WECHSLER PRESCHOOL AND PRIMARY SCALE OF INTELLIGENCE, THIRD EDITION (WWPSI-III) are essential components in the diagnosis of brain disorders. Such tests not only help clinicians establish the level of a client's intelligence but also many items relevant to neuropsychological functioning.

The neuropsychological assessment may include additional measures, such as screenings for perceptual-motor functioning such as the

BENDER-GESTALT TEST or the left-right reversal test. Memory assessments such as the BOSTON REMOTE MEMORY BATTERY or the FAMOUS FACES TEST provide useful clues regarding possible memory dysfunction. Academic achievement measures, such as the EARLY LANGUAGE MILESTONE SCALE (ELMS) or the NEW ADULT READING TEST (NART) provide useful information regarding an individual's ability to muster his or her cognitive resources to engage in academic exercises. Finally, measures such as the COGNITIVE FAILURES QUESTIONNAIRE or the WISCONSIN CARD-SORTING TEST can provide valuable information regarding specialized areas of brain functioning.

Sources of Brain Disorders

There are many possible sources of brain disorders. Although some brain disorders occur due to unknown causes, others may be endogenous (i.e., from within the person), such as tumors or genetic disorders, while others may be exogenous (i.e., from outside the person), such as infectious disease, brain injury, and lifestyle factors such as substance abuse.

Tumors   Brain tumors are either primary, the so-called true tumors, or secondary, tumors that spread from malignant primary tumors. The site of the tumor determines its direct effects. An ACOUSTIC NEUROMA, for example, found on the ACOUSTIC NERVE, is a benign tumor formed from the MYELIN cells in the vestibular area of the VESTIBULOCOCHLEAR NERVE. Direct effects of such tumors include sensorineural hearing decrease or deafness, impaired sense of balance, vertigo, and nausea and vomiting. Indirect effects can arise from a NEUROMA, the resulting swelling of the tumor, which causes impingements on adjacent nerves or decrease in blood flow to other parts of the brain. Other common brain tumors include ASTROCYTOMA, located in the cranial vault; MENINGIOMA, usually a benign tumor located in the MENINGES that causes motor, sensory, aphasic, and seizure symptoms depending on the tumor's location; MEDULLOBLASTOMA, beginning, as the name implies, in the MEDULLA or posterior fossa and causing listlessness, nausea, or headaches that may lead to a misdiagnosis of MIGRAINE; and PITUITARY TUMORS or PITUITARY ADENOMA, which are located on the PITUITARY GLAND and cause a variety of symptoms.

Infectious Disease   AIDS DEMENTIA COMPLEX (ADC) is the cluster of cognitive effects of HIV and acquired immunodeficiency syndrome (AIDS) infections. The increase of microphages and microglia in the brain as a result of the infection causes the production of NEUROTOXIN that results in markedly decreased cognitive resources, memory deficiencies, loss of motor control, and, in the latter stages, loss of activities of daily living. There are also opportunistic infections from AIDS, most notably CRYPTOCOCCOSIS, which can also result from inhaling the *Cryptococcus neoformans* fungus from infected soil. Cryptococcosis can result in a form of MENINGITIS.

Meningitis is an inflammation of the membranes covering the SPINAL CORD, called the meninges. Although the infection typically comes from a viral or bacterial infection, cancer, injury, and certain drugs can also cause the inflammation. Meningitis can result in disabling and lethal complications, including sensorineural hearing loss, EPILEPSY, dangerous brain swelling, HYDROCEPHALUS, intra-cerebral bleeding, and CEREBRAL PALSY.

Transmissible spongiform encephalopathy diseases are progressive conditions that result from infection with spiroplasmas. These infections cause production of proteins called PRIONS, which cause holes in the CORTEX giving the brain a spongelike appearance. These holes cause progressive impairment in brain functioning, including memory, personality, and movement changes. Examples of transmissible spongiform encephalopathy diseases include MAD COW DISEASE affecting livestock and its manifestation in humans, and CREUTZFELD-JACOB DISEASE (CJD), an invariably fatal disease that comes from eating the brain and spinal cord tissue of infected livestock.

Genetic Disorders   DOWN SYNDROME, sometimes referred to as MONGOLISM or Mongolian idiocy in pre-20th-century publications, is perhaps the best-known genetic disorder. This disorder is due to a whole or partial extra 21st chromosome. About one in 800 to 1,000 births leads to Down syndrome. The syndrome's physical characteristics include slanted eyes and may include a single transverse palmar crease, sometimes referred to as a simian crease owing to its similarity to the crease found in the palms of monkeys and apes.

Down syndrome manifests cognitively as mild to profound mental retardation, although there have been individuals whose intelligence has been above the deficient range.

PHENYLKETONURIA (PKU), known as cretinism in less politically correct times, results in an inability of the body to metabolize the amino acid phenylalanine to the amino acid tyrosine. If left untreated, PKU results in progressive brain deterioration, with increasing mental deficiency and seizures. However, if identified early, PKU is treatable by a diet low in phenylalanine and tyrosine. Increased awareness of PKU and aggressive efforts to identify the condition early have resulted in a marked decrease in the number of individuals who suffer the progressive brain deterioration and resulting mental retardation and seizures.

Sex-linked genetic disorders such as FRAGILE X SYNDROME and RETT SYNDROME help one understand principles of genetic transmission. In fragile X syndrome, for example, the mother passes the trait to her offspring. Their male children who receive the affected X-chromosome show more serious manifestation of the MENTAL RETARDATION or LEARNING DISABILITY (LD), social-emotional, and physical characteristics of the disorder than their female children who receive the affected X. The reason for the different level of manifestation of features is due to the presence of only one X chromosome, the affected one, in the male but the presence of two X chromosomes, one affected and one not, in the female. The unaffected X chromosome in the female can ameliorate the possible effects of the mother's genetic contribution.

Brain Injury Injuries account for many brain disorders. For example, direct injury from being struck in the skull by a baseball can also have CONTRECOUP EFFECTS from the brain ricocheting off the skull on the opposite side of the head. Concussion injuries cause subdural bleeding and death of brain tissue. Individuals with serious concussions can experience POSTCONCUSSION SYNDROME. This disorder affects 38 to 80 percent of those with concussion. Symptoms of postconcussion syndrome can include loss of consciousness (as experienced by one of the authors, Dr. Harris, following a fall off the side of a mountain); cognitive symptoms, such as increased forgetfulness and slowed reason-

ing; and social-emotional symptoms, such as emotional liability. Athletes and individuals who have received repeated concussions from blows to the head can experience so-called PUNCH DRUNK SYNDROME, characterized by DEMENTIA, slowed thinking, memory distortions, Parkinsonism, decreased coordination, impaired speech, and unsteady gait. Some affected individuals exhibit explosive, unpredictable rages.

SHAKEN BABY SYNDROME is a prevalent injury among abused children whose caregivers shake them violently, causing the skull to experience a whiplash effect resulting in retinal hemorrhage and SUBDURAL HEMORRHAGE. Most victims of this disorder are under one year of age and their neck muscles are weak. In addition, the size of their heads in proportion to the rest of their bodies makes these children particularly susceptible to more serious effects of being shaken.

Lifestyle-Related Substance abuse and addiction can have long-term brain effects. Repeated alcohol abuse over a long period of time can cause KORSAKOFF SYNDROME, WERNICKE-KORSAKOFF SYNDROME, and WERNICKE'S ENCEPHALOPATHY, characterized by anterograde amnesia, retrograde amnesia, CONFABULATION, meager context in conversation, lack of insight, and apathy. DELIRIUM TREMENS (DTs), the disorientation, confusion, agitation, and sometimes tremors following the termination of alcohol after a long period of regular alcohol consumption, occurs in 5 percent of those suffering extreme alcohol withdrawal. It is fatal in up to 35 percent of cases. Mothers who consume alcohol during pregnancy can produce offspring with FETAL ALCOHOL SYNDROME (FAS), characterized by permanent birth defects. Those birth defects include significant CENTRAL NERVOUS SYSTEM (CNS) damage, especially to the brain. The presence of alcohol impedes the development of neurons, which leads to MENTAL RETARDATION, ATTENTION DEFICIT HYPERACTIVITY DISORDER (ADHD), and behavioral problems.

Prescription medication consumption can also cause brain disorders. For example, the long-term use of antipsychotic medications such as chlorpromazine (Thorazine) can result in TARDIVE DYSKINESIA, which is characterized by tics and repetitive involuntary movements. NEUROLEPTIC MALIGNANT SYNDROME (NMS) is a life-threatening brain disorder usually caused by an adverse reaction to psychoactive medication, characterized by delirium. FETAL HYDANTOIN SYNDROME, which can include mild developmental delays, can result from a mother's taking phenytoin (Dilantin), an antiseizure medication, during pregnancy.

TOXIC ENCEPHALOPATHY results from exposure to environmental toxins such as solvents and pesticides. It results in permanent BRAIN DAMAGE and is characterized by SHORT-TERM MEMORY impairment, DEPRESSION, ANXIETY, and diminished cognitive resources.

Psychological stress results in the over-production of cortisol. Chronic overproduction of cortisol can result in or exacerbate PSYCHOGENIC HEADACHES, including migraine, TENSION HEADACHES, CLUSTER HEADACHES, high blood pressure, anxiety, and risk of STROKE.

Mixed Causes Memory disorders are often due to an interaction among several contributors. The effects of normal aging on memory have been noted for centuries. AGE-ASSOCIATED MEMORY IMPAIRMENT occurs in one-half to two-thirds of people age 50 and over. Symptoms include increasing difficulty remembering names, appointments, and other details, such as the location of the television remote control or one's keys. Minor changes in memory as the result of memory impairment are frustrating but normal.

PROSOPAGNOSIA, or difficulty remembering faces, can result from acute brain damage, but recent evidence suggests there are possible congenital factors that make certain individuals more susceptible to the effects of brain damage on facial recognition. Such loss involves damage to the TEMPORAL LOBE and the occipital lobe.

Dementia refers to the loss of cognitive abilities through brain injury beyond the normal declines due to the benign course of aging. Although disorders such as ALZHEIMER'S DISEASE result in dementia, one's lifestyle and genetic inheritance help determine the nature and extent of cognitive decline. All other factors being equal, healthier individuals who maintain healthy diet and exercise habits and positive psychological adjustment and continue to seek novelty and stimulation will frequently experience less cognitive decline than their couch potato counterparts who seek same-

ness in their environments. Even dementia due to brain events such as tumors and those due to vascular events, such as SENILE DEMENTIA, still see the marked influence of lifestyle factors and genetic inheritance.

Unknown or Disputed Causes Many disorders we presume have a basis in brain damage or brain dysfunction have either unknown or disputed causes. Some of the more widely known disorders appear below.

NEURAL TUBE DEFECTS occur when the neural tube does not close around the 28th day after conception. In SPINA BIFIDA, the vertebrae overlying the open portion of the spinal cord allow the affected area of the spinal cord to protrude through the bony opening. A fluid-filled sac surrounding the open spinal cord may develop. Other neural tube defects include ANENCEPHALY, in which the structures that become the CEREBELLUM do not close, and encephalocele, in which other brain parts do not fuse.

There is some evidence for causes or contributors to neural tube defects. Epilepsy medications taken during pregnancy, for example, are associated with a higher-than-normal risk of having children born with neural tube defects, as are FOLIC ACID deficiencies. Maternal diabetes, maternal obesity, toxins from contaminated cornmeal, arsenic, and hyperthermia may also play a role in neural tube defect development.

Alzheimer's disease is the most common source of dementia. Although the disorder is characterized by plaques and tangles in the brain, research has not yet established the precise cause or causes.

Research indicates that AUTISTIC DISORDER and related AUTISM SPECTRUM DISORDERS (ASD) have a genetic component, but the contribution of genetic endowment compared to other factors is controversial, especially in light of highly publicized increases in the incidence of these disorders. Parent groups and others outside the scientific community strongly advocate a causative role of childhood vaccines in autism, especially those containing thimerosal, and vitamin deficiencies, especially vitamin B_6.

AMYOTROPIC LATERAL SCLEROSIS (ALS), also known in the United States as Lou Gehrig's disease, is a MOTOR NEURON DISEASE that targets the neurons in the central nervous system that control voluntary muscle movement. ALS causes muscle weakness and atrophy throughout the muscular system, in most cases leading to the individual's inability to control movements. Although the precise cause is unknown, researchers are working to identify genetic mutations that may lead to a discovery of the cause.

SHY-DRAGER SYNDROME sufferers experience problems with the autonomic nervous system, including dysphagia, incontinence, hypotension, gastroparesis, erectile dysfunction, Parkinsonism, and other nonspecific symptoms.

LEARNING DISABILITY is an umbrella term that covers a wide range of academic skill deficiencies outside those caused by mental retardation and known environmental factors such as poor school attendance and deficient instruction. Although many educators and psychologists presume neurological factors underlying such learning disabilities as dyslexia, acalculia, and agraphia, there has been no single cause for those disorders.

Some other disorders with no known cause include BELL'S PALSY, which comes from an inflammation of the facial nerve due to no known reason; cerebral palsy, which is due to damage to the motor centers of the brain; migraines, which have known triggers but no specific cause; CHRONIC FATIGUE SYNDROME, a catch-all term for a constellation of poorly understood symptoms of fatigue mostly experienced by women and adults over age 40; MYASTHENIA GRAVIS, an autoimmune disease characterized by serious muscle weakness; NARCOLEPSY, characterized by excessive daytime sleepiness and falling asleep at inappropriate times and having a strong correlation with chromosome-6 factors, although the precise cause is unknown; REYE'S SYNDROME, a disorder that causes damage to the brain and liver, often associated with pediatric consumption of aspirin; and MULTIPLE SCLEROSIS and its variant, Schilder's disease, which are DEMYELINATING DISORDERS in which the immune system attacks the central nervous system.   .

brain food   In biblical times, the lentil was thought to have the power to improve the brain; by medieval days, eagle hearts or crushed lizard was thought to be the magic elixir. Asians during this period swore by ginkgo tea. By the time of France's Louis XI, hopeful savants ate gold leaf, an early Greek practice, in hopes that the substance would improve the function of the brain.

By far, the most popular brain food of all has been fish, a high-protein substance that will indeed improve health and neuron growth. However, experts warn that amounts of protein in excess of the recommended daily allowance (44 grams for women and 56 grams for men) will not boost the brain's power.

VITAMINS and minerals are also important to brain function. In recent studies, those children who were given a vitamin and mineral supplement showed improvement in nonverbal intelligence scores compared to students taking a placebo.

Scientists discovered that it is particularly important to consume enough minerals for optimum brain efficiency because most Americans are deficient in this area. Peak brain performance requires adequate levels of selenium, iron, zinc, iodine, chromium, molybdenum, boron, copper, and manganese. Because minerals are the first nutrients lost in food processing, a mineral supplement may help to make up the difference.

brain function tests   See ELECTROENCEPHALOGRAPHY; PET SCAN.

brain hemorrhage   See HEMORRHAGE, BRAIN.

brain in history   While modern thinkers today revere the brain as the most important and irreplaceable organ in the body, ancient physicians and scientists did not share such deep respect for this organ. In ancient Egypt, the heart was esteemed as the pinnacle of complexity, the seat of the soul and all mental functioning. Others at the time thought that the liver was probably the location for intellectual abilities.

By the fourth century B.C., however, medicine had made strides toward a more modern understanding of brain function, and Hippocrates identified the brain (which he thought was a gland) as the interpreter of consciousness. He was among the first to believe that the various forms of insanity originate in an unhealthy brain. On the other hand, Aristotle delegated the brain to the third-rate job of cooling the body.

By the sixth century B.C., scientists had changed their minds, now deciding that the brain was the repository of the soul, and the fourth VENTRICLE its likely home. Herophilus described the "marvelous net" (*rete mirabile*) of brain localization, a point of view later endorsed by the great anatomist GALEN. In Galen's time, the MOTOR and SENSORY NERVES had been identified and traced to the CEREBELLUM and CEREBRUM respectively.

In the time of the early Christians, scientists understood more about the complexity of the brain, believing that mental ability was located in the ventricles proceeding from the front toward the back of the head. Sensation and imagination was located in the front ventricle, they believed; reason and intellect in the next ventricle; and memory, the most selective ability, in the rearmost ventricle.

Still, agreement on neurophysiology was far from widespread. Later in the sixth century and on through the Middle Ages, physicians found themselves constantly at odds as to whether the soul was found in the brain or heart.

By about 1505, LEONARDO DA VINCI was the first to make a wax cast of the brain ventricles, using the brain of an ox. He believed that the site of sensory analysis was in fact found in the second ventricle, which had formerly been the site of reason. By 1543, the Belgian Andreas Vesalius wrote the first "modern" anatomy of the brain that was based on detailed drawings of corpses. He laid to rest the formerly popular medieval idea that the ventricles house separate mental abilities.

By the 18th century, the pseudoscience of PHRENOLOGY had become popular, in which personality traits were assigned by the shape and protuberances of the skull.

brain injury   See BRAIN DAMAGE.

brain mapping   See BRAIN SCANS.

brain scans   A type of specialized test that reveals brain structure or function using a variety of chemical, electrical, or magnetic technologies. Each type of brain scan has its strengths and weaknesses; some can distinguish the smallest structures; others can track brain function but cannot resolve structures less than half an inch apart.

Diagnostic neurology was revolutionized by the introduction of computerized scanning equipment. The most popular scans include computed axial tomographic (CAT) scanning, MAGNETIC RESONANCE IMAGING (MRI), FUNCTIONAL MRI, POSITION EMISSION TOMOGRAPHY (PET), ELECTROENCEPHALOGRAPHY, and magneto encephalography (MEG).

The computerized scanning techniques of CAT and MRI rely on two distinct methods of producing an image: CAT scans use an ultra-thin X-RAY beam, and MRI uses a very strong magnetic field. During CAT scans, an X-ray beam passes through the brain, and the intensity of the emerging beam is measured by an X-ray detector. On the scan, the brain appears as various shades of gray; bones of the skull appear white, and air appears black.

During an MRI scan, each hydrogen atom in the brain responds to the magnetic field produced by the device; a magnetic field detector measures the responses of the atoms. There is no radiation in an MRI scan, but the magnetic field may affect metallic objects such as heart pacemakers, inner-ear implants, brain aneurysm clips, or embedded shrapnel.

Both CAT and MRI scans involve taking measurements from thousands of angles; these data are then processed by computer to create a composite three-dimensional representation of the brain. Any particular slice can be selected from this representation and displayed on a TV screen; photos can also be produced from this screen.

CAT shows internal brain structures much better than conventional X-rays. It is particularly useful for diagnosing brain disorders such as STROKE, HEMORRHAGE, TUMOR, injury, abscesses, cysts, swelling, fluid accumulation, and dead tissue. MRI scans are good at imaging areas affected by stroke that cannot be seen well on a CAT scan, and to diagnose nerve fiber disorders such as MULTIPLE SCLEROSIS.

Adding to the basic MRI anatomical picture is a functional MRI (fMRI). Brain cell activity is fueled by glucose and oxygen carried in blood; when an area of the brain is active, these substances flow toward it, and fMRI highlights the areas where there is the most oxygen. The latest of these fMRI scanners can produce four images every second. Because the brain takes about a half second to react to a stimulus, this rapid scanning can clearly show activity in different parts of the brain reacting to various tasks. fMRI may turn out to be the most rewarding of scanning techniques, but it is extremely costly.

Positron emission tomography (PET) is a technique that results in similar findings as fMRI—it identifies the brain areas that are working hardest by measuring how much fuel they use. PET pictures are very clear, albeit lacking the fine resolution of fMRI. The technique also requires an injection of a radioactive marker. Although the dose is very small, no one person is usually allowed to have more than 12 scans per year (this actually equals one scanning session).

Electroencephalography (EEG) is a device that measures brain waves, showing characteristic changes according to the type of brain activity. EEG measures these waves by picking up signals via electrodes placed on the skull. The most modern EEGs take readings from many different spots and compares them, building up a picture of varying activity across the brain. Brain mapping with EEG often uses event-related potentials (ERPs), which simply means that an electrical peak (potential) is related to a particular stimulus, such as a word or a touch.

Magnetoencephalography (MEG) is much like an EEG in that it picks up signals from brain cells, but it does so by focusing on the tiny magnetic pulse they give off rather than the electric field around them. Unfortunately, the signals are usually weak and there is interference, but it has enormous potential because it is faster than other scanning techniques and can therefore chart changes in brain activity more accurately than fMRI or PET.

brain stem   Part of the REPTILIAN BRAIN, this part of the brain is an extension of the spinal cord. Located at the top of the SPINAL CORD, the brain stem connects the FOREBRAIN and MIDBRAIN to the spinal cord.

It controls such functions as heartbeat and breathing and is the source for the CRANIAL NERVES serving the eyes, ears, mouth, and other areas of the face and throat. The brain stem is one of three major divisions of the brain responsible for monitoring muscular movement and also for receiving NERVE IMPULSES through the cranial nerves. The brain stem connects with 10 of the 12 pairs of cranial nerves and controls basic functions such as breathing, vomiting, and eye reflexes. This part of the brain also acts as a conduit for messages traveling between other parts of the brain and the spinal cord.

The most primitive part of the brain, the brain stem is almost identical to the brain of a reptile, which is why it earned the nickname "reptilian brain." Evolutionary studies show that in complex animals, the brain stem was one of the first parts of the brain to develop.

From the spinal cord upward, the brain stem includes the MEDULLA, the PONS, and the midbrain. The medulla looks a bit like a thicker continuation of the spinal cord and contains the nuclei of the ninth, 10th, 11th, and 12th cranial nerves. It is responsible for relaying taste sensations from the tongue and signals to muscles controlling speech, tongue, and neck movements. The medulla also houses groups of nerve cells that regulate heartbeat, breathing, blood pressure, and digestion and relaying information about these activities via the VAGUS (TENTH CRANIAL) NERVE.

The pons is much wider than the medulla and contains bundles of nerves connecting with the CEREBELLUM lying behind the brain stem. The pons receives information from ear, face, and teeth via its nuclei for the fifth through eighth cranial nerves and also receives signals controlling the jaw, facial expression, and eye movement. The pons is also important for breathing regulation.

The midbrain is the smallest part of the brain stem, located above the pons and containing the nuclei of the third and fourth cranial nerves, which control eye movement and pupil size.

Scattered throughout the brain stem are groups of nerve cells known collectively as the RETICULAR FORMATION, which is believed to control incoming sensory information and governs such basic activities as awareness, attention, sleep, and waking, breathing, and heart rate.

The cerebellum is a separate brain organ that is attached directly to the back of the brain stem and is concerned mostly with balance and coordinated movement.

Running through the middle of the brain stem is a canal that widens into the fourth ventricle of the brain, home of the circulating CEREBROSPINAL FLUID.

The brain stem is susceptible to the same type of problems that can beset the rest of the CENTRAL NERVOUS SYSTEM; damage to different parts of the brain stem will result in different problems. Any sort of damage to the vitally important centers in the medulla can be quickly fatal; damage to the reticular formation can result in COMA. Likewise, damage to a specific cranial nerve can have particular effects; for example, damage to the seventh (facial) cranial nerve will result in facial palsy. Degeneration of the SUBSTANTIA NIGRA in the midbrain is linked to the development of PARKINSON'S DISEASE.

brain syndrome, organic   See ORGANIC BRAIN SYNDROME.

brain tissue transplants   Brain damage can be repaired by implanting brain tissue from aborted fetuses into a patient's impaired brain. Scientists agree that one of the greatest problems in treating BRAIN DAMAGE and a range of degenerative brain diseases is that up to now, brain tissue has not been able to regenerate itself. When the brain is damaged, other regions do not always take over.

Rat studies have shown that grafted brain tissue can become effective parts of the animal's brain and can even improve age-related learning impairments. Scientists have also shown improvement in some PARKINSON'S DISEASE patients after transplanting fetal brain cells to produce DOPAMINE, a key brain chemical lacking in the disease.

In 1992, a Swedish team from the University of Lund performed a fetal tissue transplant on two Americans who had destroyed their SUBSTANTIA NIGRA after injecting themselves with tainted synthetic heroin. For seven years the two had not been able to use their voluntary muscles; after receiving brain tissue from more than one fetus, both recovered enough to be able to live independently.

In the United States, scientists have implanted fetal tissue into the brains of patients with Parkinson's disease and reported that patients showed improvement in movement examinations. Scientists hope that someday they will be able to treat a range of other brain diseases with this technique.

However, the moral and philosophical issues surrounding the use of tissue implants present problems; the fact that successful transplants require the use of fetal tissue adds to the ethical and legal dilemma.

Both the Ronald Reagan and George H. W. Bush administrations banned the use of federal funds for fetal-tissue research that used tissue from aborted fetuses. President Bill Clinton lifted the ban early in his administration, and President George W. Bush has supported using federal funds for research on existing stem cell lines.

Genes and genetically altered cells also can be injected into brains to combat or reverse damage caused by degenerative diseases. The new approaches rely on the same basic strategy: using living tissue instead of drugs to supply chemicals necessary for brain function.

brain tumor   Abnormal growth in or near the brain that may or may not be malignant. These tumors are always serious because of the pressure they cause in the brain as they grow.

Abnormal growths in the brain may be primary (originating in brain tissue) such as GLIOMAS, MENINGIOMAS, ACOUSTIC NEUROMAS, and PITUITARY TUMORS, or secondary (arising from cancer cells which have spread to the brain from other parts of the body—usually the lungs or breast). Secondary brain tumors are always malignant.

Primary brain tumors are identified and classed according to their cell type, their location, and their degree of malignancy. A brain tumor's effect can be different depending on its location and its type.

While cancer in other parts of the body often spreads, primary brain tumors rarely do; if they spread, it is usually to other parts of the CENTRAL NERVOUS SYSTEM. Many brain tumors do not look like cancer cells under a microscope, and they are usually far more slow growing than other malignant tumors in other parts of the body. However, any untreated brain tumor has the potential to be fatal because of its location, if not its cell characteristics.

About 60 percent of brain tumors are gliomas, which are frequently malignant. Other primary tumors, usually benign, include meningiomas (arising from the meningeal membranes covering the brain); acoustic neuromas (on the acoustic nerve) and pituitary tumors (on the PITUITARY GLAND).

Children are prone to brain tumors located in the back of the brain, including two types of glioma: MEDULLOBLASTOMA and CEREBELLAR ASTROCYTOMA.

In the United States, about six of every 100,000 Americans will be diagnosed with a primary brain TUMOR every year; about 12,000 people will die. Tumors most often appear in people over 50, but about one in every 3,000 children die from a primary brain tumor before the age of 10. Brain tumors are the second leading cause of death in children under 15, and in young adults up to 34.

The worldwide incidence of brain tumors has been increasing steadily in the United States, the incidence of brain cancer in those over age 75 has more than doubled since 1968, and in children, brain cancer has increased by 30 percent since 1973.

While some doctors believe that what has really increased is the rate of diagnosis because of more sophisticated brain scanners, others point out that the upward surge in tumors began before some of the more sensitive equipment was in use in the late 1970s. One Canadian study found that about a third of the increase in brain tumors could be attributed to improved diagnostic technology; this leaves two-thirds or more due to a true increase of incidence.

A number of potential suspect causes have been identified, ranging from female hormones to chemical agents. Experts point out the increasing use of pesticides in this country parallel the rise in brain cancer. Other studies have implicated industrial and household chemicals, ionizing radiation (such as from X-RAYS), and electromagnetic fields (EMFs) caused by cellular telephone use, household appliances such as microwave ovens, and electronic

devices such as TVs and computers. The Environmental Protection Agency has labeled EMFs a Class B (probable) carcinogen, which places them in a category with dioxin and DDT.

But while questions have been raised about whether cellular telephones with built-in antennas cause brain cancer, there has been no proof that microwave radiation from these phones carries a health risk.

Symptoms and Diagnostic Path

Compression of brain tissue by the tumor may cause weak muscles, sensory disturbances, speech problems, and epileptic SEIZURES. Pressure also can cause HEADACHES, especially in the morning, which may get worse during coughing or straining. Pressure may also cause vomiting, visual disturbances (blurred or double vision, partial visual loss), and impaired mental processes, and hearing problems (ringing or buzzing in the ears or partial hearing loss).

Brain tumors may cause behavior changes, such as problems with speaking, thinking or remembering, sluggishness, drowsiness, or changes in personality. There also may be problems in controlling muscles, paralysis, difficulty with balance, or trouble walking.

In order to locate the tumor and determine its extent, physicians use ANGIOGRAPHY together with various types of BRAIN SCANS: CAT SCAN, MAGNETIC RESONANCE IMAGING (MRI), and X-ray studies.

Treatment Options and Outlook

Treatment of a brain tumor often depends on its classification and characteristics. For example, a medulloblastoma is usually treated with the radiation of both the brain and spinal cord because this type of tumor has a tendency to spread throughout the entire central nervous system.

Tumors are often surgically removed when possible, but too often malignant tumors are inaccessible or too extensive to be removed. In this case, survival rates are not high; less than 20 percent of these patients survive one year.

When a tumor cannot be totally removed, as much of the growth as possible will be cut out to relieve pressure on the brain, followed by chemotherapy or radiation therapy. Corticosteroid drugs can be used to reduce tissue swelling around the tumor.

Radiation is the second most common treatment for brain tumors after surgery, usually administered soon after surgery. The cells of many malignant brain tumors are readily killed by radiation, which is why this type of treatment is almost always recommended. (One possible exception is the treatment of very young children, whose developing brains may be injured by the radiation.) Most tumors do shrink from the effects of radiation, although it may take some time for swelling and dead cells to diminish so that the true size of the growth can be seen.

Another radiation technique called STEREOTAC-TIC RADIOSURGERY, or gamma knife, is used for patients with inoperable brain tumors. In this technique, the surgeon uses a small directed beam of radiation to treat areas that may be inaccessible by conventional surgery or for patients who may not be able to withstand an operation. The one-time application is an outpatient procedure that may serve as a substitute for the 20 to 30 radiation treatments normally required. Using the precisely directed beams of radiation, surgeons can focus on and destroy the diseased tissue and spare nearly all of the surrounding healthy tissue.

The key is to locate the diseased tissue and program those coordinates into a linear accelerator—the unit that emits the radiation beam. The accelerator is rotated around the target area in the patient's brain, allowing high doses of radiation to be given directly to the designated site. The procedure usually takes an entire day and is performed with a local anesthetic. A CAT scan is used to determine the exact coordinates of the diseased tissue; with that information, doctors then affix a metal ring to the head, which helps the linear accelerator focus on the target area.

At present, this type of radiation is being used for patients with various types of brain tumors, as well as brain tumors that have not responded to conventional radiation therapy. It can also be used to treat malformed blood vessels in the brain that can cause seizures and are usually inoperable under normal situations.

Chemotherapy may be used in the treatment of brain tumors, which work by interfering with various parts of the cell's cycle. Immunotherapy is also used with brain tumors. However, most chemotherapy does not easily cross the blood-brain barrier.

See also CELL PHONES AND BRAIN TUMORS.

brain waves   Patterns of brain activity traced on a sensitive electronic device called an electroencephalograph (EEG). On an ongoing basis—even during sleep—electrical signals are constantly flashing over the brain; these signals can be detected and measured by an encephalograph. Electrodes attached to the head measure the brain's electrical activity as each neuron fires a nerve impulse. This is displayed as a wavy line on the screen of an EEG machine.

Because the tissues of the body conduct electricity well, metal sensors attached to the skin of the head can detect the signals passing from the brain through the muscles and skin. The signals are amplified within the device and displayed on a monitor or paper chart. These devices show that electrical signals in the brain do not come steadily, but are produced in short bursts like a series of waves; the shape of the waves changes with the activity level of the brain.

Brain waves are measured in up to 30 cycles per second; one cycle (or one hertz) is one complete oscillation. *Brain-wave frequency* is a measurement of oscillations per second; the more there are, the higher the frequency of the wave. *Amplitude* refers to half the height from the peak to the trough in a single oscillation.

During wakefulness, the waves are fast and small; intense thoughts or walking around will produce faster, sharper, more jagged rhythms characteristic of BETA WAVES. As a person begins to feel drowsy brain cells start to fire rhythmically, every tenth of a second. These are called ALPHA WAVES. Slower pulses are called THETA WAVES. In deep sleep, the brain produces large, slow DELTA WAVES.

Measurements of brain waves can help diagnose brain abnormalities, although there are no waveforms that are clearly abnormal in and of themselves. However, the site of brain damage following STROKE may be determined by recording brain waves from different locations on the scalp. Brain-wave evaluations are especially helpful in evaluating EPILEPSY, BRAIN TUMORS, brain infections, COMA, and BRAIN DEATH. Serial brain-wave recordings can be used to trace recovery after head or brain injuries.

brain weight The weight of the human brain depends on age, stature, body weight, sex, race, blood vessel congestion, degenerative changes, and atrophy. At birth, the brain weighs about 13 ounces and makes up about 12.4 percent of the body weight. The entire brain of an adult male weighs about three pounds; a female adult brain weighs about 2.78 pounds. When factors of size and weight are considered, the size and weight of the brain in both sexes are about equal. At adulthood, the brain makes up less than 2 percent of the body's weight but uses up 20 percent of the body's energy.

Age has a considerable influence on brain weight; the brain grows rapidly during the first three years and then slows down up to the seventh year, when it is almost its full weight. After this, the increase is very gradual; prime weight is usually achieved by age 20 in males and somewhat earlier in females. From this period onward, in both sexes there is a continuous gradual lessening of the brain's weight by about a gram (0.03 of an ounce) each year.

Tall people in general have heavier brains than shorter people, but relative to their height, short people have larger heads and brains than tall people. While many people of conspicuous ability have had large brains, averages calculated for groups (such as scholarship winners) show there is really only a slight correlation between head size and intelligence.

The heaviest known normal human brain belonged to the Russian writer Ivan Turgenev, who died in 1883. His brain weighed 4.43 pounds, more than a pound heavier than the average male brain. The smallest known normal brain belonged to a woman who died in 1977; her brain weighed just 2.41 pounds.

BRAT battery A nickname for the basic psychological examination group of intelligence test, achievement test, and visual-motor integration test given to children with learning and behavioral problems. The designation originally was derived loosely from the names of the typical tests used in the basic group, including the BENDER-GESTALT TEST, WISC (WECHSLER INTELLIGENCE SCALE FOR CHILDREN), and Wide Range Achievement Test (whose acronym WRAT is pronounced "rat"). Its name emphasized the common practice in schools of referring mainly misbehaving children for psychological evaluations.

breathing center Breathing is an automatic process that is controlled by the respiratory center low in the BRAIN STEM. This breathing center sends nerve impulses to the muscles of the chest diaphragm that regulate lung expansion and contraction.

Breuer, Josef (1842–1925) An Austrian physician and physiologist who was acknowledged by Sigmund Freud and others as the principal developer of psychoanalysis. In 1880 Breuer was able to relieve the symptoms of hysteria in "Anna O" after he had induced her to recall unpleasant past experiences under HYPNOSIS. Breuer concluded that neurotic symptoms result from unconscious processes and disappear when those processes become conscious.

He later described his methods and results to Freud, and referred patients to him; together the two wrote *Studien über Hysterie* (1895), in which Breuer described his treatment of hysteria. Breuer and Freud eventually became enemies, however, over disagreements on basic theories of therapy. (See also ANNA O; FREUD, SIGMUND.)

Broca, Pierre-Paul (1824–1880) A French neurosurgeon whose study of brain lesions contributed significantly to the understanding of the origins of APHASIA (the loss or impairment of the ability to form or articulate words).

Broca founded the anthropology lab in the École des Hautes Études in Paris in 1858 and the Société d'Anthropologie de Paris in 1859, where he developed his research into the comparative study of the skulls of different races. In this work, he used original techniques to study the form, structure, and topography of the brain.

In 1861 he announced his discovery of the seat of articulate speech located in the left frontal region of the brain, since known as the convolution of Broca or BROCA'S AREA. With this discovery, Broca had provided the first anatomical evidence of the localization of brain function.

See also BROCA'S APHASIA.

Broca's aphasia An expressive language disorder that affects both written and spoken speech, producing nonfluent, labored, arrhythmic speech. However, there is reasonably good comprehension of some words, and the few words that are uttered tend to be meaningful.

Symptoms and Diagnostic Path

French surgeon Pierre-Paul Broca first diagnosed the condition in patients who had damage to BROCA'S AREA of the brain; that condition has since been named Broca's aphasia. Some experts believe that other areas of the brain can compensate for problems with Broca's area. This suggestion is based on the transient nature of Broca's aphasia symptoms, just as STROKE and brain-injured patients can learn to speak again.

Patients suffering from Broca's aphasia are able to use the organs of speech to produce sounds and even single words, but they cannot produce sentences or express thoughts. Often, patients will find one word or a short string of words and repeat them over and over in an attempt to communicate thoughts. While they may sometimes be successful in communicating, they will not be able to express themselves grammatically. Similarly, they can draw but cannot write coherent speech. In short, patients can understand speech and often can form ideas to communicate, but they cannot put words together to communicate those ideas.

The condition is usually first recognized by the physician, who then refers the patient to a speech-language pathologist, who performs a comprehensive examination of the person's ability to understand, speak, read, and write.

Treatment Options and Outlook

Sometimes a patient will completely recover from aphasia without treatment, which usually happens after a type of mini-stroke called a TRANSIENT ISCHEMIC ATTACK (TIA). In this case, language may return shortly.

Most of the time, however, language does not return so fast. While many patients have partial spontaneous recovery, some amount of aphasia typically remains. In this case, speech-language therapy can often help, especially if treatment begins early. Still, it may take up to two years to recover.

How well speech returns is linked to the cause and amount of the brain damage, the part of the brain that was damaged, and the patient's age and health, as well as the person's motivation, handedness, and educational level.

Treatment includes helping the person use remaining abilities, restore language, compensate for language problems, and learn other ways to communicate. Either individual or group treatment can work, including regional support groups called "stroke clubs." Family involvement is often a crucial component of aphasia treatment so that family members can learn the best way to communicate.

Broca's area Language center in the left CEREBRAL HEMISPHERE that controls the output aspects of language, such as speech and writing. When a person wishes to speak, the words are created in a part of the brain called WERNICKE'S AREA. The speech signals are then sent to Broca's area, which sends signals to the vocal cords, tongue, lips, and throat.

Brown-Peterson task This commonly used test of recall over delays of a few seconds features items presented to subjects (usually in threes), after which the subject engages in some interfering activity (such as counting backward) until the end of the retention interval. At that point subjects are asked to recall the items just presented.

Although recall usually declines steeply after a 30-second delay, researchers believe that the interfering task makes recall more difficult but does not completely prevent it. Patients with ALZHEIMER'S DISEASE and some with AMNESIA usually perform badly on this test.

Brown-Sequard, Charles Edouard (1817–1894) British physiologist and neurologist who made major discoveries involving the sympathetic nervous system and the SPINAL CORD and whose work foreshadowed the later discovery of NEUROTRANSMITTERS. Brown-Sequard taught at Harvard for four years and practiced briefly in New York, eventually moving to France to serve as professor of experimental medicine at the College de France. He is considered to be the founder of endocrinology.

See also BRAIN IN HISTORY.

caffeine Caffeine is a central nervous system stimulant that in moderate doses can increase alertness, reduce fine motor coordination, and, when withdrawn, can cause insomnia, headaches, nervousness, and dizziness. In massive doses, caffeine is lethal, but a person would have to drink 80 to 100 cups of coffee quickly in order to reach that level. Its stimulant effects comes largely from the way it acts on the adenosine receptors in the brain; adenosine affects the central nervous system, making one feel sleepy. Caffeine binds to these receptors instead, thereby speeding up brain activity. Caffeine also boosts the production of adrenalin, the "fight or flight" hormone that increases attention level and provides a boost in energy.

Caffeine enters the bloodstream through the stomach and small intestine; caffeine also acts at other sites in the body to increase heart rate, constrict blood vessels, relax air passages to improve breathing, and allow some muscles to contract more easily. It begins to affect the body within 15 minutes. However, it takes at least six hours for only half the caffeine to be eliminated from the body. While it may improve simple motor tasks, more complex problems involving fine motor coordination and quick reactions may be slightly disrupted.

Of course, any drug's effect depends on the amount consumed, how often, how much was absorbed by the body, and how quickly it was metabolized. However, small amounts of caffeine may not greatly affect the body; some research has shown that administering small amounts (such as two or more cups of regular coffee) did not affect performance when compared with subjects who drank the same amount of decaffeinated coffee.

Too much caffeine (and the exact amount varies from person to person) can bring on jitters, insom-

nia, and memory problems. For a habitual user, however, omitting this stimulant will have the same negative effect, in addition to dizziness and headaches. This is because regular intake of caffeine (a cup or more per day) conditions the brain to await the caffeine stimulus before it responds with wakefulness.

Caffeine may be hard to avoid. It is contained in a staggeringly large number of products in the United States; in addition to food and beverages, caffeine is found in over-the-counter stimulants, analgesics, cold preparations, antihistamines, and prescription drugs. In fact, there are more than 2,000 nonprescription drugs and 1,000 prescription drugs that contain caffeine or caffeine-type stimulants.

calcium One of the most abundant elements in the body, calcium is necessary for conducting messages from one brain cell to another. The main dietary sources of calcium are milk and dairy products, eggs, fish, green vegetables, and fruit.

During normal brain activity, the concentration of calcium in brain cells varies naturally according to a finely regulated mechanism that pulls calcium into a cell, or pushes it out with "helper" chemicals if there is too much. Too high a concentration of calcium ions can kill a brain cell if left too long.

Calcium has been indicated as a possible cause of brain disorders; high levels have been associated with memory problems. When excess calcium is blocked by drugs in the part of the brain associated with memory and learning, scientists have been able to improve memory loss in STROKE victims. Similarly, conditions that increase the level of calcium in the brain cause memory problems. At the same time, normal levels of calcium are associated with the release of a substance called CALPAIN, which seems to improve memory by improving cell-to-cell communication.

The inability to regulate levels of calcium in brain cells has been implicated in ALZHEIMER'S DISEASE.

calpain One of several brain chemicals currently being studied for their role in memory. Released by CALCIUM within neurons, calpain can alter proteins and actually change the structure of nerve terminals, letting neurons communicate more easily with each other. It could be that low calcium levels in older patients may be one reason behind the memory loss of old age.

cancer, brain See ACOUSTIC NEUROMA; ASTROCYTOMA; CRANIOPHARYNGIOMA; EPENDYMONA; GLIOBLASTOMA; GLIOMA; HEMANGIOBLASTOMA; MEDULLOBLASTOMA; MENINGIOMA; NEUROBLASTOMA; NEUROECTODERMAL TUMORS; OLIGODENDROGLIOMA; PINEALOMA; PITUITARY ADENOMAS; PITUITARY TUMOR; RETINOBLASTOMA.

Capgras, Jean Marie Joseph (1873–1950) A well-known French psychopathologist who first identified the delusional syndrome called reduplicative paramnesia (or CAPGRAS SYNDROME) that today bears his name.

Capgras and J. Reboul-Lachaux first noted the syndrome in 1923 in a female patient with a chronic paranoid psychosis who also insisted that various individuals involved in her life had been replaced by doubles. Capgras and Reboul-Lachaux called the condition *l'illusion des sosies* (the illusion of doubles).

Capgras syndrome One form of reduplicative paramnesia, this is a delusional condition also called the syndrome of "doubles," in which a patient fails to recognize well-known people or places, believing that doubles have replaced them. The delusion is often quite strong and can be deeply disturbing to family and friends whose

identity is constantly denied. Generally, the person accused as an "imposter" also is believed to have harmful intentions toward the patient.

The effect can be induced by showing patients a picture and then, a few minutes later, producing the same picture again. The patients will probably say they have seen a similar picture, but insist it is definitely not the one they are now looking at. This disorder is believed to have a psychological origin, although more recent research suggests there may be an organic cause. It is typically associated with CONFABULATION, speech disorders and denial of illness.

It was first described by Jean Marie Capgras and J. Reboul-Lachaux in 1923, who discussed a female patient with a chronic paranoid psychosis who also insisted that various individuals involved in her life had been replaced by doubles. Capgras and Reboul-Lachaux called the condition *l'illusion des sosies* (the illusion of doubles).

Capgras syndrome is one of a group of MISIDENTIFICATION SYNDROMES that can occur in psychotic patients. It also may occur as a result of brain injury. Although the precise cause of this unusual syndrome is uncertain, it may involve extensive cerebral damage, probably with extensive frontal lesions.

Frontal lesions may cause problems in the integration of different kinds of information, and when these problems are combined with perceptual and memory deficits from other brain lesions, reduplicative paramnesia or Capgras syndrome may result.

See also CAPGRAS, JEAN MARIE JOSEPH.

carbon monoxide poisoning Poisoning with a colorless, odorless gas that can cause serious brain damage and death. Carbon monoxide poisoning is the leading cause of death by poison in the United States. It causes brain damage (particularly to the BASAL GANGLIA) by interfering with oxygen to the brain. Several minutes of exposure to 1,000 ppm (0.1 percent) are enough to cause fatal poisoning.

The primary source of carbon monoxide poisoning is exposure to exhaust from car engines, but the gas is emitted from any flame or combustion device (such as kerosene heaters or stoves). Other sources

LEVELS OF CARBON MONOXIDE POISONING

Carbon Monoxide Concentration	Symptoms
Less than 35 ppm (cigarette smoke)	None, or mild headache
0.005% (50 ppm)	Slight headache
0.01% (100 ppm)	Throbbing headache
0.02% (200 ppm)	Severe headache, irritability, fatigue
0.03%–0.05 (300–500 ppm)	Headache, confusion, lethargy, collapse
0.08–0.12% (800–1200 ppm)	Coma, convulsions
0.19% (1900 ppm)	Rapidly fatal

include paint stripper (hobbyists and film processors are especially at risk). Fire victims are often affected by carbon monoxide, and burning natural gas or petroleum fuels emits the gas. Smoke from cigarettes, pipes, and cigars is another common source; smokers have a significantly higher blood level. Those who inhale secondary smoke are also exposed to and show elevated blood levels of carbon monoxide. Workers exposed to high levels in the environment are also at risk.

Symptoms and Diagnostic Path

Carbon monoxide may be either inhaled or absorbed through the skin. People exposed to carbon monoxide complain of headache, dizziness, lethargy, irritability, increased breathing rate, chest pain, confusion, impaired judgment, shortness of breath, fainting, and nausea. Patients with heart problems may experience angina or heart attacks.

Exposure to more concentrated levels may lead to impaired thinking, HYPERACTIVITY, bizarre behavior, COMA, and convulsions and may be fatal.

Chronic exposure may lead to poor memory and mental deterioration and has been linked with hearing loss.

Delayed effects (between two and four weeks after a significant exposure) may include visual loss, DEMENTIA, retardation, memory loss, lack of speech coordination, personality changes, loss of bladder control, and problems in walking).

A blood test is the best way to diagnose carbon monoxide poisoning, because symptoms are not specific.

Treatment Options and Outlook

The administration of oxygen in the highest possible concentration (100 percent) is the treatment of choice. Some experts support the use of hyperbaric oxygen chambers, which can enhance the elimination of carbon monoxide. Such treatment may be useful to patients exposed to very high levels of carbon monoxide and who are reasonably close to a chamber (found in hospitals). Survivors may suffer numerous neurological problems such as PARKINSONISM, personality problems, and memory disorders.

carotid artery Any of the four main arteries of the neck and head that supply the brain with blood. There are two common carotid arteries (left and right), each of which divides into two main branches (internal and external). The right common carotid artery arises from the subclavian artery, which branches off the heart, up the neck on the right side of the windpipe; just above the level of the larynx, it divides into two, forming the right internal and external carotid ardors. The left common carotid arises from the aorta above the heart and then follows a similar path.

The internal carotid arteries enter the skull to supply the brain with blood via its cerebral branches. At the base of the brain, branches of the two internal carotids and the basilar artery join to form a ring of blood vessels called the CIRCLE OF WILLIS. When these arteries become narrowed, they can cause a TRANSIENT ISCHEMIC ATTACK (TIA); if blocked, they cause a STROKE.

cataplexy A sudden loss of muscle tone and deep tendon reflexes leading to muscle weakness, paralysis, or collapse.

Symptoms and Diagnostic Path

Cataplexy is a recurrent condition in which a person suddenly collapses to the ground without loss of consciousness. The cataplectic patient does not lose consciousness, but lies without moving for a few minutes until normal body tone returns. It is usually provoked by any strong emotion (particularly laughter or anger). This rare cause of sudden involuntary falling is almost exclusively found among people suffering from NARCOLEPSY and other sleep disorders.

Cataplexy usually lasts for just a few seconds, and is often confused with EPILEPSY.

Treatment Options and Outlook

Cataplexy requires separate treatment from narcolepsy. The condition often can be completely controlled with imipramine or desipramine, given in gradually increasing doses.

catecholamine Any of several compounds found naturally in the body that act as hormones or as NEUROTRANSMITTERS that affect the nervous and cardiovascular systems, the metabolic rate, and body temperature. It is also implicated in the development of depression in some people. The catecholamines include such compounds as epinephrine (adrenaline), norepinephrine, and dopamine.

CAT scan (computed axial tomography) (CT scan) A quick and accurate diagnostic technique using a computer and X-RAYS passed through the body at different angles to produce clear cross-sectional pictures of the tissue being examined, allowing greater differentiation among normal soft tissues. Although MAGNETIC RESONANCE IMAGING (MRI) has become the preferred technique for brain imaging, CAT scans remain in use because they are cheaper and faster than MRI.

Still a CAT scan of the brain provides a clearer and more detailed picture than do X-rays by themselves, and it tends to minimize the amount of radiation exposure.

Before a scan is performed, a contrast dye may be injected to make blood vessels or abnormalities show up more clearly. A number of low-dose X-ray beams are passed through the brain at different angles as the scanner rotates around the patient.

Using the information produced by the scanner, a computer constructs cross-section pictures of the brain, which are then displayed on a TV screen and can reveal soft tissue, including tumors, more clearly than normal X-rays. These scans are particularly useful in scanning the brain because they sharply define the ventricles (fluid-filled spaces).

Technical advances in imaging and processing have dramatically decreased the time required to acquire data and reconstruct an image. Likewise, spatial resolution has been improved to 1 to 2 millimeters.

A CAT scan may be ordered to help evaluate an acute cranial-facial trauma, an acute stroke, suspected subarachnoid or intracranial hemorrhage, headache, or loss of sensory or motor function. A scan of the brain also can help determine if there is abnormal development of the head and neck.

The first scanner was developed as a brain research tool and was used clinically in 1973. Since then, CAT brain scans have improved the diagnosis and treatment of STROKE, HEAD INJURY, tumors, abscesses, and so forth and have superseded plain skull X-rays and PNEUMOENCEPHALOGRAPHY.

See also BRAIN SCANS.

caudate nucleus A part of the BASAL GANGLIA often referred to as the NEOSTRIATUM. The deterioration of this part of the brain results in HUNTINGTON'S DISEASE.

cell body The core of the cell that contains the nucleus, where genetic material is found.

cell phones and brain tumors A number of large studies in labs all around the world have found no increased risk for brain tumors related to cell phone use, frequency of use, or number of years of use. A few smaller studies found an increased risk of brain tumors with cell phone use, but those studies have been criticized for problems with the study design.

Studies also have found that brain tumors did not occur more frequently on the side of the head where a phone was typically used.

Unlike an ordinary phone, a cell phone does not transmit calls through a wire. Instead, its signals are encoded in radio waves that are broadcast by an antenna to a receiving tower. Often, the consumer holds the antenna close to the head. Cell phones are different from cordless phones, which broadcast much weaker radio signals to household receivers that route calls along conventional phone lines.

Like television, cell phones operate at the lowest end of the microwave portion of the electromagnetic spectrum. They conform to guidelines set by the Federal Communications Commission for acceptable emission levels of electromagnetic radiation. The signals emitted by cell phones have a frequency between 840 mH and 880 mH, located at the high end of the radio band (also called high-frequency radio waves).

Most experts do agree that there is a general lack of scientific knowledge about the health effects of the low-level radiation leaked by all sorts of household appliances. Only a few studies have been performed that explore the high-frequency radio waves generated by cell phones. It is true that at high power, high-frequency radio waves can burn the skin; although cell phones operate at low power, many brands carry warnings against pressing the antenna against the skin.

The scare began when researchers at the Medical College of Virginia found that brain tumors as well as healthy red blood cells grow faster when exposed to high-power microwave radiation. Despite the lack of further studies, most scientists expressed confidence that cellular phones will not prove harmful, and so far they never have.

The concern began when a Florida man appeared on a TV talk show to say that his wife had died of brain cancer caused by a cell phone. The tumor, he said, was where the antenna had rested; he was seeking damages from three companies involved in the phones. His assertion prompted several other claims; at the time of the lawsuit, about 10 million Americans owned such phones.

See also BRAIN TUMOR.

cells, brain See BRAIN CELLS; NEURONS; GLIA.

cellular rhythms See CIRCADIAN RHYTHM.

central nervous system (CNS) The collective term for the brain and the SPINAL CORD, which is the two-way highway for messages between the brain and the rest of the body. The CNS is responsible for integrating all nervous activities and works together with the PERIPHERAL NERVOUS SYSTEM (PNS), which consists of all the nerves that carry signals between the CNS and the rest of the body.

The CNS receives sensory information from all sensory organs in the body; analyzes this information; and triggers appropriate motor responses.

The CNS consists of neurons cells and supporting cells. Injury or disease involving the CNS usually causes permanent disability.

central nervous system depressants A group of drugs that cause sedation or diminish brain activity. These drugs include alcohol, aminoglutethimide, anesthetics, anticonvulsants, antidepressants, antidyskinetics (except amantadine), antihistamines, apomorphine, baclofen, BARBITURATES, BENZODIAZEPINES, buclizine, carbamazepine, chloral hydrate, chlorzoxazone, clonidine, cyclizine, difenoxin and atropine, diphenoxylate and atropine, disulfiram, dronabinol, ethchlorvynol, ethinamate, etomidate, fenfluramine, flavoxate, glutethimide, guanabenz, guanfacine, haloperidol, hydroxyzine, interferon, loxapine, magnesium sulfate, matprotiline, meclizine, meprobamate, methyldopa, methyprylon, metoclopramide, metyrosine, mitotane, molindone, opioid (narcotic) analgesics, oxybutynin, paraldehyde, paregoric, pargyline, phenothiazines, pimozide, procarbazine, promethazine, propiomazine, rauwolfia, scopolamine, skeletal muscle relaxants, thioxanthenes, trazodone, trimeprazine, and trimethobenzamide.

central nervous system stimulants Drugs that cause anxiety, excitation, or nervousness or that otherwise stimulate the brain and central nervous system. These drugs include amantadine, amphetamines, anesthetics, appetite suppressants (except fenfluramine), bronchodilators (xanthine-derivative), CAFFEINE, clophedianol, COCAINE, doxapram, methylphenidate, pemoline and sympathomimetics.

central sulcus The main fissure that separates the FRONTAL LOBE from the PARIETAL LOBE behind it.

centrophenoxine (Lucidril)   A drug that may improve various aspects of memory function. It is believed to remove LIPOFUSCIN deposits, the material of which "age spots" are made. Lipofuscin buildup in heart, skin, and brain cells appears with age; decreased deposits have been correlated with improved learning ability.

In some studies centrophenoxine appears to remove these deposits and repair synapses. In the bloodstream, centrophenoxine breaks down into dimethylaminoethanol (DMAE), a naturally occurring nutrient found in seafood that is normally present in the brain in small amounts. DMAE also is believed to enhance brain function.

Scientists have shown that centrophenoxine can protect the brains of animals against lack of oxygen and may be of value in treating diseases in which tissue oxygenation is lowered (such as DEMENTIA or STROKE). While centrophenoxine does not seem effective in the treatment of ALZHEIMER'S DISEASE, it may help in cases where the brain is not getting enough oxygen.

cerebellar astrocytoma   See ASTROCYTOMA.

cerebellum   This small, two-lobed, wrinkled structure actually originated as an outgrowth of the HINDBRAIN, as suggested by its position directly behind the BRAIN STEM to which it is linked, tucked under the cerebral hemispheres. Its primary function is to coordinate movement and balance, helping the body to assume postures and maintain muscle coordination. It is also responsible for certain subconscious activities and—new research suggests—for coordinating thinking as well. It is also where simple, learned motor responses (such as yanking a finger away from a hot stove) are believed to be stored.

The arrangement of nerve cells in the cerebellum is different from other parts of the brain; here, the cells are positioned with mathematical precision, much like an electrical wiring diagram.

The cerebellum is the second-largest portion of the brain, and it fits inside the skull by a process of many foldings that give it a sort of pleated look.

Latin for "little brain," the cerebellum looks very much like the CEREBRUM and makes up about 11 percent of the entire brain weight. The CORTEX (surface) of the two hemispheres is made up of many parallel ridges marked with deep ridges. Each hemisphere sports three nerve-fiber stalks from its inner side, linked to different parts of the brain stem. It is along these nerve tracts that all of the signals flash back and forth between the cerebellum and the rest of the brain.

The right and left hemispheres of the cerebellum each connect with the fibers coming from nerve tracts from the SPINAL CORD on the same side of the body and with the opposite cerebral hemisphere. Therefore, nerve impulses governing movement of the right hand start off in the left cerebral hemisphere; details about the speed and orientation of the movement are transmitted back to the left cerebral hemisphere through the right half of the cerebellum. As such, the cerebellum "updates" movement as it occurs.

Nerves in the outer edges of the cerebellum govern the ends of the arms and legs, whereas nerves embedded near the center of the cerebellum monitor the body's orientation in space and help to maintain posture in response to data about balance sent via nerve impulses from the inner ear.

The cerebellum collects information about balance and movement from other organs through its connections with the brain stem, and working together with the thalamus and BASAL GANGLIA, the cerebellum integrates movement signals sent to the MOTOR CORTEX, which transmits them to the spinal cord; from there they are sent to designated muscle groups. At the same time, the cerebellum receives impulses from the muscles and joints that are being activated, somehow compares them with instructions sent from the motor cortex, and makes adjustments via the THALAMUS. This part of the brain helps modify direction, force, rate, and steadiness of intentional movements. Movement is not initiated within the cerebellum, but it does not serve simply as a sort of transmission device, either; rather, the cerebellum continually reroutes and refines instructions for movement and may store instructions for oft-used movements and for skilled repetitive movements (those that are learned by rote).

Any damage to this part of the brain can interfere with proper posture or movement ranging from jerky eye movements of nystagmus to hand tremor or slurred speech. It may also be linked to the development of SCHIZOPHRENIA. It is this area of the brain that is impaired during excess alcohol intake, producing symptoms mimicking diseases of the cerebellum (slurred speech, jerky gait, posture and balance problems). This area is also vulnerable to STROKE, often associated with functional problems of the CRANIAL NERVES.

See also CEREBELLUM, DISEASES OF THE.

cerebellum, diseases of the The CEREBELLUM may be damaged by tumors, injuries, vascular lesions, infection, intoxicants, and metabolic diseases. The cerebellum is also involved in a number of hereditary degenerative diseases (the most common is FRIEDREICH'S ATAXIA). Malfunction in the cerebellum may also contribute to the development of SCHIZOPHRENIA.

Among the disorders that are linked with diseases of the cerebellum are ATAXIA, DYSARTHRIA, and aberrant nystagmus. In addition, MEDULLOBLASTOMA, a brain tumor of childhood, often grows in the cerebellum.

cerebral blood-flow studies Tests that measure blood flow to determine areas of blood supply. In one method for determining total cerebral blood flow, the patient inhales a mixture of 15 percent nitrous oxide and air for 10 minutes; after this, blood is drawn to measure the clearance of the gas from cerebral tissue. Another method continuously measures carotid blood flow in order to assess the capacity of cerebral collateral circulation. Regional studies can help determine areas of aberrant mental activity in the brain.

cerebral commissures The bundles of fibers connecting sites in the two hemispheres of the brain.

See also ANTERIOR COMMISSURES; CORPUS CALLOSUM.

cerebral cortex From a word meaning "bark," this outer layer of the brain is made up of cell bodies of neurons called GRAY MATTER that cover the CEREBRUM like bark on a tree. Under the pinkish-gray cortex lies the WHITE MATTER, tissue made up only of nerve fibers. Most of the work that goes on in the brain is done in the cortex.

The cortex varies in thickness from about two to four millimeters (about a quarter of an inch), lying in deep folds and creases so that many more nerve cells can be packed in tightly. If the cortex were flattened out, it would stretch out about as big as a pillowcase or a newspaper page. This large brain surface may be one reason why humans, with their wrinkled cortices, are more capable of complex thoughts than are animals, with smoother cortices.

The cortex is really what makes us human; it is the center of neurons involved in thinking, learning, remembering, and planning, and functions as a sort of control center for the rest of the brain.

It can be divided into four areas or lobes; the FRONTAL LOBE (controlling decision making, problem solving, and will), the PARIETAL LOBE (receiving sensory information), the OCCIPITAL LOBE (where vision is processed), and the TEMPORAL LOBE (hearing, memory, and language).

cerebral hemispheres The two divisions of the CEREBRUM, labeled "left" and "right," that are separated by a deep groove called the longitudinal cerebral fissure. At the base of this fissure lies a thick bundle of nerve fibers called the CORPUS CALLOSUM, which provides a structural and communication link between the two hemispheres.

The left hemisphere controls the right side of the body, and the right hemisphere controls the left, because of a crossing of the nerve fibers in the MEDULLA. Although in many ways the two hemispheres are mirror images of each other, there are important differences.

In most people, areas in the left hemisphere control speech and areas in the right control spatial perceptions.

Two major furrows called the CENTRAL SULCUS and the LATERAL SULCUS divide each cerebral hemisphere into four sections—the FRONTAL, PARIETAL, TEMPORAL, and OCCIPITAL LOBES. The central sulcus also separates the cortical motor area from the cortical sensory area.

Starting from the top of the hemisphere, the upper regions of the motor and sensory areas control the lower parts of the body, and the lower regions of the motor and sensory areas control the upper parts of the body.

Other areas in the cerebral hemispheres have also been identified; the VISUAL CORTEX is found in the occipital lobe, and the AUDITORY CORTEX is found in the temporal lobe.

cerebral hemorrhage Bleeding within the brain caused by rupture of a blood vessel.
See BRAIN HEMORRHAGE.

cerebral palsy (CP) A general term used to describe a group of movement and posture symptoms arising from nervous system damage before birth, during birth, or early in life.

In the United States, two to six of 1,000 infants develop cerebral palsy, with only a slight reduction in the number of cases over the past 30 years.

Children who are moderately disabled have a near-normal life expectancy; with special help, most who can move around and communicate effectively grow up to lead relatively independent, normal lives.

Cerebral palsy can be caused by chromosome abnormalities, inherited metabolic defects, prenatal injury or premature birth, oxygen deficiency or mechanical injury at birth, jaundice, hypoglycemia, or nervous-system infection during the first few months of life.

About 90 percent of cases occur before or at birth, most commonly due to a lack of oxygen. It is also possible that a mother's infection spreading to the fetus could cause CP. Rarely, babies with severe jaundice develop CP because the bile pigment damages the basal ganglia (nerve cell clusters in the brain that control movement).

After birth, a child could contract CP via ENCEPHALITIS or MENINGITIS or after a HEAD INJURY.

Symptoms and Diagnostic Path
The portion of the nervous system that is injured will determine the symptoms. Groups of symptoms are described as spastic (abnormal stiffness and contraction of groups of muscles), athetotic (involuntary writhing movements), or ataxic (loss of coordination and balance), depending on whether the CEREBRAL CORTEX, BASAL GANGLIA, or CEREBELLUM is the most severely affected.

The degree of disability varies from person to person and can range from simply a slight clumsiness to complete immobility. In addition, children with CP may also experience other nervous system disorders, such as hearing problems or epileptic seizures. While many of these children are also mentally retarded, some are of normal to high intelligence.

While severe nervous system damage may be noticeable at birth, it is more usual for symptoms to appear between ages two and four as the child fails to grow and develop normally. Some of the infant's muscles may be floppy; there may also be feeding problems.

In the spastic group, there are three different categories of disability: diplegia, hemiplegia, and quadriplegia. Diplegics have two limbs affected. Hemiplegics experience symptoms only on one side of the body, and the arm is usually worse than the leg. All four limbs of a quadriplegic are severely affected.

About three-quarters of all CP patients are mentally retarded with an IQ below 70; the exceptions occur mostly among those with athetotic CP; many of these patients and some people with diplegic CP are highly intelligent.

Cerebral palsy is not progressive and will not worsen with age; in fact, the conditions of the disease often improve with age and special treatment.

A physician may suspect cerebral palsy in a child whose development of motor skills is delayed. In making a diagnosis, the physician takes into account any delay in developmental milestones as well as symptoms such as abnormal muscle tone or movements, abnormal reflexes, and persistent infantile reflexes.

Making a definite diagnosis of cerebral palsy is not always easy, especially before the child's first birthday. This is why most doctors will advise waiting for the permanent appearance of specific motor problems. Most children with cerebral palsy can be diagnosed by the age of 18 months. X-rays or blood tests will not reveal CP, though the doctor may order such tests to exclude other brain diseases. Cerebral palsy is not a hereditary condition, and these tests will neither establish nor rule out a diagnosis of CP. Magnetic resonance imaging (MRI) and computed tomography (CT) scans are often ordered when the physician suspects that the child has cerebral palsy These tests may provide evidence of HYDROCEPHALUS (an abnormal accumulation of fluid in the cerebral ventricles), and they may be used to exclude other causes of motor problems. These scans do not prove whether a child has a cerebral palsy nor do they predict future function. Children with normal scans may have severe cerebral palsy, and children with clearly abnormal scans occasionally appear totally normal or have only mild physical evidence of cerebral palsy.

As a group, however, children with cerebral palsy do have brain scars, cysts, and other changes which show up on scans more frequently than in normal children. Therefore, when a scar is seen on CT scans of the brain of children whose physical examination suggests they may have cerebral palsy, the scar is one more piece of evidence indicating that the children are likely to have motor problems in the future.

Treatment Options and Outlook

Cerebral palsy is incurable, but there is much that can be done with physical and speech therapy. Physical therapy teaches the child to develop muscular control and maintain balance. Speech therapy can help improve speech; for those children who do not speak, special equipment can help them communicate nonverbally.

Parents of infants at risk (those born prematurely or during difficult births) are encouraged to take their children more frequently for routine checkups; the physician will test for any abnormalities in the baby's muscle tone and reflexes and for delay in reaching developmental milestones.

cerebral thrombosis The formation of a clot (thrombus) in a brain artery that may cause a STROKE by blocking the artery, cutting off blood and oxygen to the brain.

cerebrospinal fluid A clear fluid found in the four linked brain cavities (VENTRICLES), the central canal in the SPINAL CORD, and the space between the brain and spinal cord and the MENINGES (protective covering). The fluid fills the ventricles and flows through special ducts around the brain's outer rim before being reabsorbed by the blood; this surrounding fluid acts as a cushion to protect the brain against shock and makes turning or nodding the head effortless. This fluid also protects the spinal cord. The fluid, which contains sugar (glucose), protein, and salts, can be tested during a LUMBAR PUNCTURE to help diagnose a range of illnesses affecting the brain (such as MENINGITIS).

Excess cerebrospinal fluid that builds up during fetal development or early infancy may cause the skull to grow too large, a condition called HYDROCEPHALUS (commonly known as "water on the brain").

cerebrovascular accident (CVA) See STROKE.

cerebrovascular disease Any disease that affects an artery supplying blood to the brain, such as ATHEROSCLEROSIS (narrowing of the arteries). This type of disease may eventually lead to a CEREBROVASCULAR ACCIDENT (CVA), a sudden block or rupture of a blood vessel commonly resulting in a STROKE.

cerebrum The largest, most highly developed section that makes up 80 percent of the brain, this area is the site of most conscious (voluntary) and intellectual activities. The cerebrum contains centers for sight, sound, smell, touch, intelligence, and memory; if these parts are damaged, the senses they serve may be impaired.

The cerebrum is made up of billions of nerve cells and is divided into two hemispheres, each containing a central cavity (or VENTRICLE) filled with CEREBROSPINAL FLUID. These two hemispheres, outgrowths from the upper part of the BRAIN STEM, are called the right and left CEREBRAL HEMISPHERE. These halves are the part of the brain that is responsible for higher-order thinking and decision making.

The right side of the cerebrum controls the left side of the body, and the left side of the cerebrum controls the right side of the body. In most people (right-handed people and most left-handed ones), the so-called left brain is dominant; this is the hemisphere that focuses on word comprehension, language, speech, and numbers. The right brain focuses more on feelings and spatial relationships.

Long ago, the cerebrum functioned as part of the olfactory lobes; over time, it has grown over the rest of the brain, forming a wrinkly top layer. In sheer sophistication and size/body weight comparisons, the human cerebrum is unusual in the animal kingdom (except for certain sea mammals).

The outer layer of the cerebrum is called the CORTEX. Indentations (called fissures) divide each cerebral hemisphere into four lobes: the FRONTAL LOBE, PARIETAL LOBE, TEMPORAL LOBE, and OCCIPITAL LOBE. Functions involving memory are thought to take place within the frontal lobe, the parietal lobe, and the temporal lobe.

While scientists have come to a general understanding of the cerebrum's function, the details of its mechanism remain shrouded in mystery, and its complexity remains largely unraveled.

cerebrum, diseases of the The cerebrum, which makes up the upper bulk of the brain, can be involved in various brain malformations. It also can be vulnerable to the typical array of problems, including trauma, tumors, infections, demyelinating diseases, neurochemical disorders, and toxins.

chaining A behavioral method for helping patients with memory problems handle everyday tasks. In this method, a particular task is broken down into a series of smaller units and taught one at a time. (See also BEHAVIORAL TREATMENTS OF MEMORY DISORDERS.)

chemical brain stimulation The study of brain function in lab animals by injecting various chemicals directly into the brain or ventricular spaces. The most common studies investigate drugs that stimulate or inhibit NEUROTRANSMITTERS, which are responsible for transfer of information from one NERVE CELL to another.

The chemicals are introduced through very thin stainless-steel tubes implanted into the brain through small holes drilled into the skull. After the animal has recovered from surgery, it is subjected to a variety of behavioral tests that assess the ability to learn new tasks, regulate fluids, and so on. In a different type of procedure, glass pipettes are implanted into specific areas of the brain through which drugs are injected; while the animal remains asleep, scientists record the electrical activity of nerve cells and their response to the drugs.

chemoreceptors A cell (or group of cells) that responds to the presence of specific chemical compounds by triggering an electrical impulse in a sensory nerve. It is the chemoreceptor, for example, that allows us to tell salt from sugar, a fragrance from a stench.

child abuse, memory of Most people who were abused as children remember all or part of what happened to them, although they may not fully understand or disclose it, according to most psychologists and memory experts. This does not mean, however, that it's impossible for a memory to be forgotten and then remembered—or that a false "memory" can't be suggested and then remembered as true.

These two possibilities lie at the heart of controversy about the memory of childhood abuse and recovered memories. While experts agree more research is needed, most leaders in the field do agree that although it is a rare occurrence, a memory of early childhood abuse that has been forgotten can be remembered later. However, these experts also agree that it is possible to construct convincing pseudomemories (false memories) for events that never occurred. At this point, experts say it is impossible (without other backup evidence) to distinguish a true memory from a false one.

Experienced clinical psychologists believe that the phenomenon of a recovered memory is rare. For example, one experienced practitioner reported having a patient recover a buried memory only once in 20 years of practice. And while studies have shown that memory is often inaccurate and can be influenced by outside factors, memory research usually takes place in a lab—for ethical reasons, researchers can't subject people to a traumatic event in order to test their memory of it.

Therefore, because the issue hasn't been studied directly, it's not possible to know whether a traumatic event is encoded and stored differently from a memory of a nontraumatic event.

Some clinicians suspect that children understand and respond to trauma differently from adults, and some believe that childhood trauma may lead to problems in memory storage and retrieval. These clinicians believe that dissociation is a likely explanation for a memory that was forgotten and later recalled. (Dissociation means that a memory isn't really lost, but it can't be retrieved for a period of time.) Some experts suspect that severe forms of child sexual abuse are especially likely to lead to dissociation or delayed memory. Many clinicians who work with trauma victims believe that this dissociation is a coping mechanism to protect against a painful memory. On the other hand, critics argue that there is little or no empirical support for such a theory.

The controversy over the validity of memories of childhood abuse has raised many critical issues for the psychological community, leaving many questions unanswered. The American Psychological Association has outlined a number of areas of controversy that should be pursued, such as

- how accurate or inaccurate recollections of events may be created;
- which techniques are most likely to lead to the creation of pseudomemories;
- which techniques work best in creating the conditions under which actual events of childhood abuse can be remembered with accuracy;
- how trauma and traumatic response affect the memory process, and
- whether some people are more susceptible than others to memory suggestion and, if so, why.

The issue of repressed or suggested memories has been sensationalized by the news media to the point that the idea of a total amnesia of a childhood event is portrayed as the most common occurrence, when in fact it is extremely rare. In fact, most people who are victims of childhood sexual abuse remember all or part of what happened to them.

chlorpromazine (Thorazine) A major tranquilizer and antipsychotic drug that is used to treat SCHIZOPHRENIA and mania and to control severe ANXIETY and nausea or vomiting. Chlorpromazine also enhances the effects of painkillers and is used to treat terminally ill patients and those undergoing anesthesia. Chlorpromazine works primarily by blocking dopaminergic receptors.

Side Effects
Common side effects include dry mouth and drowsiness. Sometimes, it also causes movement abnormalities, such as TARDIVE DYSKINESIA.

choline A chemical building block of every cell, choline plays an integral role throughout the body and throughout life. It is an ingredient of the membranes surrounding cells and a precursor to molecules that relay signals between brain cells. A basic compound found in animal tissue that is essential to normal metabolism of fat, choline also has been implicated as a possible memory aid because of its ability to boost the amount of acetylcholine in the brain. So important is choline to brain function that the Institute of Medicine (IOM) in Washington, D.C., advocates eating about 0.5 gram of choline per day. Choline is found in soybeans, peanuts, potatoes, lentils, and cauliflower.

Repeated studies of administering choline to treat the memory problems of ALZHEIMER'S DISEASE patients have resulted in conflicting evidence, although most found that giving choline was not helpful. Other studies suggest choline might be useful in heading off some deterioration in the early stages of the disease.

Still other studies have suggested that egg yolk (a dietary source of choline) may be useful to patients suffering from memory problems and seems to show an improvement in alcoholics and drug addicts. The major dietary source of choline is LECITHIN; foods rich in lecithin include eggs (average size), salmon, and lean beef. While some researchers dismiss the idea that eating these foods can significantly improve memory, other scientists note at least that a "normal" level of lecithin in the diet may not be enough as people age.

Phosphatidyl choline is used by the body as part of cell membranes, including those of neurons. Nerve and BRAIN CELLS especially repair and maintain themselves with large quantities of this substance.

Research suggests that levels of choline drop as a person ages and that levels are especially low in people with Alzheimer's disease.

choline acetyltransferase (ChAT)

An enzyme in the brain that promotes a reaction that produces ACETYLCHOLINE, a NEUROTRANSMITTER involved in many functions including learning and memory, as well as the brain's control of skeletal musculature.

cholinergic

A term that refers to those brain cells that use ACETYLCHOLINE to communicate. The term also may refer to a RECEPTOR type.

cholinergic basal forebrain

Nuclei in the deep regions of the forebrain containing neurons that release the neurotransmitter ACETYLCHOLINE. The cholinergic basal forebrain includes the medial septum, which projects to the HIPPOCAMPUS; the band of Broca, which projects to the hippocampus and amygdala; and the nucleus basalis of Meynert, which projects to the neocortex and AMYGDALA. Damage to these structures of the brain is believed to contribute to organic amnesia.

cholinergic hypothesis of Alzheimer's disease

The theory that there is a link between the memory loss in Alzheimer's disease and the decrease in activity of CHOLINE ACETYLTRANSFERASE (ChAT).

ChAT is a brain enzyme that is a crucial ingredient in the chemical process that produces ACETYLCHOLINE, a NEUROTRANSMITTER linked to learning and memory. There has been a link between this change in neurochemical activity, changes in memory loss, and the physical appearance of Alzheimer brains (especially in the number of plaques).

Researchers have found a loss of NERVE CELLS in a part of the base of the brain called the NUCLEUS BASALIS; some patients with classical ALZHEIMER'S DISEASE have been shown to lose as many as 90 percent of these cells. The nucleus basalis is a major site of cholinergic neurons in the brain; its projections reach a number of brain areas associated with learning and memory.

cholinesterase inhibitors

Medications designed to enhance memory and other cognitive functions by influencing certain chemical activities in the brain, especially useful for patients with ALZHEIMER'S DISEASE.

ACETYLCHOLINE is a chemical messenger in the brain that scientists believe is important for the function of brain cells involved in memory, thought, and judgment. It is released by one brain cell to transmit a message to another. Once a message is received, various enzymes, including one called acetylcholinesterase, break down the chemical messenger for reuse.

In patients with Alzheimer's, the cells that use acetylcholine are damaged, resulting in lower levels of acetylcholine. A cholinesterase inhibitor is designed to stop the activity of the enzyme that breaks down acetylcholine. By keeping levels of acetylcholine higher, the drug may help compensate for the loss of functioning brain cells. Some types of cholinesterase inhibitors also seem to trigger the release of acetylcholine and strengthen the way certain receptors respond to it.

Three cholinesterase inhibitors are commonly prescribed for the treatment of Alzheimer's disease: GALANTINE HYDROBROMIDE (Razadyne), RIVASTIGMINE (Exelon) and DONEPEZIL (Aricept).

TACRINE (Cognex) was the first cholinesterase inhibitor to be approved (1993), but it is rarely prescribed today because of associated side effects, including a risk of liver damage.

Cholinesterase inhibitors are designed to increase levels of acetylcholine, a chemical messenger involved in memory, judgment, and other thought processes. Acetylcholine is released by certain brain cells to carry messages to other cells. After a message reaches the receiving cell, other chemicals break acetylcholine down so it can be recycled.

Alzheimer's disease damages or destroys cells that produce and use acetylcholine, reducing amounts available to carry messages. A cholinesterase inhibitor slows the breakdown of acetylcholine; by maintaining acetylcholine levels, the drug may help compensate for the loss of functioning brain cells.

Galantamine appears to stimulate the release of acetylcholine and to strengthen the way certain receptors on message-receiving nerve cells respond to it. Rivastigmine may block activity of an additional chemical involved in breaking down acetylcholine. Cholinesterase inhibitors do not stop the underlying destruction of nerve cells. Their ability to improve symptoms eventually declines as brain cell damage progresses.

Patients taking any of these three medications performed better on tests of memory and thinking than those taking a placebo, although the benefit was small and more than half of patients had no improvement. Most experts think cholinesterase inhibitors may delay or slow worsening of symptoms in some individuals for about six months to a year, although some may benefit longer.

There is no evidence that combining these drugs would be more helpful than any single medication, and combinations would probably cause more side effects.

However, there is some evidence that patients with moderate-to-severe Alzheimer's already taking a cholinesterase inhibitor might benefit a bit by adding MEMANTINE (Namenda). Memantine is a drug with a different mechanism of action, approved by the FDA in 2003 for symptoms of moderate-to-severe Alzheimer's and slightly more effective than a placebo.

Side Effects

Side effects such as nausea, vomiting, loss of appetite, and increased frequency of bowel movements might be expected with any cholinesterase inhibitor. Generally, donepezil is well tolerated. Because experience with rivastigmine and galantine is limited, it is unknown how well they will be tolerated

in the general population. Tacrine has been associated with significant liver toxicity in about half of the patients who have taken it.

cholinomimetic agents Any compound that activates cholinergic receptors, such as arecoline, nicotine, or muscarine.

chorea Involuntary, jerky movements (especially in the face and limbs) caused by dysfunction deep within the brain. Formerly called St. Vitus' Dance, these unpredictable movements are found in two diseases (HUNTINGTON'S DISEASE and Sydenham's chorea). It may sometimes appear during pregnancy or as a side effect of some drugs, in CEREBRAL PALSY or in ATHETOSIS.

chronic fatigue and immune dysfunction syndrome (CFIDS) Also known as chronic fatigue syndrome (CFS), this unexplained condition affects the brain and many body systems of more than 800,000 Americans. Characterized by debilitating tiredness, it is sometimes derisively referred to as "yuppie flu." It is also known as myalgic encephalomyelitis. Its symptoms are so debilitating that it can devastate families, destroy active lifestyles, and end fulfilling careers.

Although more people suffer from this condition than MULTIPLE SCLEROSIS, lung cancer, or AIDS, 80 percent have never been diagnosed. Yet early detection, diagnosis, and treatment are vital.

The condition first received attention in the mid-1990s after reports of about 100 cases appeared in the Lake Tahoe region of California. Initially, many physicians dismissed CFS as hypochondria or a misdiagnosed depression. Most patients were professionals in their mid-30s (especially women). Because its symptoms were so similar to other diseases, it further complicated attempts to study the condition. Without a solid definition, scientists had problems identifying its cause and seeking a cure.

Symptoms and Diagnostic Path

CFS is characterized by fatigue lasting six months or longer, together with irritability, lethargy, and an inability to think clearly. It also includes flulike symptoms such as pain in the joints and muscles, unrefreshing sleep, tender lymph nodes, sore throat, and headache.

Symptoms vary from person to person and fluctuate in severity. Specific symptoms may come and go, complicating treatment and the patient's ability to cope with the illness.

More recently, studies link the condition with physiological, rather than psychological, factors. In one study, MAGNETIC RESONANCE IMAGING scanned the brains of 259 patients in Lake Tahoe, 183 of whom were afflicted with CFS. In 78 percent of the patients, images showed tiny points of swelling on BRAIN CELLS in the central NERVOUS SYSTEM; the MYELIN SHEATH on some cells was also missing. These swellings did not appear in the same section of the brain for all patients, but researchers did discover a relationship between the region affected and the patient's symptoms. For example, patients who had vision problems also had disturbances in the OCCIPITAL LOBE of the brain—an area that processes vision.

Evidence also suggests that most patients have an active infection with herpes virus 6 (HHV-6), although scientists emphasize this does not mean the virus causes the condition. This virus is believed to infect most people in early life without producing any symptoms.

Still other studies suggest that the cause may be linked to a retrovirus in spinal fluid, known as a spumavirus or "foamy virus." Moreover, many patients suffer from irregularities in their immune systems and have abnormally low levels of hormones in the brain and endocrine glands. There is no indicator or diagnostic test that can clearly identify the disorder. Overlapping symptoms can occur with several diseases, such as fibromyalgia, Gulf War illnesses, and multiple chemical sensitivities. Lupus, hypothyroidism, and Lyme disease also have similar symptoms and will need to be ruled out when making a diagnosis.

Current diagnosis of chronic fatigue syndrome (CFS) is based primarily on whether or not the patient's symptoms fit the case definition of the condition established by the Centers for Disease Control and Prevention (CDC). Testing should be ordered to exclude other possible reasons for symp-

toms and to identify other disorders occurring at the same time. Unfortunately, there is no one all-encompassing diagnostic test that can definitively point to CFS.

Tests may include

- a complete blood count (CBC) to help rule out anemia, leukemia and other blood disorders, as well as collagen vascular disorders such as lupus
- blood chemistry test to confirm normal blood sugar, electrolytes, kidney and liver function, calcium and bone metabolism, and blood proteins.
- thyroid function studies to confirm normal thyroid function (a common cause of muscle aches and fatigue)
- sedimentation rate to reveal inflammation, infection, and collagen vascular disorders
- urinalysis to exclude infection, kidney disease, and possibly collagen vascular disorders
- antinuclear antibody (ANA)
- Lyme test (ELISA with a reflex Western Blot for borderline or positive tests)
- tilt table testing
- sleep test (polysomnography)

Medications are typically prescribed for pain, sleep problems, digestive problems such as nausea, flu-like symptoms, and (if they occur) depression and anxiety. In addition, supportive treatment aimed at helping patients relax and better cope with their condition includes mental health counseling and cognitive behavioral therapy.

Many patients with CFS also have sleep apnea and other sleep disorders, and treating sleep disorders can markedly improve symptoms and prevent secondary complications, such as weight gain, high blood pressure, and even STROKE. Patients at high risk (those with a history of snoring, apneic periods, gasping, obesity, and high blood pressure, short neck) should be strongly considered for sleep monitoring.

Complementary or alternative therapies can be helpful to some patients. These treatments may include massage, acupuncture, tai chi, and alternative food and herbal supplements (under guidelines with a physician). At the same time, daily lifestyle changes can help patients handle digestion problems, food intolerance, fatigue, thinking problems, and sleeplessness. These changes may involve different diet, modifications in exercise, and getting plenty of rest. Many patients find it helpful to consult with specialists, including a dietitian, physical therapist, occupational therapist, mental health professional, and sleep therapist.

Treatment Options and Outlook

There is no known cure for CFIDS. Until a treatment is developed that will improve all the symptoms of CFIDS or correct the underlying cause, therapy is based on symptoms.

chronic fatigue syndrome   See CHRONIC FATIGUE AND IMMUNE DYSFUNCTION SYNDROME.

cigarettes and the brain   See NICOTINE.

circadian rhythm   A daily activity rhythm that cycles over 24 hours (from the Latin *circa*, "about," and *dies*, "a day"). The best-known human circadian rhythm is the daily sleep/waking cycle. Other circadian rhythms involve body temperature, hormone levels, urine production, and levels of cognitive and motor performance.

For hundreds of years, scientists have known that plants underwent daily cycles of leaf and petal movements; more recently, the widespread circadian rhythmicity in animals has been demonstrated.

A person's rhythms are cyclical, rising and falling during certain times of the day and of the week. Although most people experience a period of peak efficiency somewhere between 11 A.M. and 4 P.M., every person's internal body clock is different. As the day progresses, a person becomes more involved in activities, but by lunch time, tiredness sets in. The daily biological cycles (body temperature, respiration, and pulse rate) alter the power of attention.

People who go to bed and wake up early learn more readily at the beginning of the day when their attention is best, while those who have a later schedule experience the opposite. Those who work a night shift probably experience different cyclical peak times than those who work a nine-to-five schedule.

What is especially striking is how a living organism will respond differently to a physiological challenge depending on its internal circadian rhythm. For example, the dose of amphetamine that will kill 78 percent of a group of rats at 3 A.M. is lethal for only 7 percent if injected at 6 A.M. or later; identical injections of lidocaine hydrochloride trigger convulsions· in only 6 percent of rodents at 3 P.M. but at 9 P.M., 83 percent of rodents experience convulsions. Similarly, allergic reactions to certain antigens tend to be more severe in the evening than during the morning hours.

Importantly, time-related variations in the effectiveness and toxic side effects of drugs are routinely found in human patients.

Years ago, scientists assumed that circadian rhythm was just a direct response to the natural sequence of day and night. However, more recent research has revealed that without such obvious time cues as regularly alternating dark and light, rhythms persist, although the period of time may deviate significantly from 24 hours and differ from one person to another. Researchers now believe that every person has an intrinsic, innate circadian rhythm ordinarily synchronized to 24 hours by recurring stimuli (such as day and night)—but not necessarily bound to those cues.

While most researchers do not believe people "learn" their rhythms, it has been shown that early experience with light and dark cycles longer or shorter than 24 hours can have a long-lasting effect on an individual's circadian rhythm.

The limits of a circadian cycle are between 20 and 28 hours; rhythms of slower frequency are called INFRADIAN RHYTHM and those of faster frequency are termed ULTRADIAN RHYTHM.

circulation and the brain   When blood pressure falls to the point where it is not high enough to pump blood to the brain, especially when a patient stands up, it causes symptoms that can include dizziness, memory loss, and fainting. If the blood does not begin flowing to the brain, the brain tissue will begin to die from lack of oxygen. Untreated this can result in coma and death.

clonidine A drug used to treat high blood pressure that works by reducing nerve impulses from the brain to the heart and circulatory system.

cluster headaches See HEADACHES.

cocaine A powerfully addictive stimulant that directly affects the brain, cocaine is an alkaloid derived from the coca plant (*Erythroxylon coca*). It produces its stimulating effects by enhancing the activity of DOPAMINE and NOREPINEPHRINE neurons. (It is dopamine that also plays a key role in the development of SCHIZOPHRENIA and PARKINSON'S DISEASE.)

Cocaine works by not only increasing the release of norepinephrine and dopamine, but also by blocking their reuptake. This overuse of the two systems takes its toll on the brain areas that normally rely on these neurotransmitter systems for function—learning and memory areas, and limbic structures. This is why heavy cocaine use leads to both emotional and cognitive disorders.

The overall effect on the brain and nervous system is to stimulate the part of the LIMBIC SYSTEM known as the NUCLEUS ACCUMBENS, where a large number of dopamine AXONS terminate, producing a feeling of euphoria. Eventually, however, the receptors become desensitized by this process, and it takes more and more cocaine to create the same sensation. Withdrawal can be just as harsh from cocaine as from opiates.

The feeling of alertness experienced by cocaine users is caused by the increasing activity of norepinephrine cells in the higher thought centers of the CEREBRAL CORTEX.

Chronic administration can result in permanent neurological damage, at least among animals; brain damage in humans is still being studied. At its worst, users can experience a frightening psychotic condition known as cocaine psychosis, which may appear similar to schizophrenia. It is believed to be related to dopamine. Scientists know that doctors treat schizophrenia by giving drugs that block dopamine receptors; cocaine, which enhances dopamine release, will worsen the condition of schizophrenia. Therefore, a cocaine psychosis may be caused by excessively high dopamine levels in the brain induced by cocaine use.

Cocaine can be snorted through the nose, smoked, or injected, or rubbed onto mucous tissues. Some users combine cocaine powder or crack with heroin (speedball). A "freebase" is an extremely dangerous form of using cocaine by smoking, which can lead to compulsive cocaine use even more rapidly. By smoking, the cocaine reaches the brain within seconds, resulting in a sudden and intense high, but the euphoria quickly disappears, leaving the user with an enormous craving to freebase again and again.

"Crack" is the street name given to one form of freebase cocaine that comes in the form of small lumps or shavings. Smoking crack produces the same debilitating effects as freebasing.

For reasons little understood, cocaine will cause psychosis selectively; cocaine poisoning is equally unpredictable. An overdose of cocaine can cause convulsions and death by depressing the brain centers that control breathing and heart activity. In these cases, death can occur so quickly that there is no time to treat the overdose. This type of cocaine poisoning has been the cause of death in several young athletes, including University of Maryland basketball player Len Bias, the first-round draft choice of the Boston Celtics in 1986.

More than 1,000 years ago, South American Indians chewed the leaves of coca plants for the energy boost it gave them. The habit was introduced by Spanish explorers into Europe, where the leaves were used to make beverages. In the United States, the original recipe for Coca-Cola used a coca leaf extract, but it was eliminated many years ago when the harmful effects of cocaine were discovered.

Cocaine was isolated from the leaves in 1860 by a German chemist, and its use was quickly taken up by Sigmund Freud, who had studied cocaine as a treatment for nervous exhaustion as a young neurologist. In 1884 he published *Über Coca,* in which he stated that a person could enjoy cocaine "without any of the unpleasant aftereffects that follow exhilaration brought about by alcohol." He believed that cocaine could cure many diseases and could also cure narcotic addiction, and he prescribed it for his close friend Ernst von Fleischl-Marxow, who was addicted to morphine. Unfortunately, Fleischl-Marxow became a cocaine addict, suffered toxic psychosis, and died. In spite of this, Freud used cocaine himself for many years, although he did finally begin to write about its newly discovered dangers.

Cocaine was eventually discredited as a medicine except for its use as a local anesthetic that can block pain without putting the patient to sleep. Procaine, a drug derived from cocaine, is still used today in eye surgery and dentistry.

Cognex   See TACRINE.

cognition   The processing of information by the brain; specifically, perception, reasoning, and memory.

cognitive development   The acquisition of intelligence, conscious thought, and problem-solving skills beginning in infancy and progressing throughout life.

Cognitive Failures Questionnaire   A test that assesses a person's susceptibility to slips of action and other failures of memory and perception. On the test, subjects are asked to assess the frequency with which they experienced specific examples of cognitive failure, such as: "Do you forget whether you've turned off the stove?" The test then gives a five-point scale ranging from "never" to "very often."

Scores from this test are not related to performance on tests of immediate and delayed memory or to perception as measured by performance on a word-identification test. The test scores are related to a person's ability to perform two tasks at the same time; the inability to pay attention and allocate processing resources effectively is associated with frequent slips of action as well as other forms of memory deficits.

Test scores are also related to forward digit span (ability to repeat back a sequence of digits in the correct order), which is involved in carrying out action sequences, such as remembering to turn off the stove.

cognitive map   A person's internal method of remembering how to find directions in unknown locations.

cognitive triage   The tendency to recall hard-to-remember items first in a series of lists of items. Scientists speculate that cognitive triage may be an unconscious adaptive strategy for getting weakly remembered items to surface first.

If the theory of cognitive triage is correct, researchers say, police officers interrogating children who have witnessed crimes might obtain more information by asking questions about critical and disturbing events first rather than starting out with easy questions in order to relax the children.

collective unconscious   A term coined by Swiss psychiatrist Carl Jung (1875–1961) to indicate a portion of shared ideas in the unconscious common to all people; also called racial unconscious or racial memory. Jung regarded the foundation of such mythical images as positive and creative (compared to SIGMUND FREUD's more negative view of mythology).

As part of his theory on the collective unconscious, Jung postulated a theory of archetypes—broadly similar images and symbols that occur in myths, fairy tales, and dreams around the world. Jung believed these archetypes were inherited from experiences in our distant past, and that they are present in each person's unconscious, controlling the way he or she views the world. Jung believed the human psyche has an inbuilt tendency to dwell on certain inherited motifs, and that the basic pattern of these archetypes persists, however much details may vary.

While Jung also believed that every person had a personal unconscious of life experiences, he felt that the collective unconscious was superior. His aim in therapy was to put the patient in touch with the profound insight of the collective unconscious, particularly through dream interpretation.

colliculus A paired structure that protrudes from the roof of the MIDBRAIN. The superior colliculus is involved in eye movements and eye-head coordination; the inferior colliculus is a relay area for auditory processing.

coma A state of unresponsive unconsciousness in which the person does not respond to external stimuli (such as a pinprick or a shout) or to inner needs (such as a full bladder). It is caused by damage or a disturbance in the parts of the brain involved in conscious activity or the maintenance of consciousness, including the CEREBRUM, upper parts of the BRAIN STEM, central regions of the brain, and the LIMBIC SYSTEM. In particular, coma will result from injury or damage to the RETICULAR FORMATION, the brain structure crucial to maintaining consciousness.

Coma may result from BRAIN DAMAGE such as that caused by brain ABSCESS, BRAIN TUMOR, or INTRACEREBRAL HEMORRHAGE. Coma could also be caused by the accumulation of toxic substances (such as in drug overdoses, acute alcohol intoxication and so on). All CENTRAL NERVOUS SYSTEM DEPRESSANTS (such as alcohol or BARBITURATES) can lead to coma when taken in overdose, and they are particularly dangerous when taken together. OPIATES (such as heroin or morphine) also can lead to coma. Coma may also result from the interruption of blood flow; inflammatory diseases such as ENCEPHALITIS or MENINGITIS may also cause coma.

A patient may remain deeply comatose but alive for many years if the brain stem is still functioning. However, once brain damage spreads to the lower brain stem, coughing, swallowing, and breathing will begin to deteriorate.

Symptoms and Diagnostic Path
A coma may occur in various degrees of severity. In mild forms, the patient may respond to stimuli by speaking a few words or moving a body part. In more severe cases, the patient cannot respond in any way. Even deeply comatose patients may continue to breathe, cough, yawn, blink, or exhibit eye movements. These automatic responses indicate that the lower brain stem, which controls these responses, is still functioning.

The depth of coma may be measured by a variety of means, such as assessments of verbal behavior, eye movements, and so on.

Treatment Options and Outlook
Coma is a medical emergency in which doctors focus on stabilizing the patient's breathing and circulation, which can rapidly reverse the coma. Help with breathing, giving fluids and blood, and other supportive care may be necessary. Emergency personnel will stabilize the person's neck in case there is a fracture.

A physician will try to identify the cause of a coma so that potentially reversible conditions are treated immediately. Surgery may be performed to repair the skull or remove a foreign object, and many patients with severe head injuries need surgery to repair or remove bleeding or bruised parts of the brain. Underlying disorders also will be treated, such as infection, diabetes, asthma, kidney failure, or liver disease. If the cause of a coma is a drug overdose, glucose, a B vitamin (thiamine), and a medication that counteracts narcotic-type drugs may be given. Medication may also be given to counteract seizures, if they are present.

Keeping a comatose patient healthy is important, and this includes preventing pneumonia and bedsores, providing a good diet, and getting physical therapy to prevent permanent muscle contractures and deformities of bones, joints, and muscles.

Sometimes the cause of a coma can be completely reversed, and the person will regain normal function. However, depending on the severity and location of the brain damage and how long the coma lasted, the patient may have permanent disabilities or may never regain consciousness. Disabilities following a coma can be physical, such as partial paralysis. There also may be changes in the patient's personality or mental ability.

People who suffer a coma from a head injury tend to recover better than those for whom illness is the cause of the coma. However, except for comas induced by drug overdoses, only a small percentage of people who are in a coma for more than a few hours make a good recovery. Age is an important factor in whether or how well a person recovers after a coma. Adults who remain comatose more than a month do not have a very good chance of ever regaining their previous level of normal function. On the other hand, children and young adults have regained normal function even after two months in a coma.

combat amnesia   Once called combat fatigue, this is a type of traumatic AMNESIA occurring after combat in which the amnesia has a straightforward origin—a distressing event during war. One method of treating combat amnesia is by the SODIUM PENTOTHAL interview, in which a slow intravenous injection of the drug relieves the patient's anxiety to the point of drowsiness. Then the injection is stopped, and the therapist can begin to question the patient about the traumatic incident. The recall at this point is often profoundly disturbing to the patient, who reaches the height of the reaction and then collapses, then often is able to pick up the story at a less traumatic point. One interpretation of this type of treatment is that the narcosis allows the patient to reinstate the extreme emotion felt during combat itself, unlocking the forgotten event.

A range of BARBITURATES, including sodium pentothal, have been used to facilitate the recall of emotionally disturbing memories.

commissures, cerebral   See CEREBRAL COMMISSURES.

commissurotomy   Cutting of the CORPUS CALLOSUM and perhaps the other cerebral COMMISSURES (anterior and posterior) as well.

See also SPLIT-BRAIN RESEARCH.

complementarity   The distribution of skills in the cerebral hemispheres so that if language is represented in one hemisphere, some nonlanguage skills will reside in the other.

computed axial tomography (CAT) scan   See CAT SCAN.

computer use and memory   Because of the computer's ability to focus attention without distraction, recent research suggests that playing computer games and using computers may influence memory and cognition, especially in the elderly. In a preliminary study in Rockville, Maryland, 50 nursing home residents in their 70s, 80s and 90s were introduced to video games modified so they would have a greater chance of success. Other than those with severe mental impairment, residents—even those with ALZHEIMER'S or PARKINSON'S disease—were able to participate and sharpen their memory skills.

concentration   See ATTENTION.

concussion   Brief unconsciousness after a blow to the head or neck, caused by a disturbance of the cell activity in the brain. An impact to the head creates a sudden movement so that the outer surface of the brain strikes the inner surface of the skull. This jolt causes aberrant neural activity that can lead to many short- and long-term problems.

A concussion produces no evidence of structural damage to the brain, although there may be cuts or bruises on the skin outside the skull. About a third of all those with concussion go on to develop a combination of symptoms called POSTCONCUSSION SYNDROME.

Research has suggested that postconcussion syndrome can include significant memory problems, dizziness, and behavior and thinking changes that can disturb patients up to a year following the HEAD INJURY. Despite sometimes significant symptoms, structural damage may not show up on brain scans.

Repeated concussions (such as damage in the boxing ring) can impair concentration and result in slowed thinking and slurred speech that may become permanent.

Symptoms and Diagnostic Path

Common symptoms immediately following a concussion include confusion, memory loss, dizziness, blurred vision, and vomiting. Partial paralysis and shock are also possible. The longer the period of unconsciousness, the more serious and persistent symptoms tend to be. During the 24 hours after the injury, symptoms may include headache, vomiting, increased pulse rate, anxiety, slurred speech, drowsiness, nausea, unequal pupil size, convulsions, unusual eye movements.

Delayed symptoms may include irritability, headaches, depression, sleep disturbances (including insomnia or difficulty waking), fatigue, poor concentration and memory, confusion, increased sensitivity to sounds, lights, and distractions, loss of sense of taste or smell, and trouble walking or coordinating use of limbs.

To diagnose a concussion, the doctor may ask questions about the accident and may conduct a neurological exam, which includes memory tests and assessments of concentration, vision, hearing, balance, coordination, and reflexes. Depending on the results of the neurological exam, your doctor may request a CT SCAN (computerized tomography, or CAT SCAN) or MAGNETIC RESONANCE IMAGING (MRI) scan.

Any loss of consciousness should be referred to a physician because of the possibility of serious bleeding within the skull that could require emergency surgery. Symptoms of serious damage may be immediately obvious or may not appear for some time.

Treatment Options and Outlook

A patient who has experienced concussion should be observed in bed for 24 hours and should not drive a car or play sports, as blackouts can occur. New symptoms (drowsiness, breathing problems, repeated vomiting, or visual disturbances) should be reported immediately to a physician because they indicate potential damage to the brain or bleeding between the skull and the outer surface of the brain.

Acetaminophen or another painkiller may be prescribed for headache. Aspirin is not generally recommended because it can contribute to bleeding. Rest and relaxation with no activities requiring concentration or vigorous movement will speed recovery within a few days.

confabulation   The production of false recollections. Confabulation is very common in psychiatric disorders and occurs especially in memories with a tinge of grandiosity. Confabulation memories also may borrow from fantasy or dream.

This problem was once thought to be a product of a person's embarrassment at losing memories, but many patients with severe AMNESIA do not confabulate. There appears to be no relationship between the severity of the amnesia and the tendency to confabulate; instead, the tendency may be related to personality traits in force before the onset of amnesia. People who are outwardly sociable but inwardly secretive are particularly prone to produce these false memories. Patients with the greatest tendency toward confabulation, however, are those with the least insight into their own memory disorder and who deny that a problem exists.

congenital brain defects   Brain defects present at birth. These defects may be caused by genetic or chromosomal problems and result in a variety of disorders such as DOWN SYNDROME, TAY-SACHS DISEASE, or CRI DU CHAT SYNDROME (all involving mental retardation). In addition, brain defects may be structural in nature; these are usually fundamental and untreatable, such as MICROCEPHALY (small head) and ANENCEPHALY (absence of the brain). Others such as HYDROCEPHALUS (water on the brain) are correctable while the fetus remains in the womb.

consciousness   The awareness of the self and of one's surroundings. This awareness depends on a combination of sensations, memories, and experiences. Consciousness relies on the proper function of the CEREBRUM (the main mass of the brain) and the reticular system in the BRAIN STEM.

Some researchers, including Endel Tulving, have postulated that there are three varieties of consciousness: noetic, autonomous, and anoetic. Noetic consciousness implies a semantic memory because it involves thinking about objects and events and relationships among them in their absence. Autonomous consciousness is self-knowing; it is related to episodic memory that recognizes events as in the personal past. Anoetic consciousness is nonknowing, but it is still consciousness because it allows appropriate behavioral responses to aspects of the environment.

Some scientists believe that the perception of consciousness occurs when NERVE CELLS fire at similar frequencies, which imposes a "global unity" on nerve cells in different brain areas.

While a person maintains consciousness, there is still a great deal that goes on without a person's awareness; this is referred to as subconscious activity. According to psychoanalysts, it is the part of the mind through which information passes on its way from the unconscious to the conscious mind. It contains feelings, thoughts, or ideas a person may be unaware of but that can be recalled.

When consciousness is impaired, the person begins to have problems with attention, concentration, and understanding; memory fails and there is a lack of direction and purpose. As the level of arousal drops, the person may pass into a state of stupor and then COMA. However, despite the common perception of "losing" consciousness, the unconscious state is more of a shift in consciousness that allows the brain to filter incoming information in a different manner.

consolidation A change in the structure of memory, other than the forgetting that occurs with the passage of time after learning.

Modern theories of consolidation can be traced to the work of Donald Hebb (1904–85), who believed that new information is first represented by a temporary trace, a specific pattern of activity within a group of interconnected neurons (which Hebb called a cell assembly). At this stage, any disruption in the pattern of activity will cause the information to be lost completely. But if the activity is maintained for enough time, structural changes in the cell will occur, causing a permanent memory trace. Once this trace is formed, there is no more need to maintain the initial pattern of activity, and the information is then in "passive storage."

Many scientists believe that the structural change underlying consolidation involves an altered pattern of synapse activity. It has been estimated that the brain has many synapses that could handle the levels of information storage in memory.

The exact way that synapses change is not known, although scientists speculate that it may involve how much neurotransmitter is released at the synapses.

context processing A mental operating system that allows a person to gather and use contextual clues to perform a wide range of mental functions. Recent research suggests that the gradual loss of the ability to gather and use contextual clues could explain why older people are less able to think clearly.

Psychologists believe that given adequate levels of the chemical messenger dopamine, the prefrontal cortex enables a person to process context for a thought, memory, or behavior. Therefore, context processing can have broad impact, affecting everything from attention and inhibition to episodic and working memory. In everyday life, context processing helps a person decide everything from which way to turn when walking down the street, to what to say based on who is listening or what an ambiguous word would mean in a particular sentence.

Researchers believe that in normal aging, declining dopamine levels start to interfere with contextual information, weakening all of the cognitive functions that depend on it.

In one study, the performance of 175 young adults aged 18 to 29 was compared to 81 older adults aged 65 to 85 on an AX-Continuous Performance Test. In the test, researchers measured how quickly and accurately participants hit a button when they saw X on a computer screen. They were told to hit the button only if X followed A, but not if X followed any other letter. This test reveals how well someone depends on context to act—in this case, responding to the cue A or "not A," with any other letter referred to as B. AY trials, in which participants responded to non-X (Y) probes after they followed A cues, would be additional "false alarm" evidence of sensitivity to context.

By comparing results from various AX, BX, and AY trials, the researchers learned that context processing correlated with the different kinds of cognitive functions tapped by the different trials. For example, participants who were primed to respond to *X* and could not hold back when they saw it after a *B* instead of an *A*, also performed worse on AX trials—the basic measure of context processing.

Moreover, when comparing the performance of young and old participants, older adults performed worse on AX and BX trials, which meant they had problems with context processing. On AY trials, the older group actually did better than the younger: they had fewer "false alarms" because their impaired context processing made them less predisposed to hit the button after they saw *A*. Interference during the test (which increases demands on context processing) accentuated age-related differences, whereas increased difficulty (which does not affect context processing) did not affect them.

Taken together, the results support the idea that there is a single, fundamental deficit in the ability to properly represent, maintain, and update task-relevant context as the underpinning for a range of age-related cognitive skills declines.

More testing is needed to determine how changes in the dopamine system, which has also been implicated in ALZHEIMER'S DISEASE, might affect cognition, including context processing.

continuous amnesia A type of PSYCHOGENIC AMNESIA in which the patient cannot recall events subsequent to a specific time up to and including the present. (See also HYSTERICAL AMNESIA.)

contrecoup effects French for "opposite blow," this term refers to HEAD INJURY damage to the side of the head opposite the point of impact. For example, a blow to the right side of the head causes the brain to crash into the left side of the inner skull. This damage is especially likely to occur in the temporal and orbital regions of the brain, and may destroy brain cells.

conversion An unconscious defense mechanism by which conflicts that would otherwise cause anxiety are instead given symbolic external expression. The repressed impulses and the defenses against them are converted into a variety of symptoms involving the nervous system, which may include paralysis, pain or loss of sensory function.

corpus callosum A bundle of white matter four inches long that contains 300 million myelinated nerve fibers. It is the main bridge between the left and right hemispheres of the brain and carries messages between them.

Some scientists believe that SCHIZOPHRENIA may be associated with abnormalities in the corpus callosum because scans and tests have found a thickened, damaged, or nonfunctioning corpus callosum in some schizophrenic patients.

Other studies of GENDER DIFFERENCES in brain structure have revealed that a man's corpus callosum is relatively smaller than a woman's. In women, the rear of the corpus callosum is larger than in men; this may explain why women use both sides of their brain for language. The smaller corpus callosum in men may also suggest that the two hemispheres in the male brain may intercommunicate less often.

See also SPLIT BRAIN RESEARCH.

corpus striatum See STRIATUM.

cortex See CEREBRAL CORTEX.

cortex, limbic See LIMBIC SYSTEM.

cortical lobes The four sections of the cerebral hemispheres devoted to processing touch (parietal), memory and hearing (temporal), vision (occipital), and speech, problem solving, voluntary movement, and emotions (frontal).

corticobasal degeneration A progressive neurological disorder characterized by nerve cell loss and shrinkage of many different areas of the brain, including the CEREBRAL CORTEX and the BASAL GANGLIA.

Symptoms and Diagnostic Path

This slow-progressive condition begins about age 60, first appearing on one side of the body but eventually affecting both sides. Symptoms are similar to those found in PARKINSON'S DISEASE: poor coordination, an absence of movements, rigidity, poor balance, and abnormal muscle postures. Other symptoms such as cognitive and visual-spatial impairments, loss of the ability to make familiar, purposeful movements (APRAXIA), halting speech, muscular jerks, and swallowing problems. Eventually, the person may no longer be able to walk.

Treatment Options and Outlook

There is no treatment that can slow the course of this disease, and the symptoms of the disease do not usually respond to therapy. Drugs used to treat Parkinson's disease-type symptoms are not effective. Occupational, physical, and speech therapy can help in managing disability.

Corticobasal degeneration usually lasts between six to eight years, ending in death by pneumonia or other complications of severe debility such as blood infection or pulmonary embolism.

corticotropin-releasing factor A chemical secreted by the HYPOTHALAMUS that stimulates the anterior pituitary to produce ADRENOCORTICOTROPIC HORMONE (ACTH). In turn, ACTH stimulates the adrenal cortex to produce glucocorticoids (primarily cortisol), which in turn stimulates the release of AMINO ACIDS. The release of corticotropin-releasing factor is an important component of the brain's response to stress.

See STRESS AND THE BRAIN.

Cotugno, Domenico (1736–1822) Italian anatomist who discovered in 1774 that the brain's cavities were not filled with "animal spirit" but with cerebrospinal fluid.

See also BRAIN IN HISTORY.

cranial nerve, eighth See VESTIBULOCOCHLEAR NERVE.

cranial nerve, 11th See SPINAL ACCESSORY NERVE.

cranial nerve, fifth See TRIGEMINAL NERVE.

cranial nerve, first See OLFACTORY NERVE.

cranial nerve, fourth See TROCHLEAR NERVE.

cranial nerve, ninth See GLOSSOPHARYNGEAL NERVE.

cranial nerve, second See OPTIC NERVE.

cranial nerve, seventh See FACIAL NERVE.

cranial nerve, sixth See ABDUCENS NERVE.

cranial nerve, tenth See VAGUS NERVE.

cranial nerve, third See OCULOMOTOR NERVE.

cranial nerve, 12th See HYPOGLOSSAL NERVE.

cranial nerves A series of 12 nerve pairs connecting directly to the brain, emerging through openings in the skull and then dividing into several major branches. All but two of the cranial nerve pairs connect with the BRAIN STEM (the lowest section of the brain). One nerve from each pair serves one side of the body, while the other nerve serves the other side.

The cranial nerves, known by a numbering system invented by the early Greek physician GALEN, include the OLFACTORY NERVE (first cranial nerve); OPTIC NERVE (second cranial nerve); OCULOMOTOR NERVE (third cranial nerve); TROCHLEAR NERVE (fourth cranial nerve); TRIGEMINAL NERVE (fifth cranial nerve); ABDUCENS NERVE (sixth cranial nerve); FACIAL NERVE (seventh cranial nerve); VESTIBULOCO-CHLEAR NERVE (eighth cranial nerve); GLOSSOPHA-RYNGEAL NERVE (ninth cranial nerve); VAGUS NERVE (10th cranial nerve); SPINAL ACCESSORY NERVE (11th cranial nerve); HYPOGLOSSAL NERVE (12th cranial nerve).

Each of the cranial nerves plays a part in at least one of the following operations: carrying motor and sensory information to regions of the head and neck; serving as the basic wiring system of the sense of vision, hearing and balance, taste and smell; and transmitting autonomic information to special glands and organs.

Some of the cranial nerves play a variety of roles. For example, the trigeminal nerve wears several hats, carrying sensations from the face, teeth, and sinuses to the brain as well as controlling several important muscles, including the strong jaw muscles used for chewing. The facial nerve sends branches to the important facial muscles of expression—those used in smiling, frowning, raising one's eyebrows, and so on. The olfactory and optic nerves carry visual and olfactory input from the eyes and nose to the brain for processing. The oculomotor nerve controls eye movements and also helps focus images on the retina. The vagus nerve, in addition to performing sensory and motor functions, sends nerve fibers to the heart, stomach, and intestines to help regulate autonomic activity.

craniopharyngioma A benign, congenital tumor of the PITUITARY GLAND that, if untreated, may cause permanent brain damage due to intracranial pressure. This very rare condition only affects one or two Americans per million yearly.

Symptoms and Diagnostic Path

This type of tumor causes symptoms by increasing the pressure on the brain, by disrupting pituitary gland function, and by damaging the optic nerve. Increased pressure on the brain causes headache, nausea, vomiting (especially in the morning), and difficulty with balance. Damage to the pituitary gland causes hormone imbalances that can lead to excessive thirst and urination, and stunted growth.

When the optic nerve is damaged by the tumor, vision problems develop that are often permanent; symptoms may worsen after the tumor is removed. This type of tumor most often affects boys and girls equally, between ages five and 10. Adults can sometimes develop this tumor.

The tumor is typically diagnosed after a thorough neurological examination, a CT scan and/or MRI scan of the brain, and endocrine hormone tests. Most patients have at least some visual defects and evidence of decreased hormone production at the time of diagnosis.

Treatment Options and Outlook

The tumor is usually surgically removed; because it is usually in a favorable location, it can often be almost completely excised. However, radiation therapy may be indicated instead of surgery. There is an 80 to 90 percent chance of permanent cure if the tumor can be completely removed with surgery or treated with high doses of radiation. However, most of the problems with hormones and vision do not improve with treatment, and sometimes the treatment may even make them worse.

A significant number of patients have long-term hormonal, visual, and neurological problems after treatment, and if the tumor is not completely removed, it may recur.

craniosynostosis The early fusion of one or more joints (sutures) between the skull bones during infancy.

Symptoms and Diagnostic Path

A baby with this condition is born without fontanelles (spaces between the plates of the skull) that allow for growth.

Craniosynostosis may appear in an infant with bone disease (such as rickets), multiple birth defects, or an abnormally small brain.

Treatment Options and Outlook

To prevent brain damage, surgical splitting of the skull bones must begin within the first few months of life.

craniotomy   Removal of part of the skull during brain surgery. In this procedure, an incision is made into the skin, and a high-speed drill is used to remove a piece of bone from the skull to expose the brain. After the operation, the piece of bone is replaced and the membrane, muscle, and skin are sutured. Patients generally experience a mild headache for a period of time after the operation.

A craniotomy is the most commonly performed surgery for removal of a brain tumor. *Crani* means "skull," and *otomy* means "cutting into."

See also BRAIN TUMOR.

cranium   The hard shell encasing the brain, which is made up of eight fused skull bones:

- the occipital bone, lying at the back of the head
- the sphenoid bone, a wedge-shaped bone at the skull base
- the parietal bones, forming a wall at the top and sides of the head
- the temporal bones forming the "temples" above the ears
- the frontal bone forming the forehead
- the ethmoid bone lying behind the nose

Creutzfeldt-Jakob disease   A very rare infectious disease of the nervous system caused by a transmissible infectious organism called a PRION that leads to a progressive dementia. It is usually distinguished from other dementias by its rapid course; it takes only months from onset of symptoms until death. CJD is much more common than its animal-related cousin, bovine spongiform encephalopathy (MAD COW DISEASE), but it gets much less attention from the media. It strikes about 250 Americans each year, usually over age 58, with a usually swift and inevitably fatal course. Although scientists believe that the disease incubates over many years, patients typically live a few months to a year after symptoms appear.

The disease is considered infectious, but not contagious—it cannot be passed from one human to another in casual contact, by hugging, kissing, or sexual intercourse. But scientists have found in laboratory tests that healthy mice contract the disease when they are injected with brain fluid from a sick mouse. Infected patients can transmit the disease to monkeys, cats, and guinea pigs. In addition, infection has been linked to brain surgery with contaminated instruments or transplantation of an infected cornea. There are also indications that there may be a genetic link.

The disease is one of a family of human and animal diseases known as the transmissible spongiform encephalopathies (TSEs). "Spongiform" refers to the way the infected brain looks, filled with holes much like a sponge.

CJD is the most common of the known human TSEs; others include kuru, fatal familial insomnia (FFI), and Gerstmann-Straussler-Scheinker disease (GSS). Kuru was first identified among Papua New Guinea tribesmen and has now almost disappeared. FFI and GSS are extremely rare hereditary diseases, found in just a few families around the world.

Animal TSEs include bovine spongiform encephalopathy; scrapie, which affects sheep and goats; mink encephalopathy; and feline encephalopathy. Similar diseases also have been identified among elk, deer, and exotic zoo animals.

While scientists know that the disease is caused by a transmissible agent, the identification of this agent is still unclear. Scientists first thought the agent was a slow virus because of the unusually long incubation period between the time of exposure and the onset of symptoms. Further research has indicated that the agent differs significantly from viruses and other conventional microbes.

Whereas viruses and other known infectious agents contain nucleic acids which contain a cell's genetic material, researchers have been unable to identify any nucleic acids in the CJD agent. Additionally, the chemical and physical procedures that inactivate most viruses have proved ineffective in stopping the CJD pathogen.

A newer theory suggests that the transmissible agent is neither a virus nor any other known infectious agent, but is instead an unconventional type of protein called a "prion," short for "proteinaceous infectious particle." Prions are thought to transform normal, benign protein molecules into infectious, deadly ones by altering the shape of the healthy molecules. They are believed to be responsible for other fatal brain diseases in animals and humans.

There are three ways to contract CJD: It can be inherited, transmitted through infection, or can simply appear sporadically.

About 10 percent to 15 percent of CJD cases are inherited as a result of a mutation in the gene coding for the prion protein. Genetic factors are thought to be responsible for the higher numbers of CJD cases in some communities in Czechoslovakia and Chile, as well as among Libyan-born Jews.

Although CJD is caused by a transmissible agent—perhaps a prion—the disease is not considered to be contagious in the traditional sense. Family members who live with CJD patients have no greater risk of getting the disease than does the general population. Very few cases of CJD have resulted from exposure to an infected individual. The only predictable way to contract CJD from an infected person has been during a medical procedure using tainted surgical instruments or human tissue. People have been infected during corneal transplants, implantation of electrodes in the brain, brain grafts, the injection of natural human growth hormone derived from cadaveric pituitaries, and after surgery with contaminated surgical instruments.

In Britain, scientists and politicians have traced a connection between BSE, or mad cow disease, and CJD. Mad cow disease was first discovered in Britain in 1986 and was traced to the practice of feeding cattle with food containing ground offal from scrapie-infected sheep. Although the rate of mad cow disease in cattle declined from its peak of 1,000 cases a week in 1992 and 1993, there were still between 280 to 300 cases per week reported in January 1996. At the same time, the incidence of CJD in Britain, though still small, nearly doubled between 1990 and 1994. On March 20, 1996, the British government stated there was a possible link between BSE and CJD after the identification of an apparently new strain of CJD discovered in 10 people under the age of 42, including some teenagers. This new strain was dubbed new variant-CJD (nvCJD). Five of the people were associated with the meat and livestock industry. British scientists decided that the most likely explanation for this unusual outbreak was that the victims had eaten beef from diseased cattle before regulations were adopted in 1989 for the disposing of potentially infectious cattle offal and forbidding the use of sheep entrails as feed.

Since it first appeared in the United Kingdom in 1986, BSE has killed about 200,000 British and European cattle, and since 1996, 98 cases of nvCJD have been suspected or confirmed in Britain, France, and Ireland. The human victims seem to have contracted the disease from eating beef contaminated with nervous system tissue, and they have had an unusual daisylike floral pattern in the brain in which an amyloid plaque core is surrounded by "petals" of spongelike tissue.

Symptoms and Diagnostic Path

Several common symptoms become evident in CJD patients as the disease runs its course. The duration of CJD from the onset of symptoms to the inevitable death is usually one year; however, shorter periods of several months are common, and longer periods of two or more years have been noted, usually in the familial form and with an earlier age of onset. The initial stage of the disease can be subtle, with ambiguous symptoms of insomnia, depression, confusion, personality and behavioral changes, strange physical sensations, and problems with memory, coordination, and sight. As the disease advances, the patient experiences a rapidly progressive dementia, and in most cases, involuntary and irregular jerking movements known as myoclonus. Problems with language, sight, muscular weakness, and coordination worsen. The patient may appear startled and become rigid. In the final stage of the disease, the patient loses all mental and physical functions. The patient may lapse into a coma and usually dies from an infection such as pneumonia, precipitated by the bedridden, unconscious state.

The patients with nvCJD become depressed and paranoid, lose the ability to walk and swallow, grow blind and comatose, and eventually die. Both diseases are incurable and, in most cases, can be diagnosed positively only after death. The latency period between exposure and nvCJD can be as short as 10 years and may be as long as 60 years.

A diagnosis of CJD should be considered when an adult patient develops a rapid dementia.

Unfortunately, confirming a diagnosis of CJD has historically been difficult, as traditional laboratory tests have been ineffective in detecting CJD. The disease does not induce a fever. The cerebrospinal fluid most often appears normal, except for an occasional elevation in the protein content. Magnetic resonance imaging (MRI), positron emission tomography (PET), and X-rays have not been helpful in diagnosing CJD. A computed tomography (CT) brain scan is usually normal, but may show some atrophy, a nondiagnostic finding seen in many other neurological conditions. The most helpful test has been the electroencephalogram (EEG), which measures brain wave activity. The EEG often shows a characteristic abnormal pattern, typically observed in later stages of the disease, but the EEG does not confirm a CJD diagnosis. Accordingly, a definitive diagnosis of CJD has traditionally required a brain biopsy or autopsy that can detect the characteristic changes in the brain tissue caused by the disease. However, a brain biopsy may sometimes produce a false negative result if the biopsied area was unaffected by the disease.

Researchers are trying to develop new diagnostic tests. One possible candidate looks for a protein marker that indicates brain cell degeneration in a patient's cerebrospinal fluid. This test would help diagnose CJD in someone who already has symptoms. Much easier and safer than a brain biopsy, the false positive rate of this test is about 5 to 10 percent.

Additional tests proposed to confirm a diagnosis of CJD include identifying the presence of the deadly prion protein or identifying the prion gene mutation. The difficulties involved in diagnosing CJD may have prevented the identification of the disease in some cases.

Because brain biopsy for diagnosing CJD is invasive, costly, and risky, it is often not performed. Moreover, some doctors may not even consider the possibility of a CJD diagnosis since the disease has been rare in the past, and the clinical symptoms of CJD can often be attributed to other ailments. Consequently, CJD may be mistaken for a variety of psychological illnesses and other neurological disorders such as ALZHEIMER'S DISEASE, PICK'S DISEASE, HUNTINGTON'S DISEASE, or brain hematomas.

The extent to which such misdiagnosis may have occurred is presently unknown.

Treatment Options and Outlook
There is no known effective treatment or cure for CJD. The disease is inevitably fatal, in up to 90 percent of patients during the first year.

cri du chat syndrome   Also known as "cry of the cat syndrome" or "5p– syndrome," this rare congenital condition is characterized by a kittenlike mewing cry caused by a small larynx. The cry usually disappears after the first few weeks of life.

"5p–" is a term used by geneticists to describe a portion of chromosome number five that is missing in these individuals. Children born with this rare genetic defect will most likely require ongoing support from a team of parents, therapists, and medical and educational professionals.

In the past, it was common to place children with 5p– syndrome in institutions with other severely retarded individuals. During the early 1980s, research revealed that those raised in family settings with the benefit of early intervention programs made remarkable progress, far exceeding the expectations of doctors who first described the syndrome.

Symptoms and Diagnostic Path
The syndrome includes MENTAL RETARDATION, poor muscle tone, heart problems, unusual facial characteristics (such as widely spaced eyes), small head, and short stature.

Most individuals with the syndrome have trouble with language. Some are able to use short sentences, while others express themselves with a few basic words, gestures, or sign language. Nearly all children with this syndrome have poor muscle tone when they are young. Other characteristics may include feeding difficulties, delays in walking, hyperactivity, scoliosis, and significant retardation. A small number of children are born with serious organ defects and other life-threatening medical conditions, although most individuals with 5p– can anticipate a normal life expectancy.

Children and adults with this syndrome are usually friendly and happy, and enjoy social interaction.

Treatment Options and Outlook

There is no treatment that can alter the chromosomal abnormality. However, most of the medical problems can be treated successfully with standard medical procedures. Early intervention programs using a variety of techniques and educational strategies that focus on enhancing physical, intellectual, sensory, and social development can greatly improve the future outlook for the child.

Since most children with the syndrome experience severe speech delay, speech and language therapy are vital. The early introduction of alternative means of communication, including sign language along with a pictorial symbol system, can enhance the child's speech development, language acquisition, and behavior. Children who cannot communicate effectively experience a great deal of frustration, and behavior problems can develop as a result.

Those most severely affected will require full-time care throughout their lives. Most people with cri du chat syndrome are capable of achieving a degree of independent self-care, but will require supervision for life. Some of those least affected by the syndrome will be able to live independently or with minimal assistance in the community. With early and consistent educational intervention, as well as physical and language therapy, children with cri du chat syndrome are capable of leading full and meaningful lives.

cryptococcosis A rare infection caused by inhaling the fungus *Cryptococcus neoformans* found in soil and bird droppings. The infection can lead to MENINGITIS, an inflammation of the coverings of the brain.

Those most susceptible to cryptococcosis are those with weakened immune systems, such as patients with AIDS.

Symptoms and Diagnostic Path

Symptoms may include low-grade fever, chest pain, and a cough, but more serious cases lead to meningitis, with symptoms of HEADACHE, stiff neck, fever, drowsiness, blurred vision, mental deterioration, and staggering gait; untreated, it can cause COMA and death.

Cryptococcosis is diagnosed from tests of spinal fluid.

Treatment Options and Outlook

If the disease has affected the brain, treatment includes a combination of the anti-fungal drugs flucytosine and amphotericin B for six weeks. Relapses can occur, however.

CT scan See CAT SCAN.

cue-dependent forgetting An explanation of forgetting that centers on problems in retrieval. With cue-dependent forgetting, the memory does not fade away, nor is it displaced by other information; instead, it merely depends on using the right cue to retrieve it.

With the right cue, the information can be retrieved from memory; if the item is "forgotten," it is because the wrong cue has been used. An example of cue-dependent forgetting is when a person cannot remember a fact until something "jogs" his or her memory.

CVA See CEREBROVASCULAR ACCIDENT.

cysticercosis Multiple brain cysts produced by the larval form of the pork tapeworm *Taenia solium*. Once the larvae have migrated from the intestine into the bloodstream, they migrate to muscle, eye, and brain, where they are associated with intense inflammation. Cysticercosis in the brain is called neurocysticercosis.

Humans become infected by ingesting tapeworm eggs in contaminated food or drinks.

Symptoms and Diagnostic Path

Neurocysticercosis often causes no symptoms at first. The most common symptom are headaches and SEIZURES. Other symptoms include mental deterioration, paralysis, lack of balance, brain swelling, giddiness, CONFUSION, and convulsions, which may be fatal. Imaging studies reveal multiple calcifications and lesions in the brain.

Symptoms can appear months or even years after an initial infection, usually when the cysts are in the process of dying. When this happens, the brain can swell and cause pressure in the brain, leading to most of the symptoms of neurocysticercosis.

This condition can be hard to diagnose and may require several different testing methods. A physician will take a detailed medical history, including travel experience and eating habits, as well as order MRI or CAT brain scans.

Treatment Options and Outlook

Broad-spectrum antiparasitic drugs in combination with anti-inflammatory drugs kill surviving organisms. Surgical removal of cysticerci may be needed to relieve pressure on the brain.

The decision to treat neurocysticercosis is based on how many brain lesions there are and the symptoms they cause. Treatment is not given if there is only one lesion, but more than one would typically require specific antiparasitic treatment. If the brain lesion has formed a hard shell around the tapeworm larvae (calcified), it is considered dead and specific antiparasitic treatment will not be helpful.

As the cysticerci die, the lesion will shrink, swelling will go down, and symptoms (such as seizures) will go away.

cytomegalovirus (CMV) Cytomegalovirus is a member of the herpes family and is one of the TORCH DISORDERS that can cause birth defects.

Symptoms and Diagnostic Path

In healthy individuals, there are usually no symptoms. However, some individuals with CMV develop mononucleosis, which has symptoms of fever and fatigue. More rarely, mononucleosis with CMV will cause swollen lymph glands, sore throat, and a swollen spleen.

CMV spreads through urine, droplets from breathing, sneezing, and coughing, and blood transfusions. According to the National Institutes of Health, children with CMV infections can release the virus in their urine for a long time, even if they do not have symptoms.

Physicians diagnose CMV with blood tests and physical exams, including palpating (feeling) the stomach area.

Treatment Options and Outlook

Treatment of CMV usually requires rest supplemented by pain medication and saltwater gargling for sore throat. Most patients with CMV recover in 4 to 6 weeks, although the fatigue may last for several months.

Between 50 and 85 percent of individuals in the United States will have a CMV infection by age 40, according to the Centers for Disease Control and Prevention.

Risk Factors and Preventive Measures

Children typically become infected with CMV in preschool, day care, and play groups, where children are not as obsessive in their hygiene (covering their mouths when they cough, washing their hands, avoiding handling objects and then putting their hands in their mouths) as older children and adults. Newborns frequently contract CMV from their infected mothers as they pass through the birth canal, consume their breast milk, and inhale droplets of respiratory moisture produced by mothers' sneezing and coughing. Premature infants and newborns in general who become infected shortly after birth are at risk for neurological and developmental disorders.

Individuals with transplants or compromised immune systems who become infected with CMV can develop disorders of the lungs, nervous system, the gastrointestinal track, and the eye, even occasionally causing blindness.

decay One of many theories of forgetting that suggests memories leave a physical trace in the brain that gradually fades away with time after a period of nonuse. (See also TRACE DECAY.)

decerebrate Absence of a functioning CEREBRUM (cerebral hemisphere), the main control center of the brain. This occurs when the BRAIN STEM (lowest section of the brain) is severed, isolating the cerebrum.

declarative memory The type of memory network responsible for memory of facts, as opposed to PROCEDURAL MEMORY, the memory for procedures—learning *what* versus learning *how.* Scientists believe that the HIPPOCAMPUS is critical to storing facts but not procedures. An amnesiac with a damaged hippocampus can still learn simple skills (such as reading reversed print in a mirror), but she can't remember anything about the training session.

Likewise, riding a bicycle involves *procedural* memory; after learning to ride the bike, people can't articulate the knowledge they have learned; all the micromovements that go into riding a bike are stored implicitly throughout the central nervous system as processes, not fact.

defense mechanism The unconscious process that provides relief from emotional conflict and anxiety. Conscious efforts often are made for the same reasons, but the true defense mechanism is unconscious. Some of the common defense mechanisms include compensation, CONVERSION, denial, displacement, DISSOCIATION, idealization, identification, incorporation, introjection, projection, rationalization, reaction formation, regression, sublimation, substitution, symbolization, and undoing.

degenerative diseases and the brain There are many degenerative diseases that can affect the brain, ranging from those that produce only slight problems to those that are rapidly fatal. These diseases include ALZHEIMER'S DISEASE, MULTIPLE SCLEROSIS, PARKINSON'S DISEASE, senile DEMENTIA, MOTORNEURON DISEASE, and HUNTINGTON'S DISEASE.

dehydroepiandrosterone (DHEA) One of the four most common steroid hormones in the body, it is produced mainly in the adrenal gland and may play a role in cognition. It is the precursor hormone to testosterone and estrogen.

Because nerve degeneration occurs most often when DHEA levels are low, some researchers wonder if DHEA may protect brain cells against ALZHEIMER'S DISEASE and other forms of SENILITY. DHEA has been shown to improve long-term memory in mice.

Proponents believe that taking DHEA supplements beginning at middle age could improve quality of life, but evidence has been inconclusive. Critics point out that taking any type of hormones on a regular basis without medical supervision could cause problems, especially in women with a history of breast cancer. DHEA is a steroid that the body converts into estrogens and androgens. Side effects can include acne, facial-hair growth in women, deepening of the voice, and mood changes.

déjà vu The sense of having already experienced an event that is happening at that moment, from the French meaning "already seen." This very common phenomenon has never been fully explained, but some scientists believe that a neurological glitch causes the experience to be registered in the memory before reaching consciousness. Other people believe déjà vu is an unconscious emotional response triggered by similarities between the current event and a past experience. Frequent occurrences of déjà vu may be a symptom of temporal lobe EPILEPSY.

Examples of déjà vu have been recorded for millennia; but while descriptions of the experience have been traced as far back as St. Augustine, no one has yet come up with the definitive theory about what causes it. Plato argued that déjà vu is a real memory of events that took place in a previous existence and that prove the theory of reincarnation. Nineteenth-century Romantic poets also believed the déjà vu experience supported the idea of reincarnation, but modern scientists believe it is a disturbance of the temporal lobe of the brain.

Other scientists suggest déjà vu is really a false memory, triggered by a current experience that has some features in common with an earlier one. They believe that memories are stored in the brain in the form of holograms and that any part of the hologram has enough information stored in it to reproduce the whole picture.

This theory helps explain how memories can be brought forward by stimulating a section of the brain and why the memory may remain even after that section is surgically removed. This fact implies that—just as with a hologram—there is enough information in any one cluster of brain cells to evoke the entire memory.

In cases of déjà vu, then, while clumps of holographic data may form entirely different memories, portions of them may be identical. This could fool us momentarily into thinking we are reexperiencing something.

Freud expressed the idea of déjà vu in relationship to consciousness and unconsciousness; a conscious experience touching on a repressed memory, he said, would set off the feeling of déjà vu. More modern psychoanalysts believe that feelings of déjà vu occur during moments of anxiety, as a means of reassurance.

delirium Acute mental confusion caused by a disordered brain function.

Symptoms and Diagnostic Path

Delirium is an acute reaction to intoxication, disturbance of body chemistry, organic mental disorder, infection, high fever, HEAD INJURY, or trauma. It is most common among the very young and the very old, especially after major surgery, or when there is a preexisting brain disturbance. Symptoms include disorientation, increased anxiety, failure to understand events, confusion, memory problems, sudden mood swings, illusions, HALLUCINATIONS, extreme excitement, panic, and violence. Symptoms are usually worse at night, either because of disturbed sleep or because the dark and quiet make visual illusions more common.

Treatment Options and Outlook

Delirium is usually reversible once the underlying condition is recognized and treated. Patients require calm and clear communication, adequate lighting, appropriate seclusion, and known attendants.

Stopping or changing medications that worsen confusion may improve cognitive functioning even before treatment of the underlying disorder. Some of these medications may include anticholinergics, painkillers, cimetidine, central nervous system depressants, lidocaine, and other medications, including alcohol and illegal drugs.

Many disorders also can contribute to confusion, and these should be treated in an attempt to lessen delirium. These may include heart failure, decreased oxygen, excessive carbon dioxide levels, thyroid disorders, anemia, nutritional disorders, infections, kidney or liver failure, and mental health problems such as depression. In fact, treating co-existing medical and mental disorders often improves mental functioning.

A person with delirium may need to be treated with medications to control aggressive or agitated behavior, especially if the behavior is dangerous. These medications include thiamine, clonazepam, DIAZEPAM, trazodone, buspirone, haloperidol, olanzapine, Risperdal, clozapine, fluoxetine, imipramine, or Celexa. Mental health counseling and behavior modification also may help some people control their behaviors.

delirium tremens (DTs)   An acute brain disorder characterized by confusion, trembling, and vivid HALLUCINATIONS, usually occurring in chronic alcoholics who stop drinking. It can be fatal in 10 to 15 percent of untreated cases. The cause of DTs is the withdrawal of alcohol after the brain and other organs have become accustomed to tolerating elevated levels of ethanol.

Symptoms and Diagnostic Path
Symptoms, which usually develop within 24 to 96 hours after drinking stops, include restlessness, agitation, trembling and sleeplessness, rapid heartbeat, fever, sweating, confusion, hallucinations, delusions, paranoia, and convulsions. Symptoms usually subside within three days.

Delirium tremens is a medical emergency. It is diagnosed on the basis of symptoms and an assessment of tests, which may include a toxicology screen (usually positive for alcohol). Blood chemistry (chem-20) may show electrolyte disturbances (especially low potassium and magnesium levels). An ECG (electrocardiogram) may show arrhythmias, and an EEG (ELECTROENCEPHALOGRAM) may rule out other reasons for seizures.

Treatment Options and Outlook
Treatment includes rest, rehydration, and sedation with vitamin injections.

DT is a potentially fatal emergency condition whose treatment goals include saving the patient's life, treating the immediate symptoms, and preventing complications. Seizures and heart problems should be treated, and depressants and sedatives may be required to reduce symptoms. Treatment may require maintenance of a sedated state for a week or more until withdrawal is complete. Diazepam can be used to treat seizures, anxiety, and tremors.

Hallucinations are treated in much the same way as any acute psychotic episode, with hospitalization as needed. Cautious use of antipsychotic medications, such as haloperidol, may be necessary.

Once the acute episode has been treated, the patient must be removed from alcohol and given treatment for alcohol use or alcoholism. This may include psychological interventions, social supports such as Alcoholics Anonymous, behavior modification, or other types of treatment. Once the immediate danger is over, long-term preventive treatment must begin.

delta waves   BRAIN WAVE pattern during deep dreamless sleep. In adults, the presence of waves during wakefulness shows the presence of BRAIN DAMAGE or BRAIN DISORDERS.

dementia   The loss of intellectual functions, such as thinking and memory, which interferes with daily function. It is not a disease in itself, but a group of symptoms that may accompany a condition, all of which produce a gradual decline in intellectual function and almost always a significant deterioration of memory.

The term *dementia* is not used to indicate a particular loss of mental function, such as occurs in amnesia, aphasia, agnosia, or apraxia. In dementia, the decline usually involves memory, other cognitive capacities and adaptive behavior without any major change in consciousness.

For centuries dementia was dismissed as SENILITY and considered an inevitable fact of aging. In fact, it is *not* a part of normal aging, but a symptom of an underlying condition.

The patient may or may not be aware of the condition, but in almost all cases the loss of memory is accompanied by defects in one or more areas of intellectual function, such as language, spatial or temporal orientation, judgment, and abstract thought. While some criteria for dementia require defects in one or more of the components of intellect, others require that the defect involve all components of intellectual function.

Dementia is a result of dysfunction of the brain, especially in those parts of the cerebrum known as the association areas, which combine perception, purposeful action and thought to enable a person to adjust and survive in his or her environment. Dementia is not the same thing as mental retardation, although a person with mental retardation may become demented upon losing intellectual abilities he or she once had. Dementia is also not the same thing as psychosis; a demented patient may or may not be psychotic, and a patient with psychosis may or may not be demented.

Although it occurs at all ages, the chance of dementia increases with advancing age; its highest rate is in the population over age 75.

Symptoms and Diagnostic Path

Loss of memory is usually the first sign, with patients repeatedly asking the same question, forgetting to turn off the stove and so on. As dementia continues, symptoms worsen, including more and more confused episodes, and more drastic impairments (such as language problems) begin to appear. Because of similar symptoms, it is often difficult to diagnose particular forms of dementia, but a number of distinct forms have been recognized.

The onset of dementia is usually gradual; it begins with mild forgetfulness, restlessness, or apathy followed by an increasing tendency to misplace things and small inconsistencies in some of the ordinary daily living tasks. Words or actions may begin to be repeated. As the dementia worsens, the cognitive dysfunction worsens and patients may begin to have problems at work, lose their way in their own neighborhoods, fail to recognize friends or family, and reverse sleep cycles.

These symptoms may be followed by hallucinations, delusions, paranoia, or inappropriate or antisocial behavior. Depending on the cause of the dementia, there may or may not be indications of organic brain disease in addition to the intellectual or behavioral changes, such as problems with balance, senses, or vision.

Proper identification of the cause of dementia is critical to treatment, since some diseases that produce dementia can be treated or reversed. (These include benign brain lesions, intoxication, infections, and metabolic and nutritional disorders.) It is likewise important to differentiate the early stages of dementia from nonprogressive cognitive changes found in normal aging—but it is not always possible. The best way to tell the difference is through a series of observations over a period of time; still, diagnoses of many of the most common dementing diseases can be confirmed only upon autopsy.

The patient's history is the most important component of the initial evaluation, and should be obtained from the patient and the family. Family members most often in contact with the patient should be interviewed first, followed by other family members, friends, and neighbors. Important objective information also can be provided by community health workers, social workers, and nurses. Previous medical records should he reviewed. A chronological account of the patient's current problems—symptoms, duration of disease, and specific intellectual and behavioral changes—should be noted. The medical history should include inquiries about relevant systemic diseases, trauma, surgery, psychiatric disorders, nutrition, alcohol, and substance abuse. A mental status exam is often part of the neurological evaluation; this is not a test of sanity, but assesses various mental functions such as memory, attention, language, and perception.

In particular, memory may be tested exhaustively, since memory problems are a prominent feature of dementia. Tests should include an assessment of a person's ability to learn both verbal and nonverbal information and the ability to recall items from the remote past. The patient may be asked to construct objects by drawing or recall these drawings later.

In addition, an assessment usually will include a battery of standardized tests of intelligence (such as the Wechsler Adult Intelligence Scale, or WAIS), memory (the Wechsler Memory Scale), language (Boston Diagnostic Aphasia Examination), and prior academic achievement (the Wide Range Achievement Test).

Lab tests may help rule out diseases with certain brain disorders, such as tumors, abscesses, strokes, fluid accumulation, heart and lung disorders, liver disease, kidney disease, infections such as AIDS or SYPHILIS. Other tests that look for these disorders might include a brain scan (magnetic resonance imaging or computerized tomography), electrocardiogram, chest X-ray, blood chemistry and urine tests and drug screening, electroencephalography (EEG), lumbar puncture, or radioisotope studies.

If all other diseases and injuries are ruled out, the patient may be suffering from ALZHEIMER'S DISEASE; there is no specific test that can uncover Alzheimer's, which is diagnosed only after all other possibilities have been exhausted. An absolute diagnosis can be made only at autopsy.

Treatment Options and Outlook

If there is a diagnosis of a curable cause of dementia, the doctor will be able to recommend the best treatment. Even if the diagnosis is one of the irreversible disorders, much can be done to help the patient and family. Careful use of drugs can lessen agitation, anxiety, and depression and improve sleeping patterns, if needed. Proper nutrition is particularly important, although special diets or supplements usually are not necessary.

Daily routines, physical activities, and social contacts are all important. Often, stimulating the individual by supplying information about time of day, place and what's going on in the world encourages the use of remaining skills and information. This keeps brain activity from failing at a faster rate. In the same way, providing memory cues helps people help themselves—these cues might include a visible calendar, a list of daily activities, written notes about simple safety measures and directions to and labeling of commonly used items.

Risk Factors and Preventive Measures

Developing interests or hobbies and becoming involved in activities that keep the mind and body active are among the best ways to avoid problems that can mimic irreversible brain disorders. Certain physical and mental changes seem to occur with age even in healthy people, but senility is by no means inevitable after age 65.

The two most common forms of dementia in old age are MULTI-INFARCT DEMENTIA and ALZHEIMER'S DISEASE, but the many different diseases capable of producing dementia can be divided into two main groups. The first group includes those disorders that appear to originate in the brain and that inevitably produce dementia. The second group includes those that begin outside the brain and affect it secondarily, and may or may not produce dementia depending on how the brain is affected—liver disease, certain metabolic disorders, and infectious disorders such as syphilis or AIDS.

Parkinson's Disease As many as 30 percent to 40 percent of people with PARKINSON'S DISEASE (a progressive, neurodegenerative condition) will develop dementia during the later course of the disease. Some Alzheimer patients develop symptoms of Parkinson's disease.

Lewy Body Dementia LEWY BODY DEMENTIA is a type of dementia similar to both Parkinson's disease and Alzheimer's disease—but also unique. Lewy bodies are protein deposits found in deteriorating nerve cells that often appear in the brains of people with Parkinson's disease. When Lewy bodies disperse throughout the brain, it causes a dementia with symptoms much like Alzheimer's disease. However, Lewy body dementia progresses differently from Alzheimer's, involving hallucinations and fluctuations in cognitive impairment.

Huntington's Disease HUNTINGTON'S DISEASE is a progressive, degenerative disease that affects the body and mind. It stems from a disorder within the brain that causes certain nerve cells to waste away. As the disease progresses, changes in personality and declines in intellect, memory, speech and judgment occur. Dementia may develop in the later stages of the disease. Huntington's is known to be caused by a genetic disorder, and the gene that causes this disease has been identified.

Creutzfeldt-Jakob Disease Dementias may occur in young or middle-aged people. CREUTZFELDT-JAKOB DISEASE is a rare and fatal brain disorder thought to be caused by a PRION. The earliest symptom of the disease may be memory impairment and behavior changes. The disease progresses rapidly with mental deterioration, involuntary movements (muscle jerks), weakness in the limbs, blindness, and eventually coma.

Pick's Disease PICK'S DISEASE is a rare brain disorder characterized by disturbances in behavior, personality and eventually memory. The disease is relentless in its progression, which may ultimately include language impairment, erratic behavior, and dementia. Because of the strange behavior associated with Pick's, people are often seen first by psychiatrists. Like Alzheimer's disease, a diagnosis is usually confirmed at autopsy.

In addition, there are a great number of reversible causes of dementia:

Drug-Related Dementia Overdose of medication or chemicals is capable of causing a dementia. Neuroactive and psychoactive drugs, opiate painkillers and the adrenocortical steroids are the most common causes. About 5 percent of dementia cases are drug-related. However, some often-used drugs may cause or aggravate dementia, including anticholinergic medicines used in the treatment of movement disorders, allergic reactions or gastrointestinal disorders; and drugs used to treat heart problems, such as high blood pressure. Almost all street drugs (from heroin to glue) can cause dementia, as can a range of common chemicals such as carbon monoxide, carbon disulfide, lead, mercury, and manganese. While all these chemicals may have irreversible or fatal effects, they are often the cause of reversible dementia.

Many medications taken by older people can cause subtle cognitive impairment, but when several drugs are taken at the same time—as often happens among the elderly—significant Alzheimer's-like problems appear: memory loss, absentmindedness, confusion, disorientation, and emotional outbursts. Alcohol use aggravates drug-related dementia.

Infections   Any infection that involves the brain is capable of producing dementia. Dementia from infections such as leptomeningitis and encephalitis, if they are treated early, can be prevented. Chronic infectious diseases such as syphilis, Whipple's disease or cryptococcus affect the brain, but the dementia can still be stopped—and sometimes reversed—at least to a degree. Chronic viral illnesses such as AIDS often produce dementia, but it is not known whether drugs that retard the AIDS process can stop or reverse changes in the nervous system that lead to dementia. The agents responsible for diseases such as Creutzfeldt-Jakob disease and progressive multifocal leukoencephalopathy do not respond to any kind of treatment. Postinfectious encephalomyelitis sometimes can result in dementia.

Metabolic Diseases   Chronic diseases of the thyroid, parathyroid, and adrenal glands and the pituitary are easily diagnosed and the resulting dementia can be reversed. A number of inherited metabolic diseases that appear in adult life, including Wilson's disease, metachromatic leukodystrophy, and neuronal storage diseases, also cause a reversible dementia.

Nutritional Disorders   Poor nutrition can lead to dementia in about 5 percent of cognitive deterioration cases. Nutrient deficiencies most closely associated with dementia include the B vitamins: thiamine (B_1), niacin (B_3), folate (folic acid), and vitamin B_{12}. Of these, folate and B_{12} deficiencies are most common. Blood tests to assess their levels are a standard part of the clinical assessment for Alzheimer's disease. The hallmark of B-vitamin deficiency dementia is memory loss with possible coordination problems (ataxia).

Although patients who have thinking problems may not eat well and could therefore have a vitamin deficiency as a result of their dementia, several studies have shown that people with both dementia and B_{12} deficiencies recover when given the vitamin by injection. Other studies have shown mental improvement when people with folate and niacin deficiencies have received supplemental vitamins. Unfortunately, only about 25 percent of those with dementia due to thiamine deficiency recover completely when given supplements; another 50 percent show partial recovery. Wernicke-Korsakoff's encephalopathy is caused by a loss of thiamine, which can lead to the irreversible Korsakoff's dementia. Thiamine deficiency is usually seen in alcoholic patients, but it also can be found among depressed people and pregnant women suffering with chronic vomiting.

Cardiovascular Disorders   High blood pressure is one of the most frequent causes of MULTI-INFARCT DEMENTIA, by causing frequent blood clots in the brain. Other causes are some forms of arteriosclerosis (a group of disorders causing thickening of artery walls), vasculitis (inflammation of blood vessels), and blood clots. The inability of the heart to pump blood efficiently also can produce dementia by single or repeated episodes of ischemia (insufficient supply of blood to the brain), which cuts off oxygen to the brain. Chronic blockage of arteries leading to the brain does not cause dementia if brain tissue has not been damaged by loss of oxygen.

Lesions   A chronic subdural hematoma (large blood clot in the space between the dura, the tough outer layer of covering of the brain [meninges] and the middle meningeal layer) can produce dementia, a not-uncommon cause of dementia in older patients. Benign tumors of the brain, especially those on the orbital surface of the frontal lobe or on the medial surface of the temporal lobe, also can cause dementia, depending on their size and location. Brain tumors cause about 3 percent of the cases of dementia. Obstructive hydrocephalus (spinal fluid on the brain) may produce dementia when certain benign lesions such as some neurofibromas press on the brain. Malignant tumors of the brain also often produce dementia; only rarely does this type of dementia respond to treatment.

Normal-Pressure Hydrocephalus This uncommon disorder is characterized by a blocked flow of cerebrospinal fluid that causes a buildup of this fluid on the brain. Symptoms include dementia, urinary incontinence, and difficulty in walking. The condition may be caused by meningitis, encephalitis, or head injury. If diagnosed early in the disease, normal-pressure hydrocephalus is treatable by surgery in which a shunt is inserted to divert the fluid away from the brain.

Depression Depressed adults are often mistakenly diagnosed as demented. Symptoms of depression include sadness, difficulty thinking and concentrating, feelings of despair and inactivity, poor concentration, and inattention. When dementia and depression occur together, which can often happen, the intellectual deterioration may be more extreme. Depression is treatable.

Delirium This state of temporary mental confusion is common in older people who have lung or heart disease, long-term infections, poor nutrition, medication interactions, or hormone disorders. Emergency treatment of delirium is vital since a serious medical illness such as bacterial meningitis may be the underlying cause. Symptoms of delirium are sometimes confused with dementia, but a person who suddenly seems to have impaired thinking, who becomes disoriented or loses consciousness is more likely to be delirious rather than demented.

Progressive Degenerative Diseases Most of the progressive degenerative diseases that cause dementia are not treatable; they originate primarily in the brain and may or may not cause other neurological signs. Alzheimer's disease is the most common of these diseases. Progressive degenerative diseases causing dementia that appear with other prominent neurological signs include diseases of the BASAL GANGLIA (Parkinson's and Huntington's diseases), cerebellar and spinocerebellar degenerations, and amyotrophic lateral sclerosis (Lou Gehrig's disease).

dementia praecox This term refers to a markedly rapid mental disintegration into senility in younger patients, which usually occurs only in very old or brain-damaged individuals.

The term *demence precoce* was first used in 1852 by Benedict Augustin Morel in his book *Etudes cliniques*. It was used 46 years later by noted psychiatrist Emil Kraepelin in his textbook *Psychiatrie* to describe the progressively degenerative mental disorder accompanied by acute or subacute mental disturbance. Kraepelin noted that dementia praecox began in late adolescence or early adulthood and that half his cases began between ages 16 and 22. He believed that the disease might be caused not only by heredity but by an organic brain disease that was degenerative and not reversible.

demyelinating disorders A group of diseases characterized by the breakdown of myelin, the fatty sheath surrounding and insulating nerve fibers that interferes with nerve function. The best-known of these is MULTIPLE SCLEROSIS; others include SCHILDER'S DISEASE and DYSMYELINATION DISEASE.

In *multiple sclerosis,* lesions appear in the brain and SPINAL CORD, causing a variety of intermittent neurological symptoms. While the cause of this demyelinating disease is unknown, some researchers believe it may involve a disruption in the body's immune system or by infection from a slow-acting virus. It generally strikes adults in their 30s and 40s, and its symptoms vary: some patients live many years with few symptoms, while others experience frequent attacks. In general, however, each new attack is followed by more severe episodes. The disease is not often immediately fatal; the average duration of life after onset is about 25 years. In the terminal stage, almost every portion of the nervous system is affected.

There is no known treatment that influences the symptoms of multiple sclerosis to any degree.

Schilder's disease, also known as encephalitis periaxialis diffusa, is a rapidly progressive sheath-destructive disorder that features widespread demyelination of the NEURONS in the cerebral hemispheres of the brain. This disease occurs more often in children and ends in death within a few years of onset.

Dysmyelination disease is best exemplified by metachromatic leukodystrophy, which results in impaired development of MYELIN in the brain along with a toughening of the brain. The disorder often appears in the fiber tracts, which should myelinate after birth. The diseased tissues contain granular material that occurs from a defect in the metabolism of fatty substances appearing in the nerves, pituitary gland, liver, testes, and kidneys and that are excreted in the urine. Symptoms, which appear in infancy, childhood, or early adult life, include convulsive seizures, optic atrophy, paralyses, and DEMENTIA, or emotional abnormalities. The disease ends in death within a few years of onset. There is no satisfactory treatment.

dendrite The branched extension of a NEURON that receives nerve impulses from other nerve cells and carries them toward the cell body.

deprenyl (Eldepryl, Jumex) A substance also known as selegiline that has been used as a treatment for PARKINSON'S DISEASE and is currently being studied for the treatment of ALZHEIMER'S DISEASE. Some researchers also are studying the drug as a life span extender and a memory enhancer.

The treatment of choice in Parkinson's disease, deprenyl also has been said to improve cognition in some patients, improving attention, memory, and reaction times. The disease has a much slower progression in newly diagnosed Parkinson patients who receive deprenyl.

Deprenyl is chemically related to phenylethylamine, a substance found in chocolate, and to amphetamine. A monoamine oxidase (MAO) inhibitor, deprenyl can correct the age-related decrease in neurotransmitters. Deprenyl is the only drug that researchers know that stimulates the substantia nigra, a tiny brain region rich in dopamine-using brain cells. (A deficiency of dopamine can result in Parkinson's symptoms.) But degeneration of the neurons in the substantia nigra also has been associated with the aging process.

Therefore, deprenyl protects against the age-related degeneration of the substantia nigra and the nervous system.

depression A sense of deep and pervading sadness caused by a collision of genetics, biochemistry, and psychological factors.

The physiological basis of depression may be found in neurons in the part of the brain responsible for human emotions centered in the HYPOTHALAMUS, a cherry-sized structure that controls basic functions such as thirst, hunger, sleep, sexual desire, and body temperature.

Each nerve cell in the brain is separated by tiny gaps called synapses; neurons communicate by sending chemical messengers across these gaps to a RECEPTOR on the other side. Each neurotransmitter has a special shape that helps it fit exactly into a corresponding receptor like a key into an ignition switch. When the neurotransmitter "key" is inserted into its matching receptor's "ignition," the cell receiving the transmitter may then fire an "action potential," the electrical impulse that travels down the axon, to release its own transmitter to the next neuron. Once the message is sent, the neurotransmitter is either absorbed into the cell or burned up by enzymes patrolling the gaps.

When there are abnormally low levels of certain neurotransmitters, messages cannot get across the gaps, and communication in the brain slows down. It appears that depression occurs if there is not enough of these neurotransmitters circulating in the brain or if the neurotransmitters cannot fit into the receptors for some reason.

While there are as many as 100 different kinds of neurotransmitters, NOREPINEPHRINE, DOPAMINE, and SEROTONIN seem to be of particular importance in depression. The pathways for these neurotransmitters reach deep into many of the parts of the brain responsible for functions that are affected in depression—sleep, appetite, mood, and sexual interest.

Scientists are not sure whether depression is directly related to abnormal levels of these transmitters or whether these neurotransmitters affect yet another neurotransmitter that is even more directly involved in depression. But it is clear that neurotransmitters are related to depression because medications that boost levels of these neurotransmitters also ease depression.

Depression appears to be far more than a simple problem with the amount of neurotransmitters in the synaptic cleft. It has become clear that it is probably influenced by a profoundly complex interplay of receptor "ignition" responses and the release of the neurotransmitter "keys." It also appears that depression depends not just on the number of neurotransmitter "keys," but also the quality and availability of the receptor "ignitions."

Symptoms and Diagnostic Path

Symptoms differ from one person to the next, major depression is almost always characterized by general feelings of sadness and a total loss of pleasure in things that once brought joy. There might be sleep and eating problems or a sense of worthlessness, a lack of interest in sex, with apathy or suicidal thoughts.

A diagnosis may begin with a brief family history with a medical workup, including tests to rule out low thyroid, mononucleosis, anemia, diabetes, adrenal insufficiency, and hepatitis.

Treatment Options and Outlook

Some of the newer antidepressants do not affect the levels of all of the neurotransmitters, while they still relieve depression, and other drugs (such as cocaine) that interfere with neurotransmitter levels do not affect depression.

Moreover, antidepressants can raise neurotransmitter levels almost immediately, but depression does not improve until weeks after drug therapy has begun.

One reason behind the antidepressants' lag time could be that antidepressants may cause a decrease in number of available receptors. When this happens, it could trigger an increase in the production of neurotransmitters. Importantly, these changes do not happen right after antidepressant treatment begins; the changes in the receptors typically can take up to several weeks. This receptor change has been reported in almost all anti-depressant drug treatment and also in ELECTROCONVULSIVE THERAPY.

As many as 90 percent of people with depression can be successfully treated, usually in 12 to 14 weeks, with a combination of antidepressant medication and counseling.

Descartes, René (1596–1650) French philosopher, mathematician, and scientist who in 1637 publicized his theory that the soul and the brain were separate. His underlying belief was that the mind is not a product of the brain.

Beginning with his famous phrase, *Cogito, ergo sum* (I think, therefore I am), he described a theory of the mind that was an immaterial substance that engages in a variety of activities, including feeling, thinking, and willing.

See also BRAIN IN HISTORY.

development of the brain   The nervous system is one of the first recognizable features of a human embryo. Only three weeks after conception, the brain's earliest form—the NEURAL TUBE—appears as a tiny sheet of cells on the back of the embryo, which is then only three millimeters long (a bit thicker than a nickel). The brain begins as a swelling at one end of the neural tube, formed by a ridge of neural tissue that rises and fuses along what will be the fetal back.

Once this occurs, the cells begin to multiply at breakneck speed, creating millions of new cells each day. The brain continues to develop along patterns roughly similar to the way the brain evolved, beginning with the BRAIN STEM. By five weeks, all three main brain regions are recognizable; by seven weeks the brain and SPINAL CORD have emerged. By 10 weeks, the FOREBRAIN has begun to overlap the brain stem, and somewhat later, the CEREBELLUM begins to grow. By 12 weeks, the brain is the size of a large pea.

BRAIN CELLS are especially active during two critical periods of fetal development—between 15 and 20 weeks after conception and again at 25 weeks. The second growth spurt persists slightly less intensively until birth.

During gestation, the brain will grow into a model about two-thirds the size of an adult brain, and is the fastest-growing structure before and shortly after birth than any other part of the body. During pregnancy, NEURONS can grow at a rate of 250,000 a minute, although half die before the baby is born. Scientists suspect this elimination of neural cells may eliminate faulty cells.

This period of brain growth is one of the most sensitive times of fetal development. Damage to developing cells may occur from maternal smoking or drinking, vitamin deficiency, prenatal exposure to chemicals, or excess heat. Illnesses of the mother during pregnancy may also severely affect fetal brain cells; studies suggest that influenza or malnutrition during pregnancy may be associated with the development of SCHIZOPHRENIA in the baby.

At birth, the brain is completely formed with every structure in place, but there is still a great deal of growth to come. Each neuron must make connections to others of its own kind, and all of the cells must be insulated with MYELIN; as the neurons branch and the cells become myelinated, the brain will enlarge and gain weight. These neuronal connections become more and more complex as the child grows. In the CORTEX itself, each cell must make as many as 10,000 connections to enable the child to speak, to perceive, and to develop coherent thought.

This process is far from an isolated exercise; the external environment, genes, and other stimulation affect a cell's connections. It is at this stage that any deprivation, whether emotional or sensory, can distort the brain's healthy growth.

Six months after birth, the child's brain weight has doubled and by age five, the child's brain is nine-tenths its adult weight.

This does not mean that a newborn baby has almost as much brain power as an adult. While its neurons are in place, the vital connections between these cells have not yet been forged.

diazepam (Valium)   One of the best-known BENZODIAZEPINE tranquilizers. With its muscle relaxant and anticonvulsant properties, diazepam is used to ease tension and anxiety and to treat EPILEPSY and insomnia.

diencephalon   An anatomical division of the brain that is part of the uppermost part of the BRAIN STEM, which includes the THALAMUS; it connects via the FORNIX to the TEMPORAL LOBES and contains the HYPOTHALAMUS, the PITUITARY GLAND, and the PINEAL GLAND.

The diencephalon (which is derived from the Greek word for "divided brain") is part of the LIMBIC SYSTEM, and is located deep within the center of the brain. It is associated with several important brain structures, including the HIPPOCAMPUS and the AMYGDALA.

dimethylaminoethanol (DMAE)   This naturally occurring nutrient is found in some types of seafood and in the human brain. Studies suggest this substance may improve memory and learning, elevate mood and increase physical energy, and act as both a mild stimulant and a sleep enhancer. It is believed to improve the brain's production of ACETYLCHOLINE, which plays an important part in memory and maintaining memory ability. Overdoses of DMAE may cause INSOMNIA, HEADACHE, or muscle tension, and while no serious adverse effects have been reported, it may deepen the depression phase in manic-depression patients.

dissociation   An unconscious defense mechanism through which emotional significance and affect are separated and detached from an idea, situation, or object. Dissociation may defer or postpone experience with some emotional impact, as in selective AMNESIA.

This splitting of the normally integrated functions of consciousness (especially identity and memory) is the defining characteristic of the DISSOCIATIVE DISORDERS, which include MULTIPLE PERSONALITY DISORDER, PSYCHOGENIC AMNESIA, psychogenic FUGUE, and depersonalization disorder.

Dissociation was first mentioned by French *alieniste* (psychiatrist) Jacques Joseph Moreau de Tours in 1845 in his book about ALTERED STATES OF CONSCIOUSNESS. The first psychological elaboration of the concept of dissociation was written in 1889 by PIERRE JANET (1859–1947) in *L'Automatisme Psychologique.*

In this book, Janet describes a syndrome he calls *desegregation,* in which associated ideas split off from consciousness and exist in parallel with the dominant stream of consciousness. Janet believed this was a pathological psychological process that occurred in HYPNOSIS, hysteria, and instances of multiple personality.

The syndrome was further discussed in *Studies on Hysteria* (1895) by SIGMUND FREUD (1856–1939) and JOSEF BREUER (1842–1925), who interpreted the famous case of ANNA O. Anna, who suffered from psychosomatic problems and dissociation, had been treated for two years by Breuer. But Breuer and Freud disagreed about the nature of Anna's absences; Breuer thought they represented a form of autohypnosis, while Freud interpreted Anna's symptoms as a defense mechanism.

Freud's theory won acceptance by clinicians over the years, although Breuer's autohypnotic explanation has won converts for its explanation of early childhood creation of multiple personality.

DMAE See DIMETHYLAMINOETHANOL.

dominant hemisphere The tendency for one brain hemisphere to control the processing of information for a particular task. "Dominant hemisphere" is often used to refer to the hemisphere controlling speech.

donepezil (Aricept) A type of medication called a CHOLINESTERASE INHIBITOR used to treat mild to moderate ALZHEIMER'S DISEASE, which has generally helped patients by improving thinking, general function, and behavior. The drug works by blocking an enzyme that destroys ACETYLCHOLINE.

One of only three drugs approved for the treatment of ALZHEIMER'S DISEASE (the other two are TACRINE and RIVASTIGMINE), donepezil is available in 5 mg or 10 mg tablets and is usually given at bedtime with or without food. Individuals with Alzheimer's have generally responded well to this drug, showing improvement in cognition, general function, and behavior. More than 3.8 million people have been treated with this drug, making it the most-often prescribed Alzheimer's drug.

The drug works by blocking an enzyme that destroys acetylcholine. Animal tests suggest that it might also make a difference in less serious memory disorders; the National Institute on Aging is embarking on a study to determine if Aricept can help people with mild cognitive impairment. Fifty percent of people over age 65 with MCI will develop Alzheimer's within five years.

Side Effects
Although many patients can better tolerate Aricept, it can cause diarrhea and vomiting, nausea, insomnia, fatigue, and anorexia. These effects are mild in most cases and usually last from one to three weeks, declining with continued use of the drug.

dopamine A chemical messenger (neurotransmitter) in the brain and a member of the class of CATECHOLAMINES that affect the nervous and cardiovascular systems, metabolic rate, and body temperature. Secreted by NEURONS in the SUBSTANTIA NIGRA, the MIDBRAIN, and the HYPOTHALAMUS, dopamine is thought to play a role in controlling movements. PARKINSON'S DISEASE, a degenerative condition characterized by muscle rigidity and tremors, is due to loss of cells in the substantia nigra that release dopamine. In fact, drugs that mimic dopamine are used to treat Parkinson's, and drugs that relieve the symptoms of SCHIZOPHRENIA may also cause Parkinson-like symptoms.

Identified in the late 1950s, this NEUROTRANSMITTER is part of the biosynthetic pathway of the neurotransmitter NOREPINEPHRINE and is believed to help regulate mood; when found in excess amounts in the LIMBIC SYSTEM, it can contribute to the development of schizophrenia.

dopamine hypothesis The theory that SCHIZOPHRENIA is the result (in part) of an excess of dopaminergic transmission in the brain. Schizophrenia can be treated in part by such drugs as CHLORPROMAZINE, a dopaminergic antagonist, which can interfere with dopamine's action.

dopaminergic Those neurons or areas of the CENTRAL NERVOUS SYSTEM that use DOPAMINE to transmit signals.

Down syndrome A congenital form of mental retardation caused by an extra chromosome, characterized by distinct physical features and developmental disabilities. Down syndrome affects people of all ages, races, and economic levels, occurring once in about every 800 to 1,000 live births. More than 350,000 people in the United States have Down syndrome.

The condition was first described in 1959 by French physician Jerome Lejeune, who discovered that instead of the usual 46 chromosomes present in each cell, there were 47 in the cells of individuals with Down syndrome. Because 95 percent of all cases of Down syndrome occur because there are three copies of the 21st chromosome, it is also referred to as "trisomy 21."

While Down syndrome is usually caused by an error in cell division, two other types of chromosomal abnormalities (mosaicism and translocation) are also implicated. Regardless of the type, all people with Down syndrome have an extra portion of the number 21 chromosome present in some of their cells.

Women age 35 and older have a significantly increased risk of having a child with Down syndrome: A 35-year-old woman has a one in 400 chance of conceiving a child with Down syndrome and this chance increases gradually to one in 110 by age 40. At age 45 the incidence is about one in 35. Since many couples are postponing parenting until later in life, the incidence of Down syndrome conceptions is expected to increase.

Symptoms and Diagnostic Path

Down syndrome is usually suspected after birth as a result of the baby's appearance. Among the most common traits are low muscle tone, a flat facial profile, an upward slant to the eyes, an abnormal ear shape, a single deep crease across the center of the palm, and an excessive ability to extend the joints. Other common symptoms include a fifth finger with one furrow instead of two, small skin folds on the inner corner of the eyes, too much space between large and second toe, and an enlarged tongue compared to the size of the mouth.

Most people with Down syndrome have some level of mental retardation ranging from mild to moderate, but most children with Down syndrome learn to sit, walk, talk, play, toilet train, and do most other activities. Because speech is often delayed, careful attention should be paid to the child's hearing, as retention of fluid in the inner ear is a very common cause of hearing and speech difficulties.

Pregnant women have access to both screening and diagnostic tests. Screening tests estimate the risk of the fetus having Down syndrome, whereas diagnostic tests tell whether or not the fetus actually has the condition. Screening tests are typically offered between 15 and 20 weeks of gestation, but they can accurately detect only about 60 percent of cases. False-positive and false-negative readings are not uncommon.

Prenatal diagnosis of Down syndrome is by chorionic villus sampling (CVS), amniocentesis, and percutaneous umbilical blood sampling (PUBS), each of which carries a small risk of miscarriage. The procedures are about 98 to 99 percent accurate. Amniocentesis is usually performed between 12 and 20 weeks of gestation, CVS between eight and 12 weeks, and PUBS after 20 weeks.

Treatment Options and Outlook

Early intervention should begin shortly after birth. These programs offer parents special instruction in teaching their child language, cognitive, self-help, and social skills, and specific exercises for gross and fine motor development. Stimulation during early developmental stages improves the child's chances of developing to his or her fullest potential. Continuing education, positive public attitudes, and a stimulating home environment also promote the child's overall development and it is important to place few limitations on potential capabilities.

Because children with Down syndrome respond well to their environment, those who receive good medical care and are included in community activities can attend school, make friends, find work, participate in decisions that affect them, and make a positive contribution to society. There is a wide variation in mental abilities, behavior, and developmental progress in these children. It may be effective to emphasize concrete concepts rather than abstract ideas. Teaching tasks in a step-by-step manner with frequent reinforcement and consistent feedback has been successful.

dreams Dreaming, the sometimes-haunting mental activity that takes place during sleep, is a state of lessened consciousness, lowered metabolism, and limited muscular activity. But scientists do not yet understand how we dream or what the biological function could be.

Some believe that dreams represent the right brain talking to itself; others believe dreams are the way the brain discharges nonproductive thoughts; still others insist dreams are the brain's creative method of solving its own problems. Sigmund Freud believed dreams were the brain's way of expressing a person's deepest desires. Finally, the more purely biological explanation is that the brain is trying to understand random firings of NEURONS during sleep.

Most scientists do suspect that dreams allow mental impressions, feelings, and ideas absorbed during the day to be sorted out; the content of dreams often closely represents the day's preoccupations, although the ideas and memories are distorted by the lack of a conscious mind.

Dreaming is believed to occur only during certain periods (the rapid eye movement, or REM stage of sleep), which last for about 30 minutes four or five times a night. Later in the sleep cycle, one spends more and more time in REM SLEEP. During this stage, blood flow and brain temperature rise, and there are sudden changes in the heart rate and blood pressure. All this may indicate the brain is restoring itself for further activity. During REM sleep, the brain is actually more active than during waking periods. This is why REM sleep is called PARADOXICAL SLEEP.

While people who are awakened during REM sleep report vivid dreams, those who awaken normally may not remember dreaming at all.

REM sleep occurs far more often in young babies and after HEAD INJURY, which may indicate the important role that dreaming plays in promoting brain development and repair. Whether dreams serve important psychological functions is still controversial.

The average person experiences about 300,000 dreams over a lifetime, spending about 20 years of life in sleep.

drugs and memory   There are a number of drugs that interfere with memory. Any medication that causes drowsiness is capable of affecting memory. Almost all psychotropic drugs can interfere with cer-

tain components of memory, including the benzodiazepines, neuroleptics, antidepressants, and lithium, although these different drug classes may not cause the same type of memory deficit. In fact, all drugs in the same class don't all cause the same type or amount of memory loss. For example, one type of antidepressant that interferes with serotonin reuptake may improve memory, compared to the tricyclic antidepressants that interfere with memory.

Neurological drugs have been less extensively studied. All the older anti-epileptic drugs are considered harmful, unlike the novel compounds Vigabatrin and Lamotrigine. Drugs used in the treatment of PARKINSON'S DISEASE should be considered as memory-enhancing, unlike the atropine derivatives, which typically induce AMNESIA.

Many substances not used in neuropsychiatry also may cause memory problems, including quinidine, naproxen, opiates, antibiotics like clioquinol or the quinolones, antihistamines, and interferons.

The best-known of all drugs that affect memory is ethanol (the alcohol contained in alcoholic beverages). Ethanol interferes with the capacity to learn, and slows down mental functions that create defective recording and storing of memory.

Other drugs that can affect memory include antihypertensives (blood pressure drugs), painkillers, insulin, beta blockers (especially those used to control glaucoma), methyldopa, seasickness patches and certain anti-epileptic drugs.

DTs   See DELIRIUM TREMENS.

dura mater   The thickest, outermost of the three membranes surrounding and protecting the brain and SPINAL CORD. It includes two layers; the inner dura extends downward between the CEREBRAL HEMISPHERES to form the falx cerebri, forward between the CEREBRUM and CEREBELLUM to form the tentorium. The inner dura is separated from the arachnoid by a thin film of fluid.

dysarthria   A speech problem caused by damage to or disease of the musculature controlling the voice apparatus; unlike APHASIA, patients with dysarthria have no problems with the speech center in the brain.

Symptoms and Diagnostic Path

Dysarthria is difficult, poorly articulated speech, such as slurring, whereas aphasia involves a problem in expressing or comprehending written or spoken language. Diagnostic tests may include a CT or MRI scan of the head, and EEG X-rays of the skull.

Treatment Options and Outlook

There is no specific treatment, although medication or surgery may restore the ability to speak by treating the underlying disease. Speech therapy may also be of help. Patients' family and friends should be encouraged to speak slowly and use hand gestures when necessary, providing enough time for patients to express themselves. Medications that are causing the problem should be stopped, if possible.

dysautonomia   A dysfunction of the autonomic nervous system (ANS). The autonomic nervous system maintains a stable internal environment, managing most bodily systems, including the cardiovascular system, gastrointestinal, urinary and bowel functions, temperature, reproduction, metabolic, and endocrine systems. This system is also responsible for the flight-or-fight response.

Symptoms and Diagnostic Path

Symptoms that may be related to problems with the ANS include absence of tears, skin blotching, excess sweating, insensitivity to pain, and excess growth. There are many disorders that cause dysautonomia, including SHY-DRAGER SYNDROME, PARKINSON'S DISEASE, mitral valve prolapse, Chagas' disease, and many other disorders.

Familial dysautonomia (FD) is characterized by widespread sensory and ANS dysfunction caused by incomplete development of sensory and autonomic brain cells. FD has been noted only in individuals of Ashkenazi Jewish extraction. Individuals with FD cannot produce overflow tears with emotional crying, and they may have an inappropriate

perception of heat, pain, and taste. Other problems experienced by individuals with FD include excessive sweating, vomiting, frequent pneumonia, speech and motor incoordination, episodic high blood pressure and low blood pressure when standing suddenly, poor growth, and scoliosis.

Treatment Options and Outlook

FD patients can be expected to function independently if treatment is begun early and major disabilities avoided.

dyskinesia   Abnormal muscular movements caused by a brain disorder, causing uncontrollable jerking or twitching. The disorder may affect the entire body or just one group of muscles. Types of dyskinesia include CHOREA (jerking movements), athetosis (writhing), choreoathetosis (a combination of jerking and writhing), tics (repetitive movements), TREMORS, or myoclonus (muscle spasms).

dyslexia   A specific reading disability characterized by poor verbal memory and problems in coping with written symbols. Research suggests that problems in encoding are the cause of a dyslexic person's problems with verbal memory. Other theories have pointed to a specific, sometimes inherited, neurological disorder, emotional disturbance, minor visual defects, or a lack of attention. Some scientists using clinical tests of many more memory measures have challenged the long-held view that verbal memory problems of dyslexic children are related to their attention span, memory strategy use, or ability to retrieve memories. But the relationship between verbal memory and reading problems is still unclear.

In a Nova University study of 122 children eight to ten years old, the dyslexic subjects differed from normals only in their ability to encode words—to store the word in memory when they hear it. Both dyslexic and normal children had the same attention spans.

While some researchers had believed that dyslexic subjects' memory problems are actually a retrieval problem (they encode the words, but then can't recall them), researchers found that both normal and dyslexic children improved at the same rate when given memory cues, indicating that retrieval is not a problem.

Symptoms and Diagnostic Path

Some 90 percent of dyslexics are male; most of the time, their intelligence is normal but the attainment of reading skills lags far behind other abilities and overall IQ. Usually dyslexic children can read musical notes or numbers much more easily than letters. While many children in the first two elementary grades make common mistakes in reversing letters or words, dyslexic children continue to make these errors. Letters are transposed ("saw" for "was") and spelling errors are common. Writing from dictation may be hard, although most can copy sentences.

Treatment Options and Outlook

Early diagnosis is critical in maintaining a child's self-esteem and to avoid any added frustrations. Specific remedial methods can help the child develop tricks to cope with the disorder, and praise for success is crucial. With the right support and training, dyslexics can usually overcome their problems.

dysmyelination disease   A rare type of MYELIN disease best exemplified by metachromatic leukodystrophy, causing poor development of myelin in the brain along with a toughening of the WHITE MATTER of the CEREBRUM and CEREBELLUM.

The disorder often appears in the fiber tracts, which should myelinate after birth. The diseased tissues contain granular material that results from a defect in the metabolism of fatty substances (sulfatides) appearing in the nerves, PITUITARY GLAND, liver, testes, and kidneys and is excreted in the urine.

Symptoms and Diagnostic Path

Symptoms, which can appear in infancy, childhood, or early adult life, include convulsive seizures, optic atrophy, paralyses, and DEMENTIA or emotional abnormalities. The disease ends in death within a few years of onset.

Treatment Options and Outlook

There is no satisfactory treatment.

dysphasia   A term used to describe a problem with the ability to select words (and/or to comprehend and read) that is caused by damage to parts of the brain that control speech and comprehension.

See also AGRAPHIA; ALEXIA; APHASIA; APRAXIA.

dystonia   Abnormal muscle rigidity resulting in painful muscle spasms, fixed posture, or strange movements. Generalized dystonia usually is caused by neurological disorders, such as PARKINSON'S DISEASE or STROKE, or may be a feature of SCHIZOPHRENIA. It may also be a side effect of ANTIPSYCHOTIC DRUGS.

Early Language Milestone Scale (ELMS) An easily administered screening instrument that provides an indication of delay in expressive and receptive language up to the age of three years.

Eccles, Sir John Carew (1903–1997) The Nobel Prize–winning Australian scientist who was one of the 20th century's pioneers in discovering and exploring how messages are transmitted in the brain and nervous system. Eccles showed that the excitement of a nerve cell causes one kind of SYNAPSE to release a neurotransmitter into the next cell that expands the pores in nerve membranes. (See NEUROTRANSMITTERS.) These expanded pores allow sodium ions to pass into the neighboring cell, reversing the polarity of electric charge, which is conducted from one cell to another as a nerve impulse.

Sir John, an Australian-born former college pole-vaulter, pursued scientific study and research in Australia, Britain, New Zealand, and the State University of New York at Buffalo, before moving to Switzerland. Sir John, who shared the 1963 Nobel Prize in physiology or medicine, tackled some of the most fundamental problems of his time, working toward an ultimate understanding of the mind and consciousness. His Nobel Prize was awarded for his discovery of the chemical means by which impulses are communicated or suppressed by nerve cells.

Sir John was born Jan. 27, 1903, in Melbourne, the son of teachers. By age 18, he had acquired an interest in the link between the action of the brain and the nature of consciousness. After graduating in medicine from Melbourne University, he went on a Rhodes Scholarship to Oxford University to study under one of the great figures in brain research, Sir Charles Sherrington, who is credited with coining the term *synapse.* After research in the 1930s with Sir Charles on switching on and off of nerve impulses, Sir John returned home. During World War II, he was involved in medical work in behalf of his country's military effort. His early work focused on cells in the spinal cord that control the action of muscles; later he moved closer to the centers of consciousness in the brain.

Sir John stood out among the scientists who produced the growing modern appreciation of the chemical mechanisms underlying the action of the brain and nervous system. He did not consider the brain and the mind to be the same thing. He believed he could explain his own body and brain, he once said, but he could not explain his own existence. The complexity of the brain so impressed Eccles that he called the mind the so-called ghost in the machine, an incorporeal essence in the body.

Sir John was knighted by Queen Elizabeth II in 1958 and held many other honors. His marriage to Irene Frances Miller, with whom he had nine children, ended in divorce after 40 years. He later married scientist Helena Taborikova.

echoencephalography A type of painless, noninvasive test that uses the transmission and reflection of ultrasonic waves to create a detailed visual image of the brain, detecting the position of the primary membranes within the brain.

Procedure

An ultrasonic transducer applied to the head just above an ear will receive echoes from the membranes around the ventricles and midline. The position of these membranes may be abnormal if the brain structures are distorted by a tumor, clot, or abnormal collection of cerebrospinal fluid in the ventricles.

Echoencephalographs have been used since the 1950s to examine patients with concussion or suspected cranial damage. In addition to the transducer, the device includes a high-voltage pulse generator, an amplifier to augment the echoes, and a processing circuit to present the echoes to the cathode ray tube. Sometimes the apparatus has two transducers so that scans are presented simultaneously from each side of the head.

Risks and Complications
There are no risks associated with the procedure.

echoic memory The registration of sounds. This form of memory lasts up to four seconds. The long-term form of echoic memory is called AUDITORY MEMORY.

Ecstasy (MDMA) An illegal stimulant drug that can kill nerve cells in the brain, also known as 3,4 methylenedioxymethamphetamine (MDMA). The drug, related to the drugs mescaline and amphetamine, is also known as "Adam," "XTC," or just "E."

Ecstasy was first synthesized and patented in 1914 by the German drug company Merck as an appetite suppressant; in the 1970s, it was given to psychotherapy patients because it helped them talk about their feelings. This practice was stopped in 1986 when animal studies showed that Ecstasy caused brain damage.

Users say Ecstasy lowers their inhibitions and relaxes them, increases awareness and feelings of pleasure, and gives people energy. However, after taking MDMA some people report side effects such as headaches, chills, eye twitching, jaw clenching, blurred vision, and nausea. Unlike the drug LSD, low doses of MDMA do not cause people to hallucinate.

Ecstasy gained national attention when it was the drug of choice at dance parties, called "raves."

In a survey taken in 2000, 8.2 percent of 12th graders, 5.4 percent of 10th graders, and 3.1 percent of eighth graders reported that they had used MDMA at least once within the year.

MDMA appears to have several effects on the brain, boosting the levels of the NEUROTRANSMITTER called SEROTONIN and then depleting it, and causing an indirect decrease in the amount of the neurotransmitter called DOPAMINE. Recent data suggest that MDMA may be toxic to the brain, according to brain scans of people who had used Ecstasy an average of 200 times over five years. In fact, those who used the drug more often had more brain damage than less frequent users. Moreover, memory tests of people who have taken Ecstasy as compared to non-drug users have shown that the Ecstasy users had lower scores. Using an imaging technique called positron emission tomography (PET SCAN), researchers found a 20 percent to 60 percent loss in healthy serotonin cells in the drug users, which could affect a person's abilities to remember and to learn. Scientists do not yet know if this damage is permanent, if those damaged cells will replace themselves, or if this loss of cells affects behavior or the ability to think.

See also AMPHETAMINES.

EEG The abbreviation for ELECTROENCEPHALOGRAM. See also ELECTROENCEPHALOGRAPHY.

effortful processing Effortful encoding and retrieval of memory. This effortful processing uses a great deal of attentional capacity and therefore disrupts—and is disrupted by—the simultaneous performance of another attention-demanding task. Effortful processing probably always requires planning, therefore it is likely to be damaged by frontal cortex lesions that disrupt the ability to plan.

Egas Moniz, António Caetano de Abreu Freire (1874–1955) A Nobel Prize–winning Portuguese neurologist and politician who performed the first LEUCOTOMY, a radical approach to the treatment of mental illnesses. (The leucotomy is similar to a

LOBOTOMY, in which the white fibers connecting the FRONTAL LOBE to the rest of the brain are cut.)

By the 1930s, he had already established a reputation for the development of cerebral ANGI-OGRAPHY as a diagnostic technique, which allowed doctors to visualize blood vessels in the brain by using radioactive tracers.

In 1935, he attended an international neurology conference where he saw a presentation on the frontal lobes of the brain and the effects of removing them from chimpanzees. His theory was that some forms of mental illness were caused by nerve cells that "stuck" and led to repeated behavior; he thought that if these cells could be destroyed, the patient might recover.

A few months after the conference, he and his assistants tried the first leucotomy by giving a patient a series of alcohol injections to the frontal lobe through holes drilled in the skull. After trying this method on six more patients, they switched to cutting the lobe with a wire. Nothing in the brain was removed, but the brain connections were severed.

The next year, he published the results of his first 20 operations on patients who had suffered from anxiety, depression, and schizophrenia. His article was well received despite the fact that his follow-up extended only to a few days after surgery.

He described the procedure in the 1936 text-book of psychosurgery, *Experimental Surgery in the Treatment of Certain Psychoses*. His work inspired American neurologists Walter Freeman and James Watts to perform the first American leucotomies.

He shared the 1949 Nobel Prize in physiology and medicine for his leucotomy work, but the procedure was generally abandoned by the 1950s, when the first of the antipsychotic drugs were introduced.

Egas Moniz served as professor of neurology at Lisbon University from 1911 until his retirement in 1944, while also pursuing a successful political career as ambassador to Spain (1917–18) and as Portugal's foreign minister at the Paris Peace Conference (1919–20).

In 1955 he was shot in the leg by a patient, which left him confined to a wheelchair. He died in 1955.

eidetic memory A very strong afterimage that allows a person to duplicate a picture mentally and describe it in detail after looking at it, similar to the idea of a "photographic memory." Among children, the ability to form eidetic images is rare (no more than 10 percent of children can), and it is even rarer after adolescence.

An eidetic person not only can imagine an object that is not there, but behaves as if it really can be seen, either with closed eyes or while looking at some surface that serves as a convenient background for the image. While a particular object can be recalled eidetically immediately after its disappearance or after a lapse of minutes, days, or years, spontaneously appearing eidetic images also have been reported. Sometimes eidetic images and the objects they represent have different colors, forms, size, position, and richness of detail, or the objects may be reproduced in almost photographic detail and fidelity.

Most experts suspect that eidetic imagery is not a different kind of visual memory, but just a greater skill in the ability to form visual images that everyone possesses to some degree.

While eidetic imagery is most likely the source of the concept of a photographic memory, there are differences in the two concepts. An eidetic image fades soon after one sees the original image and does not stay with a person over time. The image is subjective, and the details of greatest interest to the person are the ones most easily reproduced. Moreover, a person cannot form an eidetic image in one second, as a camera can snap a photo; several seconds are required to scan the picture. Once the picture has faded away, eidetic images cannot be retrieved. Those who can form eidetic images do not seem to be able to use their special ability to improve long-term memory.

Phenomena corresponding to visual eidetic images are believed to exist in other sense fields as well, but research has not uncovered much about their nature, causes, and significance.

electrical stimulation of the brain Stimulating various areas of the cortex produces a range of responses from patients; however, only stimulation of the temporal lobes elicits meaningful, integrated experiences, including sound, movement and color, far more detailed, accurate and specific than normal recall.

Stimulating one side of the brain may bring back a certain song to one patient, the memory of a moment in a garden listening to a mother calling her child to another. Interestingly, stimulating the same point in the brain elicits the same memory every time.

See also EMOTIONS AND MEMORY.

electroencephalogram (EEG) A recorded tracing of wave patterns of electrical brain activity obtained through electrodes placed on the skull.

The machine that records this activity is known as an encephalograph. The pattern of the tracings reflects the state of the patient's brain and the level of consciousness in a characteristic way.

See also ELECTROENCEPHALOGRAPHY.

electroencephalography A diagnostic method for determining the electrical activity of the brain, revealing a person's mental state, possible diseases, and level of anesthesia during surgery. It also can be used to determine BRAIN DEATH.

Procedure

On an ongoing basis—even during sleep—electrical signals are constantly flashing throughout the brain; these signals can be detected and measured by an encephalograph (EEG). Because the tissues of the body conduct electricity well, metal sensors attached to the skin of the head can detect the signals passing from the brain through the muscles and skin. The signals are amplified and displayed on a monitor or paper chart. These devices show that electrical signals in the brain do not come steadily but are produced in short bursts; the shape of the waves changes with the activity level of the brain. The tracings reveal that the electrical activity of the brain varies with the degree of alertness, depending on whether the subject is excited, relaxed, or in a deep sleep.

In normal people, there are four types of BRAIN WAVES: alpha, beta, theta, and delta waves. The EEG brain-wave patterns include ALPHA WAVES (the pri-

mary pattern of an alert adult with closed eyes); the BETA WAVES (lower, faster activity while a person is concentrating on an outside stimulus); DELTA WAVES (sleep patterns also found in infants; rarely, they are also caused by brain tumors); and THETA WAVES (dominant pattern in children ages two to five and in psychopaths; also produced by frustration).

Supplanted today by imaging studies used to detect brain pathology, the EEG is now used primarily to identify abnormal brain function that cannot be otherwise identified. It is therefore best used to evaluate transient states, such as SEIZURES; evolving conditions, such as HERPES SIMPLEX ENCEPHALITIS; or global disorders, such as DEMENTIA. Only a few EEG patterns can be used to diagnose a particular disease, but the tracings can be helpful in deciding among several disease alternatives.

Risks and Complications

This painless technique has no side effects.

embolism, cerebral A blockage of one of the arteries that supplies blood to the brain, one of the most common causes of STROKE. An embolus may be a blood clot, bubble of air or gas, bacteria, bone marrow, fat, and so on.

Symptoms and Diagnostic Path

If the embolus causes a stroke, the symptoms depend on which part of the brain has been affected; it may cause an inability to speak, inability to walk, loss of consciousness, or visual problems.

Treatment Options and Outlook

Surgery (such as balloon angioplasty) to open the blocked arteries may be tried; if surgery is not possible, drugs designed to break up blood clots, and anticoagulant drugs (to prevent the formation of clots) may be given.

Survival depends on the speed with which blood flow is reestablished; if the embolus can be removed, long-term outlook for the patient is good.

emotions and the brain Far from being a state of consciousness divorced from the physical brain, a person's emotions are produced by chemicals exquisitely intertwined with the physiological processes of the body so that in the truest sense what affects the body affects the mind and emotions, and vice versa.

The center of emotions in the brain can be found in the LIMBIC SYSTEM where the vast panoply of emotions is regulated through the release of excitatory and inhibitory NEUROTRANSMITTERS: Pleasure may be linked with chemical signals produced by the release of NORADRENALIN, and pain is associated with many neurotransmitters. Mood appears to be linked with SEROTONIN and dopamine.

In response to a variety of stimuli, emotions arise in the limbic system, traveling along neural pathways to the FRONTAL LOBES of the CORTEX, where feelings are monitored and interpreted. These two brain structures next influence the HYPOTHALAMUS, which transmits the messages that trigger appropriate physical responses.

The latest research suggests that different parts of the brain may process emotions differently. Scientists have found that the frontal lobes of the left hemisphere display more electrical activity when subjects experience positive emotions such as enthusiasm or happiness, and the frontal lobes of the right hemisphere display more electrical activity when the subjects experience negative emotions such as disgust or sadness.

While lower animals are guided by primitive instincts and may experience only rudimentary feelings, most mammals probably do have a richer range of emotional feelings. Evidence of the limbic system's so-called pleasure center was discovered in 1953 by scientists at McGill University, when a rat incessantly self-stimulated an area of the brain called the septum in the front part of the hypothalamus. Further tests revealed that not just rats, but rabbits, dogs, dolphins, monkeys, and even humans experienced intense pleasure when this part of the brain is stimulated.

The limbic system controls not just pleasure but also a wide variety of emotions with many subtle shades. Separate emotions do not exist in individual, isolated areas of the brain, however; instead, emotional reactions appear to develop from a wide range of neural pathways throughout the limbic system, working together to produce a symphony of human emotion.

encephalitis An often-fatal inflammation of the brain that can cause damage on both sides (especially the MEDIAL TEMPORAL LOBE) of the orbital FRONTAL LOBE. Many times, the MENINGES (membranes that cover and enclose the brain) are also affected.

Symptoms and Diagnostic Path

While an encephalitis attack may be so mild (headache, fever) that the patient does not notice anything amiss, more often it is a serious condition and accompanied by alarming symptoms (confusion, seizure, convulsions).

In the United States, most cases of encephalitis are caused by enteroviruses, herpes simplex virus (types 1 and 2), rabies, or viruses transmitted via the bite of an infected tick, mosquito, or other insect. Lyme disease, a bacterial infection spread by tick bite, also can cause encephalitis.

Herpes simplex encephalitis (HSE) causes about 10 percent of all encephalitis cases, more than half of which (untreated) are fatal. While about 30 percent occur during a primary herpes infection, most are caused by an earlier infection that has reactivated.

Powassan encephalitis is caused by the bite of a tick, and is fatal in up to 15 percent of cases.

In addition, four common types of mosquito-transmitted viral encephalitis are seen in the United States: equine, LaCrosse, St. Louis, and West Nile virus encephalitis.

Equine encephalitis affects both horses and humans, although it is fairly rare; fewer than 10 human cases are seen in the United States each year. There are both eastern and western types. Eastern equine encephalitis appears mostly in freshwater swamps of the eastern seaboard and along the Gulf Coast.

In humans, symptoms appear between four and 10 days, and include sudden fever, flu-like muscle pains, and headache of increasing severity. This is followed by coma; about half of infected patients die from the disorder.

Western equine encephalitis occurs in rural areas of the western and central plains states. Symptoms begin five to 10 days after infection. Children, particularly those under a year, are affected more severely and may develop permanent brain damage. Death occurs about 3 percent of the time.

LaCrosse encephalitis occurs most often in Illinois, Wisconsin, Indiana, Ohio, Minnesota, and Iowa, although it also has been reported in the southeastern and mid-Atlantic regions. Most cases affect children under age 16. Symptoms include vomiting, headache, fever, and lethargy, which appear five to 10 days after infection. Severe complications include seizure, coma, and permanent brain damage. About 100 cases of LaCrosse encephalitis are reported each year.

St. Louis encephalitis can occur throughout most areas of the country. Generally milder in children than in adults, elderly adults are at highest risk of developing severe disease. Symptoms typically appear seven to 10 days after infection and include headache and fever. In more severe cases, symptoms also include confusion and disorientation, tremors, convulsions (especially in the very young), and coma.

West Nile encephalitis is usually transmitted by a bite from an infected mosquito, although it also can occur after transplantation of an infected organ or transfusions of infected blood or blood products. It was first diagnosed in U.S. patients in 1999; 284 people are known to have died from the virus the following year. By 2003, there were 9,862 reported cases of human West Nile encephalitis, with a total of 560 deaths over five years. Symptoms resemble the flu, including fever, headache, and joint pain. Some patients may develop a skin rash and swollen lymph glands, while others may not show any symptoms at all. Elderly adults and people with weakened immune systems are at highest risk for serious complications.

A diagnosis can be determined from symptoms plus results of BRAIN SCANS, an EEG (ELECTROEN-CEPHALOGRAM), and a LUMBAR PUNCTURE (a sample of SPINAL FLUID). Blood tests may also be necessary.

Treatment Options and Outlook

Acyclovir and ganciclovir are two types of antiviral drugs currently used to treat viral encephalitis. Very mild cases of encephalitis may be managed at home, with plenty of fluids, bed rest, and painkillers to reduce fever and headache. More severe cases may require hospitalization.

Anticonvulsants may be prescribed to stop or prevent seizures; sedatives may help calm severely ill patients; antinausea drugs can help with vomit-

ing and corticosteroids can reduce brain swelling. Patients with breathing difficulties may need breathing support. Patients who have had severe brain inflammation may need physical, speech, and occupational therapy once the acute illness has passed.

See also ENCEPHALITIS LETHARGICA.

encephalitis lethargica An epidemic form of ENCEPHALITIS (inflammation of the brain) that has not been seen in major outbreaks since the 1920s. Occasional isolated cases do still occur.

About 40 percent of all patients died during the epidemics; those who survived developed postencephalitic PARKINSONISM, a movement disorder marked by symptoms of tremor, rigidity, and disturbed eye movements.

In the 1920s epidemic, the disease affected up to 5 million people, killing one-third of its victims and devastating the lives of hundreds of thousands more. Survivors were often left trapped inside bodies they could no longer control. The epidemic raged for 10 years, and then in 1928 the disease suddenly vanished as mysteriously as it had first appeared. Some doctors believe another epidemic will return in the future. Eighty years later, its cause still unknown, the disease is still one of the world's greatest medical mysteries.

In the 1960s, neurologist Oliver Sacks started working in a hospital unit occupied by survivors of the disease. Sacks knew that the virus had damaged the part of their brain that regulates movement, but he was convinced patients were mentally intact. As a last resort, he tried a revolutionary new drug called L-Dopa, and amazingly, patients seemed to recover. However, seemingly unable to cope with normal life, all the patients eventually returned to their lethargic state.

Sacks believes encephalitis lethargica may have inspired the myths of Sleeping Beauty and Rip Van Winkle, and believes that there is a history of smaller epidemics of this disease occurring over the last 500 years. If the 1920s epidemic was not a unique episode in history, many experts believe it is likely it will return again.

Symptoms and Diagnostic Path

Primary symptom is lethargy and drowsiness (hence, the popular name "sleeping sickness") together with symptoms that appear with encephalitis: HEADACHE, fever and prostration, HALLUCINATIONS, confusion, paralysis, disturbed behavior, and problems in speech, memory, and eye movement.

Treatment Options and Outlook
There is no effective treatment for this condition.

encephalomyelitis   Inflammation of the brain and SPINAL CORD that can permanently damage the NERVOUS SYSTEM. Encephalomyelitis develops as a complication in about one out of every 1,000 cases of measles, usually appearing about three days after the rash. It may also rarely appear after other viral infections, such as chickenpox, rubella (German measles), or infectious mononucleosis, or after vaccination against rabies.

About 10 to 20 percent of patients will die; those who recover may experience permanent damage to the nervous system, including MENTAL RETARDATION, EPILEPSY, paralysis, pituitary problems, loss of sensation, or incontinence.

Symptoms and Diagnostic Path
Symptoms include fever, HEADACHE, drowsiness, confusion, SEIZURES, partial paralysis, or COMA. Diagnostic tests include blood tests and magnetic resonance imaging (MRI).

Treatment Options and Outlook
There is no cure for this disease, but corticosteroid drugs can reduce inflammation, and anticonvulsant drugs can control seizures.

encephalon   The anatomical name of the BRAIN; it is rarely used.

encephalopathy   Any degenerative disease of the brain. This is a nonspecific term; there are numerous causes of encephalopathy, some of which are progressive and some reversible. Encephalopathy can range from barely discernible to so severe as to cause coma or death.

One example of a potentially reversible encephalopathy occurs with liver disease. When liver function falls to a certain point, molecules that are toxic to the brain cannot be cleared from the blood, and mental function deteriorates. If the liver condition can be improved, normal brain function may return.

Boxer's encephalopathy is an example of irreversible brain damage caused by repeated blows to the head.

In addition, various toxic substances, such as heavy metals (lead), infections, and injuries, can cause encephalopathy. WERNICKE'S ENCEPHALOPATHY is a degenerative condition caused by a lack of thiamine (B$_1$) and is most often found in alcoholics.

encoding   The process by which information is translated into electrical impulses in the brain. In order for a new memory trace (engram) to be formed, information must be translated into this code.

There are two main kinds of encoding—maintenance and elaborative encoding. *Maintenance encoding* consists of repeating word chunks over and over, which is good for recognition but usually is not enough for recall. *Elaborative encoding* may take several forms:

- reorganizing chunks by classifying and categorizing them so that they can be associated more easily with ideas already held in long-term memory
- associating chunks with images
- changing chunks for easier repetition (for example, changing them into rhymes)
- noting distinctive features of a chunk
- rehearsing and self-testing

Encoding can be understood best by looking at how a person remembers words—visually, acoustically, or semantically (having to do with meaning). Because of the multifaceted nature of words, there is some flexibility in how they can be represented in memory. If a person wanted to memorize the word *chair,* for example, the brain could devise a code based on visual, acoustic, or semantic properties (or a combination of any or all three).

endarterectomy The most commonly performed surgical technique to remove plaque from inside the carotid artery. This plaque can interfere with blood flow to the brain or be the source of particles that break off and flow to the brain. Studies show it may help those whose carotid arteries are narrowed by at least 60 percent.

Such plaque formation is a common disease called ATHEROSCLEROSIS that often occurs in the neck arteries to the brain, especially where the two branches meet. There are two carotid arteries supplying blood to the brain; if fatty plaques clog one of them, it can shut off blood flow, causing brain tissue damage and STROKE. Obstructed carotid arteries that cause no symptoms are usually diagnosed during a physical exam; the physician hears a rushing sound when holding the stethoscope to the person's neck.

Carotid endarterectomy is usually performed after TRANSIENT ISCHEMIC ATTACKS to prevent a stroke; it is sometimes performed during the first few hours of an evolving ischemic stroke.

Blockage may recur after surgery, but this is uncommon; the operation is usually successful because it eliminates further transient ischemic attacks and reduces the chance of stroke.

Procedure

In the procedure, surgeons make an incision in the neck and cut away the fatty plaque blocking blood flow. However, carotid endarterectomy is not recommended for everyone with narrowed carotid arteries. Once a possible block has been identified by a physician, more tests (ultrasounds or angiograms) must chart the extent of the problem.

While scientists have long understood that such surgery benefits people who show symptoms of, or who have suffered, a stroke, it has only recently been shown to be valuable in treating patients with no symptoms despite a severe constriction. People with no symptoms who underwent carotid endarterectomy had only a 4.8 percent chance of stroke five years later; this is significantly lower than the 10.6 percent risk for those patients who had received standard treatment for narrowed carotid arteries with no surgery. This surgery has now been shown to be superior to medical treatment in patients with arteries that are narrowed by 70 percent or more.

Risks and Complications

While the procedure has a high success rate, it also has risks. Active heart disease may make the risks of this operation too great; chronic high blood pressure should be corrected before surgery begins. Experts point out the importance of seeking an experienced surgeon to perform the surgery. An inexperienced surgeon could sharply increase a patient's risk of suffering a stroke or of dying as a result of the procedure. For that reason, the National Institute of Neurological Disorders and Stroke recommends that patients have the operation only at medical centers with complication rates of 3 percent or less.

The timing of the procedure is controversial. In the past, scientists were concerned that a sudden restoration of blood flow to the brain might cause a more serious hemorrhage; often, surgery was delayed for days or weeks after a stroke. However, many surgeons are now comfortable with operating immediately; early surgical intervention could prevent a more serious stroke.

In some people, the combined risk of diagnostic ARTERIOGRAPHY plus the surgical procedure may be higher than nonsurgical therapy such as blood-thinning medication. Risk is highest for those with acute stroke or a stroke in evolution. It is lowest for those with no stroke symptoms at the time of surgery.

endorphin One of the brain's natural OPIATES produced by the PITUITARY GLAND and involved in a wide variety of body processes, including pain control and emotions. Endorphins are chemically similar to morphine. In 1973, scientists located a variety of opiate receptors in the body where morphine acted, which led to the realization that the body must therefore produce its own opiates. This discovery led to the identification of protein molecules named endorphins (for endogenous morphines), produced by the body that also acts at these same opiate receptor sites.

While researchers are still studying the role of endorphins in the body, they have outlined their role in mood, pain mediation, euphoria, stress, and regulating intestinal contractions. Endorphins have also been implicated in the release of hormones from the pituitary gland, such as growth hormone and gonadotropin hormones, which act on the sex organs.

It is believed that both addiction and tolerance to narcotic drugs are caused by the drug's suppression of the body's own endorphins; when the narcotic drug is then stopped, the body's own stores of endorphins is depleted, and withdrawal symptoms appear because the body cannot mediate pain as well. It has been demonstrated that acupuncture and possibly some forms of meditation can control pain by stimulating the release of endorphins and enkephalins.

engram   The physical basis of memory, also known as a memory trace, this is a unit of information encoded as a pattern of lowered resistance or increased conductance to electrical impulses resulting in an increased readiness to respond to NEUROTRANSMITTERS. The engram is believed to exist in a network of nerve cells as the result of the consolidation of memory. Memories seem to be encoded in the brain's cells, which convert chemical signals to electrical signals and then are converted back to chemical signals again.

Information is carried inside a neuron by electrical pulses, but when the signal reaches the end of the axon, it must be carried across the synaptic gap by chemicals called neurotransmitters. On the other side of the synapse, another dendrite containing RECEPTORS that recognize these transmitting molecules registers the signal. If enough signals are registered, then the second cell fires an action potential. A single neuron can receive signals from thousands of other neurons, and its axon can send signals to thousands more.

When a person experiences a new event, such as meeting a new person, an engram is activated in some way, and certain brain cells light up. In order to store this memory of the new person, there must be a way to save the memory—to make new connections between neurons to create a new circuit to serve as a symbol. By reactivating the circuit, the brain can retrieve the memory. The person is

recognized when something evokes a neural pattern similar to one already stored in the brain. A picture of the person in a photo album might cause a pattern of neurons to light up that resembled the patterns joined together during the initial experience. However, the brain's circuits are not permanent; circuits break up and form new connections as knowledge is gained.

Engrams also are formed on tasks performed over and over again. To perform the task, the appropriate engram must be activated. The appropriate area of the brain then reads this engram, and the task is performed. Engrams are not constructed easily; the more complex the activity, the more rehearsals it takes to form a reliable engram and most probably a larger number of neurons is involved.

Because all memories are not stored the same way, not all memories are remembered equally well; some memories have stronger traces. What remains in long-term memory has been used many times, recalled and stored differently with different references so that the trace can be thoroughly integrated.

Every time a memory is retrieved, it appears in a different context and is altered by the new recall. The more time that has elapsed since the memory was first encoded, the greater the chance that the memory trace has been changed.

Today, scientists believe that engrams are encoded in the neurons throughout the brain. Like any circuit, electrically stimulating any neuron in an engram circuit could produce the entire memory.

enkephalin   Protein molecules that are produced in the brain, where they act as one type of the body's own (endogenous) OPIATES. They are believed to produce sedation, affect mood, and stimulate motivation. Originally believed to be the same as ENDORPHINS, they were reclassified when it was determined that they were released from different nerve endings. They are part of the endorphin peptide and, in general, activate the same opioid receptors.

enzyme   An organic compound that interacts with other substances to form a new chemical, either by synthesizing or degrading it. Brain function depends on chemical messages transmitted from cell to cell by NEUROTRANSMITTERS which depend on brain enzymes as part of their synthesis and degradation.

The enzyme CHOLINE ACETYLTRANSFERASE is important in the production of ACETYLCHOLINE, a neurotransmitter involved in learning and memory. Scientists have found low levels of this neurotransmitter in the brains of ALZHEIMER'S DISEASE patients where plaques and tangles are located.

ependymoma A common childhood tumor appearing in the CEREBRAL HEMISPHERES that may be either benign or malignant; it is usually slow growing. This type of tumor may alter the flow of cerebrospinal fluid, causing buildup of fluid in the brain (HYDROCEPHALUS).

They are the third most common brain tumor in children, with up to 30 percent occurring in children younger than age three. Half of all ependymomas occur in the first two decades of life.

Ependymomas do not usually grow rapidly, they are not invasive, and usually do not spread. In unusual cases, the risk of sudden death from large intracranial ependymomas results from increased intracranial pressure of the tumor and excess fluid pressing on the brain.

Symptoms and Diagnostic Path

Nausea and vomiting occur in about 80 percent of patients, with headache due to the local effect of pressure or increased intracranial pressure that is usually worse in the morning. There may be behavior changes, such as lethargy, irritability, diminished social interaction, and loss of appetite. There also may be problems with balance.

Treatment Options and Outlook

Ependymomas usually cannot be completely removed because of their location on the brain floor or deep in the cerebral hemisphere. The best treatment will vary depending on the tumor's location and whether it has spread. However, in general, the preferred treatment of intracranial ependymomas is aggressive surgical removal. If complete removal is impossible, treatment with radiation therapy and/or chemotherapy is considered.

Recurrence of an ependymoma depends upon how much of the tumor was removed, as well as the success of radiation or chemotherapy. Most recurrent ependymomas occur near where they were originally removed. An ependymoma can, however, spread within the central nervous system (CNS). Treatment options for an individual with a recurrent ependymoma may include reoperation, chemotherapy, and further radiation.

epilepsy A brain disorder in which clusters of nerve cells signal abnormally, causing strange sensations, emotions, and behavior, convulsions, muscle spasms, and loss of consciousness. It may be caused by a wide variety of reasons, since anything that disturbs the normal pattern of brain cell activity, such as illness or abnormal brain development, can lead to seizures.

It also can be caused by a wide variety of injuries or diseases that affect the brain, such as birth trauma, HEAD INJURY, brain infection, tumor, STROKE, drug abuse, or metabolic imbalances. In addition, it may appear for no known reason at all; there may also be an inherited predisposition to developing the disease.

About one in 200 people are affected by epilepsy; in the United States, more than one million people have the condition. The disorder, which often begins in childhood or adolescence, is sometimes outgrown.

While people with epilepsy can work, their choices of jobs may be limited; there are restrictions against obtaining a driver's license (in most states, a person must be symptom-free for several years). Unless the disease is very well controlled, most physicians advise against working in high-risk jobs, such as those involving heavy machinery or heights, and participating in sports such as skiing.

Symptoms and Diagnostic Path

Generalized seizures result in a loss of consciousness and may arise from wide areas of the brain. There are two types of generalized seizures—GRAND MAL and PETIT MAL SEIZURES. During a grand mal seizure, the person loses consciousness and may stiffen, twitch, or jerk. Breathing may stop or become very irregular; afterward, bowel and bladder control may be lost. The person may feel disoriented and confused or may have a HEADACHE and want to sleep. There is usually no memory of the event. Untreated prolonged seizures (called STATUS EPILEP-TICUS) may be fatal.

Petit mal (or "absence") seizures may involve only a brief loss of consciousness and are found primarily in children. The blank period may last from a few seconds to up to a half minute, during which the person is unaware of his or her surroundings. The person may appear to be daydreaming, and the attack may pass unnoticed. They may occur hundreds of times a day, significantly interfering with schoolwork.

Partial seizures, which may not cause unconsciousness, result from more limited BRAIN DAMAGE. Although partial seizures begin in one small area of the brain, the electrical disturbance may spread, affecting the entire brain and setting off a generalized seizure. Temporal lobe epilepsy is an example of a partial type of epileptic seizure; it may result in uncontrollable flashbacks to distant memories.

They are divided into simple (without unconsciousness) or complex seizures. Simple seizures involve an abnormal twitching movement, tingling sensation, or even HALLUCINATION of smell, vision, or taste; they occur without warning and can last for several minutes. Twitching may spread slowly from one part of the body to another on the same side; this is called Jacksonian epilepsy. These patients are aware during the event and can remember the details.

In a complex seizure, the patient may be dazed and may not respond; there may be involuntary movements such as lip smacking. The patient may not remember anything about the seizure.

Epilepsy can be diagnosed only after a person has had at least two seizures; EEGs and BRAIN SCANS are common diagnostic tests for epilepsy.

The Vagus Nerve Stimulator was approved in 1997 for those whose seizures were not well controlled by medication.

Avoiding extreme fatigue or stress and infectious diseases may all help to avoid seizures. By doing this and taking prescribed medications, people with epilepsy can reduce the frequency of the attacks. Some people discover a distracting technique that can stop a seizure once it begins.

Treatment Options and Outlook

Once diagnosed, treatment should begin right away. ANTICONVULSANT DRUGS are the first step in treating epilepsy; in almost all cases they can at least reduce the number of attacks. However, these drugs may have unpleasant side effects such as drowsiness or impaired concentration. If no seizures occur for two or three years (depending on cause), the physician may recommend reducing or stopping the drugs.

Surgery is only rarely considered if medication does not work and if there is the suggestion that only one area of the brain is responsible (usually the TEMPORAL LOBE). However, temporal lobe surgery to remove the area that produces the epileptic activity may cause a degree of memory loss. Moreover, operations on the dominant temporal lobe often interfere with the ability to learn verbal information by hearing or reading that may last for as long as three years after surgery.

In a series of operations during the mid-1950s, surgeons removed the MEDIAL TEMPORAL LOBE in 10 epileptic patients in order to lessen seizures. While the operations were successful, eight of the 10 suffered pronounced memory deficits. The most famous of these is known as HM, whose amnesic syndrome is considered to be among the purest ever studied. After the operation, HM was unable to remember anything other than a handful of events since the time of his operation and was described as living in the "eternal present."

The study revealed that AMNESIA was present only in those who had lost both the HIPPOCAMPUS and the AMYGDALA; removal of the amygdala alone did not produce amnesia.

First Aid for Seizures

Most seizures last for only a few minutes. Bystanders should let the attack run its course and not interfere with the patient, beyond checking to make sure the person is in no physical danger and can breathe. Any tight clothing around the neck should be loosened, and something soft should be placed underneath the head. The mouth should not be forced open, and objects should not be forced between the teeth.

An ambulance should be called if the seizure continues for more than five minutes, if another seizure immediately follows the first, or if the person does not regain consciousness a few minutes after the seizure ends.

epinephrine   Also known as ADRENALINE, this is a naturally occurring hormone and neurotransmitter that has been synthetically manufactured since 1900. It is one of two chemicals (the other is NOREPINEPHRINE) released by the adrenal gland in response to signals from the sympathetic division of the AUTONOMIC NERVOUS SYSTEM. The signals are triggered by exercise, stress, and emotions such as fear.

Epinephrine increases the speed and force of the heart, allowing the heart to do more work. In addition, epinephrine dilates the airways to improve breathing, and narrows blood vessels in the skin and intestine to direct blood flow to the muscles to allow them to cope with exercise.

Epinephrine also seems to be responsible for imprinting memories indelibly in long-term memory. In fact, people seem to remember better when their bodies are flooded with adrenaline. Additional research also suggests that epinephrine plays an important role in regulating memory storage; it enhances memory for many different kinds of tasks, including those that train animals using rewards as well as punishment. Some scientists suggest that hormones such as epinephrine may act as a "fixative" to lock memories of stimulating or shocking events in the brain. This could allow the brain to discard unimportant information while maintaining the important impressions we experience. It may be that these hormones act directly on the brain, or they may alter brain chemistry that allows another substance to travel to the brain and "fix" the memory.

Unfortunately, because epinephrine has a variety of unpleasant side effects on the heart and other body systems—especially in older patients—more research needs to be completed before epinephrine can be used as some sort of "memory enhancement" drug.

Epinephrine is sometimes injected as an emergency treatment for a heart that has stopped beating and is used to treat anaphylactic shock (a severe allergic reaction) and acute asthma attacks. It can be used during surgery to reduce bleeding, and when combined with a local anesthetic, it prolongs the numbing effect by slowing down the rate at which the anesthetic spreads into adjoining tissue.

Erasistratus of Chios (c. 304 B.C.–c. 250 B.C.)   The Greek anatomist and the founder of physiology who described the brain's main parts, including the MENINGES and VENTRICLES. He studied in Athens, Cos, and Alexandria, dissected the human body, and is alleged to have carried out vivisection on prisoners. He also believed that human intelligence was to be found in the brain's convolutions.

See also BRAIN IN HISTORY.

estrogen and the brain   A growing body of research suggests that the female hormone estrogen may play a protective role against memory loss and ALZHEIMER'S DISEASE and may also improve brain function. In fact, the sharp decrease in estrogen during menopause may be one reason why women are 50 percent more likely to contract Alzheimer's disease at midlife.

While the research has not yet clearly proven the role of estrogen as a brain protector, one study of 2,418 women in southern California showed that those who took estrogen supplements after menopause were 40 percent less likely to have Alzheimer's. In this study, the higher the dose of estrogen, the lower the risk of Alzheimer's. In other studies of women over age 65, women who had taken estrogen supplements continuously since menopause had significantly higher scores of verbal memory than other women.

Other studies at Columbia University suggest that estrogen may also improve brain function, boosting the level of the important brain chemical called NERVE GROWTH FACTOR (NGF) and stimulating the growth of AXONS and DENDRITES (the long projections from NERVE CELLS that allow nerves to communicate with each other).

In fact, the brain is a major target for estrogen and has plenty of estrogen receptors, especially in regions associated with learning and memory (the basal FOREBRAIN, CEREBRAL CORTEX, and HIPPOCAMPUS)—the areas most affected by Alzheimer's.

Other studies at Rockefeller University note that (at least in rats) the number of SYNAPSES (points at which nerves communicate) fluctuates during reproductive cycles. When estrogen levels are high, there are more synapses (especially in the memory centers); when estrogen levels are low, the synapses disappear.

While extensive research has also found that estrogen significantly reduces the risk of heart disease and osteoporosis, it is far from a harmless wonder drug. Estrogen supplements taken during menopause have been linked to increased risk of breast cancer.

evoked response A painless recording of electrical brain activity in response to a single, specific stimulus. This technique, which was first demonstrated in 1947, is a refined version of ELECTROENCEPHALOGRAPHY, in which the brain's activity can be analyzed to assess the function of various sensory systems. Evoked potential can reveal problems caused by tumors, inflammation, and some diseases and is used to confirm the diagnosis of MULTIPLE SCLEROSIS. The test is usually used in concert with other tests of the NERVOUS SYSTEM, such as EEGS or CAT SCANS.

The testing of each sensory system (eyes, ears, touch, and so on) takes about 30 minutes. A set of electrodes is attached to a portion of the scalp (depending on which sensory system is being tested). The patterns produced by the brain are fed to a computer, which can produce a printout of the activity after a specific period of stimulation. The amount of time between the stimulus and the response can be analyzed by the computer, which separates the information from background brain activity.

exercise and the brain Aerobic exercise can improve cognitive function, perhaps because of the increased oxygen to the brain or a rise in GLUCOSE metabolism.

Studies at the University of Pennsylvania show that a person who exercises consistently over a period of years will not show the same mental decline as someone who does not exercise. In tests of rapid decision making (such as how quickly a person could slam on the brakes if a child jumped in front of his or her car), researchers found that older men who had exercised were better at quick decision making than older men who had not. It is known that those who exercise for a long period have healthier hearts, lungs, and muscles; now scientists suspect that exercise might also slow the decline in CENTRAL NERVOUS SYSTEM processing as well. Even walking around the block has been shown to be beneficial.

There is now solid evidence that regular aerobic exercise (such as running, biking, or swimming) can ease some more moderate cases of depression by raising the level of certain brain chemicals responsible for mood—some of the same brain chemicals that are affected by antidepressants. Even a brisk midday walk for 10 or 20 minutes can help. To be most effective, a person should exercise regularly at least three times a week (five or more is better) for at least a half-hour each time. Exercise has not been shown to be effective for severe depression.

extradural hemorrhage Bleeding into the space between the external surface of the DURA (the outer layer of the protective cover of the brain) and the inner surface of the skull. A BRAIN SCAN can confirm the diagnosis.

This type of hemorrhage is usually caused by a skull fracture that ruptures the artery running over the surface of the dura. The person may briefly lose consciousness and then appear to recover. This leads to a collection of clotted blood (HEMATOMA) that rapidly enlarges, increasing pressure within the skull.

Symptoms and Diagnostic Path

The main cause of symptoms occurring a few hours to days after an accident is pressure within the skull, leading to a HEADACHE, drowsiness, vomiting, SEIZURES, and paralysis on the side of the body opposite the hemorrhage. The patient may lapse into a COMA and may eventually die.

Treatment Options and Outlook

A hemorrhage can be treated by CRANIOTOMY (drilling holes in the skull) and clipping the ruptured blood vessel. If the problem is diagnosed before serious symptoms occur, the patient's chances of recovery are excellent. This is why it is so important to seek medical care after even moderate blows to the head.

extrapyramidal system A network of nerve pathways that link nerve nuclei in the surface of the CEREBRUM (main brain mass), the BASAL GANGLIA deep within the brain, and some of the BRAIN STEM. It is a collective term for those structures involved in the central nervous control of motor function other than the pyramidal tracts and their connections.

Damage of any part of this system may interfere with voluntary movements or muscle tone and induce involuntary movements such as jerks or writhing movements. These disturbances are found in PARKINSON'S DISEASE, HUNTINGTON'S DISEASE, and some forms of CEREBRAL PALSY. The movements (called TARDIVE DYSKINESIA) can also appear as a side effect of taking some drugs, including the phenothiazines (used in treating some psychiatric disorders).

facial nerve Also known as the seventh cranial nerve; with both sensory and motor aspects, this nerve is responsible for facial expressions and taste.

See also CRANIAL NERVES.

fainting A loss of consciousness caused by a temporary lack of oxygen to the brain. Also known by the medical term *syncope,* fainting may be preceded by dizziness, nausea, or a feeling of extreme weakness.

Symptoms and Diagnostic Path

An attack is usually caused by extreme pain, fear, or stress that overstimulates the vagus nerve, which helps control breathing and circulation. A person could faint from prolonged coughing or by straining to urinate or blow a wind instrument. Another cause could be remaining in a stuffy environment with not enough oxygen.

In addition, standing still (or standing erect) for long periods of time may cause fainting due to blood pooling in the leg veins, cutting down on the amount available for the heart to pump to the brain. This is common in the elderly, those who have diabetes mellitus, and those taking drugs to treat high blood pressure.

Fainting also could be a symptom of STOKES-ADAMS SYNDROME, in which the blood flow to the brain is temporarily reduced because of an irregular heart beat, usually associated with the interruption of electrical impulses of the heart.

In some people, fainting may be associated with VERTEBROBASILAR INSUFFICIENCY, a temporary problem in speaking, or a weakness in the limbs caused by an obstruction to the blood flow in vessels passing through the neck to the brain. (This is one form of TRANSIENT ISCHEMIC ATTACK.)

Treatment Options and Outlook

A fainting episode disappears as soon as a normal blood flow to the brain is restored. This usually happens as soon as the person hits the ground because the head is then placed at the same level as the heart.

If a person does not regain consciousness within a minute or two after fainting, medical help should be obtained immediately. Repeated attacks should be checked by a physician.

Risk Factors and Preventive Measures

To head off another attack, the patient should not stand for 10 or 15 minutes after regaining consciousness. When a person senses that he or she is about to faint, the attack may be prevented by sitting with the head between the knees or lying flat with the legs raised.

Fallopio, Gabriel (1523–1562) An illustrious Italian anatomist who contributed to the early knowledge of the ear and the reproductive organs. He discovered several major nerves of the head and face and described the semicircular canals of the inner ear that are responsible for maintaining body equilibrium.

Fallopio was an anatomy professor at the University of Ferrara, the University of Pisa, and at Padua. He made most of his observations of the human body during dissection of cadavers and wrote about his findings in *Observationes anatomicae,* published in 1561.

Famous Faces Test A test of a person's ability to recall events and significant people from the past, designed by Nelson Butters, M.D., a Boston specialist in the evaluation and treatment of memory-impaired patients. The test consists of a series of photographs of famous people from the 1950s to the present. A person without memory problems should be able to identify 80 percent of the faces, such as those of Ronald Reagan, Dwight Eisenhower, Marilyn Monroe, and so on.

fatal familial insomnia   An extremely rare, genetic progressive SLEEP DISORDER that has affected just nine families in the world. It manifests itself by many symptoms due to the degeneration of the thalamus in the brain (the area responsible for sleep) and the formation of amyloid plaques, a buildup of a waxy substance made of proteins.

In one Italian family, 29 of 288 relatives over six generations are affected by the disorder. The average age of onset of the disease is 49, but this may vary with the individual.

The disease is believed to be caused by a prion, a type of mutation of a normal protein associated with brain tissue. This disease is an autosomal dominant, which means that both sexes are affected and there are no carriers. If an individual inherits the mutant gene, that individual will at some point suffer the disease.

Symptoms and Diagnostic Path
Other symptoms of this disease include the inability to produce tears or feel pain, as well as poor reflexes and dementia. The lack of sleep leads to other problems, such as hallucinations and coma.

There are four stages of the disease, beginning with a progressive insomnia that develops over about four months and includes a collection of psychiatric problems such as panic attacks and bizarre phobias. The second stage includes hallucinations, panic, agitation, and sweating, and lasts about five months. The third stage lasts about three months and involves total insomnia with weight loss. Individuals at this point look much older and may experience incontinence. The fourth stage lasts about six months and is recognized as DEMENTIA with total insomnia; it ends with sudden death.

This disease does not appear until past child-bearing years, when potentially affected individuals may have already had children who also may be affected.

Treatment Options and Outlook
There is no treatment or cure for this disease.

fetal alcohol syndrome (FAS)   A condition in which a mother's excessive drinking during pregnancy produces a specific group of physical and mental characteristics in the developing fetus. First recognized in the early 1970s, the syndrome is now considered to be one of the most common causes of MENTAL RETARDATION.

About 5,000 American babies per year are born with FAS, and a great number of others are born with "fetal alcohol effects" that include several, but not all, of the typical features of FAS.

No one knows for sure how much drinking during pregnancy is dangerous; in part, it depends on how a woman's body metabolizes alcohol. Some women consume very large amounts of alcohol without harm to their babies, while other women who drink only very small amounts have babies with the syndrome.

In particular, sudden heavy drinking—such as at just one celebration—may be the most harmful of all, according to some research, especially if the drinking occurs at a crucial time of fetal development.

For these reasons, women are advised to stop drinking altogether while they are pregnant and, if they breast-feed, until their babies are weaned.

Exactly how alcohol produces the devastating brain defects and other problems is not clearly understood. Scientists do know that alcohol consumed by the mother crosses the placenta, and while a baby's organs are still developing, they cannot break down alcohol as quickly as an adult can. As a result, the alcohol in the baby's bloodstream remains high for a much longer time.

Symptoms and Diagnostic Path
Symptoms include abnormally small head and brain, growth deficiency, deformities of face, joints,

and limbs, brain and SPINAL CORD defects, varying degrees of malfunctions in major organs (especially the heart), small wide-set eyes, short upturned nose, flat cheeks. Babies with this syndrome tend to weigh less at birth and fail to catch up later; they often suffer with HYPERACTIVITY, short attention span, poor coordination, nervousness, and behavioral problems.

Treatment Options and Outlook

There is no specific treatment for infants with FAS. Difficulties with hearing, vision, and speech become apparent as the child grows, as do delays in language and physical development. There is no cure for FAS and the progress is poor.

Risk Factors and Preventive Measures

FAS is preventable, as long as a woman does not drink alcohol while she is pregnant or trying to become pregnant. If a woman is drinking during pregnancy, the sooner she stops drinking, the better.

fetal brain development   While in the womb, the brain is the largest organ of the fetus's body; by the fifth month, it is almost the same size as the trunk. This early growth spurt of the brain is a result of the multiplication of cells, not their enlargement. Cells divide or multiply at different times in different parts of the brain.

The two hemispheres of the FOREBRAIN are the first to experience a spurt in NERVE CELL growth, which happens between the third and fourth month of pregnancy, peaking at 26 weeks. At this stage, 250,000 nerve cells are being created every minute. Most of the NEURONS, however, are formed during the second trimester; at birth, the infant's brain weighs one pound and contains about 100 billion neurons—just about the same number as in the adult brain.

GLIAL CELLS are also growing at a rapid rate in the brain, starting in the fifth month in the womb. This glial cell division peaks at birth and begins to decline within three months, although glial cells still grow until the child is two or three.

By the 10th week of pregnancy, electrical activity in certain areas of the brain can be detected, especially in areas concerned with waking and sleeping. By the 12th to 16th week the brain can direct the fetus's hands and face to move, and by two-and-a-half months, the fetus can swallow amniotic fluid. By seven-and-a-half months, the fetal brain can direct the opening of eyes and sucking of fingers.

Nutrition and Fetal Development

The mother's nutrition is critical to fetal brain development because a lack of proper nutrients can interfere with the rate of fetal cell division, resulting in a permanent reduction in the number of brain cells. Severe malnutrition during fetal development primarily affects neurons, whereas malnutrition during the early postnatal period affects glial cells.

Even if the mother suffers a nutrient deficiency for a short time, the rate of cell division in the fetal brain will increase again, but not always normally. The complex programming of brain growth and development requires that development take place in certain steps; interference during any of the steps may cause harm that is irreversible once its "developmental window" has passed. This then interferes with all stages of growth that come after it. Therefore, the earlier the period of nutritional interference, the more serious the subsequent developmental problems.

fetal hydantoin syndrome   A group of birth defects, including small head (MICROCEPHALY) in babies of women with EPILEPSY who have taken antiseizure medication derived from the chemical hydantoin. Other symptoms include MENTAL RETARDATION, growth problems, and abnormalities of nails and fingers.

field dependence   When making a perceptual judgment, the tendency to be influenced by surrounding information. This is also known as external locus of control, or field sensitivity.

field independence   The tendency not to be influenced by surrounding information when making a perceptual judgment. This is also known as internal locus of control.

See also FIELD DEPENDENCE.

fight-or-flight response   The almost instantaneous reaction of the brain to sudden fear that triggers a cascading chain of physiological reactions to prepare the body either to fight or flee from a perceived threat. This physical response triggers the sympathetic division of the AUTONOMIC NERVOUS SYSTEM to become activated, a situation that is common to all animals in reaction to threat.

The response usually begins with a visual signal that the brain interprets as a threat. This triggers fear or anger in one part of the brain, which induces the HYPOTHALAMUS to send an urgent message to the PITUITARY GLAND's anterior lobe to release the stress hormone ADRENOCORTICOTROPHIC HORMONE (ACTH) into the blood. ACTH enters the adrenal glands located on top of the kidneys, producing more stress-associated hormones (EPINEPHRINE and NOREPINEPHRINE). Due to this increase in systemic epinephrine and norepinephrine, drastic changes affect the body's blood supply; as the heart races, blood vessels supplying the skin and digestive system constrict, draining color from the skin. This shunts blood to the vital musculature where it is needed. The chest expands, widening bronchial tubes and increasing respiration rate; muscles tense, pupils dilate; the mouth grows dry; and the body sweats.

These physiological changes also occur during ANXIETY and its disorders.

fipexide   This centrally active drug has been shown in some studies to enhance the release of DOPAMINE, the NEUROTRANSMITTER related to fine motor coordination, motivation, emotions, and the immune function. In one double-blind study of 40 elderly patients with severe cognitive problems, fipexide improved cognition and performance, short-term memory, and attention. Average improvement in cognition was estimated to be 60 percent.

Fissure of Sylvius   The groove that separates the TEMPORAL LOBE of the brain from the FRONTAL and PARIETAL LOBES.

fissures, cerebral   See SULCI.

Flourens, Marie-Jean-Pierre (1794–1867)   A French physiologist was the first to demonstrate the general function of the major portions of the vertebrate brain, who proved that the brain's respiratory center lies low in the BRAIN STEM, and who pioneered the idea of nervous coordination. In 1814, Flourens began a series of experiments to discover physiological changes in pigeons after he removed certain portions of their brains. He published these findings in *Experimental Studies on the Properties and Functions of the Nervous System in Vertebrate Animals.*

Flourens discovered that the absence of the CEREBRAL HEMISPHERES at the front of the brain destroys the sense of perception but not of equilibrium. He also discovered that removing the CEREBELLUM at the base of the brain destroys the sense of equilibrium and that removing the MEDULLA OBLONGATA at the back of the brain is fatal.

As a result of these experiments, he concluded that the cerebral hemispheres are the seat of higher cognitive abilities, that the cerebellum regulates movement, and that the medulla controls breathing and other vital functions. Flourens also learned how the semicircular canals of the inner ear regulate equilibrium and coordination.

See also BRAIN IN HISTORY.

fluent aphasia   See WERNICKE'S APHASIA.

fluid balance   See THIRST.

fluid imbalances and the brain   Too much or too little water will disturb brain function by changing the osmotic balance of electrolytes (potassium, sodium chloride, calcium, and magnesium) crucial to brain function. Especially during hot weather, aging patients are particularly at risk for electrolyte-induced brain problems.

folic acid   A B vitamin found in many foods that is essential to the production of red blood cells by the bone marrow. This vitamin plays a particularly important role in the development of the fetal NERVOUS SYSTEM and formation of fetal red blood cells. Its lack during pregnancy has been linked to NEURAL TUBE DEFECTS. (Neural tube defects are a devastating birth disorder that takes place when the spinal column fails to close early in pregnancy; the condition can cause a baby to be born with part of its brain missing.)

Under the U.S. Food and Drug Administration's (FDA) folic acid fortification program begun in January 1998, manufacturers are required to add from 0.43 mg to 1.4 mg of folic acid per pound of product to enriched flour, bread, rolls and buns, farina, corn grits, cornmeal, rice, and noodle products. A serving of each product will provide about 10 percent of the daily value for folic acid.

Whole-grain products do not have to be enriched because they contain natural folate. Some of the natural folate in non-whole grain products is lost in the process of refining whole grains.

Folate also can be obtained from dietary supplements, such as folic acid tablets and multivitamins with folic acid, and from fortified breakfast cereals. An estimated 2,500 babies were born in the United States each year with this condition, and the FDA panel estimates that this number could be cut in half if women consumed the suggested daily allowance of folic acid (0.4 milligrams). The average woman ingests only 0.2 milligrams of the substance each day; the vitamin is found in green leafy vegetables, dried beans, liver, citrus juices, nuts, avocados, and cereals.

Other scientists suggest that low levels of folic acid are closely tied to psychiatric symptoms in the elderly; one study has found that elderly patients with mental disorders (especially DEMENTIA) were three times more likely to have low folic acid than others their age. Among healthy aged people, those with low folic-acid intake scored lower on memory and abstract-thinking ability. Studies have also found that low daily doses of folic-acid supplements lifted mood and relieved depression.

In other studies, scientists found that ensuring that a pregnant woman's diet is full of fruits and vegetables may dramatically reduce the risk of the child's subsequent development of NEUROECTODERMAL TUMORS in the part of the brain that controls coordination.

forebrain The largest and most expansive part of the brain is made up of two subdivisions: the telencephalon (endbrain) and the DIENCEPHALON (interbrain). Structures in the telencephalon account for about 75 percent of the weight of the entire CENTRAL NERVOUS SYSTEM and include the CEREBRAL HEMISPHERES connected by a mass of crossing fibers in the CORPUS CALLOSUM and preoptic area. The surface of the hemispheres is a layer of tissue called the CEREBRAL CORTEX, which is divided into subregions according to creases along the brain's surface (also known as SULCI). The largest subregions are the four lobes in each hemisphere (FRONTAL, PARIETAL, TEMPORAL, and OCCIPITAL).

The cerebral hemispheres are attached to the diencephalon by large bundles of fibers called the corona radiata. The major parts of the diencephalon include the THALAMUS, the subthalamus, the HYPOTHALAMUS, and the epithalamus (containing the pineal body).

fornix One of four areas of the brain associated with memory, the fornix is the bridge between the temporal lobes and the diencephalon. Some researchers believe that AMNESIA is a result of a disconnection between the fornix and mammillary bodies.

fragile X syndrome The most common cause of inherited mental impairment, ranging from learning disabilities to more severe mental retardation, with delays in speech and language development. The condition affects about one in 3,600 boys, and one in 4,000 to 6,000 girls.

Fragile X syndrome is an X-linked congenital condition caused by a chromosomal abnormality in which a male's X chromosome is malformed.

Although males are mainly affected, women are able to carry the genetic defect that is responsible for the disorder and pass it on to some of their sons, who are affected, and some of their daughters, who in turn become carriers of the defect.

Symptoms and Diagnostic Path

In addition to mental retardation, the syndrome is characterized in boys by large testicles, protruding long ears, and a pronounced nose, chin, and forehead; those affected tend to be tall and physically strong.

Girls often have milder problems with retardation and less severe or distorted behavioral or physical features.

To diagnose fragile X, two molecular DNA tests were developed in the 1990s. The southern blot analysis can determine if the gene has a full mutation and how big it is, and if there is a mixture of different cell types. The polymerase chain reaction (PCR) analysis can identify the actual number of repeats in individuals with a normal size gene or with a premutation. It is not the test of choice to diagnose a full mutation, but is still considered to be accurate.

Treatment Options and Outlook

Because the impact of fragile X is so different depending on how the child is affected, it is important to carefully evaluate a person's abilities and problems to be able to tailor a treatment plan. Special education, speech and language therapy, occupational therapy, and behavioral therapies all can help address the behavioral and mental issues these children face. In addition, medications can help deal with aggression, anxiety, hyperactivity, and poor attention span.

Freeman, Walter (1895–1972) The inventor of the LOBOTOMY and a prominent neurologist, Freeman was a scion of a well-known Philadelphia medical family who had worked for many years at St. Elizabeth's Hospital in Washington, D.C. At a conference in London in 1935, Freeman met Portuguese neurologist Antonio Egas Moniz, who had been conducting psychosurgical experiments with animals and who soon began operating on humans with a procedure called LEUCOTOMY.

After studying Moniz's book on the procedure, Freeman and his partner, James Watts, performed the first American leucotomy on a depressed patient in 1936. Impatient with the procedure and convinced he could perform it faster with a minimum of preparation, Freeman adapted the technique that he began calling lobotomy. Instead of opening the skull, he inserted an ice pick through the eye socket directly into the frontal lobe. This

allowed him to operate more quickly on far more patients, on an outpatient basis. By 1946 Freeman started performing the lobotomies "assembly-line style," operating on 10 patients a day in his office.

Based on 80 lobotomies, Freeman and Watts published their textbook *Psychosurgery* in 1942. Before the procedure eventually faded into disrepute as dangerous and inhumane, more than 40,000 lobotomies had been performed in the United States through the 1950s.

As public sentiment turned against lobotomies and the development of psychoactive drugs made them unnecessary, Freeman left Washington in 1954 and abandoned his assembly-line lobotomies. He performed his last lobotomy at the age of 72 in Berkeley.

free radicals A highly charged, potentially destructive molecule (most commonly, a species of oxygen) that is generated naturally by breathing and by the body's response to stress. While free radicals are destructive, they have a positive role to play in the body as well. Generated by the immune system, they fend off microbes and help the digestive system break down food. In the brain, they can interact with lipids, harming the brain.

While a certain amount of free radicals is necessary to maintain proper body function, high levels are toxic. Each day, the body generates thousands upon thousands of free radicals in response to ultraviolet (UV) light, smoke, and pollution. Once activated, they tear through the membrane that protects the body's cells, causing inflammation and cell breakdown.

Freud, Sigmund (1856–1939) A Viennese specialist in nerve and brain diseases who is best known for the creation of psychoanalysis and his theories on sexuality. Freud also was fascinated with the idea of memory, including the baffling questions of how—and why—we forget. It was Freud who compared memory to a magic slate: the clear celluloid receives the imprint of short-term memories, soon to be wiped clean, and the waxy cardboard underneath becomes etched with the lasting impressions.

Freud accepted the belief popularized by his contemporary, psychologist Hermann Ebbinghaus, that the brain files away all memories, but his angle of approach was wildly different. Freud studied memory not from the position of what we remember or how we remember, but on how little we remember—and why. He believed that any failure of recall had a specific cause, and since people forget things every day, he had plenty of material with which to work. For example, Freud found it implausible that childhood, filled with the richness of new experience, pleasure, and pain, should be so totally forgotten.

He argued that recalled experiences and ideas were related to other symbolically and emotionally important thoughts and feelings and that much of what a person forgets is simply repression. He believed that the lack of memories of early childhood (usually before age four in most people) was caused by repression of infantile sexuality, which peaks in the third and fourth years of life. This repression is caused by the "psychic forces of loathing, shame, and moral and aesthetic ideal demands," he said. His basic theory describes both the unconscious and conscious mind, noting that the unconscious mind can have a great effect on a person's conscious actions. We remember something, he postulated, because it is meaningful to us and significant, although that significance may be hidden.

Freud believed it was conflict, followed by repression, that made the problem of deciphering early memories so difficult. Because he thought there is nothing accidental or arbitrary about the things we forget, he believed that everyday absent-mindedness could be divided into "forgetfulness" and "false recollection" (also called a "Freudian slip," or substituting one word for another). The process that should have produced the actual memory was interrupted and the memory was "displaced" by another.

And displacement isn't simply a quirk, he argued—it followed a routine as logical as summoning up the actual memory. For example, he analyzed a number of his own "Freudian slips" in his book *The Psychopathology of Everyday Life*. When he couldn't remember the name of Rosenheim, a major railway station (translation: Rose's home), he decided that the name was lost in his memory because he had just come from visiting the home

of his sister, Rose, and the name was taken away by his "family complex." He concluded that forgotten names were associated—sometimes very indirectly—with painful and unpleasant memories. In other words, we eliminate from the conscious mind everything that makes us anxious, which, he believed, explained the loss of memories during the first four years of life.

Friedreich's ataxia A hereditary degenerative disease that damages the nervous system, characterized by the development of muscle weakness. The condition is named after the physician Nicholas Friedreich, who first described the disease in the 1860s. In Friedreich's ataxia, coordination problems are caused by degeneration of nerve tissue in the spinal cord and of nerves that control muscle movement in the arms and legs. The spinal cord becomes thinner and nerve cells lose some of their myelin sheath (the covering on all nerve cells that helps conduct nerve impulses), a process known as demyelination.

Friedreich's ataxia, although rare, is the most prevalent inherited ataxia, affecting about one in every 50,000 people in the United States. Men and women are affected equally.

Friedreich's ataxia is an autosomal recessive disease, which means the patient must inherit two affected genes, one from each parent, for the disease to develop. A person who has only one abnormal copy of a gene for a recessive genetic disease such as Friedreich's ataxia is called a carrier. A carrier will not develop the disease but could pass the affected gene on to his or her children. If both parents are carriers of the Friedreich's ataxia gene, their children will have a one in four chance of having the disease and a one in two chance of inheriting one abnormal gene that they, in turn, could pass on to their children. About one in 90 Americans of European ancestry carries one affected gene.

Symptoms and Diagnostic Path

Symptoms usually begin between the ages of five and 15 but can, on rare occasions, appear as early as 18 months or as late as age 30. The first symptom to appear is usually difficulty in walking (gait ataxia). This gradually worsens and slowly spreads to the arms and then the trunk. Foot deformities such as clubfoot, involuntary bending of the toes, hammer toes, or foot inversion (turning inward) may be other early signs.

Over time, muscles begin to weaken and waste away, especially in the feet, lower legs, and hands, and deformities develop. Other symptoms include loss of tendon reflexes, especially in the knees and ankles. There is often a gradual loss of sensation in the extremities, which may spread to other parts of the body. Slowness and slurring of speech develops, and the person is easily tired. Rapid, rhythmic, involuntary movements of the eyeball (nystagmus) is common. Most people with Friedreich's ataxia develop scoliosis (a curving of the spine to one side), which, if severe, may impair breathing.

Other symptoms that may occur include chest pain, shortness of breath, and heart palpitations. These are caused by various forms of heart disease that often accompany Friedreich's ataxia, such as cardiomyopathy (enlargement of the heart), inflammation of the walls of the heart (myocarditis), formation of fibrous material in the muscles of the heart (myocardial fibrosis), and cardiac failure. Heart rhythm abnormalities such as fast heart rate and heart block are also common.

About 20 percent of people with Friedreich's ataxia develop carbohydrate intolerance and 10 percent develop diabetes mellitus. Some people lose hearing or eyesight.

The rate of disease progression varies from person to person, but generally within 15 to 20 years after the appearance of the first symptoms the person is confined to a wheelchair. In later stages of the disease, individuals become completely incapacitated.

Most people with Friedreich's ataxia die in early adulthood if there is significant heart disease, which is the most common cause of death. However, some people with less severe symptoms of Friedreich's ataxia live much longer.

Doctors diagnose Friedreich's ataxia by performing a careful clinical examination, including a medical history and a thorough physical examination. Tests may include

- electromyogram (EMG), which measures the electrical activity of muscle cells

- nerve conduction studies, which measure the speed with which nerves transmit impulses

- electrocardiogram (EKG), which gives a graphic presentation of the electrical activity or beat pattern of the heart

- echocardiogram, which records the position and motion of the heart muscle

- magnetic resonance imaging (MRI) or computed tomography (CT) scan, which provides a picture of the brain and spinal cord

- spinal tap to evaluate the cerebrospinal fluid

- blood and urine tests to check for elevated glucose levels

- genetic testing to identify the affected gene

Treatment Options and Outlook

As with many degenerative diseases of the nervous system, there is currently no effective cure or treatment for Friedreich's ataxia. However, many of the symptoms and accompanying complications can be treated to help patients live a normal life for as long as possible. Diabetes can be treated with diet and medications such as insulin, and some of the heart problems can be treated with medication as well. Orthopedic problems such as foot deformities and scoliosis can be treated with braces or surgery. Physical therapy may prolong use of the arms and legs. Scientists hope that recent advances in understanding the genetics of Friedreich's ataxia may lead to breakthroughs in treatment.

Genetic testing is available at some specialized laboratories and can help with clinical diagnosis, prenatal diagnosis, and carrier status determination. Genetic counselors can help explain how Friedreich's ataxia is inherited. Psychological counseling and support groups for people with genetic diseases may also help patients and their families cope with the disease.

frontal aphasia   See BROCA'S APHASIA.

frontal lobe   Front part of the brain. One of the roles of the frontal lobe is concerned with intellectual functioning, including thought processes, planning, organizing, behavior, and memory. The frontal lobe is also an important center of voluntary and planned motor behaviors, such as voluntary movement of eyes, trunk, and the many muscles used for speech. The motor speech area (BROCA'S AREA) is usually in the frontal lobe of the left hemisphere, no matter which hemisphere is dominant.

The front part of the frontal lobe is called the prefrontal cortex. It is important in higher thinking functions, also called executive function. The back part of the frontal lobe helps to modify movements.

frontal lobotomy   See LOBOTOMY; LEUCOTOMY.

functional magnetic resonance imaging (fMRI)   A modification of the technique of MAGNETIC RESONANCE IMAGING (MRI), which uses radio waves and a strong magnetic field instead of X-rays, to provide clear and detailed pictures of internal organs and tissues. Functional magnetic resonance imaging (fMRI) is a relatively new procedure that uses MR imaging to measure the rapid and minute metabolic changes that take place in an active part of the brain.

Procedure

The fMRI exam follows the same procedure as an MRI exam and begins with the patient lying on a moveable table in the examination room. Small coils are attached to the body to detect radio waves. The table moves into the MRI unit. Depending on the disorder being investigated, the patient may be asked to perform certain tasks, such as reading, listening to music, or speaking during the exam.

Although experts know the approximate areas in the brain where speech, sensation, and memory are found, their precise locations vary from one person to the next. An fMRI can help a radiologist explore the brain's anatomy and figure out what part of the brain is handling sensation, speech, or movement. This information can be critical when planning surgery, radiation therapy, or other treatments.

Risks and Complications

There are no known risks of the exam.

fundus   Cortical valleys of brain tissue that lie beneath the outer layer of the brain that according to research, may help coordinate problem solving and other complex types of thinking.

The new research, using PET SCANS, suggests that more demanding and complex cognitive functions rely on cortical fundal activity to a higher degree than do less demanding processes. The research found that these cortical valleys showed the most activity during especially complex problem-solving and memory tasks, and yet these areas make up only about 8 percent of the entire CORTEX.

Because fundal cells handle short-range communications in the brain, some scientists suggest that these NEURONS may also function as a central point where related lines of information converge to make complex thinking possible.

fusiform gyrus   A band of tissue that runs lengthwise along the base of each side of the brain. Recent research suggests that parts of the fusiform gyrus show distinctive electrical responses to patterns of letters; one part of the fusiform gyrus responds comparably to all types of letter strings but not to illustrations or visual patterns. Another part is activated only during presentations of actual words.

The two parts of the fusiform gyrus play a part in the brain's visual system that specializes in word recognition, some researchers believe. While the first site in this part of the brain perceives separate letters in an array and in meaningful arrangements of those letters, the second appears to form visual meanings of words or to help retrieve memories of word meanings based on emotional qualities of a word or on its context in a sentence.

This whole process of word recognition takes about a fifth of a second to complete.

See also READING.

GABA The abbreviation for *gamma-aminobutyric acid*. This is an AMINO-ACID NEUROTRANSMITTER released by nerve terminals in the brain and SPINAL CORD. GABA is known as an inhibitory neurotransmitter, for its action is to inhibit the electrical activity of the neuron it is released upon. GABAergic systems shape the activity of other transmitter systems through the inhibition or reduction in firing rate of target neurons. BENZODIAZEPINE drugs boost the activity of GABA, and anticonvulsant drugs decrease its activity. It is believed that GABA helps control anxiety.

Some research indicates that patients with HUNTINGTON'S DISEASE may have too few GABA-producing NERVE CELLS in the areas that coordinate movement. Huntington's is associated with involuntary movement and mental problems.

galantamine hydrobromide (Razadyne) ALZHEIMER'S DISEASE medication that appears to work by boosting the level of ACETYLCHOLINE, a brain chemical important in memory, learning, and function. Patients with Alzheimer's have low levels of acetylcholine, and many experts believe that the loss of this chemical interferes with a patient's ability to remember and think.

Razadyne is the newest member of a class of medications called acetylcholinesterase inhibitors, all of which block the action of acetylcholinesterase, an enzyme that breaks down acetylcholine. None of these drugs cure the disease, although improvement may be noted in some patients. All Razadyne and the other drugs can do is to maintain patients at their current level of functioning for as long as possible.

It is designed to be used with patients who have mild to moderate Alzheimer's. The drug may be prescribed as soon as the diagnosis is made, because the earlier treatment starts, the better the effect may be.

Side Effects
The most common side effects are a temporary nausea, vomiting, diarrhea, loss of appetite, and weight loss. However, some people experience a slowed heart rate, which may lead to fainting.

Serious stomach problems can occur in people taking medications such as nonsteroidal anti-inflammatory drugs (NSAIDs) or those at risk for stomach ulcers.

Galen (A.D. 129–199) The great Greek physician of the second century A.D. who established some basic (albeit slightly garbled) theories of the brain and body that were practiced for the next 1,500 years. He was born the son of a gifted architect in the city where the healing shrine of the god Asclepius was located. At the medical school that was connected with the shrine, Galen observed many of the treatments for a variety of diseases and eventually became chief physician for the gladiators in 157. Galen based his anatomy on the dissection of lower animals such as the African monkey. His important contributions included the discovery of seven pairs of CRANIAL NERVES and the discovery that the brain controls the voice.

Gall, Franz Joseph (1758–1828) German anatomist and physiologist who dissected the brain, established the basis of modern neurology, and was the first to ascribe particular functions to various areas of the brain. Gall is also the cofounder of PHRENOLOGY, the practice of assessing a person's intellect and personality from shape of the skull. He was also the first to identify the GRAY MATTER of the brain with NEURONS and the WHITE MATTER with GANGLIA (conducting tissue).

Gall was convinced that mental functions were to be found in specific areas of the brain (localization); these theories were shown to be correct when French physician Pierre-Paul Broca demonstrated the speech center of the brain in 1861. Unfortunately, he enlarged on these theories and assumed that the surface of the skull reflected the development of the various brain regions lying underneath. It was later found that the thickness of the skull varies and so does not reflect the underlying brain.

gamma-aminobutyric acid (GABA)   See GABA.

gamma hydroxybutyrate (GHB)   A colorless, odorless, slightly salty central nervous system depressant that contains some of the same ingredients as floor stripper and industrial cleaners. As a recreational drug, it was once limited to large warehouse scenes such as "raves," but it has gradually become a drug of choice at teenage parties around the country.

GHB provides a feeling of euphoria, but it can have variable effects in different people; a dose that makes one person feel euphoric can make another person sick. Some who take the drug can lose control within minutes and lose consciousness. The U.S. Drug Enforcement Agency has linked GHB to 58 deaths since 1990, with at least 5,700 overdoses recorded since that time.

Possible symptoms of GHB use include dizziness, drowsiness, dependence, vomiting, seizures, and coma. Treatment of overdose is difficult because it is hard for emergency room doctors to detect the drug.

GHB was first developed as a general anesthetic, but since it did not work very well to prevent pain, its use as an anesthetic declined. The observation that GHB might help release growth hormone then interested some athletes and bodybuilders, who took the drug because they thought it might increase muscle development. First available as a dietary supplement, GHB was not regulated by the U.S. Food and Drug Administration (FDA). Eventually, after numerous reports that GHB caused illness, the FDA in 1990 reclassified the drug as an illegal substance. The only use for which it is approved is for the treatment of narcolepsy.

GHB has been grouped with other drugs, such as Rohypnol, in the "date-rape drug" category, because it can be easily slipped into a drink and given to an unsuspecting victim, who often does not remember being assaulted afterward. GHB is especially dangerous when combined with alcohol.

Although it can be made in the laboratory, it is also produced normally in the brain through the synthesis of a neurotransmitter called GABA. Some of the greatest concentrations of GHB are found in the areas of the brain called the SUBSTANTIA NIGRA, the THALAMUS, and the HYPOTHALAMUS. When GHB is ingested, it affects several different neurotransmitter systems in the brain, increasing ACETYLCHOLINE and SEROTONIN levels, and slowing DOPAMINE activity, especially in the BASAL GANGLIA. The effects on the dopamine system may depend on the size of the dose.

The FDA lists GHB as a Schedule 1 drug, like heroin, which means it has a high potential for abuse; its possession has been illegal since February 18, 2000.

ganglia   Groups of peripheral neuron cell bodies in which nerve signals are processed.

gender differences   For hundreds of years, scientists have searched for differences between the brains of men and women. Early research showing that male brains were larger than female brains was used to "prove" that male brains were superior. Even today, a great deal of controversy remains about the differences in the brains of men and women from an anatomical and functional point of view. Studies that have looked at differences in the brains of males and females have focused on total brain size and the HYPOTHALAMUS.

Almost all studies show that a male brain is bigger than a female brain at birth, when the average male brain is between 12 percent and 20 percent larger than that of females. Male head circumference is also slightly larger. However, when the size of the brain is compared to body weight at this age, there is almost no difference between males and females, so female infants and male infants who weigh the same will have similar brain sizes.

In adults, the average brain weight in men is about 11 percent to 12 percent more than the average brain weight in women, but a man's head is also about 2 percent bigger than a woman's. Of course, men typically weigh more than women, and absolute brain size may not be the best measure of intelligence.

In addition, many behavioral differences have been reported for men and women. For example, some studies suggest that women are better in certain language abilities and men are better in certain spatial areas. As a result, many studies have tried to find differences in the right and left cerebral hemispheres to suggest that male and female brains are different, but few of these experiments have found meaningful differences. In fact, there are many similarities between the cerebral hemispheres of men and women.

The hypothalamus is one area of the brain with well-documented differences between men and women. Two areas of the hypothalamus (the preoptic area and the suprachiasmatic nucleus) have clear differences. The hypothalamus is involved in mating behavior, and in men the preoptic area of the hypothalamus is greater in volume, in cross-sectional area, and in the number of cells. In men, this area is about 2.2 times larger than in women, and it contains twice as many cells. Apparently, the difference in this area becomes obvious only after a person is four years old, when there is a decrease in the number of cells in this nucleus in girls. The exact function of this nucleus in behavior is not fully known.

The suprachiasmatic nucleus of the hypothalamus is involved with circadian rhythms and reproduction cycles. The only difference between women and men in this area is one of shape: in males, this nucleus in spherical; in females it is more elongated. However, the number of cells and volume of this nucleus are the same in men and women. It is possible that the shape of the suprachiasmatic nucleus influences the connections that

this area makes with other areas of the brain, especially the other areas of the hypothalamus.

Behavioral and neurological differences between men and women require further study. However, current evidence suggests that differences in many cognitive behaviors (such as MEMORY) may be related more to differences between individuals than to gender.

While some differences in the brain appear to be the result of sex hormones, others are simply structural in nature—it is clear that male brains tend to be bigger and heavier than female brains. Of course, this does not mean that intellectual capacity is likewise more advanced in males.

This is because the brain operates through electrical and chemical processing, not through the physical storage of facts; therefore, the actual size of the brain should have no bearing on intellect.

Beyond that, the issue of male-female brain differences is extremely controversial. There are other structural differences in the brain between men and women as well, although it is not clear what these may mean. First of all, females tend to have a left cortical dominance while males usually have a right cortical dominance. This is why, scientists believe, women appear to be predisposed toward better verbal abilities; they usually speak earlier and more clearly, learn languages more easily, and can repeat tongue twisters better. They also have better fine-motor control (and therefore tend to have better penmanship). On the other hand, men typically are inclined to outperform women in spatial functions, such as negotiating a maze.

The CORPUS CALLOSUM (fiber network joining the left and right hemispheres) is proportionately much larger in a female brain. For hundreds of years, doctors noted that women seemed to recover more quickly and more completely from BRAIN INJURIES than did men. More recently, scientists have discovered that this is possible because the bridge that joins the two hemispheres is more closely connected in women, allowing one side of the brain to better compensate for damage to the other. Moreover, brain hemispheres in both men and women become more and more specialized with each year of life from birth until puberty; after this, the corpus callosum becomes thinner and thinner. Because women generally reach puberty first, their brains tend to be less specialized than men and therefore are able to recover more quickly from BRAIN DAMAGE. Men are also far more likely to suffer from DYSLEXIA, stuttering, AUTISM, and HYPERACTIVITY.

This thicker "bridge" between the two hemispheres might also explain the mystery of "women's intuition," according to Dr. Jerre Levy of the University of Chicago. Dr. Levy suggests that this close connection between the two hemispheres in women makes it easier for them to integrate the details and subtleties of a situation.

Of course, scientists emphasize that the skill differences between men and women due to brain configuration are only slight. In fact, they emphasize that only a small part of the difference between men and women in any one skill is due to the structure and chemical makeup of their brains. The rest—probably as much as 80 percent—of the differences reflect a person's expectations, encouragement, education, and environment.

genetic disorders of the brain A number of genetic disorders can affect the brain and its function. These include inherited chromosomal abnormalities resulting in mental retardation (such as TAY SACHS DISEASE or DOWN SYNDROME), degeneration of brain tissue (such as HUNTINGTON'S DISEASE) and structural problems, such as ANENCEPHALY (absence of the brain), MICROCEPHALY (very small head), or HYDROCEPHALUS (water on the brain).

ginkgo biloba This extract from the oldest known species of tree (also known as a maidenhair tree) seems to be able to increase the flow of nutrients and oxygen to the brain. As the extract increases circulation, it also boosts the production of ADENOSINE TRIPHOSPHATE (ATP), an energy-carrying molecule, and streamlines the brain's ability to metabolize GLUCOSE. It also appears to prevent platelet clumping in arteries and serves as a powerful ANTIOXIDANT.

It is widely used to treat memory problems in Germany and France, and studies have documented the safety and efficacy of ginkgo in treating patients with mild to moderate Alzheimer's, although experts agree that more research is needed and the treatment does not result in big improvements.

Extracts are made up of flavone glycosides, several terpene molecules unique to the tree, and organic acids. Scientists believe the special terpenes improve circulation in the brain, and extracts are thought to have both antiinflammatory and antioxidant properties.

Side Effects

Few side effects are associated with the use of ginkgo as a dietary supplement, although it does reduce the ability of blood to clot, potentially leading to more serious conditions, such as hemorrhaging. This risk of hemorrhage may increase if ginkgo biloba is taken in combination with other anticoagulants, such as aspirin.

glia cells See GLIAL CELLS.

glial cells A supportive type of brain cell that protects and feeds NEURONS, outnumbering them 10 to one—the brain contains more than 100 trillion glial cells. Some of the glial cells seem to act as a sort of bed for neurons. Unlike neurons, glial cells do not generate electrical impulses, but they do play an important supportive role in maintaining efficiency along the brain's nerve network. They help to form a covering to protect the large neurons in the SPINAL CORD; MYELIN is placed around the axons of some neurons by a particular type of glial cell, and AXONS covered by this myelin sheath conduct impulses up to 12 times faster than those without it. The areas of the brain that contain myelin-covered axons are called the WHITE MATTER, because the myelinated axons look white. In addition, some glial cells may get rid of dead neurons.

There are three types of glial cells—astrocytes, oligodendrocytes, and microglia. Astrocytes are involved with neurotransmission and neuronal metabolism; oligodendrocytes help produce myelin, the insulating material around neurons; and microglia are part of the immune system.

glioblastoma A fast-growing, highly malignant type of BRAIN TUMOR. Glioblastoma multiforme is a type of GLIOMA, a tumor arising from the GLIAL CELLS within the brain. Most glioblastomas develop within the CEREBRUM (the main mass of the brain). This type of brain tumor occurs in 10 out of a million people in the United States each year.

The most common primary brain tumor of adults and the third most common of preteens, it occurs most often in those between ages 48 and 60, affecting twice as many men as women and whites more often than non-whites.

It is a rapidly spreading tumor with tentacles that invade nearby tissue, resembling a butterfly pattern of distribution throughout the WHITE MATTER of both CEREBRAL HEMISPHERES. The spread of this tumor outside the brain and SPINAL CORD is rare.

While glioblastomas may occur in any part of the cerebral hemispheres, they are most common in the FRONTAL, TEMPORAL, and PARIETAL LOBES.

Its cause is unknown, and although there have been cases of this type of tumor appearing in the same family, research has not yet found a hereditary link. Some research has suggested a possible link to a type of rare virus. Males with type A blood appear to be at higher risk, as are children who swallow lead or BARBITURATES; occupational chemical factors have also been associated with this type of tumor, such as those employed in rubber-manufacturing industries or who are exposed to vinyl chloride or pesticide sprays.

However, some factors have been excluded as a possible cause, including using birth control pills, smoking, alcohol use, prior HEAD INJURY, or exposure to dental X-RAYS.

Symptoms and Diagnostic Path

Because the tumor can grow so quickly, doubling its size every seven to eight days, the primary symptom is related to the compression of brain tissue by the tumor. Because the skull cannot enlarge to accommodate the increased pressure, it causes an "all-over" HEADACHE that is worse in the morning, together with vomiting (although not usually nausea). Other symptoms may include weak muscles, sensory disturbances, speech problems, SEIZURES, visual disturbances, and impaired mental processes.

Checking for a suspected brain tumor involves a fairly standard procedure, including a basic neurological exam testing eye movement and pupil reaction, observation of walking pattern, repeat rapid alternating movements, heel-to-toe walking, heel-to-shin movements, balance with feet together and eyes closed, sensation by pin prick, and smelling. Other tests may evaluate concrete and abstract thinking.

This may be followed by a set of plain skull X-rays together with some combination of scanning procedures. In order to locate the tumor and determine its extent, physicians may use ANGIOGRAPHY together with CT SCANNING, MAGNETIC RESONANCE IMAGING (MRI), ELECTROENCEPHALOGRAMS (EEG), RADIONUCLIDE BRAIN SCAN (RN), or POSITRON EMISSION TOMOGRAPHY (PET).

Treatment Options and Outlook

The tumor is surgically removed when possible, but too often this type of tumor is inaccessible or too extensive to be removed. In this case, survival rates are not high; less than 20 percent of these patients survive one year. When a tumor cannot be totally removed, as much of the growth as possible will be cut out to relieve pressure on the brain, followed by chemotherapy or radiation therapy. Corticosteroid drugs can be used to reduce tissue swelling around the tumor.

Laser microsurgery may be able to remove (by vaporization) some tissue past the tumor border in order to try to remove microscopic tumor infiltrates without damaging normal tissue too much. However, glioblastomas can never be totally removed because cells too small for the surgeon to see are present in the surrounding area. With luck, aggressive surgery can reduce the number of tumor cells so that chemotherapy or radiation therapy can be more effective. If the tumor recurs, a second or even third surgery may be performed.

Radiation is the second most common treatment for brain tumors after surgery, usually administered soon after the operation. The cells of many malignant brain tumors are readily killed by radiation, which is why this type of treatment is almost always recommended. (One possible exception is the treatment of very young children, whose developing brains may be injured by the radiation).

Most tumors do shrink from the effects of radiation, although it may take some time for swelling and dead cells to diminish so that the true size of the growth can be seen.

After radiation has reduced the number of tumor cells, chemotherapy is given to try to destroy any that remain. Chemotherapy may also be given at the same time as radiation.

Other possible treatments include brachytherapy (also called interstitial radiation or "seeding") in which radioactive pellets are implanted directly into the tumor during surgery. Brachytherapy is used primarily in recurrences when the tumor is confined to one side of the brain and measures less than six centimeters (about the size of a golf ball).

Other research is investigating the use of different types of radiation (such as neutrons), intraoperative radiation, and so on. Immunotherapy is also being studied, using drugs such as interferon, levamisole, interleukin-2, and thymosine in conjunction with chemotherapy or radiation therapy in the hopes of stimulating the body's own immune system.

There is also a whole range of new drugs being tested, plus better methods of drug delivery.

Long-term survival with this type of tumor is not very good. With surgery alone, median survival is 17 weeks; with radiation, 37.5 weeks; and with chemotherapy, 50 to 60 weeks. Chemotherapy increases the number of long-term survivors (those who live more than a year) from 4 percent to 20 percent; a few patients do survive for five years or more.

The Association for Brain Tumor Research maintains a current list of specialists in the glioblastoma field, who will agree to review medical records for a consultation fee.

glioma   A general name for a variety of brain tumors (see BRAIN TUMOR) arising from GLIAL CELLS within the brain. About 60 percent of all brain tumors that originate within the brain are gliomas; there are about two to four new cases per 100,000 people each year in the United States.

Symptoms and Diagnostic Path

Compression of brain tissue by the tumor may cause weak muscles, sensory disturbances, speech problems, and epileptic seizures. Pressure also can cause HEADACHES, vomiting, visual disturbances, and impaired mental processes.

In order to locate the tumor and determine its extent, physicians use ANGIOGRAPHY together with various types of BRAIN SCANS: CT SCANNING, MAGNETIC RESONANCE IMAGING (MRI), and X-RAY studies.

Treatment Options and Outlook

The tumor is surgically removed when possible, but too often it is inaccessible or too extensive to be removed. In this case, survival rates are not high; less than 20 percent of these patients survive one year. When a tumor cannot be totally removed, as much of the growth as possible will be cut out to relieve pressure on the brain, followed by chemotherapy or radiation therapy. Corticosteroid drugs can be used to reduce tissue swelling around the tumor.

Radiation is the second most common treatment for brain tumors, usually administered a few weeks after surgery. The cells of many malignant brain tumors are readily killed by radiation, which is why this type of treatment is almost always recommended. (One possible exception is the treatment of very young children, whose developing brains may be injured by the radiation.) Most tumors do shrink from the effects of radiation, although it may take some time for swelling and dead cells to diminish so the true size of the growth can be seen.

See also ASTROCYTOMA; OLIGODENDROGLIOMA; EPENDYMOMA; and GLIOBLASTOMA.

glioma of the optic nerve   A type of GLIOMA commonly found in children.

Symptoms and Diagnostic Path

This tumor causes blindness in one eye because of the pressure on the optic nerve; sometimes, the tumor extends to the third ventricle of the brain.

Treatment Options and Outlook

The usual treatment is radiation therapy, because this type of glioma is sensitive to radiation, or surgical excision. However, if the tumor extends into the third ventricle, the chances for survival are not good.

glossopharyngeal nerve Also known as the ninth cranial nerve, this nerve is mainly responsible for taste and throat sensations.

See also CRANIAL NERVES.

glucose A simple sugar that is the primary source of energy for the brain. Because glucose is not stored within the brain, a continuous supply is essential. If the brain is deprived of glucose for 10 to 15 minutes, irreversible brain damage can occur.

Free glucose is not found in many types of food (except for grapes), but it is a part of both sucrose and starch, both of which break down and form glucose after digestion. Glucose is stored in the body in the form of glycogen; its concentration in the blood is maintained by a variety of hormones (especially insulin and glucagon).

If the blood-glucose concentration falls below a certain level, symptoms of low blood sugar (hypo-glycemia) may occur. These symptoms include dizziness, apprehension, and fainting; in severe cases, COMA and death may follow. On the other hand, if there is too much glucose in the blood, hyperglycemia (the primary symptom of diabetes) may result.

glucose utilization scan See PET SCAN.

glutamate An amino acid found in every cell in the body, it is also used in the nervous system as a "fast excitatory" neurotransmitter. Glutamate is important in the proper function of the HIPPO-CAMPUS, among other brain areas; an imbalance will cause epileptic seizures, memory disorders, or both.

Glutamate is the best known of a group of excitatory amino acids that plays an important part in initiating and transmitting signals in the brain. Almost half of the brain's neurons use glutamate as a primary transmitter.

Normally, glutamate is bound tightly in the cells, and only tiny amounts are allowed into the spaces between brain cells at any one time. But new research suggests that abnormal glutamate activity may also be responsible for BRAIN DAMAGE following lack of oxygen from injury, STROKE, or SEIZURE. When the brain is deprived of oxygen and some of the cells that store glutamate shut down, glutamate comes flooding out of the cells; in such high levels, it kills brain cells—just five minutes of excess glutamate is enough to kill cells.

grand mal seizure The most severe type of EPILEPSY in which a person cries out and falls to the floor unconscious, jerking uncontrollably from muscle contractions. The seizure may last for a few minutes, and unconsciousness may last for some time afterward. The person may not remember anything about the seizure upon awakening. Sometimes, people experience warning symptoms before a grand mal attack.

gray matter Parts of the brain and SPINAL CORD that include mostly closely packed, interconnected nuclei of NERVE CELL bodies (instead of the AXONS that make up WHITE MATTER). Gray matter in the brain is primarily found in the outer layers of the CEREBRUM (the main mass of the brain) and in some deeper areas of the brain. Gray matter also makes up the inner core of the spinal cord.

growth hormone A hormone that promotes growth of the long bones and increases protein synthesis, both produced and stored in the PITUITARY GLAND. The release of growth hormone is controlled by the growth hormone releasing factor and the hormone somatostatin. The release of too much growth hormone can result in gigantism before puberty, and acromegaly (increase in size of hands, feet, and face) in adults. Lack of this hormone in children can produce dwarfism.

Guillain-Barré syndrome A rare disease of peripheral nerves characterized by numb, weak arms and legs. The condition usually appears 10 to 20 days after a respiratory infection that triggers an allergic response in the peripheral nerves, inflaming and destroying the MYELIN nerve sheath. The condition is also known as acute idiopathic polyneuritis or ascending paralysis.

In 1976, an epidemic occurred in the United States following mass vaccination against swine flu, but further evaluation showed the vaccination did not cause the flurry of cases. Two-thirds of cases occur after a viral infection that may be a form of herpes (such as Epstein-Barr virus), or it may follow flu, a cold, or other minor infection. The syndrome may also appear with conditions such as Hodgkin's disease.

Occasionally, Guillain-Barré is associated with medical procedures and 5 to 10 percent occur after operations.

A severe attack of Guillain-Barré is a medical emergency and may require a stay in intensive care; a few patients need artificial ventilation during the illness. Generally, recovery begins after a few months, and most people recover completely without specific treatment, although there is permanent weakness in about 10 percent of cases. Others may suffer from repeated attacks of the disease. The mortality rate is 3 to 4 percent.

Symptoms and Diagnostic Path

A few days to a week or so after infection, or one to four weeks after an operation, symptoms appear, including tingling sensations in fingers and toes and general muscle weakness. A sensation of weakness can spread from legs to arms and face; in severe cases, weakness turns into paralysis and may affect respiratory muscles. Muscles controlling eye or facial movements, speaking, chewing, or swallowing may also be affected. About 3,500 cases occur every year in the United States and Canada.

The disease is diagnosed by a variety of tests (such as ELECTROMYOGRAPHY), analysis of cerebrospinal fluid extracted by LUMBAR PUNCTURE (spinal tap), and a physical exam.

Treatment Options and Outlook

Patients are treated in the hospital with supportive care; mechanical ventilation may be necessary. Some patients benefit from plasmapheresis (removal of plasma and damaging antibodies from the blood) during the first few weeks of a severe attack; this may improve the chance for a full recovery. Once the condition has stabilized, rehabilitation will include whirlpool baths to relieve pain and retrain movements, physical therapy, and training with adaptive devices.

habituation A decrease in the intensity of a behavioral response because a stimulus has been presented so often that it is no longer consciously noticed. Perhaps the most common form of learning, habituation enables humans and other animals to ignore unimportant stimuli and focus on those that are rewarding or important for survival.

Habituation is the very first learning process found in infants, who learn, for example, to ignore harmless household noises.

Haller, Albrecht von (1708–1777) Swiss biologist and the father of experimental physiology who showed that the sensation of touch depends on nerves and that nerves activate muscles. Von Haller also traced nerves from the body's limbs to the brain's CEREBRAL CORTEX. While serving as professor of medicine at the University of Göttingen, he wrote the eight-volume landmark in medical history: *Physiological Elements of the Human Body.*

See also BRAIN IN HISTORY.

hallucination Seeing, hearing, touching, smelling, or tasting something that does not actually exist.

hallucinogenic mushrooms Mushrooms are a kind of fungus that come in many varieties, from edible to toxic and/or hallucinogenic. The hallucinogenic mushrooms, which include the psilocybin/psilocin and *Amanita muscaria* mushrooms, can alter or produce false perceptions of sight, sound, taste, smell, or touch. Some toxic substances in these mushrooms can cause severe illness and even death, and most hallucinogenic substances are illegal.

The hallucinogenic properties of certain mushrooms have been known for centuries, as seen in mushroom sculptures from ancient ruins in Central and South America suggesting that these mushrooms were used by native people during religious ceremonies. The Aztecs used the term *teonanacatl* meaning "flesh of the gods" to describe hallucinogenic mushrooms. Historians believe that Aztec spiritual leaders used these hallucinogens to induce an altered state of consciousness that they believed would allow them to communicate with their gods and other spirits.

Psilocybin/Psilocin

Mushrooms that contain the hallucinogens psilocybin and or psilocin belong mainly to the genera Psilocybe, Stropharia, Conocybe, and Panaeolus. The word *psilocybin* comes from the Greek words *psilo* ("bald") and *cybe* ("head"). Some specific mushrooms containing psilocybin and or psilocin include

- *Psilocybe mexicana*
- *Stropharia cubensis*
- *P. semilanceata*
- *P. pelliculosa*
- *Panaeolus subbalteatus*
- *P. cyanescens*
- *P. baeocystis*

Both psilocybin and psyilocin produce yawning, inability to concentrate, restlessness, increased heart rate, and hallucinations. These symptoms may appear 30 to 60 minutes after the mushroom is eaten, and can last for about four hours.

Their chemical structure is similar to the neurotransmitter SEROTONIN. In fact, the primary effect of psilocin is on the receptors for serotonin. There is also evidence that psilocybin reduces the reuptake of serotonin by brain cells, allowing this neurotransmitter more time to act in the brain.

Amanita Muscaria

Also known as "fly agaric" because of its ability to attract and kill flies, this mushroom does not contain psilocybin or psilocin. Its hallucinogenic chemicals include muscimol and ibotenic acid. It is related to other deadly mushrooms, including *A. virosa* ("Destroying Angel"), *A. verna,* and *A. phalloides* ("Death Cap"), all of which are deadly and contain toxins that destroy cells in the liver and kidneys.

The muscimol in these mushrooms produces feelings of euphoria, hallucinations, muscle jerks, drowsiness, sweating, pupil dilation, and increased body temperature. Symptoms appear 30 to 90 minutes after ingestion, and are most intense after two or three hours. People who eat these mushrooms usually fall into a deep sleep. Some people describe the effects of eating *A. muscaria* as similar to being intoxicated by alcohol.

Muscimol and ibotenic acid appear to act on the GABA neurotransmitter system; muscimol activates GABA receptors on brain cells. The GABA neurotransmitter system is one of the brain's major inhibitory systems, therefore muscimol acts to inhibit the activity of neurons in the brain.

hallucinogens   A class of drugs that cause HALLUCINATIONS by interfering with the normal chemical balance of the brain, mimicking the naturally occurring OPIATES that affect the LIMBIC SYSTEM.

There are four main groups of hallucinogens, each containing drugs derived from plants: the *indole alkaloid derivatives* (including LSD, harmatine, ibogaine, and psilocybin); *piperidine derivatives* (atropine, belladonna, and scopolamine); *phenylethylamines* (amphetamines and mescaline); and *cannabinols* (cannabis, or marijuana).

Most hallucinogens, including LSD, stimulate the SYMPATHETIC NERVOUS SYSTEM, boosting pulse rate and blood pressure resulting in sweating and palpitations. Others (such as the cannabinols) reduce stomach acid secretion and have a calming effect on the brain.

Hallucinogens also have an intense effect on the brain's limbic system, influencing mood and emotions and suppressing centers controlling memory and higher functions such as judgment. This combination of limbic system effects (which can cause violent mood swings) together with loss of judgment can be dangerous.

Particular effects depend on the type of drug and the dose; some emphasize feelings while others influence fantasies. Effects may also depend in part on the user's personality, and those unused to drugs may experience ANXIETY, depression, or nausea. Those who have used drugs often report euphoria and irrational thoughts or mystical experiences that may be confused with a higher state of consciousness. While not normally addictive, hallucinogens may trigger a psychological dependence.

handedness   A person's preference for using the right or the left hand; 90 percent of healthy adults use the right hand for writing, and most (66 percent) favor the right hand for most other activities requiring coordination. The rest are either left-handed or ambidextrous (able to use either hand). Handedness has no correlation to gender, and if the brain becomes damaged before age 12, it is possible to switch handedness.

Handedness is related to the two hemispheres of the brain, each of which controls movement and sensation in the opposite side of the body. The dominant hemisphere in right-handed people is always the left one, but oddly enough, this is true for left-handers as well, although a few have dominant right hemispheres. Some display no dominance at all. Scientists suspect that some language disorders such as DYSLEXIA and stuttering are more common in left-handed people and may be related to a problem in developing cerebral dominance.

Scientists believe that a tendency toward the right or the left hand is inherited, although it is possible to force a left-handed child to use the right hand. In early centuries, a left-handed person was considered to be unlucky at best and evil at worst (indeed, the word *sinister* comes from the Latin word for "left"). While this is no longer true today, so many people are right-handed that the pressure to conform is very high, especially in cultures that reserve the left hand for cleaning the anal area after defecating.

It is not clear whether handedness is related to special abilities, and while the left brain is related to verbal ability and local reasoning and the right to emotional and spatial ability, there is no evidence that more artists are left-handed or more writers are right-handed. In fact, about 60 percent of left-handed people, like right-handers, process speech in the left hemisphere, while the other 40 percent use both sides of the brain. This is one indication that each of the brain's hemispheres has the potential for processing any function. It often takes advantage of this potential following BRAIN INJURY from trauma or STROKE. However, there is some evidence that there are disproportionately large numbers of left-handers at both the upper and lower extremes of intelligence. A few scientists suspect that the CEREBRUM evolved into two almost identical parts to provide a sort of "back-up" brain in case of accidents.

The right brain does seem to be critically involved in appreciating and interpreting spatial relationships and visualizing complex three-dimensional shapes, in addition to recognizing faces.

Harvey, William (1578–1657) The British physician who discovered the secret of blood circulation and who also believed that sensory nerves sent sensations to the brain and that motor nerves worked muscles. A graduate of the University of Padua medical school, he was a member of the Royal College of Physicians, and served as physician extraordinary to James I of England. He was one of the doctors in attendance at the death of the king in 1625. He was also appointed personal physician to Charles I.

See also BRAIN IN HISTORY.

headaches Pain in the head or front of the face that can range from mild to extremely severe. One of the most common medical complaints, each year headaches affect as many as 24 million Americans seriously enough for them to miss work. While most headaches do not represent a life-threatening condition, they can significantly interfere with the activities of daily living. Headaches that may represent a more serious medical problem are those that appear suddenly, that are extremely severe, or that change in pattern or severity of pain.

The many different causes for headache are diagnosed according to how they occur, together with their severity, onset, and location. There are many types of headaches as well, including: tension headaches, vascular headaches, cluster headaches, toxic headaches, hypertensive headaches, and headaches caused by trauma or disease.

Tension Headaches

These common headaches are set off by severe muscle contractions caused by stress or exertion. People who are so anxious that they grind their teeth or hunch their shoulders may find that the strain can travel to the nerves in the brain, producing constant pain. Many people report this pain as a kind of tight band around the forehead, affecting both sides of the head. Tension headaches occur most often in the front of the head, although they may also appear at the top or the back. Eyestrain caused by coping with a great amount of paperwork can cause a tension headache that builds up during the day.

Tension headaches respond very well to over-the-counter drugs such as aspirin, ibuprofen, or acetaminophen, or by massaging the tense muscle groups responsible for the pain. Those who often get tension headaches should consider taking stress breaks throughout the day.

Vascular Headaches

Vascular headaches can be divided into four subcategories. The first is the *migraine,* the most debilitating of all headaches, which causes a profound throbbing pain that is often accompanied by nausea and vomiting. Researchers thought that migraines were caused by abnormally dilated blood vessels in the head, but more recently they have found the pain is caused by electrochemical activity in the brain that is usually caused by stress, hunger, fatigue, sensory overload, hormone fluctuations, or addiction withdrawal. Some people with migraines see spots, auras, flashes, or blank spots right before a migraine strikes. Migraines are almost always limited to one side of the head. People who place a great deal of stress on themselves are more likely to suffer with treatment-resistant migraines.

TYPES OF HEADACHES

Symptoms	Type	Cause
Pain on both sides of head	Tension headache	Muscle contraction
Agonizing pain on one side of head; nausea or vomiting	Migraine	Stress, hunger, fatigue, addiction withdrawal, sensory overload, hormone fluctuation
Less pain than migraine; stuffy sinus	Cluster	Same as migraine
Dull head pain	Hypertensive	High blood pressure
Head pain	Toxic	Food or chemicals, allergies
Pain with weakness, loss of balance, numbing	Injury/disease	Infection, anemia, trauma, neurological problems

Migraines are treated by prescription drugs that affect the brain's chemistry, such as ergotamine, methysegide, and verapamil. Migraines also respond to antidepressants (especially the SELECTIVE SEROTONIN REUPTAKE INHIBITORS such as Prozac), not because the patient is depressed but because the drugs normalize the brain's level of SEROTONIN, which is believed to be askew in migraine patients.

Cluster headaches are milder cousins of the migraine that do not announce their onset with visual disturbances, do not cause nausea, and do not last very long. They usually occur in two or three episodes in one day, lasting between 10 minutes to a few hours each time. Unlike migraines, cluster headaches include the sensation of a stuffy sinus. Cause and treatment are the same as for migraines.

Cluster headaches are treated by the same type of prescription drugs used to treat migraines—drugs that affect the brain's chemistry, such as ergotamine, methysegide, and verapamil.

Toxic headaches are caused by chemical fumes (such as carbon monoxide) or by chemicals in food such as chocolate, cheese, or citrus fruits. They also may be caused by allergies or weather changes. Medical tests can determine whether a person's headache is of toxic origin.

Hypertensive headaches are caused by high blood pressure, characterized by a dull pain that is easily relieved by bed rest.

Headaches Caused by Trauma/Disease

This type of headache can be the most difficult to diagnose. The headaches may be caused by a wide range of problems, including sinus infections or infection in the blood or lymph system; a neurological problem in the brain, eyes, ears, teeth, face, or spine; anemia; or trauma caused by blows, tumors, or blood clots. They may be particularly severe or accompanied by numbness, balance problems, or weakness.

head injury   Even the mildest bump on the head is capable of damaging the brain; research suggests that 60 percent of patients who sustain a mild BRAIN INJURY continue to have a range of symptoms called POSTCONCUSSION SYNDROME as long as six months after the injury. These symptoms can result in a puzzling interplay of behavioral, cognitive, and emotional complaints that can be difficult to diagnose. Although research is still limited, studies have found that symptoms following even the mildest head injury can linger, causing ongoing discomfort and destroying personal lives.

The fact that head injury can have effects throughout the body has been known for at least the past 3,000 years; the Edwin Smith Surgical Papyrus written between 2,500 and 3,000 years ago contains information about 48 cases in which eight people describe head injuries that affect other parts of the body.

Symptoms and Diagnostic Path

Symptoms following head injury may be due both from the direct physical damage to the brain and also to secondary factors, such as lack of oxygen, swelling, and vascular disturbance. A penetrating injury may also cause a brain infection. The kind of injury the brain receives in a closed head injury is determined by the type of accident; whether or not the head was unrestrained upon impact; and the direction, force, and velocity of the blow. If the head is resting upon impact, the maximum damage will be found at the impact site; a moving head will cause a "contrecoup" injury where the damage will be on the side opposite the point of impact.

Both kinds of injuries can cause swirling movements throughout the brain, tearing nerve fibers and causing widespread vascular damage. There may be bleeding in the CEREBRUM or SUBARACHNOID SPACE leading to HEMATOMAS. Swelling may raise intracranial pressure and may block oxygen to the brain.

After a head injury, there may be a period of impaired consciousness followed by a period of confusion and impaired memory with confusion, disorientation, and impairment in the ability to store and retrieve new information. For some reason, the physical and emotional shock of the accident interrupts the transfer of all information that happened to be in the short-term memory just before the accident; this is why some people can remember information several days before and after the accident, but not information right before the accident occurred.

There may be a temporary AMNESIA following head injury that often begins with memory loss over a period of weeks, months, or years prior to the injury, diminishing as recovery proceeds. Permanent amnesia, however, may extend for just a few seconds or minutes before the accident; in very severe head injuries, however, the permanent amnesia may also cover weeks or months before the accident.

A small minority are plagued by symptoms, including HEADACHE, dizziness, confusion, and memory loss which may continue for months.

Until recently, diagnostic tools were not sensitive enough to detect the subtle structural changes that can occur and sometimes persist after mild head injury. Typically, CT SCANS have yielded negative results from this group of patients. But studies involving MAGNETIC RESONANCE IMAGING (MRI) and brain electrophysiology indicate that contusions and diffuse injuries associated with mild head injury are likely to affect those parts of the brain that relate to memory, concentration, information processing, and problem solving.

CT Scans While CT scans are widely available in emergency rooms to help in the diagnosis of neural hematomas, many experts believe these scans may not pick up the subtle damage following a mild head injury.

MRI Many researchers believe MRI is more sensitive in diagnosing many brain lesions beyond a basic hematoma. For example, MRI is more sensitive in detecting the diffuse axonal or shearing injury and contusions often seen in mild head injury.

Quantitative EEG (qEEG) In many patients, neither CT scans nor MRI can detect the microscopic damage to white matter that occurs when fibers are stretched in a mild, diffuse axonal injury. In this type of mild injury, the axons lose some of their covering and become less efficient, but MRI detects only more severe injury and actual axonal degeneration. Mild injury to the white matter reduces the quality of communication between different parts of the cerebral cortex. A quantitative EEG is different from a regular electroencephalogram in that the signals from the brain are played into a computer, digitized, and stored. EEG can measure the time delay between two regions of the cortex and the amount of time it takes for information to be transmitted from one region to another.

Evoked Potentials This electrophysial technique of measuring evoked potentials (EPs) generally is not useful in patients with less-serious mild head injury. EPs are not sensitive enough to document any physiologic abnormalities, although a patient may be having symptoms. If testing is done within a day or two of injury, an EP may pick up some abnormalities in brain stem auditory evoked potentials.

Neuropsychological Testing Neuropsychological tests may show positive results when imaging tests and neurologic exams are negative. In some patients with persistent symptoms following mild head injury, neuropsychological tests are part of a comprehensive assessment. The tests can also provide information when litigation is an issue.

Future Tests PET (positron emission tomography), which evaluates cerebral blood flow and brain metabolism, may provide useful information on functional pathology. Single-photon emission computerized tomography (SPECT) is less expensive than PET and might provide data on cerebral blood flow after mild head injury.

Treatment Options and Outlook

Only a small percentage of patients with mild head injury are hospitalized overnight, and instructions they receive upon leaving the emergency room usually do not address behavioral, cognitive, and emotional symptoms that can occur after such an injury.

Patients who do experience symptoms are advised to seek out the care of a specialist; unless a family physician is thoroughly familiar with medical literature in this newly emerging area, experts warn that there is a great chance that patient complaints will be ignored.

hearing The sense of hearing occurs when the ears convert sounds into electrochemical signals that travel to the brain's TEMPORAL LOBES (the "hearing centers") where sounds are interpreted.

Sound waves travel through the outer ear tunnel to the eardrum, the gateway to the middle ear. Sound waves vibrate the eardrum, which in turn vibrates a sequence of tiny movable bones (the hammer, anvil, and stirrup [or malleus, incus, and stapes]). Sound vibrations also reach the inner ear via the skull bones. As the vibrating stapes plunges in and out of the oval window leading to the inner ear, waves are sent through fluid-filled membrane chambers including the cochlea of the inner ear. In turn, this stimulates the organ of Corti, a tunnel surrounded by rods with thousands of sensitive hairs attached to nerve fibers. When the hairs vibrate, the nerves send signals corresponding to the pitch and volume of the sound, through the ACOUSTIC NERVE (or eighth cranial nerve) to the BRAIN STEM.

In the brain stem, nerve fibers from both sides of the head cross, taking signals up through the CEREBRAL HEMISPHERES to the tops of the temporal lobes to be analyzed. This way, signals from each ear reach both temporal lobes, which means if one lobe is damaged, the patient will not necessarily be functionally deaf in one ear.

Signals arriving from both ears help pinpoint the location of sound. Humans are capable of detecting sound waves with frequencies ranging from a low of 20 cycles per second to a high of 20,000 cycles per second.

Any sound loud enough to cause physical pain is capable of damaging a person's hearing; in addition, some diseases or drugs can cause deafness. Central hearing loss is caused by damage or impairment of the nerves of the CENTRAL NERVOUS SYSTEM, either in the pathways to the brain or the brain itself. This type of hearing loss may result from congenital brain abnormalities, tumors, or lesions in the central nervous system, STROKES, or some types of medications.

Hebb, Donald (1904–1985) A Canadian neuroscientist who revived the idea that memories are stored as patterns of newly connected neurons. In his book *The Organization of Behavior* (1949), Hebb speculated that the new circuits might be made during a learning situation, when one neuron tends to fire another, strengthening the synapse between them.

Two neurons that tend to be active at the same time will form a new connection automatically; if they are already weakly connected, the synapse between them will be stronger, and if not, an entirely new synapse will be made. This has come to be called the HEBB SYNAPSE.

Hebb's theory also includes ideas about long-term potentiation (LTP), which explains how when an axon of one cell excites its neighbor cell repeatedly or consistently, some growth process or metabolic change takes place in both cells. This increased synaptic efficacy may last for weeks.

While today the idea does not seem unusual, in the early 1940s when Hebb came up with the notion, there was no evidence to believe that experience caused any kind of physiological change in the brain.

Hebb's rule If two neurons fire at the same time, they increase the strength of the connection between them. The rule is named for Canadian neuroscientist Donald Hebb, who explored the idea of long-term potentiation in his book *The Organization of Behavior* (1949). (See also HEBB, DONALD.)

Hebb synapse The name given to a synapse strengthened by a link formed when two connected neurons fire together. It also refers to a new synapse formed if there is no connection between firing cells.

The idea, formulated in 1949 by Canadian neuroscientist Donald Hebb, is part of his learning theory that explains how neurons are connected to form neural assemblies that are integrated into still larger structures called phase sequences. (See also HEBB, DONALD.)

hemangioblastoma A rare type of tumor of the SPINAL CORD (also known as Lindau's tumor) that consists of blood vessel cells usually developing in the form of cysts in the CEREBELLUM or the MENINGES. The tumors are usually found in children and young adults.

In von Hippel-Lindau disease, hemangioblastomas (especially in the cerebellum) are associated with renal and pancreatic cysts, tumors in the retina, cancer of the kidney cells, and red birthmarks.

Symptoms and Diagnostic Path
Symptoms include HEADACHE, vomiting, incoordination, and rapid involuntary eye movements (nystagmus).

Treatment Options and Outlook
The tumor is slow growing and is normally clearly differentiated from the surrounding brain tissue; it can usually be removed surgically. In most cases, this surgery completely cures the condition.

hematoma A collection of clotted blood caused by bleeding from a ruptured blood vessel that may occur anywhere in the body; however, it is most serious when it presses on the brain (such as a EXTRADURAL HEMATOMA or a SUBDURAL HEMATOMA). Hematomas are usually caused by an injury that ruptures a blood vessel under the skull; they may be fatal unless treated promptly.

hemiballismus The irregular, uncontrollable movements of an arm or a leg on one side of the body caused by disease in the BASAL GANGLIA. The movements are unpredictable, and they may be so severe that they injure the person or other people.

hemispatial neglect The tendency for a patient with BRAIN DAMAGE (usually to the right side of the brain) to ignore one side of space; the side ignored is almost always the left side.

hemispherectomy The surgical removal of half of the human brain as a way to treat severe SEIZURES that do not respond to any other treatment. The procedure is most successful when performed on children because the growing brain is capable of taking over many of the functions of the missing lobe. Many children who have had the operation show surprisingly intact cognitive function.

Once the CORTEX is removed, the skull fills with CEREBROSPINAL FLUID to take up the empty space.

When the operation was first performed in the 1940s, few patients survived. However, by the mid-1980s, advances in BRAIN SCANS and new methods to stop bleeding made the procedure far safer, although it still carries a risk of COMA or death. Today, several dozen hemispherectomies are performed on children in the United States each year, as a treatment for Rasmussen's ENCEPHALITIS and certain forms of EPILEPSY (those that destroy the cortex but do not cross over from one hemisphere to the other).

It is possible to survive such a profound insult to the brain because surgeons are careful not to remove areas that control basic bodily functions, such as the DIENCEPHALON (controlling emotion and body function), the CEREBELLUM (which coordinates movement), or the BRAIN STEM (overseeing breathing, heart rate, and so on).

hemispheres of the brain See CEREBRAL HEMISPHERES.

hemisphericity The tendency for one hemisphere of the brain to be dominant, no matter what the task.

hemorrhage, brain   Bleeding within the brain caused by rupture of a blood vessel.

See also EXTRADURAL HEMORRHAGE; INTRACERE-BRAL HEMORRHAGE; SUBDURAL HEMORRHAGE.

heroin and the brain   Researchers in the 1970s discovered that OPIATES like heroin are effective because the brain contains built-in opiate receptors whose selective activation by opiates kills pain. Researchers realized the only reason the brain had such an opiate system must be that the brain was capable of producing its own opiates—which they subsequently discovered and named ENDORPHINS.

Endorphins may be released during powerful emotions, during childbirth, during pleasurable activities, or during exercise.

But when a person adds external opiates to the brain, the body's own production of the endorphins drops. The body requires more and more endorphins to achieve the same degree of pleasure, and the withdrawal pains worsen; finally, withdrawal can cause intense physical pain, HALLUCINATIONS, and even death.

Herophilus of Chalcedon (335–280 B.C.)   The father of anatomy, Herophilus was an Alexandrian physician who performed public dissections of human cadavers.

Herophilus practiced medicine during one of the brief periods in Greek medical history when it was acceptable to dissect humans. He spent his time studying the VENTRICLES of the brain. As early as 300 B.C., Herophilus believed that the brain was the central part of the NERVOUS SYSTEM and associated nerves with movement and sensation. He traced the sinuses of the DURA MATTER (the tough membrane covering the brain) to their junction, where he classified the nerve trunks as either motor or sensory.

Herophilus was a proponent of Hippocrates' doctrine of medicine based on balancing the four humors of the body—blood, phlegm, choler, and melancholy. He also emphasized the importance of medications, diet, and exercise. He wrote at least nine books, including discussions of anatomy and the cause of sudden death, all of which were lost

in the destruction of the library of Alexandria in A.D. 272.

See also BRAIN IN HISTORY.

hindbrain   One of the three major sections of the brain, also known as the rhombencephalon, part of which exits into the SPINAL CORD at the base of the skull. The hindbrain is made up of the metencephalon (including the PONS and CEREBELLUM) and the myelencephalon (the MEDULLA OBLONGATA). The pons and medulla oblongata transmit all signals between the spinal cord and the higher parts of the brain and contain clusters of cranial nerve nuclei that connect the nerves going to and from the face and head; it also governs automatic functions such as heart rate and breathing. Because of the shape and position of the pons and medulla at the brain base, they are referred to as the BRAIN STEM, although this term usually also includes structures in the MID-BRAIN and lower DIENCEPHALON.

hippocampus   A structure located beneath the TEMPORAL LOBE that may be the site of learning ability. This ridge, a part of the LIMBIC SYSTEM, is named for its curving shape, which reminded ancient scientists of a seahorse. The paired structure found on each side of the brain links nerve fibers involved in touch, vision, sound, and smell with the limbic system.

The hippocampus receives NERVE CELL input from the CORTEX and appears to consolidate information for storage as permanent memory. It appears to be particularly important in learning and remembering spatial information. The hippocampus is related to memory because of its response to repetitive stimulation; its SYNAPSES change according to previous experience, which may form the structural basis of memory itself. But because research shows that a person with a damaged hippocampus can still retain long-term memory, it is not likely that this part of the brain is the primary storehouse for this type of memory.

A damaged hippocampus interferes with the ability to form new memory, but only the conscious memory or recall of facts and events is lost. The ability to learn both mental and physical skills remains intact, nor is there damage to the memory used in immediate recall (that is, matters to which a person is paying current attention).

In addition, the hippocampus does not play a vital role in storing older memories but is profoundly important in the short-term memory of contextual information (such as the series of clues a person would recall when trying to find a parked car in a crowded lot). It is also important in converting new sensory information into a form that can be preserved elsewhere in the brain.

Other research into the action of the hippocampus has found that people use different areas of their brains to perform different types of memory tasks. Using PET SCAN (POSITRON EMISSION TOMOGRAPHY), researchers monitored changes in blood flow in the volunteers' brains as they provided endings to words flashed before them. Areas of increased blood flow revealed the brain regions used during the various tasks.

When subjects drew upon memories of previous lists to complete the fragment "mot-," the right hippocampus showed an increased blood supply. This means that subjects were using this part of the brain to remember the word, even though researchers had always attributed such verbal processing to the left brain. If the subjects did not search their brains for a word they had already seen and instead gave the first word that came to them, blood flow did not increase to either side of the hippocampus.

Sometimes, subjects spontaneously recalled words from the lists even if they did not remember having seen the words before. Psychologists call this phenomenon *priming,* and it prompted increased blood flow to the visual cortex.

Still other studies found that monkeys that learned to recognize objects 16, 12, eight, four, and two weeks before surgery damaged their hippocampus forgot what they had learned two to four weeks before the damage, but they recalled early learning better. Normal monkeys remembered more recent learning better than older memories.

Both the NEUROTRANSMITTER GLUTAMATE and the inhibitor neurotransmitter GABA (GAMMA AMINOBUTYRIC ACID) are important in the proper function of the hippocampus; an imbalance in either of these transmitters will cause epileptic seizures, memory disorders, or both. (Patients with EPILEPSY usually demonstrate memory problems as well.)

The most common cause of damage to the hippocampus is ANOXIA (loss of oxygen) to the brain during a difficult birth and delivery; most patients with idiopathic epilepsy suffered from anoxia at birth, which damaged the hippocampus. One reason why memories may be so vulnerable to the loss of oxygen is that hippocampus cells are the quickest to die when oxygen to the brain is cut off.

Hippocrates (460–377 B.C.) The fourth-century B.C. Greek physician popularly known as the father of medicine. In his writings, Hippocrates noted that madness is the result of too much "moistness" in the brain. This belief was based on the then-popular belief that human health was based on the four "humors" (earth, fire, air, and water).

Interestingly, the idea of an excess moistness appears to be curiously accurate in the case of schizophrenic patients; recent research suggests that SCHIZOPHRENIA patients have larger fluid-bearing VENTRICLES than normal patients.

hologramic brain The theory that any part of the brain contains the entire mind, just as any part of a hologram holds the entire image.

hormones Chemicals made of protein produced and released by a gland, they circulate through the bloodstream until they reach target cells, which they stimulate into activity. Hormones control the rate and the way that various reactions in the body happen. The PITUITARY secretes nine hormones into the blood that control targeted tissues.

hot tubs Women who use hot tubs or saunas during early pregnancy nearly triple their chances of giving birth to babies with SPINA BIFIDA or brain defects, according to research. One study, which surveyed 22,762 women, was designed to explore other issues relating to childbirth and did not include detailed questions about hot tubs and saunas. Nevertheless, the findings showed that women who used a hot tub during the first two months of pregnancy were 2.8 times more likely to bear a child with birth defects than were women with no exposure to heat. The study found no such effect for electric blankets. (Saunas and hot tubs already carried warnings against using during pregnancy.)

These findings support what was already known about the detrimental effects of heat on animal pregnancy.

human prion diseases   Diseases primarily affecting the nervous system that are characterized by microscopic holes and pits in brain tissue (spongiform degeneration) and an abnormal form of a protein called a PRION. Prions are a normal component in brain tissue, but mutant forms of these proteins become deformed and resist being broken down into normal proteins, instead building up in the brain.

The prion diseases can be spontaneous (sporadic), transmitted by infection (acquired), or inherited. Sporadic prion diseases include CREUTZFELDT-JAKOB DISEASE (CJD) and familial insomnia. Inherited types of prion diseases include classic CJD, fatal familial insomnia, and Gerstmann-Sträussler-Scheinker syndrome. Acquired types of prion diseases include new variant CJD, classic CJD, and KURU.

hunger   An uncomfortable feeling caused by the need for food (unlike APPETITE, which is a pleasant sensation felt when expecting a meal).

Hunger occurs when the stomach is empty and blood GLUCOSE (the primary sugar that the body uses for food) is low. Special sugar receptors in the HYPOTHALAMUS monitor the blood levels of glucose; when these levels drop, sugar receptors stimulate eating by causing the stomach to contract. When pronounced, these contractions produce hunger pains.

In the past, NEUROLOGISTS thought feelings of hunger and fullness were controlled by just two areas in the hypothalamus called the feeding center and the satiety center, but today we know that a person's hunger is affected by many different brain regions; at least 25 NEUROPEPTIDES all over the brain affect food intake.

Researchers at Rockefeller University in New York City discovered that two chemicals in the brain are responsible for causing some types of food cravings: neuropeptide Y causes carbohydrate cravings in rats, and galanin seems to underlie a desire for fatty foods. The more of these chemicals the body produces, the stronger the drive to eat those particular foods. Hormones and the amount of glucose used by cells moderate the amount of neuropeptide Y production. Scientists hope that once the neurochemical signals for hunger are better understood, doctors may be able to deal with appetites for fats and sugars.

Huntington's disease (HD)   An inherited disorder that causes abnormal involuntary movements (CHOREA) and progressive mental impairment, including memory loss. The disease slowly diminishes the affected individual's ability to walk, think, talk, and reason. Eventually, the person with HD becomes totally dependent upon others for his or her care. Huntington's disease profoundly affects the lives of entire families: emotionally, socially, and economically.

Named for Dr. George Huntington, who first described this hereditary disorder in 1872, HD is now recognized as one of the more common genetic disorders. More than a quarter of a million Americans have HD or are at risk of inheriting the disease from an affected parent. HD affects as many people as hemophilia, cystic fibrosis, or muscular dystrophy.

It is caused by the degeneration of the CAUDATE NUCLEUS in the BASAL GANGLIA (paired nerve-cell clusters in the brain) and of the frontal association NEOCORTEX.

In 1993, the gene was isolated and a direct genetic test developed which can accurately determine whether a person carries the HD gene. However, the test cannot predict when symptoms will begin. In the absence of a cure, some individuals at risk elect not to take the test.

Since the discovery of the gene that causes HD, scientific research has accelerated and much has been added to the understanding of Huntington's disease and its effects upon different individuals.

The origins of this brain atrophy are unknown, but some scientists believe the damage may be caused by a buildup of natural chemicals that flood the bundles of NEURONS within the FOREBRAIN, killing them and causing the progressive memory loss, angry rages, and muscle spasms that mark the disease.

The two main chemicals believed responsible for the nerve-cell degeneration are quinolinic acid and GLUTAMATE. These two play essential roles in normal concentrations (quinolinic acid is a breakdown product of TRYPTOPHAN and glutamate is a NEUROTRANSMITTER and metabolic agent). But too much of either chemical kills certain cells, and both bind to the receptor site for a chemical called NMDA. Researchers have found that the brains of Huntington's disease patients had 93 percent fewer NMDA RECEPTORS, indicating that the cells with those receptors had died. In two other studies, researchers found decreased number of receptors for five other chemicals in the brains of Huntington's patients.

Symptoms and Diagnostic Path

Symptoms usually appear between the ages of 35 and 50, although in rare cases they appear during childhood. This is a genetic disorder with an autosomal pattern of inheritance; each child of an affected parent has a 50 percent chance of developing the condition. Huntington's is found in about five out of every 100,000 Americans.

The jerky movements usually affect the face, arms, and trunk, causing random grimaces, twitches, and general clumsiness. These changes usually occur first, followed in several years by dementia beginning with personality and behavior changes, irritability, problems making decisions, memory loss, and apathy. Language tends to remain normal for a much longer period than it does in other cortical dementias. Psychotic disorders may also become apparent, including both manic-depressive psychosis and schizophreniclike HALLUCINATIONS.

Today, offspring of affected parents can take a test to discover whether they have inherited the abnormal gene responsible for the condition.

Treatment Options and Outlook

There is no known cure for Huntington's disease, but drugs like CHLORPROMAZINE can lessen the jerky movements. Most people with Huntington's disease live for about 15 years after the onset of symptoms, although some have lived as long as 30 years.

Researchers suggest that some cells may be more vulnerable to damage from glutamate and quinolinic acid because they contain more NMDA receptors. It is hoped that finding a way to block those receptors might slow the disease; however, selective NMDA-block has not been effective. Although there is no treatment available to stop the progression of the disease, the movement disorders and psychiatric symptoms can be controlled by drugs.

Hydergine (ergoloid mesylates) This extract of ergot, a fungus that grows on rye, is a widely used treatment for all forms of dementia in the United States, and has been approved by the U.S. Food and Drug Administration as a treatment for Alzheimer's disease. Some doctors also may prescribe it to combat brain aging in healthy people.

Its effectiveness in reducing symptoms of senility have been well established. Scientists think it works by interfering with dangerous forms of oxygen (called free radicals), enhancing brain cell metabolism and increasing blood supply and oxygen to the brain. Some scientists believe it may boost memory by mimicking the effect of nerve growth factor, a substance that stimulates dendrite growth in the brain.

hydrocephalus Also known as "water on the brain," this is an excess of CEREBROSPINAL FLUID within the skull (usually under increased pressure). This condition is often associated with other abnormalities present at birth, especially SPINA BIFIDA.

The condition is diagnosed with CAT SCANS or MRI, which show the location and nature of an obstruction.

Untreated, the condition will progress to extreme drowsiness, severe BRAIN DAMAGE, and SEIZURES, which may be fatal within a few weeks.

Hydrocephalus is caused by the excessive formation of cerebrospinal fluid, by a circulation block of this fluid, or both. It may be present at birth, or it may develop following severe HEAD INJURY, brain hemorrhage, infection (such as MENINGITIS) or a brain tumor (see TUMORS, BRAIN).

Symptoms and Diagnostic Path

If present at birth, the symptom is an enlarged head that continues to grow at an excessively fast rate because the skull bones are not rigid and expand to accommodate the fluid. Other features include leg rigidity, EPILEPSY, irritability, lethargy, vomiting, and absence of REFLEXES.

If the condition occurs in late childhood or in adulthood, the skull cannot swell, and the symptoms will be caused by a rising pressure within the skull; this is characterized by HEADACHE, vomiting, loss of coordination, and deteriorating mental function.

Treatment Options and Outlook

Usually, excess fluid will be drained away by a shunt from the brain to another part of the body (such as the lining of the abdomen), where it will be absorbed. The shunt (or tube) is inserted into the brain through a hole in the skull; sometimes, the shunt will be left in place indefinitely.

In older children and adults, treatment may be for underlying cause only.

hyperactivity A behavior pattern in which a person is constantly moving around and making rapid, often disorganized, motions. A general term, hyperactivity is used loosely to refer to a wide range of behaviors and is considered to be part of a wider complex of behaviors called ATTENTION DEFICIT HYPERACTIVITY DISORDER (ADHD). Some experts may use the term *hyperkinesis* to refer to this phenomenon.

Hyperactivity may affect as many as 5 to 10 percent of children in the United States and is four to five times more common in boys.

It is important to realize that some symptoms of hyperactivity are present at some time in almost all children and that overactivity in itself does not indicate hyperactivity. But when other causes are ruled out and the intense behavior continues past age four—and appears significantly different from other children's behavior—it may be reasonable to think of the child as hyperactive.

In many cases, hyperactivity fades away in adolescence, while others experience a transmutation of symptoms into sluggishness, depression, and moodiness. Occasionally, all symptoms of hyperactivity continue into adulthood.

Some research suggests that hyperactive children may have a subtle form of brain damage. Scientists also know that there appears to be a genetic component to the problem and that hyperactive children appear to be more likely to have hyperactive fathers. Children who have MENTAL RETARDATION, CEREBRAL PALSY, or TEMPORAL LOBE EPILEPSY are also more likely to be hyperactive.

Because stimulant drugs appear to ease the symptoms of hyperactivity, this suggests that the condition may be caused by an underaroused MIDBRAIN, which is unable to control movements or activity. Stimulant drugs appear to work by inducing this area of the brain to suppress extra activity.

Scientists have found that adults suffering from hyperactivity since childhood display markedly reduced metabolism in brain regions regulating motor activity and attention. It is suspected that stimulants increase metabolism in this area.

Symptoms and Diagnostic Path

Symptoms include continual overactivity that often worsens in group situations; it may not appear during a physical exam in the doctor's office. There appears to be a lessened need to sleep, with impulsive and reckless behavior. Hyperactive children are often irritable, emotionally immature, and aggressive; they have a shortened attention span and do not conform to orderly routines.

Hyperactivity may lead to antisocial behavior and learning problems, although IQ is usually normal. It is unclear whether the behavior is part of the disorder or is simply a result of the child's poor attention span.

Treatment Options and Outlook

Stimulant drugs such as amphetamine or Ritalin appear to be effective, and behavior therapy and counseling of child and parents also may be helpful.

More controversial are special diets that exclude certain additives, artificial colorings, preservatives, and so on.

hyperbilirubinemia   See KERNICTERUS.

hyperkinetic syndrome (hyperkinesis)   Another term for HYPERACTIVITY, now generally called ATTENTION DEFICIT HYPERACTIVITY DISORDER (ADHD).

hypnosis   A trancelike psychological state of altered awareness characterized by extreme suggestibility and certain physiological attributes. Hypnosis was once believed to be a form of sleep, but an EEG tracing during hypnosis does not show normal BRAIN-WAVE patterns typical of sleep. A hypnotized person functions at a level of awareness other than the ordinary conscious state, characterized by receptiveness and responsiveness in which inner experiences are given as much significance as external reality. While hypnotized, a person can think, act, and behave as well or better than during ordinary awareness, probably because of heightened attention. It is not possible to hypnotize someone who does not want to be hypnotized.

hypoglossal nerve   The 12th cranial nerve, this "undertongue" nerve transmits motor signals from the brain to the tongue; poking out the tongue and using the tongue to talk both involve this nerve.

See also CRANIAL NERVES.

hypoglycemia   A deficiency of glucose in the blood, causing weakness, confusion, and sweating. Because BRAIN CELLS require an adequate amount of sugar to maintain metabolic activity, a drop in the blood-sugar level can lead to brain-function problems. Insulin (a hormone secreted by the pancreas) helps maintain normal levels of blood sugar; too little insulin and the level will rise; too much and the level will fall. Diabetics are at particular risk for brain problems resulting from low blood

sugar; excess amounts of insulin can cause blood sugar to plummet, triggering a seizure.

Even a slight decrease in blood sugar, however, can alter brain function and trigger memory problems in almost anyone. It is not just diabetics who can get too much insulin—stress or nerves can activate the production of this hormone, as can eating too much sugar. One way to avoid this is to eat another food (such as peanut butter) during high-sugar meals; this helps slow the stomach's emptying and helps the body absorb sugar.

See also GLUCOSE.

hypothalamus   The cherry-sized part of the brain involved in pleasure, body temperature, and sleep is situated behind the eyes and beneath the THALAMUS. The hypothalamus controls the SYMPATHETIC NERVOUS SYSTEM (part of the AUTONOMIC NERVOUS SYSTEM, which controls body organs) and is responsible for the FIGHT-OR-FLIGHT mechanism.

Other groups of nerve cells within the hypothalamus control body temperature; some are sensitive to heat and some to cold so that when the blood flowing to the brain fluctuates in temperature, the hypothalamus induces temperature-regulating mechanisms such as shivering or sweating.

The hypothalamus receives information from sense organs about the GLUCOSE level in the blood and the body's water levels, stimulating the urge to eat or drink. The hypothalamus also regulates sleep, sexual behavior, and mood and emotions.

The hypothalamus also coordinates nervous control of the endocrine systems, connecting neuronally to the PITUITARY GLAND via the hypophyseal tract, thereby controlling hormonal secretions from the gland. In this way, the hypothalamus can convert nerve signals into hormonal signals.

Because of its many responsibilities, damage to this part of the brain can have wide-ranging consequences. Impaired hypothalamic function can result in hormonal disorders, malfunctioning temperature regulation, and increased or decreased appetite for sleep, food, and sex. Disorders involving the hypothalamus are usually linked to a brain hemorrhage or a pituitary tumor. In addition, LAURENCE-MOON-BIEDL SYNDROME is believed to be associated with a malfunctioning hypothalamus.

hypothyroidism Underactivity of the thyroid gland. Severe hypothyroidism can cause depression and DEMENTIA because of a drop in metabolic activity; borderline hypothyroidism (subclinical hypothyroidism) can cause memory disturbance, poor concentration, and mental confusion.

Symptoms and Diagnostic Path
Patients with a severe lack of thyroid hormone may appear unclean and disheveled, and over-drugged. There may be generalized tiredness, muscle weakness, cramps, a slow heart rate, dry flaky skin, hair loss and a deep, husky voice, thickened skin, weight gain, and goiter. The severity of the symptoms depends on the degree of thyroid deficiency. Mild deficiency may cause no symptoms; severe deficiency may produce all of the symptoms. Those with the borderline problem also may experience cold hands and feet, menstrual problems, dry skin, thin hair, and low energy levels.

A simple test for hypothyroidism is to take the temperature immediately upon awakening (while still in bed); temperature below 97.8°F. may indicate hypothyroidism. It also can be diagnosed by measuring the level of thyroid hormones in the blood.

Treatment Options and Outlook
Treatment includes replacement therapy with the thyroid hormone thyroxine; in most cases, hormone therapy must be continued for life. Once replacement therapy has begun, most or all of the symptoms with this disorder can be reversed; however, treatment may not cure goiter, which may require surgery.

hypoxia Lack of oxygen to the cells of the brain, which may be caused by the interference or block of blood or the oxygen it carries. Hypoxia may occur during drowning, childbirth, or choking. Hypoxia during birth is one of the primary causes of CEREBRAL PALSY and may be related to LEARNING DISABILITIES.

hysterical amnesia A type of psychogenic amnesia that involves disruption of episodic memory, hysterical amnesia is quite different from loss of memory associated with injury or disease. Unlike organic-based AMNESIA, this type of forgetfulness is sharply restricted to specific emotionally important groups of memories. In general, it can be understood in relationship to a patient's needs or conflicts, such as the need to escape a particularly distressing argument.

In addition, hysterical amnesia may extend to basic knowledge learned in school (such as arithmetic), which is never seen in organic amnesia unless there is an accompanying aphasia or dementia. Hysterical amnesia almost always can be treated successfully by procedures such as HYPNOSIS.

A normal, mentally healthy person is assumed to be integrated within a unified personality. But under traumatic conditions, memories can become detached from personal identity, making recall impossible. Modern accounts of hysterical amnesia have been heavily influenced by Sigmund Freud who attributed it to a need to repress information injurious to the ego. According to this theory, the memory produces a defense reaction for the individual's own good. This explains why hysterical amnesia occurs only in the wake of trauma and is consistent with the high incidence of depression and other psychiatric disorders in those who subsequently develop psychogenic memory problems.

See also FREUD, SIGMUND; FUGUE.

idebenone A molecule found in the heart that plays an important role in the production of ADENOSINE TRIPHOSPHATE (ATP).

imaging techniques There are a wide range of techniques that have been developed to allow physicians to look at the living brain, including the X-RAYS, computer-augmented techniques such as CAT SCANS, MAGNETIC RESONANCE IMAGING (MRI), ULTRASOUND SCANNING, PET SCANS, and so on.

While X-rays are still being used to view the skull following trauma, this method is less effective in visualizing the soft tissues of the brain. Instead, CAT and MRI scans are particularly valuable in diagnosing disorders of the brain, whereas PET scans have been extremely helpful in visualizing brain activity.

immune system A collection of cells and proteins that protect the body from bacteria, viruses, and fungi. The AUTONOMIC NERVOUS SYSTEM has primary responsibility for controlling the body's immune system, which fights infections by producing antibodies or immunoglobulins (protective proteins).

More and more researchers are coming to believe that there may be a link between people's vulnerability to infectious disease and their state of mind. The term *psychoneuroimmunology*—from *psycho* (the mind), *neuro* (nerve cells or the nervous system), and *immuno* (the immune system)—is the study of how one's beliefs and emotions influence one's brain chemistry and state of health. Coined by Dr. Robert Ader of the University of Rochester in 1975, psychoneuroimmunology is a controversial discipline that may hold promise if researchers can discover how the mind, the brain, and the immune system communicate.

A range of studies have linked depression, separation and loss, and stress with poorer health. Prolonged stress impairs the function of the immune system, and when the immune system is depressed, infection can take hold.

Both the brain and the immune system communicate through chemical signals. Moreover, studies have found that the HYPOTHALAMUS not only transmits emotional signals but also regulates the immune system.

Research by NEUROPSYCHOLOGIST Candace Pert at the National Institute of Mental Health has shown that infection-fighting white cells, like BRAIN CELLS, can both send or receive a wide variety of messages and can make and release hormones. Moreover, her work has also shown that the thymus and the spleen—two of the main structures used by the immune system—are connected by an especially intricate network of nerve cells to and from the brain.

indomethacin An anti-inflammatory drug used to treat arthritis that may be helpful in treating ALZHEIMER'S DISEASE.

infantile amnesia The term used to describe the almost universal phenomenon of memory loss for events before age three and a half—except for memories of sibling birth or hospitalization. The reason why is not yet understood.

Psychoanalyst SIGMUND FREUD wrote in 1919 that this type of childhood AMNESIA was caused by the REPRESSION of infantile sexuality, but later researchers suggested that infants construct a record of their experience that is organized differently from the record of later experiences; this would mean that adults could no longer access information acquired during early childhood.

Many modern memory researchers say infantile amnesia is due to the lack of early development of various mental abilities (such as language) used to cue memory. Scientists argue that these developmental changes in memory are linked with specific maturational changes in the brain; they also propose that the hippocampus is the key region undergoing this change.

Studies have shown that babies can recognize people and places they have been to before, but their memories aren't permanent. When something is out of sight, they have no idea that it still exists. Not until nine months of age will an infant look under a pillow to find a toy that she has seen someone hide there. When the toy disappeared—even though she saw where it went—her memory of the toy also disappeared. Some researchers believe this is a kind of error very similar to those made by adult amnesics. Other researchers believe that memories do exist but are difficult to retrieve because they were stored before an infant could talk, when the baby relies more on its senses.

However, new research by Emory University psychologists JoNell Adair Usher and Ulric Neisser found that going to the hospital or the birth of a sibling are memorable events that can be remembered as early as age two. Other events, even those as important as a death in the family or a move, are not recalled in adulthood unless they occur at a somewhat later age.

infantile neuroaxonal dystrophy (INAD) A rare inherited neurological disorder that affects axons, the part of a nerve cell that carries messages from the brain to other parts of the body and causes progressive loss of vision, muscular control, and mental skills. While the basic genetic and metabolic causes are unknown, INAD is caused by an abnormal buildup of toxic substances in nerves that communicate with muscles, skin, and the conjunctive tissue around the eyes.

Symptoms and Diagnostic Path

Symptoms usually begin within the first two years of life, with the loss of head control and the ability to sit, crawl, or walk, accompanied by deterioration in vision and speech. Some children may have seizures. Distinctive facial deformities may be obvious at birth, including a prominent forehead, crossed eyes, an unusually small nose or jaw, and large, low-set ears. The first symptoms may be slowing of motor and mental development, followed by loss or regression of previously acquired skills. Rapid, wobbly eye movements and squints may be the first symptoms, followed by floppiness in the body and legs (more than in the arms).

Electrophysiology (nerve conduction velocities) may help diagnose the disease, although diagnosis is usually confirmed by tissue biopsy of skin, rectum, nerve, or conjunctive tissue to confirm the presence of characteristic swellings in the nerve axons.

Treatment Options and Outlook

There is no cure and no treatment that can stop the progress of the disease. Treatment is aimed at easing symptoms; doctors can prescribe medications for pain relief and sedation. Physiotherapists and other physical therapists can teach parents and caregivers how to position and seat their child and how to exercise arms and legs to maintain comfort. INAD is a progressive disease, and once symptoms begin, they will get worse over time. Generally, a baby's development starts to slow down between the ages of six months to three years.

For the first few years, a baby with INAD will be alert and responsive, despite being increasingly physically impaired, but eventually, because of deterioration in vision, speech, and mental skills, the child will lose touch with its surroundings. Death usually occurs between the ages of five to 10 years.

Risk Factors and Preventive Measures

INAD is an autosomal recessive disorder, which means that both parents must be carriers of the defective gene that causes INAD to pass it on to their child. Researchers continue to search for the defective gene that causes INAD in hopes of developing drugs that can stop the disease.

infection Bacteria, fungi, or viruses can attack the brain or other parts of the CENTRAL NERVOUS SYSTEM and can cause considerable damage, although the body's immune system can usually successfully fight off these challenges. These infections may include ENCEPHALITIS, RABIES, MENINGITIS, POLIOEN-CEPHALITIS, and POLIOMYELITIS.

An infectious agent may invade the entire nervous system, while others may attack selective regions of the brain. Organisms also may directly infect the brain following head trauma or from an infected ear or sinus. The blood may carry other infections to the brain or by following the nerves.

Infections also may physically affect the brain, causing pus, inflamed blood vessels, excess fluid, and inflammation.

Symptoms and Diagnostic Path

Infections in the brain tend to produce inflammation, nausea, photophobia, fatigue, confusion, vomiting, fever, convulsions, and partial paralysis. Infections in the meninges may produce a stiff neck. Specific infections such as rabies may produce fear of water and hyperactive behavior.

Treatment Options and Outlook

Treatment depends on the cause of the infection. Antibiotics may cure bacterial infections, but there is no cure for many of the viral conditions.

inflammation of the brain See ENCEPHALITIS; INFECTION; MENINGITIS.

infradian rhythm Rhythms that occur over a period of time longer than a day. The monthly cycle of ovulation and menstruation is a good example of infradian rhythms in humans. These longer-than-normal rhythms are more difficult to study than daily (circadian) rhythms. Many animals exhibit seasonal swings in hormone levels by certain behavioral events, but in humans there is less outward appearance of small changes in hormonal levels.

The mechanism that controls the infradian reproductive cycle in humans is not well understood, although there seems to be a relationship between circadian rhythms of body temperature and the infradian reproductive cycle. (An increase in body temperature at awakening of 0.4°F or more above the average temperature of the five preceding days indicates that ovulation is taking place.)

intelligence The ability to understand ideas and their relationships and to reason about them. An extremely complex function of the brain, intelligence consists of the capacity for general knowledge, memory, learning, attention, comprehension, judgment, abstract thinking, language, orientation, perception, and association.

Scientists have tried to quantify intelligence and developmental level by a number of tests with many different psychological methods. The most common include the WECHSLER ADULT INTELLIGENCE SCALE–FOURTH EDITION (WAIS-IV), the WECHSLER INTELLIGENCE SCALE FOR CHILDREN–FOURTH EDITION (WISC-IV), the STANFORD-BINET INTELLIGENCE SCALE: FIFTH EDITION, the Denver II and the EARLY LANGUAGE MILESTONE SCALE (EMS), and the Central Linguistic Auditory Milestones Scale (CLAMS).

Interestingly, while more and more scientists disagree about the notion of general intelligence, scientists at the University of California at Irvine have shown that intelligent brains appear to solve problems by conserving rather than expending energy. In the studies, PET SCANS chart the rate at which the brain burns GLUCOSE; as subjects puzzle out mental tests, the scans track the level of cerebral activity. Studies with volunteers scoring high on IQ tests show reduced energy use in areas of the brain uniquely activated by tests; other tests with these subjects record sharp drops in overall brain activity after one or two months of daily practice in a video game.

However, glucose efficiency appears to provide only a partial picture of the intelligent brain. Highly intelligent subjects showed a jump in brain activity when moving from an easy version of a task to a difficult version. On the other hand, moving from the difficult version to an easier memory task resulted in a drop in brain activity.

interneuron Small intercommunicating neurons in the brain that connect major pathways. Neither purely sensory nor purely motor, interneurons are local nerve cells whose processes are confined within a small, restricted area. The largest number of interneurons are found in the CEREBRAL CORTEX.

When a baby is born, the interneurons are not connected; as a result of experience, learning, and repetition, the interneurons weave synaptic links with countless programmed pathways in other parts of the brain.

intracerebral hemorrhage Bleeding within the brain from a ruptured blood vessel, one of the three main incidents that can cause a STROKE. Each year, this type of hemorrhage strikes one out of every 2,500 Americans—usually older people with untreated high blood pressure or ATHEROSCLEROSIS (fatty deposits causing narrowed arteries).

Unlike most SUBDURAL and EXTRADURAL HEMORRHAGES in which bleeding occurs between the surface of the brain and the skull, an intracerebral hemorrhage can occur spontaneously, without any injury to the head. The blood seeps outward from the rupture, forming a round or oval mass that may grow to a few inches in diameter, disrupting brain tissue as the blood volume increases. Usually the rupture is found in the main mass of the brain (CEREBRUM), although it may occur in other brain structures, such as the BRAIN STEM or CEREBELLUM.

Symptoms and Diagnostic Path

Symptoms include sudden HEADACHE, weakness, confusion, and loss of consciousness. Over a period of minutes or hours, other symptoms resulting from disturbed brain tissue include speech problems, paralysis, or one-sided weakness.

Treatment Options and Outlook

Surgery is not usually possible because of the difficulty of reaching the rupture. Treatment usually involves life support and attempts to reduce blood pressure.

Only about 25 percent of patients survive, especially if the hemorrhage is large. However, if the patient survives, recurrent bleeding from the same site does not usually occur.

intracranial pressure (ICP) A measure of pressure depending on the amount of brain tissue, intracranial blood volume, and CEREBROSPINAL FLUID within the skull. Normally, a person's ICP fluctuates depending on the position of the body and the head, but it is usually considered to be less than or equal to 15 mm/Hg.

The volume and pressure of the brain tissue, blood, and cerebrospinal fluid is usually considered to be in a state of equilibrium. Because the skull does not allow much room for expansion, an increase in any of these three will alter the volume of the other two. Normally, the brain undergoes constant minor changes in blood volume and cerebrospinal fluid during changes in posture, blood pressure, internal pressure due to coughing, sneezing, or straining or fluctuations in arterial blood-gas levels.

Moreover, a range of brain problems (including STROKE, HEAD INJURY, inflammation, BRAIN TUMOR, or intracranial surgery) change the relationship between the volume and pressure within the skull. An increase in ICP may reduce cerebral blood flow, which is usually accompanied by a slow, bounding pulse and breathing problems. Such changes in blood pressure, pulse, and breathing give important clues to the existence of an increased ICP. Eventually, a consistently high ICP can cut off blood flow. Exquisitely sensitive to lack of blood flow, the BRAIN CELLS will die if the flow is cut off for more than three to five minutes.

Elevated ICP is most often associated with head injury, but it can also occur as a side effect of a range of other conditions, including brain tumors, SUBARACHNOID HEMORRHAGE, and toxic and viral brain inflammations.

Symptoms and Diagnostic Path

In the initial phase of increased pressure, the brain and its components can adjust their volume to allow for the expanding volume, but after a certain point the brain simply cannot continue to compensate for the high pressure.

At this point, the patient may show changes in consciousness, with slowed heartbeat and breathing changes. The earliest sign of increasing ICP is lethargy, with slowed speech and a lag in responding to verbal directions. The patient may become more and more sleepy or exhibit sudden changes in condition (such as shifting from quiet to restlessness). As the pressure continues to increase, the patient may begin to react only to very loud or exaggerated stimuli, indicating a probably serious problem in brain circulation and the onset of COMA. As the condition worsens, the patient's arms and legs become flaccid and reflexes disappear.

Treatment Options and Outlook

Immediate action is necessary to reduce the size of the brain by reducing swelling, decreasing the volume of cerebrospinal fluid, or lowering blood volume. This can be done by administering corticosteroids and osmotic diuretics, reducing the restricting fluids, draining cerebrospinal fluid, controlling fever, and reducing metabolic demands.

Profound coma with pupils fixed and dilated and impaired breathing usually leads to death.

Iowa Test of Basic Skills   A set of group-administered, paper-and-pencil tests that measure basic academic skills in grades K through nine. The tests cover vocabulary, reading, language, spelling, capitalization, punctuation, usage, work and study skills, visual materials, reference materials, concepts in mathematics, problem solving and compu-

tation, listening, word analysis, science, and social studies. For older students (grades nine to 12), the Iowa Tests of Educational Development may be used, which focus on more sophisticated material and skills. Any of these tests may be scored either by hand or by computer. The "Iowas" are used to identify strengths and weaknesses in basic skills, to evaluate classroom instruction, and to monitor a student's progress from year to year.

IQ tests   A group of tests of varying reliability that purport to assess an individual's general intelligence and developmental level. It is difficult to reproduce results using any of the IQ tests (especially among young people), and all fail to completely correct for the known effects of cultural and educational background, interest, motivation, and effort. In addition, some mental disorders (especially SCHIZOPHRENIA and DEPRESSION) may appear to lower IQ scores. Whether this occurs because these disorders actually lower intelligence or because the disorders impair motivation is not known.

Still, IQ tests are the only way of estimating intelligence, and they can be useful, providing their limitations are taken into consideration. The most common tests include the WECHSLER ADULT INTELLIGENCE SCALE–FOURTH EDITION (WAIS-IV), the WECHSLER INTELLIGENCE SCALE FOR CHILDREN–FOURTH EDITION (WISC-IV), the STANFORD-BINET INTELLIGENCE SCALE: Fifth Edition, the Denver II and the EARLY LANGUAGE MILESTONE SCALE (ELMS), and the Central Linguistic Auditory Milestones Scale (CLAMS).

J

Janet, Pierre (1859–1947) A French psychiatrist and philosopher, one of the most famous figures in psychology, who explored the realm of the unconscious mind. A professor of philosophy at the Liceum of Le Havre in 1881 at age 22, he volunteered to work at the local asylum, where he conducted research.

He included his studies of the highly hypnotizable hysterical female patients there in his book *L'Automatisme Psychologique* (Psychological automatisms) (1889). There he described systems of associated ideas that have been split off from consciousness and exist in a parallel life along with the dominant stream of consciousness. Calling this desegregation (or DISSOCIATION), he noted that the gaps between the parallel streams of consciousness gradually widen, and secondary existences are created. He believed this pathological process could be found in hysteria, HYPNOSIS, and MULTIPLE PERSONALITY DISORDER.

Janet invented the term *abaissement du niveau mental* (lowering the level of consciousness, or ALTERED STATES OF CONSCIOUSNESS) to describe the weakening control of consciousness prior to dissociation. While Janet believed this altered state of consciousness was found not just in dissociation but also in multiple personality, trances, and automatic writing, Swiss psychoanalyst Carl Jung adopted the term to describe SCHIZOPHRENIA. Jung believed that Janet's *abaissement* was the root of schizophrenia. Jung became a student of Janet in 1902 in Paris and was influenced by Janet throughout his life.

While Janet wrote widely in French, very few of his works have been translated into English.

jet lag Interruption of the body's sleep-wake cycles causing fatigue and mental confusion as a result of flying across different time zones. The human body is regulated by a biological clock that sets the pace for everyday rhythms of sleep, activity, temperature, cortisol, and melatonin release on a 24-hour cycle (called the CIRCADIAN RHYTHM). When an air traveler flies across several time zones, the person's day—as timed by an external clock—is longer or shorter than 24 hours, depending on the direction of the flight.

Jet lag tends to be worse when flying eastward, which shortens the traveler's day; it is also more likely to affect people over age 30 who normally follow a specific daily routine.

Symptoms and Diagnostic Path

Most of the traveler's circadian rhythms are not able to adjust, causing jet lag when the flight is over. People with jet lag have the urge to sleep during the day, feel awake at night, are generally tired, and have problems with physical and mental activity. Memory may also be affected.

Treatment Options and Outlook

The capacity for the human hormone MELATONIN to modulate the circadian rhythm has led to its use in the treatment of sleep disorders associated with jet lag.

It is also possible to somewhat modify the symptoms of jet lag by staying away from heavy meals and drinking plenty of nonalcoholic fluids during the flight.

The body may take a few days to readjust after traveling to a new time zone—about a half-day to a day for each time zone crossed. This adjustment can be eased by taking a stopover on a long journey and by resting after the flight.

Risk Factors and Preventive Measures

People who expect to be flying east should try to go to bed earlier than usual for a few days before

176

the flight; people flying west should do the opposite. If possible, travelers should try to arrive in the new time zone in the early evening and go to bed early.

Jordan Left-Right Reversal Test   A paper-and-pencil test for children aged five to 12 to measure the frequency of transpositions (reversals of letters, numbers, or upside down) among groups of numbers and letters and to identify words with similar errors. Children with perceptual errors often miss the real transpositions while identifying others. The test may be given to individuals or groups and is scored by hand. Scores are sometimes used as a kind of developmental screening test or diagnostic assessment for children believed to have learning disabilities.

Joseph disease   See MACHADO-JOSEPH DISEASE.

jugular vein   One of three veins on each side of the neck that carry deoxygenated blood from the head to the heart. The largest of the three is the internal jugular, which arises at the base of the skull, travels down the neck alongside the CAROTID ARTERIES and passes behind the collarbone, where it joins the subclavian vein—the large vein draining blood from the arms. Because the jugular lies deep in the structures of the neck, it is rarely injured.

kernicterus A rare disorder caused by the buildup of bilirubin (bile pigments) from destruction of the blood cells in the newborn. The bilirubin buildup damages the BASAL GANGLIA deep within the brain, leading to kernicterus. Untreated kernicterus causes BRAIN DAMAGE and MENTAL RETARDATION in newborns (especially premature infants).

Without treatment, the infant will probably die by the end of the first week of life; those who survive may be deaf and may suffer from uncontrollable writhing movements and spasticity (muscle stiffness). This may be followed by mental retardation, bizarre eye movements, speech problems, and SEIZURES.

Symptoms and Diagnostic Path
Jaundice in the first few days of life, together with listlessness and arched back and neck.

Treatment Options and Outlook
Prompt treatment of jaundice (by resting under special lights or temporary weaning from mother's milk) will completely prevent kernicterus. There is no cure for the brain damage that arises from untreated kernicterus.

ketoconazole (Nizoral) An antifungal drug used to treat severe fungal infections of the brain (as well as other organs). To avoid nausea, this drug should be taken with food. Other possible adverse effects include rash and (rarely) liver damage. Taking this drug with alcohol increases the chance of liver damage; taking with tobacco products decreases the drug's effect. The drug may also trigger an increased sensitivity to light.

Kohs Block Design Test A type of intelligence test for children or adults with a mental age of three to 19 years, especially handicapped people with defects of language or hearing, disadvantaged children, or those who are not native English speakers. In the test, the person is given a variety of colored blocks with which to copy designs shown on a series of cards. The person is tested not only on success in copying the design, but also in attention, adaptive behavior, and self-criticism. This test may be included in other tests, such as the Merrill-Palmer Scales of Mental Development.

Korsakoff, Sergey Sergeyevich (1854–1900) A Russian psychiatrist who may have been the first to recognize that AMNESIA does not necessarily have to be associated with DEMENTIA. Korsakoff noted a severe but specific amnesia for recent and current events among alcoholics with no problems in intelligence or judgment. This observation, now called KORSAKOFF SYNDROME, is found in a number of brain disorders in addition to problems resulting from alcoholism and appears to be caused by damage in a relatively localized part of the brain.

See also WERNICKE-KORSAKOFF SYNDROME.

Korsakoff syndrome Also known as Korsakoff psychosis, this condition was first described in cases of chronic alcoholism. The main feature of the syndrome is a problem in recent memory that may be so severe patients can store new information for only a few seconds; there is therefore no continuity between one experience and the next.

It is also the second stage in WERNICKE-KORSA-KOFF SYNDROME, which is believed to be caused by the interaction of chronic alcohol abuse and a thiamine deficiency brought on by the poor diet typical of chronic alcoholics.

Korsakoff syndrome occurs in a wide variety of toxic and infectious brain illnesses, as well as in association with nutritional disorders such as a deficiency of the B vitamins. It also has been observed among people with cerebral tumors, especially those involving the third ventricle. While it's often a temporary sign of a brain disorder, it can be chronic over many years. Even if the person's condition does improve, however, recent memory may not be strong, especially related to time sequence.

Symptoms and Diagnostic Path

People with Korsakoff syndrome seem to be incapable of learning new information. In addition, patients almost always experience RETROGRADE AMNESIA from a few weeks past to as much as 15 or 20 years before onset of the disorder. However, there are usually islands of memory amidst this amnesia, and how well a person can remember seems to depend to a great extent on circumstances. A woman patient may recognize her husband when he walks in the door, but as soon as he leaves she may insist she is not married.

Typically, patients are disoriented in place and time, and may underestimate their age by many years. Some patients remember experiences they never had, and may deny their memory problems. Otherwise, they seem to be intelligent and may show little personality change.

Treatment Options and Outlook

Korsakoff syndrome can be treated if the person stops drinking and follows a healthy diet with vitamins. Doctors are not sure if extra thiamine causes any improvement after brain damage has occurred, but added vitamins may help prevent further damage.

About a quarter of patients make a very good recovery within two years; about half partially recover, but they may need help to manage their lives; another quarter do not recover and may need long-term care.

This disease is likely to continue to progress if the person continues to drink heavily and does not eat well.

kuru A rare, progressive, ultimately fatal brain infection that occurs in some natives of the New Guinea highlands, caused by a virus spread by cannibalism. The disease is caused by a slow virus with an incubation period of up to 30 years, which has now virtually disappeared.

Kuru belongs to a class of infectious diseases called transmissible spongiform encephalopathies (TSEs), also known as PRION diseases. The hallmark of a TSE disease is an abnormal protein molecule that clumps together in brain tissue. Other TSEs include CREUTZFELDT-JAKOB DISEASE and fatal familial insomnia in humans, Bovine Spongiform Encephalopathy in cattle (also known as mad cow disease), SCRAPIE in sheep and goats, and chronic wasting disease in deer and elk.

Symptoms and Diagnostic Path

Symptoms include progressive movement disorders and eventually DEMENTIA.

Treatment Options and Outlook

There is no treatment.

language Most linguistic processing takes place in the dominant hemisphere of the brain (usually the left hemisphere, although in a few people the right hemisphere is dominant). The two most important areas for language in the dominant hemisphere are BROCA'S AREA and WERNICKE'S AREA. Broca's area is found in the rear of the FRONTAL LOBE near the face and tongue portions of the MOTOR CORTEX, and Wernicke's area is located in the TEMPORAL LOBE. These two areas are linked by a bundle of nerve fibers called the arcuate fascinulus and also are connected to the visual, auditory, and motor areas.

Spoken language travels to the AUDITORY CORTEX, where nerve fibers carry those sounds that have been translated into electric pulses to Wernicke's area, where they are consciously recognized as words. In much the same way, visual information about the shapes and combinations of letters pass from the eye through the VISUAL CORTEX and VISUAL ASSOCIATION AREAS to Wernicke's area, where the information is interpreted as words. In WERNICKE'S APHASIA, the patient cannot comprehend spoken or written language because of a problem in this area, although the person may still produce language.

Language production takes place in Broca's area, which signals the appropriate portions of the motor cortex (such as the hand muscles for writing) to produce language. BROCA'S APHASIA is therefore not a disorder of comprehension, but of articulation–the person understands written and spoken language but cannot speak or write normally.

When the various language areas are used together, it becomes possible, for example, to read a prepared text to an audience. In this case, the written words would first travel to Wernicke's area via the visual cortex, and these impulses would then travel to Broca's area and on to the motor cortex

for articulation. In cases of a conduction aphasia caused by disruption of the arcuate fasciculus, the link between language comprehension in Wernicke's area and language production in Broca's area malfunctions. Patients with this condition will have trouble reading aloud or repeating phrases they have heard.

While one hemisphere is dominant for language, this does not mean that the other hemisphere has nothing whatsoever to do with the process. Scientists have discovered areas in the opposite (usually right) hemisphere that are analogous to language centers in the left and that appear to be responsible for imbuing communication with emotion. This is where the normal intonation and rhythm of human language are coordinated. The right-side equivalent of Wernicke's area interprets this important aspect of speech. Other right-brain functions in language include the analysis of facial expression and responding to the emotional content of music. In APROSODIA, damage to these right-brain regions results in a curiously flat, emotionless speech or problems in appreciating the emotional qualities of speech or gestures.

language areas of the brain The areas of the brain associated with language reception, comprehension, processing, and production are still not fully understood, but functional brain scans have helped explain how the brain interacts with language.

Even further divisions can be made, based on exactly what aspect of these processes an area controls; for example, the motor portion of speech production versus the cognitive task of sentence planning. While the original data on locations of functional areas in the brain were based on studying patients with language problems and then looking at their brains after death, functional imaging technology has allowed assignments of function to be based on data from normal individuals (those without damage to their brain). Being able to base data on healthy brains is much more exact, since damage to one area of the brain could have multiple effects on a vast number of functions.

Broca's Area

Most studies agree that this area of the frontal lobe in the dominant hemisphere is primarily related to speech production. BROCA'S AREA is usually associated with maintenance of a list of words and parts of words used in producing speech and their associated meanings. It has been linked to articulation of speech and semantic processing (assigning meanings to words).

The original area described in 1861 by PIERRE-PAUL BROCA to be the "seat of articulate language" has now been further studied and subdivided by functional imaging studies (fMRI and PET) into smaller subsections that each participate differently in language tasks. Semantic processing has been linked to the upper portion of the area, while articulation falls within the center of Broca's original region of importance.

Broca's area is not simply a speech area; it is associated with the process of articulation of language in general. It controls not only spoken but also written and signed language production.

M1-Mouth Area

This area of the brain is responsible for controlling the physical movements of the mouth and articulators used to produce speech. Part of the motor cortex, it controls the muscles of the face and mouth just as the rest of the motor cortex controls various other parts of the body's movement. It is not involved with the cognitive aspects of speech production, though it is located near Broca's area and is activated in speech tasks along with Broca's area.

Wernicke's Area

This semantic processing area is associated with some memory functions, especially the short-term memory involved in speech recognition and production, as well as some hearing function and object identification. WERNICKE'S AREA is most often associated with language comprehension, the processing of incoming written or spoken language.

This distinction between speech and language is key to understanding the role of Wernicke's area to language. It does not simply affect spoken language, but also written and signed language. Wernicke's area works with Broca's area, Wernicke's handling incoming speech and Broca's handling outgoing speech.

Auditory Cortex

The areas of the brain responsible for recognizing and receiving sound are closely linked with language processing. In spoken language tasks, without correct auditory input, language comprehension cannot happen. As people speak or read words aloud, there is also evidence that they listen to themselves as they are speaking in order to make sure they are speaking correctly. Areas around the auditory cortex near Wernicke's area have also been suggested to be involved in short-term memory, specifically a "loop" in which language heard is continuously repeated in the brain in order to maintain that language in the memory.

Visual Cortex

The area responsible for vision, also known as the STRIATE CORTEX, is important in reading words and recognizing objects as an initial step in naming objects. The visual areas of the brain are usually among the first parts of the brain activated in reading and object-naming activities for speech tests in fMRI and PET scans. Other than this primary visual area located in the OCCIPITAL LOBE, another set of areas associated with vision are located in the PARIETAL LOBE, above the visual cortex. This region is associated with object naming and word reading, and is thought of as supplementary to the primary visual cortex. The visual cortex, along with the auditory cortex, is one possible first step on the path to language comprehension.

language delay   A lag in the development of communication skills, progressing more slowly than would be expected based on age, environment, or specific deprivation or disease. A child with a

LEARNING DISABILITY is likely to have LANGUAGE delays. Language delay includes the diagnostic subgroups of language disorder, language and learning disability, MENTAL RETARDATION, and AUTISM.

language processing disabilities Children with this problem, one of the most common types of LEARNING DISABILITY, may have trouble with any aspect of LANGUAGE, such as

- hearing words correctly
- remembering verbal material
- understanding the meaning of words
- communicating clearly

The child with this problem has trouble with the spoken word, which usually interferes with reading and writing when the child first starts school. This learning problem may range from mild to extremely severe—so difficult that the child may find that coping with reading and writing is like learning a foreign language. They may be slow in learning to speak and speak in brief sentences, and their memory for verbal directions is poor.

Many children with this problem may speak in a garbled fashion because their brains may have trouble sorting out the right sounds; these children may pronounce *elephant* as "efelunt." They may have a poor grasp of grammar and trouble with word sequencing in a sentence, and may confuse words that sound alike. These types of errors usually get worse if they must speak in public or before an authority figure.

Lashley, Karl (1890–1958) A pioneering psychologist and brain researcher who conducted extensive investigations from the 1920s through the 1950s into brain mass and learning. This memory expert devoted the greater part of his career to the search for the part of the brain that stores engrams (memory traces). In his search for the location of memory, he assumed that memory can be found in one place.

Lashley believed that if learning involves the construction of specific connections between

behavior and events, and if memory is the impact of that connection on behavior, then that connection ought to be found in a specific location in the cerebral cortex. To test his assumption, he trained rats to run mazes, cut out snippets of their brain tissue, and then set the rats loose in the mazes again. But after operating on hordes of rats, Lashley could not find one single place in the brain where the memory of the maze existed.

Not surprisingly, the more bits of brain he cut away, the more problems the rats had running the maze—but it didn't seem to matter *what* portion of the brain he cut out. Eventually Lashley gave up trying to map the location of memory in the brain, believing that memory existed everywhere, disseminating like smoke throughout the folds and fissures of the brain.

He served as professor at the University of Chicago (1929–35) and at Harvard University (1933–35); he also served as director of the Yerkes Laboratories of Primate Biology in Orange Park, Florida, from 1942.

See also ENGRAM.

lateral geniculate bodies The region of the brain into which the optic nerve first feeds its signal.

lateralization The functional asymmetry of the two individual cerebral hemispheres of the brain, despite the fact that both halves typically work as a coordinated unit.

While many scientists traditionally refer to the left hemisphere as dominant, in fact both halves have important roles to play in brain function.

The most typical example of lateralization is a person's HANDEDNESS—whether a person favors the right or left hand, which is often related to the lateralization of other functions such as speech. For example, people who are right-handed almost always have primary speech function in the left hemisphere, which controls the right hand; while this is also true for most left-handers, they are more likely to have speech function primarily in the right or distributed equally in both hemispheres.

In the mid-1800s, French neurosurgeon PIERRE-PAUL BROCA identified a particular area of the left hemisphere that plays a primary role in speech production. Shortly afterward, German neurologist CARL WERNICKE identified another part of the left hemisphere primarily concerned with language comprehension.

Most humans have left hemisphere specialization for language abilities. The only direct tests for speech lateralization are too invasive to use on healthy people, so most of what we know in this area comes from clinical reports of people with brain injuries or diseases. Based on these data, and on indirect measures, it is estimated that 70 percent to 95 percent of humans have a left-hemisphere language specialization. That means that some unknown percentage of humans (5 percent to 30 percent) have different patterns of specialization.

However, the neurological mechanisms underlying language abilities are extremely complicated. For instance, some language functions (like prosody—the emotional content of speech) are specialized in the right hemisphere of people with left-hemisphere language specializations. Yet there is still a great deal about brain lateralization that we simply do not understand.

Clarifying the relationship between handedness and functional brain specializations, and learning more about the developmental and neurobiological mechanisms that underlie these relationships, may help experts better understand a wide range of issues such as dyslexia, stuttering, brain research, developmental neurobiology, and the origins of language.

lateral preference   The development of a preference for one side of the body. Also known as lateralization, this preference develops very early in life, and is expressed most prominently in HANDEDNESS (the dominant hand that a child uses for activities such as writing or throwing a ball).

In some cases, lateralization is not clear, and an individual will express a mixed lateral preference—writing with one hand, for example, and throwing a ball with the other.

Laurence-Moon-Biedl syndrome   A very rare inherited disorder believed to be caused by a prob-

lem with the HYPOTHALAMUS (the area of the brain that helps regulate hormone balance).

Symptoms and Diagnostic Path

Characterized by MENTAL RETARDATION, obesity, retinitis pigmentosa, abnormal number of fingers or toes, or absence of secondary sexual characteristics.

There is some confusion in the medical literature about the difference between Bardet-Biedl syndrome and Laurence-Moon syndrome. Some researchers still believe that Bardet-Biedl syndrome is a subdivision of Laurence-Moon-Biedl syndrome.

Treatment Options and Outlook

There is no treatment.

L-dopa   See LEVODOPA.

lead poisoning and the brain   Lead poisoning can be the cause of significant brain damage; it can be found anywhere there are old buildings, old paint, lead pipes—even in vegetable gardens that receive lead-contaminated runoff. Alarmingly, *one out of six American preschoolers* is considered to be lead poisoned (or 3 million children under age 6 in 2005). The brain is most sensitive to lead during the first six years of life, when the brain cells are rapidly developing. Nearly 1 million U.S. children have lead levels in their blood that are high enough to cause irreversible damage to their health.

Lead can be ingested from dust, soil, and lead-based paint flecks in old homes. In fact, more than 80 percent of homes built before 1978 have lead paint, and the older the house, the more likely it is to contain lead-based paint. In public playgrounds and in yards, the dirt where children play may contain high lead levels. Decades of peeling exterior building paint, air emissions from leaded car exhaust, and pollution from smelters and other industries are significant sources. The highest levels of lead in soil usually are found close to foundations of homes painted with exterior leaded paint.

In addition, lead is still found in low levels in some drinking water as a result of lead-based solder on old water pipes. The Environmental Protection Agency estimates that drinking water is the source of about 20 percent of Americans' lead exposure. Even after lead pipes were banned, leaded solder was legal for use on drinking water lines until the 1980s and is still for sale in hardware stores. Faucets and plumbing fittings may legally contain up to 8 percent lead. The greatest risk is to infants who are fed formula mixed with contaminated water.

Lead-glazed pottery that has not been properly fired also can allow lead to leach into whatever comes into contact with it, and lead can be found in some folk remedies, "health foods," and cosmetics.

Because young children often crawl and like to mouth objects, they are more likely to ingest lead; moreover, a child's smaller body size means a higher dose of lead per exposure. At the same time, a child is not as capable of clearing lead from the body, so the body's concentration builds up.

Chronic exposure can lead to a motor neuropathy that looks identical to AMYOTROPHIC LATERAL SCLEROSIS; acute exposure features disturbances of higher brain function, DELIRIUM, mania, SEIZURES, and blindness.

Lead poisoning is unfortunately one of the most common and preventable childhood health problems today. Even very small exposures can produce subtle but dangerous health effects. In 1991, the Centers for Disease Control lowered the amount of lead it considers dangerous in children from 25 microliters to 10 micrograms per deciliter of blood (mcg/dl).

In late July 2007, Mattel, Fisher-Price, and other toy manufacturers learned that more than 22 million of their toys manufactured in China contained unacceptable levels of lead. According to Consumer Product Safety Commission scientists, the levels of lead in those Chinese-manufactured toys posed health risks to children by ingestion of the lead paint the manufacturers used but also by handling the toys. The major toy manufacturers decided to recall all toys containing more than 0.06 percent lead. The resulting massive recall of Chinese-manufactured toys due to high levels of lead included such popular items as: Dora the Explorer characters, Big Bird and Elmo, and die-cast "Sarge" automobiles from the movie *Cars*.

Shortly after the first massive toy recall on August 2, 2007, Cheung Shu-hung, co-owner of Lee Dur Industrial, a Chinese toy manufacturer, hanged himself in a toy warehouse.

Lead, like most heavy metals, is a NEUROTOXIN, which means that it will impair both physical and mental function and development. For many years, people assumed that children would have to ingest large amounts of lead before being harmed. Today, most experts believe even small exposures (the amount released by raising and lowering a window painted with lead paint in the presence of a child) can result in subtle developmental and intellectual delays.

Lead poisoning causes the most damage to the brain, nerves, red blood cells, and digestive system. Lead interferes with the GABA-ergic neurotransmission. A cumulative poison, it remains in the kidneys for seven years and in the bones for more than 30 years.

Symptoms and Diagnostic Path

Unfortunately, there may be no symptoms of lead poisoning until the damage has already been done. Because lead's effects vary from one child to another, it is almost impossible to predict how an individual child will fare. While the symptoms of severe lead poisoning are obvious, repeated exposures to small amounts can also cause poisoning but may not be as easily detectable. There may be no visible symptoms of lead poisoning in this instance which would alert parents to seek medical care.

Symptoms of low levels of lead poisoning include low IQ scores, decreased attention span, poor hearing, speech delays, and other developmental problems. The body absorbs about 10 to 15 percent of the ingested metal; the rest is slowly excreted. Most of the absorbed lead is stored in the child's bones, with smaller amounts deposited in bone marrow, brain tissue, and red blood cells. If the lead poisoning continues, it will accumulate to toxic levels. Lead is excreted very slowly from the body, so it builds up in tissues and bones and may not even produce detectable physical effects, although it can still cause mental impairment. If they do appear, early symptoms include listlessness, irritability, loss of appetite and weight, constipation, and a bluish line in the gums, followed by clumsiness, vomiting and stomach cramps, and a general "wasting away."

The Centers for Disease Control and Prevention (CDC) recommends testing every child at 12 months of age and, if resources allow, at 24 months. Screening should start at six months if the child is at risk of lead exposure (for example, if the child lives in a home built before 1960 that has peeling or chipping paint). Decisions about further testing should be based on previous blood-lead test results and the child's risk of lead exposure. In some states, more frequent lead screening is required by law.

The CDC in 1991 identified a number of reasons for testing a child for lead poisoning, including

- child lives or regularly visits a house built before 1960 that is being renovated or that has peeling, chipped paint
- sibling or classmate is being treated for lead poisoning
- child lives with someone whose hobby includes exposure to lead, such as making pottery or stained glass, working in auto repair or bridge or highway construction
- child lives near industry likely to release lead
- child received treatment for foreign object in ear, nose, or stomach
- child often swallows nonfood items
- any child under six with unexplained developmental delays, hearing problem, irritability, severe attention deficit, violent tantrums, or unexplained anemia

The test identifies how many micrograms of lead are found in one deciliter of the child's blood. Based on what is known today, children should have less than 10 micrograms per deciliter (10 µg/dl) of blood lead concentration. If higher levels are found, certain steps can be taken.

At 10–19 µg/dl, a child has mild lead poisoning and should be retested in a few months. The home and all the places the child spends time should be checked for lead sources, and identified lead hazards should be controlled. Frequent wet cleaning and handwashing will help reduce lead dust. Good nutrition can help the child fight lead.

A blood lead level between 20 and 44 means the child has moderate lead poisoning. Sources of lead in the child's environment must be removed, and the child may need chelation therapy to remove lead from the body. Chelation therapy means the child is given a drug capable of binding lead and reducing its acute toxicity. All drugs have potential side effects and must be used with caution.

A blood lead concentration of 45–69 is severe lead poisoning. A child with this concentration needs both medical treatment and lead removed from the environment.

A blood lead level greater than 70 is an acute medical emergency. The child may stay in the hospital for treatment and not be released until he or she can return to a safe, lead-free home.

A child with elevated blood lead levels or enough absorbed lead in the body to show symptoms will probably require hospitalization. Treatment usually includes the administration of medicines (called chelating agents) to help the body rid itself of lead. In mild cases, the chelating agent penicillamine may be used alone; otherwise, it may be used in combination with edetate calcium disodium and dimercaprol. Chelation therapy has its risks, however, and must be properly monitored to avoid kidney damage. In acute cases, stomach pumping may be necessary.

Treatment Options and Outlook

If untreated, the toxic lead levels in a child's body can lead to serious cognitive complications, including MENTAL RETARDATION. Babies exposed to high levels of lead before birth reveal impaired attention span, hearing, language ability, and intelligence. After birth, the affected infants may recover, but only if they are no longer exposed to lead. If lead exposure continues, their cognitive performance will continue to be affected for at least the first five years of life.

In addition, some researchers suggest that there may be an association between exposure to lead and pre- and postnatal hyperactivity, behavior disorders, and attention deficit disorder.

While lead poisoning is almost always a chronic problem, it is possible—albeit extremely rare—to suffer from an acute case of lead poisoning when a large amount of lead is taken in by the body over a short period of time. This is generally found among adult drinkers of bootleg whiskey. Acute

LEAD POISONING GUIDE

The following recommendations have been provided by the U.S. Centers for Disease Control

Lead Levels	Complications	Treatment
0–9 mcg/dl	None	Annual checks until age six
10–14 mcg/dl	Borderline (possible test inaccuracy); risk for mild developmental delays even without symptoms	Nutrition, housecleaning changes will bring level down
15–19 mcg/dl	Risk for IQ decrease; no symptoms usually noticed	Test for iron deficiency; nutrition, housekeeping changes will lower level
20–44 mcg/dl	Risk for IQ impairment increases; usually no symptoms	Complete medical evaluation; eliminate lead; drug treatment possible
45–69 mcg/dl	Colic, anemia, learning disabilities	Remove from home until lead is removed; drug treatment
70 mcg/dl	Vomiting, anemia, critical illness	Immediate hospitalization; lead removal

mcg/dl = micrograms per deciliter of blood

poisoning symptoms include metallic taste in the mouth, abdominal pain, vomiting, diarrhea, collapse, and COMA. Large amounts directly affect the nervous system and cause HEADACHE, convulsions, coma, and sometimes death.

Risk Factors and Preventive Measures

The most effective way to protect children from lead poisoning is to prevent lead from building up in blood, tissues, and bones. While many products contain lead, it is most often associated with paint; until about 40 years ago, *all* house paint contained some. Lead was added to paint because it helped the paint dry more quickly and gave it a shiny, hard finish. In fact, the more lead in a can of paint, the better and more expensive the product—some paints were as much as 50 percent lead.

By the late 1970s, the government began to regulate the amount of lead in paint, but nothing was done about the lead-filled paint already on the walls in millions of older homes and schools throughout the United States. It is this lead-based paint that causes most of the lead poisoning in children. More than three-fourths of American homes built before 1980 (57 million dwellings) still contain lead paint, and 14 million housing units have high levels of lead in dust or chipping paint—3.8 million of them housing young children. If a house was built before 1950, it is almost guaranteed that its paint contains the toxic substance; if it was built between 1950 and 1978, there is a 50 percent chance of lead paint.

HOW TO REDUCE A CHILD'S LEAD EXPOSURE

- To reduce lead paint and dust temporarily, clean floors, windowsills, and window wells at least twice a week with a trisodium phosphate detergent, available at hardware stores. Sponges used for this purpose should not be used for anything else.

- Move cribs and playpens away from chipped or peeling paint, mantels, windowsills, and doors. Replace or strip baby furniture that may be decorated with lead paint.

- Wash the child's hands, face, bottle nipples, and toys often.

- Children and pregnant women should not be in the area while lead paint is being removed.

- Do not buy large-size canned foods and juices, as lead-soldered seams can leach into food; avoid imported brands.

- Feed children plenty of calcium, iron, and protein, with plenty of milk, breads, low-fat foods, and green leafy vegetables. These foods diminish lead's effects in the body.

- Limit the amount of dirt tracked in the home.

- Avoid storing acidic food (such as orange juice and tomatoes) in ceramic or crystal containers, which may contain lead glaze.

- Lead levels in the home water supply should not exceed 15 parts per billion; for high levels, consider a water-treatment device to remove lead from tap water.

- Never boil water to eliminate lead; boiling only concentrates lead.

- Allow water to run on cold for a few minutes before using; never cook with hot water from the tap (especially when making baby food) because lead leaches more quickly into hot water.

- If your soil tests high in lead, cover with clean soil and seed or sod.

To prevent further lead poisoning, parents should keep children away from peeling or chipping paint and chewable surfaces painted with lead-based paint, especially windows, window sills, and window wells. Parents should wet-mop and wet-wipe hard surfaces, using trisodium phosphate detergent (found at hardware stores) or automatic dishwasher soap and water. Hard surfaces should not be vacuumed because this is believed to scatter dust. If inspection shows that a house had lead-based paint, the family should not renovate or attempt to remove the paint themselves. Work should be done by someone who knows how to protect workers, the family, and the environment. The family should not be in the home during renovations or paint removal.

Parents should wash children's hands and faces before meals and wash toys and pacifiers frequently. Children should eat regular, nutritious meals, since more lead is absorbed on an empty stomach. Children's diets should contain plenty of iron, such as that found in liver, fortified cereal, cooked beans, spinach, and raisins. Calcium is also important (including that found in foods like milk, yogurt, cheese, and cooked greens).

If soil around the home is likely to be contaminated (if a home was built before 1960 or near a major highway), parents should plant grass or other ground cover. If lead-based paint is the source of soil contamination, most lead will be near painted surfaces such as exterior walls. In such cases, parents should plant bushes next to the house to keep children away. If the soil is contaminated with lead, parents should provide a sandbox with a solid bottom and top cover, and clean sand for children to play and dig in.

If the lead content of tap water in the home is higher than the drinking water standard, parents should let the water run for several minutes (until the temperature changes) before using. Only fully-flushed water from the cold-water tap should be used for drinking and cooking. To conserve water, parents should collect drinking water in bottles at night after water has been fully flushed from the tap. This procedure will help if the source of lead is from the home's plumbing, but it will not help if the city water supply is contaminated.

Parents should not store food in open cans (especially imported cans), nor in pottery that is meant for decorative use, or in lead crystal or china.

If members of the family work with lead, they should make sure children are not exposed to any lead-contaminated clothing or scrap material brought home.

The average blood level of lead in the general population has been gradually dropping during the past 20 years since lead was eliminated from gasoline—but an estimated 7 million tons of lead remain in the soil.

During renovation of an older home, experts should ascertain whether or not there is a lead problem and, if so, how to handle the situation. Because children who live near factories that melt metal may also have a lead-poisoning problem, it is important for parents who live near these factories to find out if lead is being released from the stacks by checking the EPA's Toxics Release Inventory, available at public libraries.

learning   A general term for a category of changes whereby behavior or information is acquired or modified; learning begins as soon as a baby is born.

The learning process is believed to rely on the creation of new pathways from the synaptic connections established among the vast network of NEURONS in the brain. A SYNAPSE is the junction between one neuron and the next.

As people learn, their synapses undergo functional changes. For example, if someone is learning to play the violin, the neural signals from their brain to the muscles they are using travel through existing pathways. But the person's movements are slow and uncoordinated while they are learning. With more practice, the same signals are passed more and more often. These neural pathways begin to change; more connections are made; the pathways are becoming more efficient. As new, faster, more coordinated pathways develop, the budding musician can eventually move fingers and hands more quickly and precisely. Eventually, the person can play accurately without looking at the position of the hands on the instrument.

In autopsies of children, scientists found that new babies have fewer connections between their neurons, but the number quickly increases as children age, indicating that the child has learned more about the world.

The ability to learn is vulnerable to injury to those areas of the brain that process learning. For instance, ALZHEIMER'S DISEASE causes a depletion of ACETYLCHOLINE, a neurotransmitter used by the brain for, among other functions, the processing of learning and memory. This depletion of acetylcholine causes problems in learning and memory.

See also DYSLEXIA AND MEMORY; LEARNING DISABILITY.

learning disability (LD) A neurobiological disorder in which a person's brain works or is structured differently, affecting one or more of the basic processes involved in understanding or using spoken or written language. Such a disability may result in a problem with listening, thinking, speaking, reading, writing, spelling, or doing mathematical calculations. Experts believe that children with learning disabilities have a problem with the way the brain handles information that hinders the normal learning process.

Learning disabilities affect one in seven people and represent a national problem of enormous proportions. In fact, learning disabilities constitute the most-often-assigned special education classification. Every year, 120,000 additional students are diagnosed with learning disabilities, a diagnosis now shared by 2.4 million schoolchildren in the United States. Many thousands more are never properly diagnosed or treated, or do not get treatment because they are not considered eligible for services. The most common learning disability is difficulty with language and reading.

All children learn in highly individual ways. Children with learning disabilities simply process information differently, but they are generally of adequate or above-average intelligence. Sometimes overlooked as "hidden handicaps," learning disabilities are often not easily recognized, accepted, or considered serious once detected. The impact of the disability, which often runs in families, ranges from relatively mild to severe. Learning disabilities can be lifelong conditions that, in some cases, affect many parts of a person's life: school or work, daily routines, friendships, and family life. In some peo-

ple, many overlapping learning disabilities may be apparent, while others may have a single, isolated learning problem that has little impact on other areas of their lives.

Learning disabilities are not the same as MENTAL RETARDATION, AUTISM, deafness, blindness, or behavioral disorders. Nor are learning disabilities caused by poverty, environmental factors, or cultural differences. Learning disabilities are not curable, but individuals can learn to compensate for and even overcome areas of weakness. Attention deficits and hyperactivity sometimes appear with learning disabilities, but not always.

Common learning disabilities include:

- **Dyslexia**—a language-based disability in which a person has trouble understanding words, sentences, or paragraphs.
- **Dyscalculia**—a mathematical disability in which a person has a very difficult time solving arithmetic problems and grasping math concepts.
- **Dysgraphia**—a writing disability in which a person finds it hard to form letters correctly or write within a defined space.
- **Auditory and Visual Processing Disabilities**—a sensory disability in which a person has difficulty understanding language despite normal hearing and vision.

More than one in six children will encounter a problem in learning to read during the first three years in school. Currently, more than 2.8 million school-age children receive special education services as students with learning disabilities, which represents about 6 percent of all children in public schools. However, these statistics do not include the tens of thousands of students who attend private and religious schools, nor does it include the scores of students who may have serious problems with learning, but who may not meet the criteria established by school districts to receive special education services.

Experts do not know exactly what causes learning disabilities, but they are assumed to be disorders of the central nervous system triggered by many different factors. These may include heredity, problems during pregnancy or birth, and incidents after birth.

The fact that learning disabilities tend to run in families indicates that there may be a genetic link. For example, children who lack some of the skills needed for reading, such as hearing the separate sounds of words, are likely to have a parent with a related problem. However, a parent's learning disability may take a slightly different form in the child. A parent who has a writing disorder may have a child with an expressive language disorder. For this reason, it seems unlikely that specific learning disorders are inherited directly. Instead, what is inherited might be a subtle brain dysfunction that can lead to a learning disability.

There may be an alternative explanation for why LD might seem to run in families. Some learning difficulties may actually stem from the family environment. For example, parents who have expressive language disorders might talk less to their children, or the language they use may be distorted. In such cases, the child lacks a good model for acquiring language and therefore may seem to be learning disabled.

LD problems also may be caused by illness or injury during or before birth, the mother's use of drugs and alcohol during pregnancy, untreated RH incompatibility with the mother, premature or prolonged labor, or lack of oxygen or low birth weight.

Throughout pregnancy, the fetal brain develops from a few cells into a complex organ made of billions of specialized, interconnected nerve cells called neurons. During this process, things can go wrong that may alter how the neurons form or interconnect.

In the early stages of pregnancy, the fetal brain stem forms. This is the part of the brain that controls such basic functions as breathing and digestion. Later, a deep ridge divides the cerebrum (the thinking part of the brain) into two halves, a right and left hemisphere. Finally, the areas involved with processing sight, sound, and other senses develop, as well as the areas associated with attention, thinking, and emotion.

As new cells form, they move into place to create various brain structures. Nerve cells rapidly grow to form networks with other parts of the brain. These networks allow information to be shared among various regions of the brain.

Throughout pregnancy, fetal brain development is vulnerable to disruptions. If the disruption occurs early, the fetus may die, or the infant may be born with widespread disabilities and possibly mental retardation. If the disruption occurs later, when the cells are becoming specialized and moving into place, it may leave errors in the cell makeup, location, or connections. Some scientists believe that these errors may later show up as learning disorders.

Scientists have found that mothers who smoke during pregnancy may be more likely to bear smaller babies who tend to be at risk for a variety of problems, including learning disorders. Alcohol also may be dangerous to the fetus's developing brain, distorting the developing neurons. Heavy alcohol use during pregnancy has been linked to FETAL ALCOHOL SYNDROME, a condition that can lead to low birth weight, intellectual impairment, HYPERACTIVITY, and certain physical defects. Any alcohol use during pregnancy may influence the child's development and lead to problems with learning, attention, memory, or problem solving. Drugs such as cocaine (especially crack cocaine) seem to affect the normal development of brain receptors that help to transmit incoming signals from skin, eyes, and ears. Because children with certain learning disabilities have trouble understanding speech sounds or letters, some researchers believe that learning disabilities (as well as ADHD) may be related to faulty receptors. Current research points to drug abuse as a possible cause of receptor damage.

After birth, learning disabilities may be caused by head injuries, nutritional deprivation, poisonous substances, or child abuse. New brain cells and neural networks continue to be produced for a year or so after the child is born, and these cells are vulnerable to certain disruptions too.

Some environmental toxins may result in learning disabilities, possibly by disrupting childhood brain development or brain processes. Cadmium and lead, both prevalent in the environment, are becoming a leading focus of neurological research. Cadmium, used in making some steel products, can get into the soil, then into food. Lead was once common in paint and gasoline, and is still present in some water pipes. A study of animals sponsored by the National Institute of Health showed a connection between exposure to lead and learning difficulties. In the study, rats exposed to lead experienced changes in their brain waves, slowing their ability to learn. The learning problems lasted for weeks, long after the rats were no longer exposed to lead.

In addition, there is growing evidence that learning problems may develop in children with cancer who had been treated with chemotherapy or radiation at an early age. This seems particularly true of children with brain tumors who received radiation to the skull.

The 2004 Individuals with Disabilities Education Improvement Act (IDEIA) revisions represent an attempt to make federal handicapped education legislation compatible with No Child Left Behind (NCLB). The addition of the word *Improvement* to the title signifies the NCLB concept of constant progress. The new act also adds reading fluency as an area of manifestation of LD. Although the previous IDEA legislation required documentation of "a severe discrepancy between potential and achievement," the 2004 revisions introduced the requirement of demonstration of failure to respond to appropriate "research-based interventions" over a reasonable amount of time. Such definition revision represents a change from a psychometric to an instructional identification model. Previously, the psychoeducational evaluation served the gatekeeper function for Learning Disabilities eligibility.

The IDEIA revisions now place the burden of identifying students who are eligible for LD placement on the Student Assistance Team (sometimes known as the Child Study Team or as some similar name), which must monitor the application of research-based interventions over a suitable period of time before declaring students placement-eligible. Early reports from school districts employing the revised eligibility definition indicate confusion regarding what practices constitute "research-based interventions" and what period of time is suitable to require for monitoring such interventions. Given the already-present preference of many education personnel to place rather than to not place and the increasingly litigious nature of the relationship between parents who want their children classified as LD and school districts, early

reports indicate increases of 25 to 50 percent in LD identification. School district special education and school psychological personnel contacted in preparation of this section also expressed frustration that the IDEIA revisions leave some areas so vague that litigation will be necessary to clarify them, such as

- Does the terminology requiring interventions (plural) mean that, even if the application of one intervention demonstrates conclusively there is a learning disability, must school districts continue with additional interventions, delaying the provision of needed special education and related services?

- How long is a reasonable amount of time to demonstrate failure to respond to research-based interventions? If an obvious LD emerges immediately, must the Student Assistance Team delay special education to satisfy minimum time requirements?

- What is a research-based intervention? Many education publications offer opinion-based rather than research-based interventions, leaving only a precious few interventions with any research base. How much research support must an intervention have to qualify as a research-based intervention under the law?

- How do school districts reconcile the IDEIA requirements of providing "research-based interventions" over a reasonable period of time, with that of proceeding in a "timely manner" in identifying eligible students?

- What role, if any, does the school psychologist play in identifying learning disabilities? Under the IDEIA revisions, the school psychoeducational evaluation is no longer directly necessary for LD classification.

- How does the requirement of demonstration of failure to respond to research-based interventions by the Student Assistance Team reconcile with parents' rights to have the results of an outside psychoeducational evaluation considered? School psychologists outside school systems are in a position to evaluate cognitive and academic functioning but not the failure to respond to research-based interventions over a reasonable amount of time.

Parents and professionals should gather information and discuss concerns about a child who is struggling with learning problems. The child's parents should arrange for a comprehensive school psychological evaluation, which can only take place with the parent's written consent. Evaluations can help identify the child's relative strengths and difficulties and help determine whether the student is eligible for special assistance in school.

When parents and school staff agree, the public school system must provide an evaluation to determine if a student is entitled to special education services. Evaluations can be arranged for free through the school system, or through private clinics, private evaluators, hospital clinics, or university clinics. However, some school districts may not automatically accept test results from outside sources. Parents should check with their school district before seeking evaluation services from private facilities.

The actual diagnosis of learning disabilities is made using individually administered standardized tests that compare the child's level of ability to what is considered normal development for a person of that age and intelligence. Test outcomes depend not only on the child's actual abilities, but on the reliability of the test and the child's ability to pay attention and understand the questions.

Each type of LD is diagnosed in slightly different ways. To diagnose speech and language disorders, a speech therapist tests the child's pronunciation, vocabulary, and grammar and compares them to the developmental abilities seen in most children that age. A psychologist tests the child's intelligence. A physician checks for ear infections, and an audiologist may be consulted to rule out auditory problems. If the problem involves articulation, a doctor examines the child's vocal cords and throat. In the case of academic skills disorders, academic development in reading, writing, and math is evaluated using standardized tests. In addition, vision and hearing are tested to be sure the student can see words clearly and can hear adequately. The specialist also checks to see if the child has missed much school. It is important to rule out these other possible factors. After all, treatment for a learning disability is very different from the remedy for poor vision or missing school.

ADHD is diagnosed by checking for the long-term presence of specific behaviors, such as excessive fidgeting, losing things, interrupting, and talking. Other signs include an inability to remain seated, stay on task, or take turns. A diagnosis of ADHD is made only if the child shows such behaviors substantially more than other children of the same age.

If the school fails to notice a learning delay, parents can request an outside evaluation at public expense. After confirming the diagnosis, the public school is obligated to provide the kind of instructional program the child needs.

Parents should stay abreast of each step of the school's evaluation, and they may appeal the school's decision if they disagree with the findings of the diagnostic team. Parents always have the option of getting a second opinion.

Symptoms and Diagnostic Path

There is a great paradox regarding the identification of students as learning disabled. On the one hand, the earlier a learning disability is detected, the better chance a child will have of succeeding in school and in life. However, because the establishment of a learning disability diagnosis requires a severe discrepancy between potential and achievement and more recent IDEIA provisions require multiple research-based interventions, a learning disability may not be reliably discernable in younger children. Parents are encouraged to understand the warning signs of a learning disability from as early as preschool, since the first years in school are especially crucial for a young child. Yet there is no one indication of learning disabilities. Although most children have an occasional problem with learning or behavior, a consistent pattern of the following problems may suggest the need for further testing.

Preschool

Does the child have trouble with

- learning the alphabet
- rhyming words
- connecting sounds and letters
- counting or learning numbers
- being understood when speaking to a stranger

- using scissors, crayons, or paint
- reacting too much or too little to touch
- using words or using phrases
- pronunciation
- walking up and down stairs
- talking (identified as a "late talker")
- remembering names of colors
- dressing

Elementary School

Does the child have trouble with

- learning new vocabulary
- speaking in full sentences
- understanding conversation rules
- retelling stories
- remembering information
- playing with peers
- moving from one activity to another
- expressing thoughts
- holding a pencil
- handwriting
- handling math problems
- following directions
- self-esteem
- remembering routines
- learning
- reading comprehension
- drawing or copying shapes
- deciding what information presented in class is important
- modulating voice
- neatness and organization
- meeting deadlines
- playing age-appropriate board games

Adulthood

Does the adult have trouble with

- remembering new information
- organization

- reading comprehension
- getting along with peers or coworkers
- finding or keeping a job
- sense of direction
- understanding subtle jokes
- making appropriate remarks
- self expression
- following directions
- reading, writing, spelling, and math
- self-esteem
- using proper grammar
- meeting deadlines

Symptoms may appear in only one skill area, such as reading or writing, in many people with learning disabilities. The following is a brief outline of warning signs for possible learning disabilities in specific skill areas.

Attention

- has short attention span
- is impulsive
- has difficulty conforming to routines
- is easily distracted

Auditory

- does not respond to sounds of spoken language
- consistently misunderstands what is being said
- overly sensitive to sound
- has trouble differentiating simultaneous sounds

Language

- can explain things orally but not in writing
- has trouble telling or understanding jokes or stories
- misinterprets language
- does not understand what is said
- responds in an inappropriate manner, unrelated to what is said
- responds only partially to what is said

Math

- has problems with arithmetic, math language, and math concepts
- reverses numbers
- has problems with time, sequencing, or problem solving

Memory

- learns information presented one way but not another
- trouble memorizing information
- unable to repeat what has just been said

Movement

- performs similar tasks differently each day
- has trouble calling phone numbers or holding a pencil
- has poor coordination, is clumsy
- is unaware of physical surroundings
- has a tendency to self injury

Organization

- has trouble following a schedule
- is often late
- has trouble learning about time
- has difficulty organizing belongings

Reading

- poor reading ability or poor comprehension
- may misread information
- has problems with syntax or grammar
- confuses or reverses similar letters or numbers
- has problems reading addresses, small print, and/or columns

Social

- has trouble with social skills
- misinterprets nonverbal social cues
- experiences social isolation
- does not use appropriate eye contact
- is socially imperceptive

Thinking

- acquires new skills slowly
- has trouble following directions
- confuses right/left, up/down, under/over, behind/between
- gets lost in large buildings
- seems unaware of time or sequence of events

Writing

- has problems writing down ideas
- has problems organizing thoughts on paper
- reverses or omits letters, words, or phrases when writing
- has problems with sentence structure, writing mechanics
- may spell the same word differently in a single paper
- may read well but not write well (or vice versa)

It is also important to understand what is *not* included in the LD category. For example, attention deficit disorder (ADD) and ATTENTION DEFICIT HYPERACTIVITY DISORDER (ADHD) are not learning disabilities, but there is a 20 percent probability that someone with ADD or ADHD also has one or more learning disabilities. In clinical jargon, there is 20 percent "comorbidity" between ADHD and LD. Other conditions that are not considered to be learning disabilities include AUTISM, blindness and deafness, emotional problems, hyperactivity, illiteracy, mental retardation, "slow learner," physical disability, or juvenile delinquency.

"LD" covers a range of possible causes, symptoms, and treatments. Partly because learning disabilities can show up in so many forms, it is difficult to diagnose or to pinpoint the causes.

Not all learning problems are necessarily learning disabilities; many children are simply slow to develop certain skills. Because children show natural differences in their rate of development, sometimes what seems to be a learning disability may simply be a delay in maturation. For a problem to be diagnosed as a learning disability, specific criteria must be met. These criteria appear in the *Diagnostic and Statistical Manual of*

Mental Disorders (DSM), and can be divided into three broad categories: developmental speech and language disorders, academic skills disorders, and "other," a category that includes certain coordination disorders and learning handicaps not covered by the others. Each of these categories includes a number of more specific disorders. In addition, the law requires a severe discrepancy between potential and achievement or failure to respond to appropriate research-based interventions in one or more of the following:

- basic reading skill
- reading comprehension
- mathematics calculation
- mathematics reasoning
- written expression
- oral expression
- listening comprehension
- reading fluency (added with the 2004 IDEIA revisions)

Speech and language problems are often the earliest indicators of a learning disability. People with developmental speech and language disorders have trouble producing speech sounds, using spoken language to communicate, or understanding what other people say. Depending on the problem, the specific diagnosis may be

- developmental articulation disorder
- developmental expressive language disorder
- developmental receptive language disorder

With a developmental articulation disorder, children may have trouble controlling their rate of speech, or they may lag behind others of the same age in learning to make speech sounds. These disorders are common, appearing in at least 10 percent of children younger than age eight. Fortunately, articulation disorders can often be outgrown or successfully treated with speech therapy.

Some children with developmental expressive language disorder have problems expressing themselves in speech: they may call objects by the wrong names, speak only in two-word phrases, or be unable to answer simple questions.

Some people have trouble understanding certain aspects of speech; this is developmental receptive language disorder. This explains the toddler who does not respond when called by name or the worker who consistently cannot follow simple directions. While hearing is normal, these individuals cannot make sense of certain sounds, words, or sentences. Because using and understanding speech are strongly related, many people with receptive language disorders also have an expressive language disability.

Of course, some misuse of sounds, words, or grammar is a normal part of learning to speak. It is only when these problems are not resolved that there is any cause for concern.

Academic Skills Disorders Students with academic skills disorders often lag far behind their classmates in developing reading, writing, or arithmetic skills. The diagnoses in this category include

- developmental reading disorder
- developmental writing disorder
- developmental arithmetic disorder

Developmental reading disorder (also known as dyslexia) is quite widespread, affecting 2 percent to 8 percent of elementary school children. The ability to read requires a rich, intact network of nerve cells that connect the brain's centers of vision, language, and memory. While a person can have problems in any of the tasks involved in reading, scientists have found that a significant number of people with dyslexia cannot separate the sounds in spoken words. For example, a child might not be able to identify the word *cat* by sounding out the individual letters, c-a-t, or to play rhyming games. Fortunately, remedial reading specialists have developed techniques that can help many children with dyslexia acquire these skills. However, there is more to reading than recognizing words. If the brain cannot form images or relate new ideas to those stored in memory, the reader will not be able to understand or remember the new concepts. This is why other types of reading disabilities can appear in the upper grades, when the focus of reading shifts from word identification to comprehension.

Writing, too, involves several brain areas and functions. The brain networks for vocabulary, grammar, hand movement, and memory must all work well if the child is to be able to write well. A *developmental writing disorder* may be caused by problems in any of these areas. A child with a writing disability, particularly an expressive language disorder, might be unable to compose complete, grammatical sentences.

Arithmetic involves recognizing numbers and symbols, memorizing facts such as the multiplication table, aligning numbers, and understanding abstract concepts like place value and fractions. Any of these may be difficult for children with *developmental arithmetic disorders.* Problems with numbers or basic concepts are likely to show up early, whereas problems that appear in the later grades are more often tied to problems in reasoning.

Many aspects of speaking, listening, reading, writing, and arithmetic overlap and build on the same brain capabilities. So it is not surprising that people can be diagnosed as having more than one area of learning disability. For example, the ability to understand language underlies the ability to learn to speak. Therefore, any disorder that interferes with the ability to understand language will also interfere with the development of speech, which in turn hinders learning to read and write. A single problem in the brain's operation can disrupt many types of activity.

"Other" Learning Disabilities   There are additional categories of learning disabilities, such as motor skills disorders and specific developmental disorders not otherwise specified. These diagnoses include delays in acquiring language, academic, and motor skills that can affect the ability to learn, but do not meet the criteria for a specific learning disability. Also included are coordination disorders that can lead to poor penmanship, as well as certain spelling and memory disorders.

Attention Disorders   Nearly 4 million school-age children have learning disabilities; of these, at least 20 percent have a type of disorder that leaves them unable to establish and maintain attention and concentration. Some children and adults who have attention disorders are easily distracted or appear to daydream constantly. Children with this problem may have a number of learning difficulties.

In a large proportion of affected children (mostly boys) the attention deficit is accompanied by hyperactivity, such as running into traffic or toppling desks. Hyperactive children cannot sit still: They blurt out answers, they interrupt, they cannot wait their turn. Because of their constant motion and explosive energy, hyperactive children often get into trouble with parents, teachers, and peers. By adolescence, physical hyperactivity usually subsides into fidgeting and restlessness, but the problems with attention and concentration often continue into adulthood.

At work, adults with ADHD often have trouble organizing tasks or completing their work. They do not seem to listen to or follow directions. Their work may be messy and appear careless.

While attention disorders (with or without hyperactivity) are not considered learning disabilities in themselves, because attention problems can seriously interfere with school performance, they often accompany academic skills disorders.

Treatment Options and Outlook

Although a diagnosis is important, even more important is creating a plan for getting the right help. Schools typically provide special education programs either in a separate all-day classroom or as a special education class that the student attends for several hours each week. Some parents hire trained tutors to work with their child after school. If the problems are severe, some parents choose to place their child in a special school for the learning disabled.

Planning a special education program begins with systematically identifying what the student can and cannot do. The specialist looks for patterns in the child's gaps, such as the failure to hear the separate sounds in words or other sound discrimination problems. Special education teachers also identify the types of tasks the child can do and the senses that function well. By using the senses that are intact and bypassing the disabilities, many children can develop needed skills. These strengths offer alternative ways the child can learn.

After assessing the child's strengths and weaknesses, the special education placement committee develops an individualized educational program (IEP). The IEP outlines the specific skills the child needs to develop as well as appropriate learning activities that build on the child's strengths. Many effective learning activities engage several skills and senses. For example, in learning to spell and recognize words, a student may be asked to see, say, write, and spell each new word. The student may also write the words in sand, which engages the sense of touch. Many experts believe that the more senses children use in learning a skill, the more likely they are to retain it.

An individualized, skill-based approach often succeeds in helping where regular classroom instruction fails. Therapy for speech and language disorders focuses on providing a stimulating but structured environment for hearing and practicing language patterns. For example, the therapist may help a child who has an articulation disorder to produce specific speech sounds. During an engaging activity, the therapist may talk about the toys, then encourage the child to use the same sounds or words. In addition, the child may watch the therapist make the sound, feel the vibration in the therapist's throat, then practice making the sounds before a mirror.

Assistive technology Learning disabilities cannot be cured, but with the help of certain tools, a child with a learning disability can work around difficulties with reading, writing, numbers, spelling, organization, or memory. Complex, high-tech tools and devices—assistive technology—can help people work around specific deficits.

Tools for people with learning disabilities can be as simple as highlighters, color coded files or drawers, audio books, tape recorders, calculators, or a different paper color or background color on a computer screen. Sometimes, standard technologies (such as voice recognition systems) can be adapted or designed to help people with learning disabilities perform everyday tasks. Complex assistive technology includes computers that "talk" to help people with reading and writing difficulties, speech recognition systems that translate oral language into written text, "talking" calculators that assist people with math difficulties, and software that predicts words for people with spelling difficulties.

Researchers are also investigating nonstandard teaching methods. Some create artificial learning conditions that may help the brain receive information in nonstandard ways. For example, in some language disorders, the brain seems abnormally slow to process verbal information. Scientists are testing whether computers that talk can help children learn to process spoken sounds more quickly. The computer starts slowly, pronouncing one sound at a time. As the child gets better at recognizing the sounds and hearing them as words, the sounds are gradually speeded up to a normal rate of speech.

The term *learning disability* was coined by psychologist Samuel A. Kirk in 1963 to describe children who experience difficulty acquiring academic skills despite normal intelligence. He proposed this term because of his discomfort with the widespread use in an educational setting of medical terms such as DYSLEXIA, congenital word blindness, and minimal brain dysfunction. There were other common descriptors such as reading retardation and six-hour retardation. Although the term has become widely accepted, there has been a great deal of controversy about the exact definition and methods of assessment and identification of the condition.

The term has provided a focal point for legislation and advocacy that has resulted in far-reaching changes in the nature of public and postsecondary education in the United States. At the same time, the term *learning disabilities,* the range of potential learning problems that it includes, and the broad and rapidly changing field that it describes, all continue to be controversial. In fact, there is still no consensus on the definition of learning disabilities or on what the category should include or exclude, and the coming years are likely to see continuing debate on the fundamental issues of definition, classification, diagnosis, and treatment.

According to the National Joint Committee on Learning Disabilities, the term refers to a group of disorders marked by significant difficulties in listening, speaking, reading, writing, reasoning, or mathematical abilities. These disorders are presumed to be caused by central nervous system dysfunction, and may occur at any time. Although learning disabilities may appear at the same time as other handicapping conditions (such as deafness, blindness, mental retardation, or serious emotional disturbance), they are not caused by these conditions.

The primary legal definition of a learning disability, according to Public Law 94-142 (as amended by the Individuals with Disabilities Education Improvement Act) indicates: a disorder in one or more of the basic psychological processes involved in understanding or in using spoken or written language. This may include an imperfect ability to listen, think, speak, read, write, spell, or to do mathematical calculations. The term includes such conditions as perceptual handicaps, brain injury, minimal brain dysfunction, dyslexia, and developmental aphasia. The term does not include children who have problems primarily caused by visual, hearing, or motor disabilities, or mental retardation, emotional disturbance, or by environmental, cultural, or economic disadvantage.

Most definitions suggest that learning disabilities are permanent, affect a range of language and mathematics functions, and are caused at least in part from problems within the central nervous system. In addition, definitions of LD have generally focused on two key identifying factors: discrepancy and exclusion.

Discrepancy means that a child with a learning disability exhibits a significant gap between aptitude and performance. In many states, diagnosis of a learning disability depends on a very strict statistical measurement of this discrepancy between achievement and aptitude. The 2004 IDEIA reauthorization added the concept of failure to benefit from research-based educational interventions.

Exclusion means that a learning disability is not caused by some other handicapping condition, such as physical impairment or social status. A child who struggles to learn because she cannot see, or because he comes from a disadvantaged background, is not considered to have a learning disability if these are the primary factors in the learning problems.

The discrepancy formulation for learning disabilities, the requirement of failure to benefit from research-based educational interventions, and the role that exclusion of other conditions plays have become subjects for increasing debate in recent years. Many researchers have proposed redefining the concept of learning disabilities to focus on specific language and thought processing problems that may be identified by appropriate testing, without necessarily involving the question of aptitude or intellectual potential.

Some experts have argued that the exclusionary element in definitions of LD has led to the underidentification or misdiagnosis of individuals who come from poverty or from minority cultural, racial, or ethnic backgrounds. They argue that the difficulties such children have in learning are more likely to be ascribed to their backgrounds and upbringing than to a potential learning disability, and that approaches to diagnosis that depend on aptitude/achievement discrepancies are also likely to underrepresent such individuals.

Treatment for learning disabilities is extremely important if the child is to be successful. In fact, 35 percent of students with untreated learning disabilities fail to finish high school. Most students with learning disabilities were not fully employed one year after graduating from high school. Adolescents with untreated learning disabilities are at higher risk for drug and alcohol abuse. One study showed that up to 60 percent of adolescents in treatment for substance abuse had learning disabilities. Even though learning disabilities cannot be cured, there is still cause for hope. Because certain learning problems reflect delayed development, many children do eventually catch up.

Of the speech and language disorders, children who have an articulation or an expressive language disorder are the least likely to have long-term problems. Despite initial delays, most children do learn to speak. For people with dyslexia, the outlook is mixed. But an appropriate remedial reading program can help learners make great strides. With age, and appropriate help from parents and clinicians, children with ADHD become better able to suppress their hyperactivity and to channel it into more socially acceptable behaviors.

People with learning disabilities who have not been diagnosed or properly treated experience serious, lifelong negative consequences, including low self-esteem, delinquency, and illiteracy. Thirty-five percent of students identified with learning disabilities drop out of high school: This does not include students who drop out without being identified as having learning disabilities. Of adults with severe literacy problems, 50 to 80 percent have undetected or untreated learning disabilities. Fifty percent of young criminal offenders tested were found to have previously undetected learning disabilities; when offered educational services that addressed their learning disability, the recidivism rates of these young offenders dropped to below 2 percent.

See also APHASIA.

lecithin   Called "nature's nerve food," this is the major dietary source of CHOLINE, the brain chemical implicated as a possible aid to improving memory. Repeated studies of administering lecithin to treat the memory problems of ALZHEIMER'S DISEASE patients have resulted in conflicting evidence, although the majority found it was not helpful. Other studies suggest it might be useful in heading off some deterioration in the early stages of the disease.

Although it is available in supplemental form, many researchers do not believe lecithin can offer significant memory improvement. Still, according to the U.S. Food and Drug Administration, lecithin is not toxic and has no side effects. It is found in the cells of all animals and plants and helps build the insulation around nerves called the MYELIN SHEATH.

left brain-right brain   Many people believe that the left side of the brain is the home of logical thought and the right brain controls intuition. While this concept has grown astronomically popular during the past 20 years, the separation of abilities between left and right brains is not nearly so straightforward in actuality.

It is true that the left hemisphere does tend to be responsible for such analytical functions as understanding language, speech, computing, and judgment. The right hemisphere tends to be involved with more imaginative tasks, such as recognizing faces, visualizing images, and reconstructing songs. But both hemispheres are much more alike than they are different, and almost every mental process a person undertakes actually requires the cooperation of both hemispheres.

It was not until the 1960s that Dr. Roger Sperry published his research on the functional differences between the brain's two hemispheres based on his studies of epileptics whose hemispheres had been surgically severed.

Leonardo da Vinci (1452–1519)   Artist and scientist who in 1505 made the first wax cast of the brain's ventricles using the brain of an ox. Leonardo shifted the supposed site of sensory analysis in the brain to the second ventricle, where earlier researchers had thought the seat of reason could be found.

leucotomy   A surgical procedure invented in 1935 in which nerve tracts connecting the frontal association CORTEX with deeper structures are severed. The term is derived from the Greek words meaning "white" and "to cut," alluding to the fact that the white fibers connecting the FRONTAL LOBE to the rest of the brain are cut.

The first United States leucotomy was performed in 1935 in Washington, D.C., by American neurologists Walter Freeman and James Watts. Because the term *leucotomy* referred specifically to severing specific fibers, *lobotomy* was preferred as a more general term for any psychosurgical procedure involving the cutting of the lobe's nerve fibers.

While a leucotomy was a type of major brain surgery in which the skull was opened, Freeman developed a less severe "transorbital lobotomy" using an ice pick-like instrument through the eye socket to pierce the brain; a few quick jabs damaged enough brain tissue to tranquilize the patient. For his first patients, Freeman used an ice pick from his own kitchen.

The development of this lobotomy technique was an attempt to treat severe mental illness, but it led to the mass BRAIN DAMAGE of thousands of institutionalized psychiatric patients in the 1940s and 1950s, causing harmful personality changes. Lobotomy is now used only as a last resort.

levodopa   Also known as L-dopa, this drug is used in the treatment of PARKINSON'S DISEASE, a neurological disorder caused by a deficiency of the neurotransmitter DOPAMINE in the brain. Unlike many drugs, L-dopa can be absorbed into the brain, where it is converted into dopamine. It is usually given together with an enzyme such as carbidopa, in order to boost the amount of L-dopa available to the brain by reducing the amount that is first broken down by the liver. This allows for a lower dose of L-dopa, which can reduce the risk of adverse effects.

Side Effects

These adverse effects may include nausea and vomiting, nervousness, low blood pressure, and agitation. Prolonged use of L-dopa can worsen these side effects.

Unfortunately, L-dopa does not permanently cure Parkinson's disease, and there is still no real treatment for Parkinson's.

Lewy body dementia A dementing illness associated with protein deposits called Lewy bodies—abnormal brain cells that are distributed in varying degrees throughout all areas of the brain. This condition, also called dementia with Lewy bodies, describes several common disorders causing dementia. This is the second most common cause of dementia after ALZHEIMER'S DISEASE.

The name for the disease comes from the presence of abnormal lumps that develop inside nerve cells, called Lewy bodies. The condition is also known as diffuse Lewy body disease, cortical Lewy body disease, senile dementia of Lewy type or Lewy body variant of Alzheimer's disease.

Lewy body dementia was first described in 1961 and has been more often diagnosed over the past five to 10 years. Sometimes it occurs alone as the presenting illness, and sometimes it occurs simultaneously with Alzheimer's or PARKINSON'S DISEASE. It is very similar to Alzheimer's disease, characterized by progressive loss of memory, language, calculation, and reasoning as well as other higher mental functions.

Several key areas of the brain undergo degeneration in this form of disease, beginning with an area in the brain stem called the substantia nigra (as also occurs in Parkinson's disease). Normally,

the substantia nigra contains nerve cells responsible for making the neurotransmitter DOPAMINE. In both Parkinson's disease and Lewy body dementia, these cells die. Remaining nerve cells contain abnormal structures called Lewy bodies, which are a hallmark of the disease. Shrinkage of the brain is particularly seen in the temporal lobe, parietal lobe, and the cingulate gyrus.

The cause of this form of neurodegenerative disease is uncertain, although there appears to be a genetic component. Genetic studies are beginning to show a group of different genes that may contribute to the development of LBD.

Symptoms and Diagnostic Path

People with Lewy body dementia may have problems with short-term memory, word-finding difficulties, problems sustaining a line of thought and locating objects in space. They also may experience symptoms of anxiety and depression. The condition may cause acute episodes of confusion that vary from hour to hour. Because the "confusion" is not there all the time, it may seem as if the person is pretending to be confused.

Hallucinations are an early characteristic of this condition, and may occur at any time, but are often worse during the times of acute confusion. The most common hallucinations are visual, and often involve people, usually in the same place (such as a man standing by a certain door). Some patients see colored patterns or shapes. These hallucinations are not always distressing to patients, and many people learn to distinguish between real and unreal images; in fact, some people come to enjoy the hallucinations. On the other hand, many patients experience visual hallucinations together with unpleasant persecution delusions.

Some patients develop the features of Parkinson's disease (rigidity, tremor, stooped posture, slow shuffling movements), followed later by the fluctuating cognitive performance, visual hallucinations, memory loss, and a progressive dementia. Others experience the cognitive symptoms first and go on to develop Parkinsonian features later in the disease.

An important feature that helps to distinguish LBD from Alzheimer's disease is the presence of striking fluctuations in cognitive performance during the early stages of the disease. For example, one day a patient may be able to hold a sustained conversation, but on the next day he may be drowsy, inattentive, or mute. The basis of these fluctuations is not clear.

There are no specific diagnostic tests for the disease. Detailed psychological tests may help confirm the pattern of dementia. Brain scans may show generalized brain atrophy. In most patients the main diagnostic problem is to distinguish LBD from the more common Alzheimer's disease. LBD is suspected in those with fluctuation in mental ability, hallucinations, and spontaneous parkinsonism.

Treatment Options and Outlook

There is no cure for Lewy body disease, but it is sometimes possible to treat some of the symptoms. For example, the depression that often accompanies the disease usually responds to antidepressants. Occasionally unpleasant hallucinations may be reduced with medication.

In almost all patients, the disease is relentless and progressive; eventually, patients become profoundly demented and immobile, and usually die from pneumonia or another illness after an average of seven years from the onset of symptoms. A small proportion of patients have a rapidly progressive illness, becoming profoundly demented within months.

Risk Factors and Preventive Measures

Risk factors for developing the disease have not been identified. In the genetic cases of Lewy body disease, families inherited it as an "autosomal dominant" disease. This means that if a person carries the gene, he or she will eventually develop the disease. The children of such a person have a 50 percent chance of inheriting the illness.

limbic system   A network of ring-shaped structures in the center of the brain's NEO-CORTEX perched on top of the BRAIN STEM, associated with emotion and behavior—especially motivation, gratification, memory, and thought. It is also responsible for controlling body temperature, blood pressure, and blood sugar.

It is the complexity of emotions as mediated by the limbic system, together with a sophistication of sensory and motor systems, that leads to the profoundly complex behavior that is uniquely human. While much is still to be learned, scientists do know that the limbic system and the HYPOTHALAMUS are deeply interconnected with emotional feelings and with certain types of basic primitive behaviors such as eating, drinking, and sexual activity.

The limbic system developed early in evolution, which is not surprising considering that this area governs such basic survival necessities as fear, aggression, hunger, and sexual desire. The neural function and connectedness of the limbic system are fundamentally similar in all mammals. This extensive system includes a range of substructures such as the HIPPOCAMPUS, cingulate gyrus, and AMYGDALA. Because it contains the mechanisms that make an organism warm blooded, it is known as the mammalian brain.

The structures of the limbic system receive input from all the senses, but in most animals (and to some degree in humans) the sense of smell plays an especially important part in this system. Other parts of the brain that connect closely with the limbic system include the association areas of the CEREBRAL CORTEX, which is involved in higher thought processes, and midbrain structures such as the RETICULAR FORMATION (awareness, attention, and so on).

It is possible to recognize this sensory influence on emotions when considering how strong an impact a sentimental song or an odor reminiscent of childhood can have.

The effects of the limbic system are widespread, including the formation of tears and sweat, heart rate, hormone release and motor activity (such as facial expressions). Most of the messages sent by the limbic system end up in the hypothalamus, located beneath the THALAMUS, at the midline of the CENTRAL NERVOUS SYSTEM. Connected directly to the PITUITARY GLAND below, it controls the body's hormones and regulates instinctive behavior and the AUTONOMIC NERVOUS SYSTEM.

The most common symptoms of damage to this area of the brain include abnormalities of the emotions, including inappropriate crying or laughing, easily provoked rage, unwarranted fear, anxiety and depression, and excessive sexual interest.

lithium An ANTIPSYCHOTIC medication used primarily to treat bipolar disorder (MANIC DEPRESSION). Lithium is an element of the periodic table that readily forms salts. Prescribed since 1973 in the United States, it was heralded as the first effective treatment for manic depression. While scientists are not quite sure how this drug works, they believe it may help correct chemical imbalances in neurotransmitters (SEROTONIN and NOREPINEPHRINE) that influence emotion and behavior. While lithium can have a mild antidepressant effect, it is primarily effective by controlling the "high" of mania. Lithium can also be effective in the treatment of major DEPRESSION and can boost the effectiveness of other antidepressants when these drugs do not quite work on their own.

Lithium bromide was used as a sedative since the early 1900s but fell into disfavor in the 1940s when some heart patients died after using it as a salt substitute. Almost immediately thereafter, Australian psychiatrist John Cade discovered that lithium salts were extremely effective in treating manic depression. Eventually, lithium's popularity grew and by the late 1960s it was widely prescribed in other parts of the world. However, it remained restricted as an experimental drug in the United States until 1971.

Unfortunately, lithium does not work well for everyone; it is most effective for those who have had no more than three episodes of mania. About 20 percent of people will have complete remission of mania from taking lithium, and the rest will have varying degrees of relief. Some will experience fewer episodes of mania; those that do occur are shorter and less severe—and patients will feel more stable in between manic episodes.

Lithium will only work when it is maintained at the correct level in the bloodstream, making regular blood tests necessary. For some people, lithium may just stop working.

Side Effects

More common and less dangerous side effects may include thirst and frequent urination. Some people also gain weight during the first few months they take lithium. Signs of lithium toxicity include sluggishness, unsteadiness, tremor, muscle twitching, vomiting, or diarrhea. Severe cases of lithium toxicity can cause lasting BRAIN DAMAGE or death. Lithium toxicity can occur not only with a direct overdose but also if a patient's salt and water metabolism becomes imbalanced (such as by an infection that causes anorexia or fluid loss).

lobectomy An operation that involves cutting out a lobe of the brain.

lobotomy A psychosurgical procedure that involves cutting the nerve fibers of the lobe of the brain. It was used in the 1940s and 1950s as a way of permanently tranquilizing difficult psychiatric patients by destroying their brain. The term was first used by American neurologist Walter Freeman and surgeon James Watts to replace LEUCOTOMY, a more specific term referring to cutting certain white fibers in the brain. A leucotomy involved opening the skull and major brain surgery.

Having observed that the optimum results were achieved when the lobotomy induced drowsiness and disorientation, Freeman and Watts decided to see if they could use this information to judge how an operation was proceeding; they began to perform lobotomies under local anesthetic. Now they could speak to the patient while cutting the lobe connections and gauge whether they were being successful. They asked patients to sing a song or to perform arithmetic, and if they could see no signs of disorientation, they chopped away some more until they could. Initial professional reaction to the 1936 operations was outwardly not promising, drawing outraged responses from psychoanalysts and many psychiatrists. Privately, however, the technique aroused great interest, although in keeping with the medical tradition of discretion, these reservations were not voiced to the public at the time. Ten years later, however, everybody would declare that they had always opposed the lobotomy. Critics referred to the "offhand manner" in which the operation was described. For the time being, Freeman and Watts could not obtain coveted access to the many thousands of inmates of asylums. They remained in Washington, doing what work they could.

However, the introduction and wide acceptance around this time of such therapies as sodium amytal (the "truth drug") and insulin-coma shock therapy soon began to create a climate in which the lobotomy might seem more acceptable. Freeman was a neurologist, and neurologists had traditionally taken the view that there were physical causes for mental illness that required physical treatment. Psychiatrists, on the other hand, had argued that mental disorder was exclusively a problem of the mind. The two groups had bickered over whose property madness was, and the psychiatrists were initially Freeman's greatest opponents. But in the face of soaring mental hospital populations and the lack of rapid cures, both sides began to adopt increasingly extreme therapies. It was not long before the superintendents of mental institutions, faced with overcrowding and limited mental health budgets, began to adopt lobotomy. The economic arguments were very strong: a lobotomy could be performed for $250, while it could cost $35,000 or more a year to maintain a patient in hospital.

Psychosurgery began to gain in popularity in the United States, though in Europe its acceptance was more limited. Basing their work on the Freeman-Watts system, American neurosurgeons rapidly developed myriad variations.

Until 1945 Freeman had never actually performed a lobotomy himself, but had always worked in tandem with Watts. What Freeman wanted to develop was a version of the operation that could be performed not just by neurosurgeons, but by anyone, anywhere, in a few minutes.

During the winter of 1945, Freeman tried to develop a transorbital approach to lobotomy by practicing on corpses. Watts cooperated, believing that ultimately he would do the surgery, and Freeman would assist. Freeman put a special hammer-shaped head on the ice pick, which allowed it to be pushed and pulled more easily, and it was this instrument that was used in the first transorbital lobotomies in America in a procedure that became known as the "ice pick lobotomy."

Armed with his new tool, Freeman was convinced that a transorbital would be a simple surgical procedure which would not require a neurosurgeon. He decided that he would operate on the first living patient without telling Watts, whom he hoped would be impressed enough to offer his encouragement afterwards. Secretly he operated on a series of patients, to whom he explained that the technique had been used successfully in Italy for a number of years. He did not dwell on his own lack of surgical experience. He anesthetized patients with three rapid bursts of electric shock, and then drew the upper eyelid away from the eyeball, exposing the tear duct. The sharp point of the ice pick was placed in this, and a light tap with a hammer drove the ice pick into the brain. When it was about two inches inside, Freeman would pull the ice pick about 30 degrees backward, as far as he could without cracking the skull, and then move it up and down in another 20-degree arc in order to cut the nerves at the base of the frontal lobes. The procedure took only a few minutes.

After operating on 10 patients, he told Watts, who was deeply distressed to see the perfunctory, brutal nature of Freeman's operation. He angrily threatened to break with Freeman if he continued, and within months Watts had left their joint practice. Freeman began to visit mental hospitals in other states where he could practice his technique, although he was continually angered by finding himself given the most deteriorated patients to operate on. He wanted transorbital lobotomy to be performed on people who were just developing signs of mental disorder.

By the early 1950s, concerns about the effects of the lobotomy began to grow. Postoperative infections and deaths were common; autopsies showed that large areas of brains, not selected nerves, were utterly destroyed. There had still been no reliable studies of the effects on patients other than Freeman's optimistic data. Though some patients did continue to pursue their professional and private lives after the operation, it was impossible to state that this was because of the surgery, and it was impossible to judge "recovery" in many. The inert, emotionless, inhuman quality of many lobotomized began to revolt the public. As early as 1951, even the Soviet Union, where psychiatric abuse was rife, had stopped performing the lobotomy on the grounds that it produced unresponsive people.

Lobotomy was finally seen for what it was: not a cure, but a way of managing patients.

In 1952, chlorpromazine, the first of the new generation of revolutionary tranquilizers for schizophrenia and depression, was tested in France. After this, Freeman would be known as the "ice pick lobotomist," and his clientele rapidly diminished, along with his reputation. By 1954, psychopharmacology had hit America, and the manufacturers of the biggest-selling tranquilizer, Thorazine, could not keep pace with demand.

The development of this lobotomy technique led to the brain damage of thousands of institutionalized patients in the 1940s and 1950s, including the retarded young Rosemary Kennedy, sister of President John F. Kennedy.

locus coeruleus   Latin for "blue area," this is an area in the BRAIN STEM related to physiological responses to stress through the synthesis and release of the NEUROTRANSMITTER NOREPINEPHRINE. Stimulants (such as amphetamines and cocaine) increase the user's alertness by simulating norepinephrine and sometimes raising the concentration of norepinephrine at the SYNAPSES.

long-term memory   A type of memory consisting of many layers (or processes) of memory that lasts indefinitely. In long-term memory, a person stores an indefinite number of chunks in interconnected semantic networks. Long-term memory is very active in consolidation and association.

What a person chooses to store in long-term memory is probably closely tied to the emotions, and in fact the limbic system, which mediates emotion in the brain, is highly involved in memory function. Because humans generally seek pleasure and shun pain, we tend to repeat something that is rewarding (remember it) and avoid what is painful (forget it).

The amount of information each of us possesses is amazing, according to psychologist and memory expert Elizabeth Loftus. She notes that long-term memory records as many as 1 quadrillion separate bits of information; hypnosis and certain drugs are able to uncover stored information from early childhood, which can demonstrate how deeply information can be recorded. And on repeated recall tries, people usually can remember more material than they did on the first attempt. In addition, this ability to recall long-ago memories from childhood while under the influence of certain drugs or hypnosis illustrates the huge capacity, and permanent nature, of long-term memory.

Many researchers divide long-term memory into three types—procedural, semantic, and episodic memory. Procedural memory is the ability to remember how to do something (such as ride a bike or write a letter). Semantic memory involves remembering factual information, such as the capital of North Dakota or multiplication tables, with no connection to where or when we learned the information. Episodic memory involves remembering personal events, such as a first kiss or where one learned how to ride horseback.

Long-term memory differs from short-term memory in more than the length of time that a memory is able to be retrieved. The nerve changes involved in long-term memory may be different; the process is not easily disrupted and its capacity is virtually unlimited. Retrieval from short-term memory is automatic, whereas retrieval in long-term memory is not easy or always automatic.

The evidence of the physiological difference between short- and long-term memory is bolstered by the fact that some diseases or drugs may affect one type of memory while leaving the other type intact. For example, one patient with a defective short-term memory (he could not remember more than two digits at a time) had a normal long-term memory—his retention of everyday events was not diminished. And the famous research subject HM, whose long-term memory was lost when his frontal lobes were destroyed, still retained old memories recorded in long-term memory. His short-term memory was also intact; he just couldn't form any new long-lasting memories. In other words, he could not transfer any information from his short-term memory into long-term memory.

Information reaches long-term memory by going through short-term memory; therefore, the amount of information that is remembered depends on the ability of the short-term memory to code information into long-term memory.

LSD (lysergic acid diethylamide) A chemical that alters a user's mood, thoughts, or perceptions, one of a class of drugs known as hallucinogens or psychedelics. These drugs may cause auditory, visual, or sensory hallucinations, paranoia, or dreamlike states.

LSD was first produced from a fungus that grows on rye and other grains in 1938, by Sandoz, a Swiss pharmaceutical company, which intended it to help stimulate circulation and respiration.

LSD is a very powerful, water soluble, odorless, colorless, and tasteless drug in which a dose as small as a single grain of salt can produce some effects. Psychedelic effects are produced at slightly higher doses. The effects of LSD also depend on a user's mood and expectations of what the drug will do and last several hours.

The behavioral effects that LSD can produce include

- feelings of "strangeness"
- vivid colors
- hallucinations
- confusion, panic, psychosis, anxiety
- emotional reactions like fear, happiness, or sadness
- distortion of the senses and of time and space
- "flashback" reactions months or even years later
- increases in heart rate and blood pressure
- chills and muscle weakness

Tolerance to the effects of LSD develops quickly, and users must increase their intake of LSD to get the same effects.

The exact brain pathways that are affected by LSD are not completely known, but LSD has a chemical structure that is very similar to the NEUROTRANSMITTER called SEROTONIN. It is thought that the effects of LSD are caused by stimulation of serotonin receptors on neurons, perhaps in the brain area called the raphe nuclei. However, it is still not clear what produces all the effects of LSD.

L-tryptophan A precursor of SEROTONIN, one of the brain's NEUROTRANSMITTERS.

lucid dreaming The ability to "wake up" inside one's dream without physically waking. An EEG of a lucid dreamer shows waking waveforms superimposed on REM (dream-state) waveforms. The body is still asleep, however.

lumbar puncture (LP) The medical term for a spinal tap, this is a diagnostic procedure to withdraw and examine the CEREBROSPINAL FLUID (CSF). The procedure was introduced at the end of the 19th century as a way to diagnose neurologic disorders.

As other tests have become more sophisticated, the LP is no longer automatically performed in the analysis of all types of CENTRAL NERVOUS SYSTEM disorders. However, it is still used to help diagnose central nervous system infection, tumors in the SUBARACHNOID SPACE, MULTIPLE SCLEROSIS, GUILLAIN-BARRÉ SYNDROME, and neuroimmunologic disorders.

LPs also can be used to inject drugs into the spinal fluid, including a variety of chemotherapy drugs for the treatment of cancer, and can be used to inject a local anesthetic without causing loss of consciousness. They also can be used to insert a dye that will show up on X-RAY pictures of the SPINAL CORD (called MYELOGRAPHY).

Procedure

In the 20-minute procedure, the patient lies sideways with knees drawn up, pulling the vertebrae apart. The skin at the base of the spine is anesthetized with a local anesthetic, and a hollow needle is then inserted between two of the vertebrae in the lower part of the spinal canal to remove some cerebrospinal fluid. After the needle is removed, the puncture site is covered.

Risks and Complications

Some patients experience a mild HEADACHE that wears off soon after the procedure.

lysergic acid diethylamide See LSD.

Machado-Joseph disease (MJD) A genetic disorder of the central nervous system that cripples and paralyzes. It affects all races and many ethnic groups, and is often misdiagnosed as MULTIPLE SCLEROSIS, PARKINSON'S DISEASE, or spino-cerebellar degeneration. MJD is also known as Joseph disease, spino-cerebellar ATAXIA, type 3 or SCA/3, a common hereditary ataxia.

Symptoms and Diagnostic Path
The earlier the disease appears, the more severe the form it will take, but typically symptoms can begin any time from early adolescence to about age 70. This progressive disease gets worse as time goes on.

There are several types of MJD depending on when symptoms appear. Type I MJD begins between ages 10 and 30 and progresses quickly, with severe muscle rigidity. Type II begins between the ages of 20 and 50 and may develop more slowly, with spastic gait and exaggerated reflexes. Type III has the slowest progression, and begins between ages 40 and 70 years of age; it features muscle twitching and atrophy along with unpleasant sensations such as numbness, tingling, cramps, and pain in the hands, feet, and limbs.

In addition, almost all patients have vision problems, including blurred or double vision, color/contrast visual problems, or uncontrollable eye movements. Some MJD patients also experience symptoms much like Parkinson's, including slow movement, rigidity or stiffness, tremor or trembling, and impaired balance and coordination.

MJD can be diagnosed from the symptoms of the disease and by taking a family history, but a definitive diagnosis can only be made with a genetic test.

Life expectancy ranges from the mid-30s for those with severe forms of MJD to a normal life expectancy for those with mild forms. For those who die early from the disease, the cause of death is often aspiration pneumonia.

Treatment Options and Outlook
There is no known cure for the disease at this time. Symptoms of Parkinson's can be treated with levodopa therapy for many years. Spasticity may respond to treatment with antispasmodic drugs, such as baclofen, or with Botulinum toxin. (However, botulinum toxin should be used as a last resort due to the possibility of side effects, such as swallowing problems.)

Speech problems can be treated with medication and speech therapy. Wearing prism glasses can help correct blurred or double vision, but eye surgery is only briefly helpful due to the progressive degeneration of eye muscles.

Physiotherapy can help patients cope with walking problems, and patients may find walkers and wheelchairs useful. Other problems, such as sleep disturbances, cramps, and urinary dysfunction, can be treated with medications and supportive medical care.

mad cow disease (bovine spongiform encephalopathy) A chronic, degenerative disease affecting the central nervous system of cattle. In humans, "mad cow disease" is known medically as new-variant CREUTZFELDT-JAKOB DISEASE (v-CJD). Humans are believed to get the new variety of the condition by eating beef contaminated with bovine spongiform encephalopathy (BSE). About 200 cases of v-CJD have been identified worldwide, including three in the United States.

Scientists have known for some time of classical CJD, a slow degenerative disease of the central nervous system causing progressive dementia, memory loss and degeneration of the brain. It occurs sporadically worldwide at a rate of one case per million people each year. On March 20, 1996, 10 cases of a new form of CJD were discovered and labeled variant CJD. All of the v-CJD patients got sick in 1994 or 1995. The variant form differed from the sporadic classical form of CJD in that affected individuals were much younger than were the classical CJD patients. Typically, CJD patients are more than 63 years old. The average patient age for the onset of variant CJD is 28, ranging from 14 to 52. In addition, the course of the disease in the v-CJD patients averaged 13 months, whereas classical CJD cases average 6 months. In addition, patients with v-CJD showed a different pattern of electrical activity in the brain from classical CJD. Although brain pathology was recognizable as CJD, the pattern was different, with large clumps of PRION protein plaques.

All victims of v-CJD ate beef or beef products in the previous 10 years, but none had knowingly eaten brain material. One of the affected individuals had been a vegetarian since 1991. Two significant studies published in the October 2, 1997, edition of *Nature* made it seem likely that the BSE agent is highly likely to be the cause of v-CJD.

The vast majority of v-CJD in humans have been detected in the United Kingdom, although there have been two patients in France and one in Ireland. There have been three cases of v-CJD as of 2008 in the United States.

Mad cow disease belongs to the family of diseases known as the transmissible spongiform encephalopathies (TSEs) caused by a transmissible agent which is not yet fully characterized, but which many believe to be a prion. It is believed that British cattle became infected from improperly rendered animal scraps processed into cattle feed. In the 1970s and early 1980s, animal rendering services in Britain allowed animal meat and bone scraps to be transformed by a more gentle process into bone meal used for animal feed. It appears that sheep infected with scrapie, one type of TSE, were butchered and rendered into bone meal, which was then fed to cattle as a protein supplement. Within several years, herds of cattle were affected by BSE.

The disease only affected cattle until two young dairymen became afflicted by the apparent variant form of Creutzfeldt-Jakob disease.

Following the outbreak of mad cow disease in Britain, the practice of feeding animal products to other animals as supplements was banned. Since that time the number of cattle infected with BSE has dropped. However, in July 2000 two new cases of mad cow disease were discovered in two separate herds in western and central France, and 224 exposed cows were slaughtered. New cases of the disease are expected to appear in France until 2002, five years after authorities took rigorous measures to prevent more outbreaks, because mad cow disease has an average incubation period of five years.

There have been more than 188,535 cases of mad cow disease reported in cattle around the world since it was first diagnosed in 1986 in Great Britain. BSE has had a substantial impact on the livestock industry in the United Kingdom, where 95 percent of all cases have occurred; however, it has also been confirmed in cattle in Austria, Belgium, Canada, Czech Republic, Denmark, Falkland Islands, Finland, France, Germany, Greece, Hong Kong, Israel, Italy, Japan, Liechtenstein, Luxembourg, Oman, Poland, the Netherlands, Republic of Ireland, Slovakia, Slovenia, Sweden, Switzerland, Thailand, and the United States.

The TSE diseases share a number of characteristics. They all cause a progressive fatal neurological illness with a prolonged incubation period of months or years, affecting only the central nervous system—but without setting off any immune response in the victim. They are all caused by similar uncharacterized agents that produce spongiform changes in the brain, which many experts believe may be prions. In humans, the TSEs include CJD, variant CJD, Gerstmann-Straussler syndrome, fatal familial insomnia, and kuru.

Cause

The cause of mad cow disease as well as other TSEs and the CJDs has not yet been proven. In addition to prions, some experts think the diseases could be caused by an unconventional virus or a virino ("incomplete" virus). Scientists do know that whatever causes mad cow disease is smaller than most viruses and highly resistant to heat, ultraviolet light, ionizing radiation and common disinfectants that normally inactivate viruses or bacteria. It also triggers no immune or inflammatory response and has not been observed under the microscope.

Symptoms

Early symptoms of v-CJD include anxiety, paranoia and restlessness; as the disease progresses over two years, patients experience dementia and loss of physical control, followed by death.

Diagnosis

In the past, doctors and researchers diagnosed the brain disorder by examining patients' brains, often after death. In 1997, however, scientists found an abnormal form of the prion protein, which is the signature of v-CJD, in the tonsils of a deceased patient. Since then, researchers have collected a large number of lymph tissue samples.

Prevention

The United States began import restrictions in 1989 and active surveillance in 1990. The Food and Drug Administration (FDA) established regulations on August 4, 1997, that prohibit feeding most mammalian proteins to ruminants such as cows and goats. They neglected to ban byproducts of ruminants, which can be fed to pets and other ruminants (pigs) and poultry. A proposal to stop using cow blood, restaurant scraps, and poultry litter was never implemented.

Classical CJD remains rare in the United States, and fewer than 50 cases were reported each year until recently (the recent rise may be more attributed to increased awareness of the disease rather than to a true increase in frequency).

magnetic resonance imaging (MRI) Also called NUCLEAR MAGNETIC RESONANCE (NMR), this diagnostic scanning technique provides high-quality cross-sectional images of the brain without using X-RAYS or other types of radiation. For many, it has become the preferred technique for brain and SPINAL CORD imaging. (In fact, only the lower cost and faster imaging time for CAT SCANS keep that technology popular for most brain imaging.)

MRI brain scans have several advantages over CAT scans; first, they can easily scan on several planes. In addition, the GRAY and WHITE MATTER differences are more easily defined in an MRI scan. The lack of signal from bone gives MRI an advantage over CAT scans for infarctions in the BRAIN STEM.

MRI is an expensive technique that requires considerable skill to operate; however, the extremely high quality of current images exceeds any other imaging technology. As new computer programs are being developed, imaging time is being shortened and the introduction of paramagnetic "contrast" agents should further enhance imaging and may help shorten scanning time.

Procedure

Painless devices containing coils that send and receive radio waves are positioned near the part of the body being studied. The examination table will move into the MRI unit to record the images transmitted by the coils.

The technology is based on an interaction between radio waves and nuclei within the body in the presence of a powerful magnetic field. The machine's powerful electromagnet first aligns the nuclei of atoms of hydrogen, phosphorus, or other elements and then knocks them out of position by radio waves. When they realign with the magnetic field, they produce a radio signal that can be detected and transformed into a computer-generated image.

Risks and Complications

There is no known danger with MRI, other than the effect of the electromagnetic field on metal such as implants or metal clips, on magnetic credit-card strips, analog watches, and so on. It cannot be used in patients with pacemakers and some aneurysm clips.

magnetite A natural magnetic material, commonly known as lodestone, magnetite is found in the brains of certain animals, from homing pigeons to whales; the animals use the internal magnets to help orient their sense of direction. Recently, scientists at the California Institute of Technology in Pasadena have found magnetite crystals in tissues of the human brain as well.

Brains contain an average of 7 billion crystals of iron magnetite, each either a millionth of an inch or 10 millionth of an inch in width. The total weight of the crystals in the brain is about a millionth of an ounce.

Researchers do not yet know how the magnetite relates to the human nervous system, although some scientists suspect it might provide a ·clue to the effects of electromagnetic fields (EMFs) and disease. EMFs have been linked to certain disorders such as cancer, but in the past critics have questioned this possibility because they believed the human body contains no magnetic material.

malnutrition For proper function, the brain must have the correct amount of food, including glucose, vitamins, minerals, and other essential chemicals. For example, the fuel the brain uses is glucose, which is produced from eating carbohydrates or other foods that can be converted to glucose. To grow new connections or add myelin, a fatty sheath to axons, the brain must manufacture the right proteins and fats. It does this by digesting proteins and fats in food and using the resulting amino acids and fatty acids to make the new brain proteins and fats. Without the correct amount and balance of particular building blocks, the brain will not work properly. Too little or too much of the necessary nutrient can affect the nervous system.

Vitamin and mineral deficiencies can be caused by

- starvation
- poor diet
- poor absorption of vitamins and minerals
- damage to the digestive system
- infection
- alcoholism

The brain of a human fetus grows rapidly from the 10th to 18th week of development, so it is important for the pregnant woman to eat nutritious foods during this time. The brain also grows rapidly just before and for about two years after birth. Malnutrition during these periods of rapid brain growth may have devastating effects on the nervous system and can affect not only neurons, but also glial cell development and growth, which can affect myelin development. Babies born to mothers who had poor diets may have some form of mental retardation or behavioral problems, and children who do not eat well in their first few years of life may develop problems later. Often the effects of malnutrition and environmental problems, such as emotional and physical abuse, can combine to create behavioral problems. Therefore, the exact causes of behavioral disorders are difficult to determine.

Some effects of malnutrition can be repaired by a proper diet, so not all of the effects of poor diets are permanent. Researchers believe that the timing of malnutrition is an important factor in determining if problems will occur. This means that missing out on a particular nutrient at the time when a part of the brain is growing and needs that nutrient will cause a specific problem there.

Scientists have just begun to understand how changes in particular nutrients alter the brain and how these neural changes then affect intelligence, mood, and the way people act. Experiments that investigate this nutrition-brain-behavior interaction, particularly those that study the effects of malnutrition, are difficult for several reasons. There is a link between poor nutrition and environmental factors, so that changes in behavior may be due not just to poor nutrition but to other factors such as education, social, or family problems.

It is difficult to alter only one substance in the human diet. Therefore, it is difficult to determine if a particular vitamin or mineral has a certain effect on behavior. For ethical reasons, experiments in which a person is not allowed to eat a particular nutrient cannot be done, so much of the data comes from animal experiments. Studies in humans are generally limited to examining the effects of famine and starvation, situations where many nutrients are missing.

People respond to different diets in different ways. In other words, there is a large individual variation in the body's response and need for different nutrients. A change in diet may have a placebo effect. The placebo effect occurs because a person thinks something will have an effect. In other words, if a person thinks a change in diet will affect behavior, it may actually affect behavior even if the nutrients are not causing the change. Therefore, experiments must have a placebo control and be performed in a double-blind manner, where neither the experimental subject nor the experimenter know who has received an altered diet.

Malpighi, Marcello (1628–1694) Italian anatomist and pioneer microscopist who was the first to study brain cells by microscope. He concluded that most living materials are glandular and that even the largest organs are composed of tiny glands.

While little is known of his childhood, Malpighi earned doctorates in both philosophy and medicine and taught theoretical medicine at the University of Pisa in 1656. He returned to Bologna in 1659, where he continued to conduct microscopic research and to teach, despite the hostile reception he received from many of his colleagues. As a result of the lack of understanding of his colleagues, he accepted a professorship in medicine at the University of Messina in Sicily in 1662, returning after four years to Bologna, where he continued the microscopic study of the brain in addition to other organs.

In the last 10 years of his life, he was beset by tragedy and failing health. In 1684, scientific opposition reached fever pitch, and his villa was burned, his instruments shattered, and his papers destroyed. In an effort to support the scientist, Pope Innocent XII invited him to Rome in 1691 to be his personal physician, where further honors were showered upon him. He died in Rome three years later.

mammillary bodies Part of the uppermost portion of the BRAIN STEM; this top surface of the DIENCEPHALON forms the floor on which the mammillary bodies lie. The mammillary bodies may be related to memory function. They are generally considered nuclei of the hypothalamus—part of the LIMBIC SYSTEM. If they are related to memory, it is in some vague, emotional way. Most researchers believe mammillary bodies are related to primitive temperature regulation.

manic-depressive disorder See BIPOLAR DISORDER.

mapping the brain The task of mapping the brain's regions and assigning functions to separate areas is an immense, ongoing task in the field of NEUROLOGY. As early as the 1860s, scientists began to locate specific areas of the brain by noting specific personality or behavior changes in people with EPILEPSY with damage to certain brain areas. Monitoring behavior electrically later enabled scientists to map the motor and sensory areas in both cerebral hemispheres.

During the 1920s, Canadian surgeon WILDER PENFIELD probed the motor, sensory, and "psychic" areas by touching certain areas of the exposed brain with two- and three-volt currents fired from an electrode tip. When Penfield touched certain areas, he sparked an activity in remote but functionally related brain regions connected to them.

Scientists have also been able to study the brain by stimulating electrodes implanted deep within the brain and by watching the living brain at work through PET SCANS. PET scans allow scientists to watch the brain's use of sugar and to relate this to specific mental or physical activities.

In addition, it is possible to tag brain cells to find which nerve connects to which, tracing their passage through the brain.

marijuana The world's most commonly used hallucinogenic drug that is derived from a plant (Cannabis sativa) contains delta-9 tetrahydrocannabinol (THC). Marijuana is usually smoked like a cigarette or in a pipe, but it also can be cooked into baked goods such as brownies or cookies, or brewed like a tea. THC is also contained in hashish, which is the resin from the plant. Hashish is usually smoked in a pipe. Other names for marijuana include grass, reefer, pot, weed and muggle.

THC acts on cannabinoid receptors, which are found on brain cells in many places throughout the brain, including areas involved in MEMORY (the HIPPOCAMPUS), concentration (CEREBRAL CORTEX), PERCEPTION (sensory portions of the cerebral cortex), and movement (the CEREBELLUM). When THC activates cannabinoid receptors, it interferes with the normal functioning of these brain areas.

In low to medium doses, marijuana causes relaxation, reduced coordination, low blood pressure, sleepiness, disruption in attention, and an altered sense of time and space. In high doses, it can cause hallucinations, delusions, impaired memory, and disorientation. The effects of marijuana begin in one to 10 minutes and can last from three to four hours.

Scientists have known for a long time that THC interacted with cannabinoid receptors in the brain, but they did not know why the brain would have such receptors. In 1992, scientists discovered anandamide, the brain's own THC, but they are not yet sure what the function of this chemical might be in a normal brain.

Use of cannabis may impair or reduce short-term memory and comprehension, alter the sense of time, and reduce ability to perform tasks requiring concentration and coordination. The substance's negative effects on memory have been recorded for some time; in 1845 French psychiatrist Moreau de Tours noted that hashish could gradually weaken the power to direct thoughts at will. More recent studies suggest that the most obvious problem with memory occurs within three hours of smoking, with a direct effect on the hippocampus, the memory center of the brain. Some researchers suggest marijuana may affect the way a person processes and remembers different kinds of information. It appears to interfere with cholinergic transmission, resulting in problems in retrieving words and making it difficult to recall numbers; the ability to store new memories also seems to be affected. Some scientists believe the chronic use of marijuana may cause the same kinds of memory effects as those experienced in patients suffering from brain infections, KORSAKOFF SYNDROME, and ALZHEIMER'S DISEASE.

Other studies suggest marijuana may interfere with memory because it increases the number of intrusive thoughts.

Experiments have shown that THC can affect two neurotransmitters: NOREPINEPHRINE and DOPAMINE; SEROTONIN and GABA levels may also be altered. Experts do not agree about whether marijuana use can produce addiction and whether it causes long-term mental problems. While there have been no documented fatal overdoses produced by marijuana, there is a high level of tar and other chemicals in marijuana; smoking the drug causes similar health problems to cigarette smoking. There is a bigger risk of lung problems and lung cancer later in life due to marijuana smoking.

medial temporal lobe   An area of the brain important in memory formation. Direct evidence of the importance of this area of the brain comes in the wake of neurosurgery to remove parts of the TEMPORAL LOBE as a treatment for EPILEPSY.

In a series of operations during the mid-1950s, surgeons removed the medial temporal lobe in 10 epileptic patients in order to lessen SEIZURES. While the operations were successful, eight of the 10 suffered pronounced memory deficits. The most famous of these was known as HM, whose amnesic syndrome is considered to be among the purest ever studied. After the operation, HM was unable to remember anything other than a handful of events since the time of his operation and was described as living in the "eternal present."

The study revealed that AMNESIA was present only in those who had lost both the HIPPOCAMPUS and the AMYGDALA; removal of the amygdala alone did not produce amnesia.

meditation and the brain   Meditation is used in an attempt to achieve tranquility, clear headedness, and relaxation by learning to focus on a single mental task (such as visualizing an object, contemplating a word or sound, or paying attention to the breath).

Basically, meditation's effects occur as a result of alteration of the brain waves. Different BRAINWAVE patterns reflect different states of consciousness. Rapid BETA WAVES are associated with normal arousal; slower ALPHA WAVES indicate a relaxed, meditative state; THETA WAVES, which are still slower, represent drowsiness or deep reverie; DELTA WAVES, the slowest of all, occur during sleep.

Meditation slows and deepens the brain-wave pattern from beta to alpha or (in advanced stages) even to theta, which produces a mildly altered state of consciousness.

medulla   One of three parts of the BRAIN STEM, the medulla looks like a thickened extension of the SPINAL CORD and contains the nuclei of the ninth through the 12th CRANIAL NERVES, receiving and relaying taste sensations from the tongue and relaying signals to speech muscles and in tongue and neck movements. It is situated in the skull, above the PONS and below the spinal cord. The medulla also contains the groups of nerve cells that control the automatic activities of the heartbeat, breathing, blood pressure, and digestion, sending and receiving information about these automatic functions via the VAGUS NERVE. It is also responsible for coughing, sneezing, and gagging.

medulla oblongata   Full name of the MEDULLA.

medulloblastoma   A malignant tumor of the CEREBELLUM (a part of the brain located in the lower rear portion of the cranium), one of the most common type of BRAIN TUMOR found in children. About 50 percent of these tumors are confined to the connecting bridge between the two halves of the cerebellum; the rest actually invade the cerebellum or the BRAIN STEM. The cause of a medulloblastoma is unknown.

Most medulloblastomas occur between the ages of four and eight, with a peak incidence around age five and one-half. Boys of this age are twice as likely as girls to have this type of tumor, but the sexual difference lessens with age. Several hundred cases of medulloblastoma are diagnosed each year in the United States.

Symptoms and Diagnostic Path

Among infants, the only sign is usually increased head size. After age 18 months, the most common symptoms are vomiting and HEADACHE just after awakening (caused by increased pressure within the skull). Other symptoms include irritability, sluggishness, personality change, and impaired attention and memory. Because the cerebellum controls and coordinates activities such as walking and speech, these activities may be affected as the tumor grows; an "ataxic gait" (stumbling, uncoordinated movements) is a common initial symptom. Depending on the exact location of the tumor, there may be muscle weakness, spasticity,

reflex change, limp muscles, stiff neck, imperfect eye coordination, or RAPID EYE MOVEMENTS.

Medulloblastomas are diagnosed with non-invasive tests such as CAT SCANS and MAGNETIC RESONANCE IMAGING (MRI). SPINAL TAPS are never performed if increased intracranial pressure is suspected because of the danger of severe brain damage.

Treatment Options and Outlook

Medulloblastomas can block the normal flow of SPINAL FLUID, and shunting to remove this fluid may be necessary to decrease the intracranial pressure before the tumor is removed. Surgery can remove most of the tumor, increasing the effectiveness of chemotherapy or radiation. While there is a link between the extent of the excised tumor and subsequent survival, this type of tumor can never be completely removed because stray cells too small for the surgeon to see are almost always present in the surrounding area.

Since the 1920s, radiation therapy has been used to destroy tumor cells that remain after surgery. Irradiation of the entire brain and spine begins about a week after surgery because the tumor may spread throughout the CENTRAL NERVOUS SYSTEM. While this treatment is associated with long-term side effects, some hospitals report up to a 70 percent five-year survival rate for patients whose tumor has apparently been completely removed followed by radiation. High-risk patients also may benefit from chemotherapy.

Poor growth is often the consequence of radiation therapy caused by possible damage to the HYPOTHALAMUS; 80 percent of children treated with radiation have a decreased amount of growth hormone. Radiation damage to the spine may also cause shortness or curvature. The endocrine system may also be damaged. Many children less than four treated with radiation and/or chemotherapy also suffer some degree of decreased intellect, with problems in reading, writing, and short-term memory. Older children suffer less intellectual damage.

melatonin   A hormone released by the PINEAL GLAND that induces sleep and influences CIRCADIAN RHYTHMS; experts now believe an abnormal level of melatonin may also suppress mood and mental quickness. The human body is regulated by a biological clock that sets the pace for everyday rhythms of sleep, activity, temperature, and cortisol and melatonin release. Most people maintain a certain flexibility in their biological clock, allowing them to synchronize their system to environmental changes. But experts suspect that some people do not synchronize their clocks so easily. It could be that some people are out of step with the world's 24-hour rhythm, so that melatonin is released too early (causing early-evening sleepiness and early-morning awakening) or too late (causing insomnia and trouble waking up). Normally, melatonin is produced in the dark during sleep, and its production peaks during the winter months.

During the day, melatonin levels are low; at sunset, the cessation of light triggers neural signals that stimulate the pineal gland to begin releasing melatonin. This rise continues for hours, eventually peaking around 2 A.M. in normal, healthy young people and about 3 A.M. in elderly patients. After this, it begins a steady decline to minimal levels again by morning. The delay in timing and decrease in amount of melatonin appears to be a part of the aging process; interestingly, the maximum amount of melatonin released in the bloodstream of the elderly is only about half of that in young adults. This decrease is so predictable that some experts have proposed blood melatonin levels as a measure of biological age. This reduction in melatonin among the elderly may be part of the reason for the sleeping problems and daytime fatigue many senior citizens report.

The melatonin cycle appears to regulate many neuroendocrine functions. When the timing or intensity of the melatonin peak is disrupted by aging or jet lag, for example, many physiological and mental functions are affected. Some of these functions include cognitive ability, memory, and judgment.

There has been some research investigating the possibility of melatonin's ability to slow down the aging process in animal studies. It is being investigated as a treatment to prevent ATHEROSCLEROSIS, reduce triglyceride levels, improve cellular immunity, and increase lifespan. It is also linked with depression; recent research at the University of California at San Diego found that some women who are depressed as a result of PMS (premenstrual syndrome) have lower amounts of melatonin when they sleep. In other studies, manic depressives were found to be extremely sensitive to light; exposure to it caused their melatonin levels to plummet. In addition, the pineal gland appears to be particularly important in the development of SEASONAL AFFECTIVE DISORDER (SAD); treatment of SAD by special lights may ease depression by readjusting the circadian rhythms, thereby normalizing the secretion of melatonin by the brain.

Scientists are studying the possibility of using melatonin as a treatment for conditions including jet lag, cancer, sleep disturbances, stress, and poor memory. In some studies, melatonin appears to inhibit tumor growth and may be of value in untreatable cancer patients whose disease has spread. There has even been some suggestion that melatonin may help to overcome the negative health consequences of electromagnetic fields.

memantine (Namenda)   It was approved to treat moderate to severe ALZHEIMER'S DISEASE. Classified as an "uncompetitive low-to-moderate affinity N-methyl-D-aspartate (NMDA) receptor antagonist," it is the first Alzheimer drug of this type approved in the United States. It appears to work by regulating the activity of glutamate, one of the brain's specialized messenger chemicals involved in information processing, storage, and retrieval.

memory   Traditionally understood as the storage and retrieval of information, memory is really not so much a retrieval as an active construction, an abstraction that refers to a process—remembering. Memory has not been located in any one place in the brain but is believed to function at the levels of NEURONS scattered in a weblike pattern throughout the brain. In fact, there is no firm distinction between how a person remembers and how a person thinks.

In the brain, neurons connect with other cells via junctions called synapses. When a neuron sends an electrical signal down its axon, the signal triggers the release of NEUROTRANSMITTERS (special signaling substances) that diffuse across the synapses between cells, attaching themselves to RECEPTORS on the following NERVE CELL. When the neurotransmitter binds to the receptor, this chemical transmission stimulates (or inhibits) the electrical activity of the second neuron; in this way, neurons communicate. The human brain contains about 10 billion of these nerve cells joined together by about 60 trillion synapses.

Bits and pieces of every experience are not stored in one place but are sent out to different regions of the brain: Memories of sound are found in the AUDITORY CORTEX, memories of the appearance settle into the VISUAL CORTEX. Each neuron represents a small bit of the memory, and all the scattered fragments of memory remain physically linked. To be recalled, the memory is called up by the LIMBIC SYSTEM, which pulls different aspects of each memory from the fragments scattered throughout the CORTEX through electrochemical signaling. Consolidation of information into a thought or image seems to require correlated nerve-cell signaling in different parts of the brain.

The backbone of memory could be the parts of the brain cells that receive electric impulses—the DENDRITES, the wisps at the tip of the brain cell that receive signals from the axon terminals of preceding neurons.

Researchers have generally agreed that anything that influences behavior leaves a trace (ENGRAM) somewhere in the nervous system. As long as these memory traces last, they can theoretically be restimulated, and the event or experience that established them will be remembered.

It could be that the HIPPOCAMPUS (part of the limbic system) retrieves a memory using a single moment or sensation to trip off recall of the others: The smell of perfume or the feel of a soft sweater brings with it the memory of *mother*. Each time the memory is called up, the hippocampus strengthens the connections between the various elements of each perception.

Where Is Memory?

Little is known about the physiology of memory storage in the brain. Some researchers suggest that memories are stored at specific sites, and others say that memories involve widespread brain regions working together; both processes may in fact be involved. Theorists also propose that different stor-

age mechanisms exist for short-term and long-term memories, and that if memories aren't transferred from one to the other, they will be lost.

Several brain structures are involved in the process of memory, including the hippocampus, hypothalamus, THALAMUS, and TEMPORAL LOBES. Damage to any one of them can cause memory problems.

The hippocampus plays a vital role in transforming short-term memories into permanent ones, which makes this part of the brain crucial to learning. It was in the hippocampal area that the best-documented link to memory was discovered with the patient HM, an epileptic whose temporal lobes were destroyed to alleviate seizures. After surgery, HM was unable to learn any new information and showed symptoms of a classic amnesic syndrome. From these data, scientists realized that an intact hippocampus was essential for normal memory function. Further research has shown that removing the left temporal lobe causes verbal memory deficits and removing the right lobe impairs nonverbal memory (such as remembering mazes, patterns or faces).

However, memory problems following damage to the hippocampal structures do not occur only after surgery; injury following a stroke also can cause a profound short-term memory problem.

The thalamus is one of the main parts of the DIENCEPHALON, and is involved in many cases of memory disorder in WERNICKE-KORSAKOFF patients. One of the best-known cases of thalamic damage and memory problems is NA, a man who was stabbed in the thalamic region at age 22 and suffered extensive memory problems as a result. Other cases of thalamic tumors have been reported, which can lead to a rapidly developing dementia.

But permanent memories are also stored elsewhere in the brain. Another region, an almond-size bit of tissue known as the AMYGDALA, seems to be crucial in forming and triggering the recall of a special type of memory tied to strong emotion, especially fear. The hippocampus allows a person to remember having been afraid; the amygdala evidently calls up the feelings that go along with each such memory.

Animal studies indicate that structures in the brain's limbic system have different memory functions. For example, one circuit through the hippocampus and thalamus may be involved in spatial memories, whereas another, through the amygdala and thalamus, may be involved in emotional memories. Research also suggests that "skill" memories are stored differently from intellectual memories.

In general, memories are less clear and detailed than perceptions, but occasionally a remembered image is complete in every detail. This phenomenon, known as eidetic imagery, is usually found in children, who sometimes project the image so completely that they can spell out an entire page of writing in an unfamiliar language that they have seen for a short time.

False Memory

This system of recalling memory from consolidating bits of information from all over the brain almost guarantees that people may not always remember accurately. It is quite possible that people may assemble accurate snippets inaccurately. For example, if someone witnessed a car running a red light and someone else later mentions that car running the stop sign, the witness may very possibly reconstruct the memory as a car running a stop sign. Unfortunately, it may be impossible to tease out accurate memories in such a case because there is no structural difference between a memory of a true event and a false one.

One of the most famous cases of false memory was reported by the psychologist Jean Piaget. He reported that his earliest memory was of his nurse defending him against a potential kidnapper at age two. He distinctly recalled sitting frightened in the baby carriage while the nurse fought off the man (incurring a scratch on her face in the process), and the police officer chasing away the kidnapper with his short white baton. Piaget was even able to describe the officer's uniform in detail. His family was relieved that the nurse prevented his kidnapping and rewarded her with a gold watch.

Thirteen years later, the nurse returned the gold watch to the family accompanied by a letter in which she confessed that she had made up the entire event. She said she had made up the story because she wanted to raise the family's opinion of her, and secure her position. Piaget used this false memory to emphasize the role of others' influ-

ences on one's memories. He noted that the nurse frequently had recounted the story in his presence, and others then had repeated the story in his hearing, thus creating the memories he had adopted as his own. Piaget noted that even in his old age those memories persisted as clear events even though he knew them to be false.

Many individuals report vivid childhood memories only to later learn that they are false. Maybe they recall Aunt Mary, who actually died before they were born, or they recall residing in a home the family moved from before they were born. Sometimes this phenomenon occurs with adults: Dr. Harris distinctly recalls wrecking his van after being shot. He vividly recalls the van's windshield exploding and blood splattering the seats. Actually, he struck his head very hard when he had a head-on collision with an inebriated driver a state trooper was trying to stop. When Dr. Harris visited the garage to sign over his wrecked van to the insurance company, he saw that the windshield was intact and there was no blood on the seats.

The same state trooper happened to respond to a traffic accident that Dr. Harris witnessed a year later. The state trooper told Dr. Harris that his first words were that he "had been shot" when the officer helped remove him from the van.

Because the origin of a memory (called "source memory") deteriorates more quickly than other aspects of the memory, it is highly prone to suggestion. While not everyone is considered to be suggestible, certain conditions—such as severe emotional stress—can render these people more sensitive to suggestion. This is particularly so during therapy, when comments by a therapist may be internalized and later recalled as actual memory according to psychologist and memory expert Elizabeth Loftus, Ph.D.

HYPNOSIS is especially capable of creating instead of retrieving memories, according to psychiatrist David Spiegel, M.D., of Stanford University. This problem of "false memory" becomes especially important during litigation of repressed memories in abuse cases.

Types of Memory

Memory is a biological phenomenon with its root firmly in the senses. In fact, there are many different types of memories: visual, verbal, olfactory, tactile, kinesthetic, and so on. While people often think of memory as a single phenomenon, in fact there are two distinct mechanisms corresponding to different mental processes—voluntary and involuntary memory. The smell of grandmother's perfume may trigger an involuntary memory if the sensation comes by surprise; it will appear as a voluntary memory if a person chooses to search for it.

If a person's earliest memory is of nestling in the arms of a mother, the person's visual system identified the objects in space—this shape is a sweater, this shape is the mother's face, this is its color, this is its smell, this is how it feels—binding them into the experience of being held by mother. Each of these separate sensations then travels to the hippocampus, which rapidly integrates the perceptions as they occur into a single, memorable experience. The hippocampus then consolidates information for storage as permanent memory in another brain region.

About 60 percent of Americans have primarily a "visual" memory, easily visualizing objects, places, faces, and the pages of a newspaper. The others seem better at remembering sounds or words and the associations they think of are often rhymes or puns.

In addition, some researchers believe there are at least three different types of memory subsystems—sensory, short-term, and long-term memory (although other researchers believe long-term memory is made up of several different types of remembering). While most people think of long-term memory when they say *memory,* in fact these researchers believe information must pass through the first two systems before it can be stored in long-term memory.

Formation of a memory begins with registration of information during perception; the data are then filed in a short-term memory system that seems to be very limited in the amount of material it can store at one time. Unless it is constantly repeated, short-term memory is lost within minutes and is replaced by other material.

The next stage of memory formation is the transference of important material to long-term memory—called consolidation—where the process of storage involves associations with words or meanings, with the visual imagery evoked by it, or with other sensory experiences, such as smell or sound.

People tend to store material on subjects they already know something about because the information has more meaning to them. This is why a person with a normal memory may be able to recall in detail many facets about one subject. In addition, people remember words that are related to something they already know because there is already a file in their memory related to that information.

The final stage of memory is retrieving (or recall), in which information stored on the unconscious level is brought up into the conscious mind at will. How reliable this material is, researchers believe, depends on how well it was encoded during stage two.

While most people speak of having a bad memory or a good memory, in fact most people are good at remembering some things and not so good at remembering others. When a person has trouble remembering something, it is generally not the fault of the entire memory system—just an inefficient component in the memory system.

For example, if a person wanted to remember where he had placed his keys, first he must have become aware of where he put them when he walked in the door. He registers (takes notice of) what he has done by paying attention to the action of putting his keys down on the hall table. This information is consolidated, ready to be retrieved at a later date.

If the system is working properly, he can remember exactly where he left his keys. If he has forgotten where he puts his keys, one of several things could have happened:

- He may not have registered clearly to start with.
- He may not have consolidated what he registered.
- He may not be able to retrieve the memory accurately.

Research indicates that older people have trouble with all three of these stages but are especially troubled with registering and retrieving information.

There are many factors that go into how well a memory is formed, including how familiar the information is and how much attention has been paid. Good health also plays a major part in how well a person performs intentional memory tasks. When mental and physical conditions are not in peak condition, the entire memory system functions at a slower pace. Attention (a key to memory performance) is diminished and long-term memory weakens. Ideas and images are not likely to be registered as strongly, and memory traces become fainter, making them harder to retrieve or file into long-term memory. In fact, patients who frequently become ill have significantly more memory problems than those who stay in good health, according to a survey of 1,000 subjects by the National Center of Health Statistics.

Techniques available for improving memory generally invoke teaching association techniques that show people how to improve their coding systems. For example, a person might visualize a well-known street and then think of each building as representing a new fact.

People with high IQs usually have good memories, although some people have exceptionally good memories that seem to be unrelated to their intellectual functioning. There are even some people with MENTAL RETARDATION who have profoundly intense memories for specific types of information—the so-called idiot savants.

Research into the biochemical basis of memory itself was first begun during the 1950s, when studies suggested that the complex molecule RNA (ribonucleic acid) served as a chemical mediator for memory. Rat studies showed that when animals were trained to do certain tasks, RNA in certain cells changed. Blocking the rats' RNA did interfere with long-term memory, although no change was apparent in short-term memory. In addition, it appears that active learning that involves the use of memory causes the brain to produce increased amounts of RNA, which in turn increases the amount of protein production. Swedish researchers have discovered that the brains of rats undergoing a learning experience have produced up to 40 percent more RNA than the brains of control rats who had not learned anything.

Today, other memory-enhancing chemicals being studied include CALPAIN, NOREPINEPHRINE, d-amino-d-arginine vasopressin (DDAVP), and ADRENALINE.

Calpain seems to be able to digest protein and unblock receptors, facilitating neuronal communication. Calpain is naturally activated by release of calcium from internal stores in the cells, which leads scientists to wonder if calcium deficiency may decrease enzyme activity in older people, leading to memory loss.

Norepinephrine, a neurotransmitter associated with stress, also appears to be linked to memories (especially memories associated with stress).

Adrenaline appears to be a key to locking memories in place in the brain because rats who cannot produce adrenaline have poorer recall ability than those who can produce the hormone, and rats who get a booster shot of adrenaline after learning something can remember the information better. This may support the idea that hormone deficiency in older people contributes to memory loss. Adrenaline also boosts attention.

Scientists theorize that hormones like adrenaline act as fixatives, locking up memories of exciting or shocking events. This allows the brain a way to remember important information while discarding trivial bits.

Studying Memory

In order to study memory, traditional researchers have used drugs or surgery on animals to affect parts of the brain and then used behavioral tests to measure those effects.

Today, new imaging methods such as X-RAY computerized tomography and MAGNETIC RESONANCE IMAGING (MRI) allow more precise views of these damaged animal brain sections. PET SCANS (POSITRON EMISSION TOMOGRAPHY) have allowed scientists to study the human brain as it functions for clues to the relationship between brain structure and function.

memory, active working   A type of short-term MEMORY that enables a person to hold information in mind while manipulating or using it. For example, when adding several numbers together, a person might hold the amount "carried" in active working memory while adding a new row of numbers. When learning this skill, children typically are taught to write the "carried" amount above the next number, because they are not yet able to perform this operation mentally.

Research suggests that remembering gets easier with age because using these processes becomes more automatic after extended use and practice. Active working memory also allows a person to return to earlier steps in a problem-solving sequence so the process can be integrated. Because it has a limited capacity, this kind of memory is linked to attention.

Active working memory is critical to success at school, at home, and in personal relationships, and it is a fundamental component in the process of reading and writing. It enables reflection on past events and helps monitor the passing of time. Individuals who have ADHD or a learning disability that includes difficulties with impulsivity and attention may find it difficult to use active working memory effectively.

memory, disorders of   There is a wide range of specific impairments to memory that can occur from an astonishingly large number of causes, ranging from organic (brain dysfunction) to psychogenic (psychological).

Disorders of memory can be caused by a problem at any of the three stages of memory (registration, long-term memory, and recall). Most problems involve an inability to recall past events because of a failure at the retention or recall state (see AMNESIA). A person who cannot store new memories suffers from anterograde amnesia, while a pronounced loss of old memories is called retrograde amnesia. These two forms of amnesia may appear together or alone.

Sometimes, however, the problem occurs at the registration stage (for example, depressed people cannot remember because their preoccupation with uncomfortable thoughts and feelings gets in the way of paying attention).

Problems with memory is one of the most common symptoms of impaired brain function; these memory defects may be transitory (such as those after an epileptic SEIZURE) or long term, such as after a severe HEAD INJURY.

In addition, memory problems may be the result of an organic problem in the brain. These problems could include ALZHEIMER'S DISEASE and the DEMENTIAS, in which cognitive functions are progressively

lost. In the early stages of Alzheimer's, there is usually a selective amnesia caused by degenerative processes in the parietemporal-occipital association NEOCORTEX, the CHOLINERGIC BASAL FOREBRAIN, and the LIMBIC SYSTEM structures (such as the HIPPOCAMPUS and AMYGDALA).

Organic amnesia (or global amnesia) is a memory disorder featuring very poor recall and recognition of recent information (anterograde amnesia) and very poor recall and recognition of information acquired before brain damage occurred (RETROGRADE AMNESIA). It is caused by lesions in various brain regions, including the hippocampus and amygdala, by bursting ANEURYSMS, and so on.

HUNTINGTON'S DISEASE, an inherited disorder causing involuntary movements, also causes cognitive problems and memory deficits. Huntington's is caused by the increasing atrophy of the CAUDATE NUCLEUS in the BASAL GANGLIA and the frontal association neocortex.

KORSAKOFF SYNDROME causes a form of organic amnesia resulting from chronic alcoholism, probably related to thiamine deficiency and poor diet. PARKINSON'S DISEASE is a progressive motor disorder that may also include cognitive problems and poor memory arising from dysfunction of the SUBSTANTIA NIGRA.

Postencephalitic amnesia is caused by a viral infection of the TEMPORAL LOBES of the brain; while the term covers various viruses, the herpes simplex virus is most commonly the cause. The amnesia in these patients is probably caused by destruction of the hippocampus and amygdala; retrograde amnesia is probably caused by the destruction of the temporal association neocortex.

SCHIZOPHRENIA, the most common form of psychosis, affecting 1 percent of the population, has also been linked to memory disorders. However, it is unclear to what extent the memory problems depend on a certain subtype of schizophrenia and to what extent they are the result of the effects of an inability to pay attention to external events.

BRAIN TUMORS are abnormal growths that destroy brain tissue and put pressure on nearby brain structures. Those tumors causing particular memory problems similar to Korsakoff syndrome are often found on the floor of the third ventricle near the

DIENCEPHALON. But memory deficits are likely to show up in a wide variety of brain tumors.

memory distortions Memory can be affected by a person's interests or values so that an experience is remembered the way a person *wants* to remember it. In other words, memories can be changed to fit what we want them to be or how we think they ought to be.

This theory can be tested by asking someone to repeat as many as possible of the following words that are read aloud: dream, awake, tired, bed, night, rest, sound, slumber, snore. Most people will also recall the word *sleep,* although that particular word does not appear on the list. People recall that word because most of the words on the list are related to sleep, and it seems as if that word *ought* to be on the list.

Distortion is of particular importance in the courtroom, where a leading question may cause a witness to "remember" something that did not exist. For example, asking "What color was the victim's sweater?" may cause a witness to remember a sweater that was not even worn. Statements that imply a conclusion may cause a person to remember the conclusion as if it had happened. Madison Avenue ad agencies often use this aspect of distortion to promote products without directly making false claims.

memory for crime See AMNESIA AND CRIME.

memory for events Failure of reality monitoring shows that people sometimes cannot distinguish in memory between what they have really perceived and what they have only heard about or imagined. Memory for events tends to be incomplete; in everyday life situations, if an event is not very unusual, people probably will not pay much attention to it or may simply fail to see what is going on. However, if the event is dramatic, observers are more likely to pay attention—but if the event is at all frightening or emotional, stress can make their subsequent recall less reliable.

It is possible to alter a person's memory of a witnessed event, either through leading questions or subsequent misleading information. Once an alteration has occurred in a person's memory, resurrecting the original memory as it was first experienced is almost impossible.

The vacant slot hypothesis holds that the original information was never stored, so that false information after the event was simply popped into a "vacant slot" in the memory representation. However, many leading experts in the field, including witness expert Elizabeth Loftus, reject this hypothesis on the grounds that 90 percent of subjects who are tested immediately after witnessing an event and aren't exposed to postevent information can correctly recall the event.

Those who believe the coexistence hypothesis state that both the original memory and the false postevent memory coexist, as two competing alternatives. When asked about the event, witnesses usually respond with the false version because it is the more recent memory and is therefore more accessible. This hypothesis suggests that even if a person produces a false memory, the original is recoverable.

The demand characteristics hypothesis is similar to the coexistence hypothesis in that it also holds that both memories exist—but this theory argues that the memories are equally accessible. People produce the false memory because that is the one they think is what is demanded of them, not because it is more or less accessible. When Loftus tested this theory by asking subjects after witnessing an event to recall both the original and false memory versions, however, very few subjects could comply.

The substitution hypothesis explains that false information after an event replaces or transforms the original memory, which then is irretrievably lost. This theory, which is supported by Loftus's research, assumes a destructive updating mechanism in the brain; it assumes that subjects would have remembered the correct information if their knowledge had not been interfered with by false postevent information.

Finally, the response bias hypothesis claims that misleading information after the event biases the response but has no effect on the original memory. This theory argues that in most experiments, people have forgotten the original information by the time it is tested, and when they respond with false data they are not remembering incorrectly but are simply choosing the wrong answer.

memory for faces The memory of a face activates a region in the right part of the brain that specializes in spatial configurations. But recent research has found that the brain systems that learn and remember faces are found in a completely different place from those that learn and recall manmade objects. While the face memory is stored in the part of the brain responsible for spatial configurations, the memory of a blender, for example, activates areas that govern movement and touch.

Scientists believe the difference in remembering types of information lies in how the brain acquires knowledge. The theory says that memories are stored in the very same systems that are engaged with the interactions—in the case of the blender, the memory is found in the same part of the cortex that originally processed how the blender felt and how the hands operated it.

Other studies have shown that it is often easier to recognize someone's face than to remember the name that belongs to that face. This is because recognition requires a person to choose among a limited number of alternatives, but remembering requires a far more complex mental process; therefore, it is usually easier to recognize a person than remember the person's name. The following quiz will illustrate the difference.

Recall
Who was president of the United States during the Civil War?

Recognition
Who was president of the United States during the Civil War?
  (a) Robert E. Lee
  (b) Abraham Lincoln
  (c) Ulysses S. Grant

memory for languages In order to maintain memory for language, a person must experience the language in written or verbal form; otherwise, active vocabulary will shrink, although passive understanding will be maintained. Recognition and recall of a language both depend on proficiency, exposure, and practice.

The best way to do this is to listen to the radio or tapes, read books or newspapers and read at least once a week in the language to be maintained.

Although it is harder to learn a foreign language later in life, the more previous knowledge of the language, the more references there will be to facilitate new learning.

Vocabulary can be actively increased by putting the words in context and reviewing them often for several weeks.

memory for music Even as a young child, Mozart could memorize and reproduce a piece of music after having heard it only once. Since he learned to read music and started composing at almost the same time, it is believed that he visualized the sounds on the musical staff as well as on the keyboard and mentally re-created the notes of the melody. He could play a piece immediately after hearing it, which crystallized the memory when the trace was freshest.

While few musicians can perform to the level of Mozart, they can mentally hear whole pieces of music, enabling them to rehearse anywhere—even far from their instruments.

Certain strategies can boost one's memory for sounds and music. One should concentrate on the sounds, analyze them and dwell on them. When hearing a piece of music, one should study in particular the transitions between movements, because they act as cues for what will follow. By rehearsing the links, the associations between musical elements will be strengthened.

memory for names In everyday memory, remembering other people's names seems particularly problematic. In fact, poor memory for names appears to be quite common. While most people seldom forget the names of objects, names of individuals are often forgotten; it appears that memory for proper names is different from memory for common nouns. Memory for names is a particularly difficult and embarrassing everyday problem for those who have suffered brain damage.

In fact, one study found that when subjects were given a brief history of a named individual and then asked to repeat this information, recall of first names and surnames was poorer than the recall of information about place names, occupations, and hobbies. Furthermore, research suggests that last names tend to be harder to remember than other names, probably because they are less common. Recent studies have found that 13 percent of people age 18 to 44 have trouble sometimes or frequently remembering names, compared with 35 percent for ages 45 to 54, 48 percent for ages 55 to 64, and 51 percent at ages 75 and above.

Experts say that people forget a name because they haven't paid enough attention or rehearsed the name enough to register it, or they were tense, preoccupied, or distracted as they heard the name. It is not clear, however, why proper names are organized differently from object names, or why they are particularly susceptible to age and stress. While it is true that names of new people we meet are hard to remember because we often aren't paying enough attention during the introduction, even well-known names elude us from time to time. Scientists suggest that our memory systems treat proper names more like the vocabulary of a foreign language than the words of our mother language.

Fortunately, research also has discovered several methods to help people with this problem, including external aids such as wearing name tags or keeping a notebook with photos and names of certain people likely to be encountered during the day. External aids have strengths and weaknesses, and there are several other options.

Rote learning is sometimes used to treat amnesia patients. In rote learning, success and reinforcement are combined with a slowly increasing distribution of practice: The new name is presented followed by testing after a short time and then gradually increasing the interval of repeating the name and testing as learning proceeds. However, this method is rarely effective for severe amnesics.

There are two main groups of internal strategies, or "mnemonics"—verbal techniques (such as alphabetical searching and first-letter cueing) or the VISUAL IMAGERY METHOD.

Among the various memory strategies included in visual imagery, the face-name association method was designed specifically for learning names. Research has indicated that amnesic patients can learn some paired associations if they are based on a logical association (that is, if they rhyme or are phonetically similar). In research with Korsakoff patients, subjects who were taught the face-name method (select a distinctive feature, transform the person's name into a noun, and then link the feature with the noun) were able to learn names.

A simpler type of visual imagery is simply to turn the name to be remembered into a picture, which is then drawn on a card. For example, Bill Smith could be drawn as a blacksmith with a long, rounded nose like a duck's bill. This type of system does not require mental imagery, and a person doesn't need to have any distinctive features.

However, research suggests that imagery is probably of limited value in a patient's day-to-day life. It works best when only the names of those who are regularly contacted are taught.

memory for numbers To remember a number, a person's eyes first register the individual numbers; once this visual sensory input enters the brain, the information is retained just long enough to be remembered briefly. Selected bits of information may enter long-term memory if the numbers are rehearsed or repeated over and over, or if there is a strong sensory or emotional component to the number.

Remembering numbers is probably one of the hardest memory chores—but it can be solved by using any of several memory strategies. For example, the number 8005552943 might be difficult to memorize, but by grouping the numbers, the task is much easier. Instead of the long series of 8005552943, by writing it as a telephone number, suddenly it becomes (800) 555–2943, a fairly simple number to maintain in short-term memory.

Other, more complicated techniques have been developed to memorize long strings of numbers, such as employing a simple phonetic alphabet with just 10 pairs of digits and sounds to represent the numbers to be remembered.

Some researchers believe that short-term memory for numbers also can be improved through aerobic exercise. While researchers aren't sure why, they suspect it may be linked to the increase in oxygen efficiency or a rise in GLUCOSE metabolism. Good examples of aerobic activities include walking, cycling, swimming, jogging, and racquet sports done three times weekly for 30 minutes at a time.

memory for objects   In everyday life, memory for objects involves both object identification and object location. Humans identify and classify objects by relying on memory representations—to recognize what the objects are and to what category they belong. We must remember where objects are in our vicinity, not just what they are.

However, forgetting or misplacing objects happens every day. We may forget an object's location because we are feeling absentminded—it was put in an out-of-the-way place and we can't remember where that place is. Its loss might be attributed to being put in several different places lately, and we can't remember which place we put the object last (updating errors). Or the object may be lost because of a detection failure—it was put in its proper place, but it hasn't been detected there.

memory for odors   Of all the senses, smell is most directly linked to memory because scent perceptions are recorded in the limbic system, which is considered to be the seat of emotions. In addition, smells are encoded exactly as they are without needing to be processed verbally in order to be retrieved.

Research has found that those born between 1900 and 1929 associate their childhood with fragrances of nature, including pine, hay, horses, sea air, and meadows. Those born between 1930 and 1979 remember the smell of plastic, scented markers, airplane fuel, VapoRub, Sweet Tarts, and PlayDoh.

Other research suggests that the happiness of a person's childhood influences which smell triggers childhood memories. The one in 12 subjects studied who reported having unhappy childhoods were most likely to remember somewhat unpleasant odors in connection with their youth, including mothballs, body odor, dog waste, sewer gas, and bus fumes.

memory for places   Information about location, orientation, and direction is encoded in spatial memory, which is used to remember places and how to find our way, and to locate objects and remember to find things. In each case, the problem is to locate something (either oneself or an object) within a spatial layout.

In looking at individual differences in memory for places, such as the ability to read a map or find one's way in a strange environment, scientists testing students have discovered that those with "a good sense of direction" are those who can benefit from experience and acquire an accurate cognitive map. In addition, subjects with a good sense of direction also rated themselves as better at giving and following directions, remembering routes as a passenger, liking to read maps and finding new routes.

It is not clear whether a sense of direction is a particular ability that affects performance on a variety of spatial tasks, or whether a good sense of direction is a grouping of different abilities (such as good visualization, visuospatial memory, spatial reasoning, and so on) that reinforce each other.

In a study of the ability to use maps, researchers discovered large individual differences based on different acquisition strategies. Good learners allocated their attention, used visuospatial imagery to encode patterns and spatial relations, tested their own memory to find out how they were doing, and focused on areas they hadn't learned. Poor learners tried to learn the whole map at once, used no imagery, relied on verbal rehearsal of named elements, and did not evaluate their own memory. According to some researchers, maps are stored mentally in the form of a network of propositions instead of a visual image.

There are two kinds of spatial information—stored and computable. Stored spatial information is already stored in memory as a proposition (that is, Paris is in France). The knowledge that Paris is north of Marseilles is not stored directly but can be deduced logically from a set of propositions. New information also can be figured out by analysis of existing knowledge, such as finding a new route to a destination.

To remember places one visits, one must look at the scene with interest, identifying anything that is peculiar, and dwell on strong images, flashing back to them occasionally for the job of mentally traveling back there. The more one involves the senses, the stronger the memory trace will be.

memory for rote movements   New studies suggest that the cerebellum may house the memory of rote movements, such as touch typing or violin fingering. Interestingly, this is the same part of the brain that controls balance and coordination.

memory for stories   It appears that there is a general rule allowing the meaning of stories (the most important, most relevant facts) to be preserved in memory, along with a few specific details that also are stored for a fairly short period of time. (The exception to this is material that has been deliberately memorized; in this case, verbatim memory can persist as long as a person lives, although it may take many repetitions to acquire this lifetime memory.)

In one study of students who had years ago memorized certain famous writings (the 23rd Psalm, the Preamble to the Constitution, and Hamlet's soliloquy), the students revealed similar characteristics in what they remembered using very long-term verbatim memory.

There were very few constructive errors—either recall was perfect or it completely failed. For Hamlet's speech and the Preamble, most people showed a marked primacy effect; they could recall about the first 20 words and then memory completely broke down. Recall of the psalm did not show such a strong primacy effect, probably because its rhythmic structure made recalling the entire thing easier.

Researchers conclude that recall is organized in terms of surface structure, since the breakdown of memory occurred at syntactic boundaries. The surface units are remembered as associative chains, and if a part of the chain is broken, the rest is usually lost.

memory for taste   While all of the senses of a human being can evoke memory, taste is one of the most powerful aids to remembering, partly because the olfactory fibers make an immediate connection with memory structures in the brain—they interact directly with the HIPPOCAMPUS and AMYGDALA, whereas vision requires several intermediate cell connections.

memory for voices   While it is not unusual to be able to identify the voice of a friend not heard for many years over the telephone, identification of once-heard voices is not nearly as good. In one study, subjects were 98 percent correct in identifying the familiar voices of coworkers, but much less for strangers. And the memory for the unfamiliar voices decreases rapidly as time passes.

In addition, accuracy of voice recognition is reduced if the voice is whispering. Even the determination to remember an unfamiliar voice does not help recall after two or three days.

memory trace   See ENGRAM.

meninges   The three membranes that cover and protect the brain and SPINAL CORD, guarding against shocks, knocks, and vibrations. The tough leathery outer membrane (DURA MATER) lines the inside of the skull, draping loosely around the spinal cord. Next comes the arachnoid mater, an elastic web-like substance that is separated by the fluid-filled arachnoid space from the innermost membrane, called the pia mater. The pia mater lies directly next to the brain and is much thinner; it closely follows the bumps and wrinkles on the brain's surface.

Infection of the meninges is called MENINGITIS; tumors of the meninges are called MENINGIOMAS.

meningioma   Although these benign tumors of the MENINGES are not specifically tumors of the brain, they are classified as such and grow from the middle layer of the meninges. These tumors usually attach themselves to the outside layer (DURA MATER) of the meninges.

Constituting 15 to 20 percent of all brain tumors, about one new case per 100,000 is diagnosed each year in the United States among patients of all ages. This type of tumor is slow growing, sometimes becoming quite large before ever causing symptoms. These tumors are quite rare in children and in African Americans of any age; they occur most often in middle-aged women.

Symptoms and Diagnostic Path

Symptoms vary depending on the size and location of the tumor. HEADACHE is the most common symptom of this type of tumor, although not all tumors will trigger one. A tumor in the FRONTAL LOBE may produce progressive weakness of one area of the body, SEIZURES, or mental changes (such as drowsiness, listlessness, dullness, or personality change). A tumor in the dominant side of the brain (the left side in most righthanded people) can produce speech difficulties such as APHASIA, the loss of the ability to smell, visual problems, loss of bladder control, or ANOMIA (problems in recognizing and naming objects).

A tumor in the nondominant TEMPORAL LOBE may cause no symptoms at all except for seizures.

A tumor in the PARIETAL LOBE may trigger seizures or astereognosis (inability to identify an object by touching it). The tumor may spread to underlying bone. In children, it can thicken and swell an area of the skull, if the bone is still soft.

Meningiomas can be detected by BRAIN SCANS (CAT or MRI), X-RAY, ELECTROENCEPHALOGRAPH (EEG) and by ARTERIOGRAPHY.

Treatment Options and Outlook

Because these tumors are often quite sharply distinct from underlying brain tissue, they can often be completely removed by surgery. If complete excision is not possible, they may be partially removed; because they are so slow growing, it could be many years before further surgery is necessary. Neither radiation therapy nor chemotherapy is indicated for meningiomas because they do not respond very well to this type of treatment.

If a tumor is discovered accidentally during X-rays following a HEAD INJURY or because of an odd lump on the head, the surgeon may opt to do nothing but monitor the tumor—especially if the patient is old or in ill health.

The "abortion pill" mifepristone (RU-486) has shown promise in treating tumors of the brain, among other things; in 1994 a meningioma patient won approval to take the pill, which had been banned in the United States. Approval for this use came after the patient testified before Congress that it was his only available treatment.

Complete recovery is possible after surgery, and may take two years or more. However, like other tumors, meningiomas can recur if all the cells were not removed. While the overall recurrence rate is about 20 percent, a patient's individual risk depends on the location of the original tumor. It is also possible that recurrent symptoms are not caused by a reappearance of the tumor but by damage done to the brain from the original growth.

Because these tumors do not spread, they will recur in the same area as the first tumor. If the original surgery was successful, chances are very good that subsequent surgery will also be successful.

meningitis An acute infection and inflammation of the MENINGES (the membranes that cover the brain and SPINAL CORD) that can cause symptoms of DEMENTIA. About 2,600 people get this disease every year in the United States and 10 to 15 percent die despite treatment. Meningitis usually results from infection by a variety of microorganisms; while viral meningitis is fairly mild, bacterial meningitis is dangerous and can cause dementia and death. In about 8 percent of cases, the disease progresses so rapidly that death occurs during the first 48 hours, despite early treatment with antibiotics. Rarely, some yeasts can also cause meningitis.

Organisms that go on to infect the brain usually travel through the bloodstream from an infection somewhere else in the body although some may be caused by HEAD INJURY.

The most common forms of bacterial meningitis include neonatal meningitis, hemophilus meningitis, meningococcal meningitis, and pneumococcal meningitis.

Among the most common problems associated with meningitis are MENTAL RETARDATION, ear and hearing problems, EPILEPSY, HYDROCEPHALUS, LEARNING DISABILITIES, and movement or coordination problems. Because damage is not always noticeable immediately, children who have had meningitis (especially neonatal meningitis) should be checked by a NEUROLOGIST for two years after recovery to identify damage.

Symptoms and Diagnostic Path

Meningitis symptoms include fever, severe HEAD-ACHE, vomiting, confusion or drowsiness, stiff neck, and sometimes SEIZURES. All of these symptoms may not develop early in the condition.

To diagnose the disease, a physician will examine the head, ears, and skin (especially along the spine) for sources of infection, together with samples of pus from the middle ear or sinuses, X-RAYS of chest, skull, and sinuses (or a CT SCAN to detect abscess or deep swelling). The definitive diagnosis is made by analyzing SPINAL FLUID extracted by lumbar puncture for low GLUCOSE level and increased white-blood-cell count.

Treatment Options and Outlook

Meningitis is a medical emergency treated with large doses of antibiotics. The most important thing to remember about the treatment of meningitis is speed—suspicious symptoms should be reported as soon as possible. In some cases, treatment for brain swelling, shock, convulsions, or dehydration may be necessary.

Risk Factors and Preventive Measures

There are two MENINGOCOCCAL VACCINES available in the United States: meningococcal polysaccharide vaccine (Menomune), available since the 1970s, and meningococcal conjugate vaccine (Menactra), licensed in 2005. Both can prevent four types of meningitis, including two of the three types most common in the United States and a type that causes epidemics in Africa. Although these vaccines cannot prevent all types of the disease, they do protect many people who might become sick if they did not get the vaccine. Both vaccines work well, and protect about 90 percent of those who get one of them.

Menactra is expected to give better, longer-lasting protection and should be more effective at preventing the disease from spreading from person to person. It is currently recommended for all children at their routine preadolescent doctor checkup

(11 to 12 years of age). Anyone who never got Menactra should be given a dose as recommended at high school.

The vaccine is also recommended for other people at increased risk for meningococcal disease, including college students living in dormitories, microbiologists routinely exposed to meningococcal bacteria, U.S. military recruits, and anyone traveling to or living in a part of the world where meningococcal disease is common, such as parts of Africa. It is also recommended for anyone with a damaged or absent spleen, anyone with an immune system disorder, or anyone who might have been exposed to meningitis during an outbreak.

Menactra is the preferred vaccine for people 11 to 55 years of age in these risk groups, but Menomune can be used if Menactra is not available. Menomune should be used for children two to 10 years old, and at-risk adults over age 55. Menomune may be recommended for children three months to two years of age under special circumstances.

meningitis, hemophilus Once the most common and dangerous type of bacterial MENINGITIS in children up to age 10; however, the introduction of a vaccine to protect infants from hemophilus infection has prevented many new cases.

Before the vaccine was introduced, meningitis accounted for approximately 50 percent to 65 percent of cases of invasive Hib (*Hemophilus influenzae* type B) disease, and was the most common type of bacterial meningitis in infants. Hearing impairment or brain problems occurred in 15 percent to 30 percent of survivors, and the fatality rate was 2 percent to 5 percent, despite effective antimicrobial therapy. Before the vaccine, the peak age of invasive Hib disease was six to seven months; 60 percent of cases occurred in children less than 12 months of age, and 90 percent occurred in children less than five years of age.

Today, four different vaccines for Hib are licensed in the United States. The vaccine is not routinely recommended for children over five years of age, because very little Hib disease occurs after that age. One dose of Hib vaccine could be considered for children at high risk of invasive Hib disease, such as children without a functional spleen.

The number of reported cases has dropped precipitously since the vaccine was produced, particularly since 1990. In 1995, only about 259 invasive hemophilus cases were reported among children under the age of five.

Symptoms and Diagnostic Path

Onset of symptoms may be gradual, beginning with fever and lack of energy, followed by headache, vomiting, stiff neck, drowsiness, and mental confusion.

Treatment Options and Outlook

Antibiotics such as ampicillin or a third-generation cephalosporin or chloramphenicol are used to treat hemophilus meningitis. Those in close contact with children who have the disease should receive rifampicin to prevent secondary cases.

Risk Factors and Preventive Measures

Menomune and Menactra are the two vaccines currently used to prevent the four types of preventable meningitis. Although no vaccine is 100 percent effective, these two achieve about 90 percent effectiveness.

meningitis, meningococcal A type of bacterial MENINGITIS that is more common in older children and young adults, caused by *Neisseria meningitidis.* While slightly less serious than other types of bacterial meningitis, it is still capable of causing death (about 13 percent of patients die), although its damage in survivors is not as long lasting.

Symptoms and Diagnostic Path

Symptoms usually begin suddenly, with high fever, lack of energy, HEADACHE, and vomiting, with possible stiff neck, shoulders, and joints. Within 24 to 48 hours, the patient becomes sleepy and confused and may fall into a COMA. There may be convulsions, and about half of patients may have a rash of small red spots or irregular bruising lesions scattered over the whole body. Young children may be irritable and restless during the early stages.

Treatment Options and Outlook

Certain antibiotics are very effective in eliminating the germ from the nose and throat; penicillin is the drug of choice. People who have been in close contact with a patient diagnosed with meningococcal meningitis (household members, intimate contacts, health care personnel performing mouth-to-mouth resuscitation, day care playmates) should be considered for preventive treatment. Such people are usually advised to obtain a prescription for a special antibiotic (either rifampin or ciprofloxacin) from their physician. Casual contact in a regular classroom, office, or factory setting is not usually significant enough to cause concern.

Risk Factors and Preventive Measures

Currently available vaccines achieve about 90 percent effectiveness in preventing the four preventable forms of meningitis. These vaccines include meningococcal polysaccharide vaccine (Menomune) and meningococcal conjugate vaccine (Menactra). Menomune has been available for more than 30 years, while Menactra is less than five years old.

meningitis, neonatal A particularly dangerous type of bacterial MENINGITIS that may affect as many as 40 or 50 out of every 100,000 newborns. If the disease is contracted during the first week of an infant's life, it is fatal 50 percent of the time; half of the survivors will have BRAIN DAMAGE.

Infants often pick up the disease during delivery from their mothers, from the birthing staff, or from equipment in the delivery room. Premature or low-birth-weight babies are particularly at risk because of an immature immune system.

Neonatal meningitis is usually caused by either *Streptococcus group B* or *Escherichia coli* bacteria.

Symptoms and Diagnostic Path

Infants may show no signs of disease or infection, other than irritability, poor appetite, and fluctuating temperature. Any unexplained fever or sign of infection in newborns—especially those at risk for meningitis—should be treated with suspicion.

Treatment Options and Outlook

Neonatal meningitis in newborns is usually treated with intravenous antibiotics such as penicillin or ampicillin.

High doses of penicillin given intravenously is the treatment of choice for pneumococcal meningitis, but other antibiotics may be used in patients who are allergic or resistant to penicillin or in the case of an uncertain diagnosis. Patients must be treated with antibiotics as soon as possible, especially because of the recent emergence of penicillin resistance in strains of pneumococci from many countries. Treatment lasts for up to two weeks in order to best prevent complications or recurrence. Severe cases will need careful monitoring in an intensive care unit and may need artificial ventilation for breathing support.

About half of survivors will have some degree of lasting brain damage, which may include deafness, weakness, or EPILEPSY. Some of these complications are mild and will slowly improve after several weeks or months, but many patients are left permanently disabled.

Risk Factors and Preventive Measures

A pneumococcal vaccine is available but offers relatively poor protection in many high-risk patients.

Menactra is the preferred vaccine for people 11 to 55 years of age in these risk groups, but Menomune can be used if Menactra is not available. Menomune should be used for children two to 10 years old, and at-risk adults over age 55. Menomune may be recommended for children three months to two years of age under special circumstances.

See also MENINGITIS, HEMOPHILUS; MENINGITIS, MENINGOCOCCAL; and MENINGITIS PNEUMOCOCCAL.

meningitis, pneumococcal　The less-common but most-dangerous of all types of bacterial MENINGITIS. Caused by the *Streptococcus pneumoniae*, it can strike anyone from infants to adults, usually after a respiratory infection or HEAD INJURY.

Symptoms and Diagnostic Path

Symptoms usually begin suddenly with high fever, lack of energy, HEADACHE, and vomiting, with possible stiff neck, shoulders, and joints. Within 24 to 48 hours, the patients become sleepy and confused and may fall into a COMA. There may be convulsions. This type causes a death rate of more than 30 percent and leaves survivors with extensive, lasting BRAIN DAMAGE.

Treatment Options and Outlook

High doses of penicillin given intravenously is the treatment of choice for pneumococcal meningitis, but other antibiotics may be used in patients who are allergic or resistant to penicillin, or if the diagnosis is uncertain. Patients must be treated with antibiotics as soon as possible, especially because of the recent emergence of penicillin resistance in strains of pneumococci from many countries. Treatment lasts for up to two weeks in order to best prevent complications or recurrence. Severe cases will need careful monitoring in an intensive care unit and may need artificial ventilation for breathing support.

About half of survivors will have some degree of lasting brain damage, which may include deafness, weakness, or EPILEPSY. Some of these complications are mild and will slowly improve after several weeks or months, but many patients are left permanently disabled.

Risk Factors and Preventive Measures

A pneumococcal vaccine is available but offers relatively poor protection in many high-risk patients.

meningocele　A form of SPINA BIFIDA, this is a protrusion of the MENINGES (protective covering) of the SPINAL CORD. It is caused by a congenital problem with the spine. A meningocele is less serious than myelocele (protrusion of the spinal cord and the meninges).

meningococcal vaccines　See MENINGITIS, MENINGOCOCCAL.

mental illness　A general term describing problems with one or more functions of the mind, such as perception, memory, or emotion. Mental illness is different from subnormality, in which a person fails to develop normal intellectual capabilities.

Mental illness is broadly divided into neurosis, in which the patient can appreciate reality, and psychosis, in which the ability to appreciate reality is missing. Neuroses appear to be related to environment, upbringing, and personality, whereas psychoses appear to be problems caused by complex biochemical brain disease.

mental retardation Below-average intellectual functioning abilities as determined by intelligence quotient (IQ) testing, and low adaptive functioning at home or in a work environment. An individual is considered to have mental retardation if IQ is below 70–75, there are significant limitations in two or more adaptive skill areas, and the condition is present from childhood.

Mental retardation affects 6.2 million to 7.5 million people in America. It is 10 times more common than cerebral palsy and 28 times more prevalent than neural tube defects such as spina bifida. Mental retardation can affect people of all racial, ethnic, educational, social, and economic backgrounds; one out of 10 American families is directly affected by mental retardation.

Mental retardation can be caused by any condition that impairs development of the brain before birth, during birth, or in the childhood years. Several hundred causes have been discovered, but in about one-third, the cause remains unknown. The three major known causes of mental retardation are DOWN SYNDROME, FETAL ALCOHOL SYNDROME, and FRAGILE X SYNDROME.

Genetic conditions These conditions are caused by abnormal genes or from other disorders of the genes caused during pregnancy by infections, overexposure to X-rays, and other factors. More than 500 genetic diseases are associated with mental retardation, such as

- PKU (PHENYLKETONURIA): a single gene disorder caused by a defective enzyme.
- Down syndrome: a chromosomal disorder that happens sporadically, caused by three chromosomes at what is assumed to chromosome pair 21. Down syndrome is referred to as trisomy 21 by doctors.
- Fragile X syndrome: a single gene disorder located on the X chromosome that is the leading inherited cause of mental retardation.

Problems during pregnancy Alcohol, drugs, or smoking during pregnancy can cause mental retardation. Other risks include malnutrition, certain environmental contaminants, and illnesses of the mother during pregnancy, such as toxoplasmosis, cytomegalovirus, rubella, and SYPHILIS. Pregnant women who are infected with HIV may pass the virus to their child, leading to future neurological damage.

Problems at birth Although any unusual stress during birth may injure the infant's brain, prematurity and low birth weight are more likely to predict serious problems than any other conditions.

Problems after birth Childhood diseases such as whooping cough, chicken pox, measles, and Hib disease (which may lead to MENINGITIS and ENCEPHALITIS) can damage the brain, as can accidents such as a blow to the head or near drowning. Lead, mercury, and other environmental toxins can cause irreparable damage to the brain and nervous system.

Poverty and cultural deprivation Children in poor families may become mentally retarded because of malnutrition, disease-producing conditions, inadequate medical care, and environmental health hazards. Also, children in disadvantaged areas may be deprived of many common cultural and day-to-day experiences provided to other youngsters. Research suggests that such understimulation can result in irreversible damage and can serve as a cause of mental retardation. This type of mental retardation is often called cultural-familial retardation.

Symptoms and Diagnostic Path

Intelligence testing alone is only one measure of functioning ability. A person with limits in intellectual functioning who does not have limits in adaptive skill areas may not be diagnosed with mental retardation. "Adaptive skill areas" are those daily living skills needed to live, work, and play in the community. They include communication, self-care, home living, social skills, leisure, health and safety, self-direction, functional academics (reading, writing, basic math), community use, and work. Adaptive skills are assessed in the person's typical environment across all aspects of an individual's life.

Many individuals have been diagnosed with mental retardation, particularly at a young age, who are later diagnosed with profound learning disabilities but with average or above-average intelligence. For this reason, most psychologists working with young children speak in terms of developmental delays rather than mental retardation.

The effects of mental retardation vary considerably among people, just as the range of abilities varies considerably among people who do not have mental retardation. About 87 percent will be mildly affected and will be only a little slower than average in learning new information and skills. As children, their mental retardation is not easy to see, and may not be identified until school age. As adults, many individuals with mental retardation will be able to lead independent lives in the community.

The remaining 13 percent of people with mental retardation (those with IQs under 50) will have serious limits in function. However, with early intervention, a good education, and appropriate support as an adult, all can lead satisfying lives in the community.

People with mental retardation may have trouble communicating, interacting with others, and being independent. They may not comprehend the importance of health and safety issues. Not all skills are necessarily impaired, and individuals with mental retardation may learn to function independently in many areas. However, education programs, providing skilled assistance and ongoing support, are necessary for determining appropriate living and work environments.

While the term *mental retardation* still exists as a clinical diagnosis, contemporary usage is moving towards terms such as *developmental disabilities*, which some believe do not carry the same negative connotations or misuse. In the past, those who were retarded were traditionally divided by IQ scores into *educable, trainable,* and *custodial;* today, the more commonly used terms include *mild, moderate, severe,* or *profound,* based on the level of functioning and IQ. Individuals with mental retardation are not a homogenous group, but have widely differing levels of functioning.

- **Mild retardation**—This classification is used to specify an individual whose IQ test scores lie between 50–55 and 68 or 69, and corresponds to an educators' label of "educable retarded." The individual is capable of learning basic academic subjects. Many people with mild retardation are able to live and work independently.

- **Moderate retardation**—This classification is used to specify an individual whose IQ test score is between 35–40 and 50–55; it corresponds to the earlier label of trainable retarded. These individuals can usually learn functional academics and vocational skills. They often achieve coached employment goals and live with limited assistance.

- **Severe and profound mental retardation**—This classification applies to individuals with IQ scores below 35. These are the most seriously impaired of the mentally retarded, often characterized by physical and sensory impairment as well as mental retardation. They can sometimes achieve supported employment goals; more typically they can function at the level of sheltered employment. They generally require significant assistance with daily living skills.

Mental retardation is diagnosed primarily on the basis of intelligence testing, but affected individuals often demonstrate other brain problems such as attention deficits, movement problems, and perceptual difficulties. Dexterity and coordination may also be limited.

The first step is to administer standardized intelligence tests and a standardized adaptive skills test. Next, an expert should describe the person's strengths and weaknesses in intellectual and adaptive behavior skills, emotions, physical health, and environment. These skills can be assessed by formal testing, observations, interviews, and interacting with the person in daily life.

Risk Factors and Preventive Measures

It is possible to prevent some forms of mental retardation. During the past 30 years, significant advances in research have prevented many cases of mental retardation. For example, every year in the United States, about 250 cases of mental retardation due to PKU are prevented by newborn screening and dietary treatment. Newborn screening and thyroid hormone replacement therapy prevent 1,000 cases of mental retardation due to congenital hypothyroidism, and more than 1,000 cases of mental retardation from Rh disease and severe jaundice are prevented by using anti-Rh immune globulin to prevent Rh disease. The Hib vaccine prevents another 5,000 cases of mental retardation caused by Hib diseases, and 4,000 cases of mental retardation due to measles encephalitis can be prevented because of the measles vaccine. Countless cases of mental retardation caused by rubella during pregnancy are prevented, thanks to the rubella vaccine.

Removing lead from the environment reduces brain damage in children, and child safety seats and bicycle helmets reduce head trauma. Early intervention programs with high-risk infants and children have shown remarkable results in reducing the predicted incidence of subnormal intellectual functioning.

Finally, early prenatal care and preventive measures before and during pregnancy increase a woman's chances of preventing mental retardation. Pediatric AIDS is being reduced by AZT treatment of the mother during pregnancy, and dietary supplementation with folic acid reduces the risk of neural tube defects. Research continues on new ways to prevent mental retardation, including research on the development and function of the nervous system, a wide variety of fetal treatments, and gene therapy to correct the abnormality produced by defective genes.

mental status examination   A diagnostic assessment to determine if a patient knows basic information such as where he is, the date, and general level of functioning (intellectual, emotional, and social) after trauma. The examiner observes general appearance, attitudes, and behavior and tries to assess orientation by asking "What is your name?" or "What day is it?" The examiner tests mental grasp by asking a person to complete a basic mental task, such as counting backward.

mesencephalon   See MIDBRAIN.

Mesmer, Franz Anton (1734–1815)   An Austrian physician whose system of treatment (known as MESMERISM) was the forerunner of modern-day hypnosis. While still a student at the University of Vienna in 1766, Mesmer discovered the work of the Renaissance mystic physician Paracelsus. He tried to uncover a link between astrology and human health as a result of planetary forces transmitted through a subtle invisible fluid. By 1775, Mesmer began to teach that a person may transmit universal forces to others in the form of "animal magnetism" and based his therapeutic sessions on those beliefs. During these sessions, several people sat around a vat of dilute sulfuric acid while holding hands or touching iron bars sticking out of the solution.

Three years later, his beliefs became increasingly unpopular with other physicians and he was forced to leave Austria for Paris, where he continued to maintain a lucrative practice in mesmerism. However, here too physicians did not accept his beliefs. In 1784 King Louis XVI appointed a special scientific commission, which included U.S. statesman and inventor Benjamin Franklin, guillotine inventor J.I. Guillotin, and chemist A.L. Lavoisier, to investigate Mesmer's methods.

Their report found there was no scientific basis in his methods, noting that his cures were probably the result of a patient's own beliefs and imagination. However, the French Revolution ended his Parisian practice and sent him into exile in London.

Still, those he had taught continued to practice his beliefs. Among his former students was the Marquis de Puysegur of Buzancy, who treated a young peasant who went into a state that would be today described as a hypnotic trance. Because it was like sleep but more like sleepwalking, Puysegur called the state "artificial somnambulism"; the term later became associated with a highly hypnotizable person. But despite the peasant's alertness during the trance, when he awoke he had no recollection of what had happened. Puysegur had discovered post-hypnotic amnesia, which had never before been described, and took the peasant to Paris to meet Mesmer just before Mesmer left for London.

After Mesmer died in 1815, his followers were known as mesmerists and their technique was known as mesmerism.

mesmerism   Also known as animal magnetism, this 18th-century system of treatment was the forerunner of modern-day hypnosis. Mesmerism was named for Austrian physician Franz Anton

Mesmer who developed the practice while trying to uncover a link between astrology and health as a result of planetary forces transmitted through a subtle invisible fluid. By 1775, Mesmer began to teach that a person may transmit universal forces to others in the form of "animal magnetism" and based his therapeutic sessions on those beliefs. During these sessions, several people sat around a vat of dilute sulfuric acid while holding hands or iron bars sticking out of the solution. After he died in 1815, his followers were known as mesmerists and their technique was known as mesmerism.

One of his followers, Abbe Faria, renamed somnambulism *lucid sleep* and criticized Mesmer's theory that some sort of fluid transferred from the operator to the patient. He was one of the first to understand that the ability of a person to enter lucid sleep depended more on the patient than on the mesmerist. During the 19th century, mesmerism was renamed *hypnotism* after the Greek god of sleep (Hypnos), and the practice began to receive attention from the medical community of the time.

See also MESMER, FRANZ ANTON.

metacognition   The awareness and knowledge of an individual's own mental processes; the ability to think about thinking. Metacognition refers to a person's understanding of what strategies are available for learning and what strategies are best used in which situations. Ordinarily, these abilities develop in childhood; children learn that mental activities go along with decision making. They know when they know something and when they do not.

Metacognition skills are directly related to reading, writing, problem solving, and any process that requires error monitoring. Students must be able to examine how they learn best and learn what resources they can draw upon in order to set and achieve academic goals.

methylphenidate hydrochloride (Ritalin)   A CENTRAL NERVOUS SYSTEM stimulant that increases nerve activity in the brain by triggering the release of neurotransmitters. It reduces drowsiness and increases alertness by its action on the RETICULAR ACTIVATING SYSTEM in the BRAIN STEM and midbrain. It is often given as part of a treatment program for ATTENTION DEFICIT HYPERACTIVITY DISORDER (ADHD). About 3 percent to 5 percent of the general population has the disorder, which is characterized by agitated behavior and an inability to focus on tasks.

Ritalin has effects similar to, but more potent than, caffeine—but weaker than amphetamines. It has a notably calming effect on hyperactive children and a "focusing" effect on those with ADHD.

Scientists think ADHD occurs in part because certain receptors in the brain involved in focusing attention and reining in impulsiveness fail to respond to dopamine and norepinephrine, the brain's natural neurotransmitters. It is the interaction between these chemicals and the brain's receptors that helps most people stick with tedious chores or rein in inappropriate impulses. Researchers think that drugs like Ritalin boost the level of these brain chemicals and stimulate the inhibitory receptors—which is why a stimulant drug can increase inhibition. The drugs enter the body quickly, curing nothing but helping a child focus on the important work of learning.

Although the drug clearly reduces the symptoms of ADHD, and many students have been taking the drug for years, no studies have continued long enough to see if it has a lasting effect on academic performance or social behavior. Moreover, a positive response to Ritalin does not automatically mean a child suffers from ADHD. Stimulants can temporarily sharpen almost anyone's focus.

First introduced in the 1940s, Ritalin is usually prescribed as a part of a treatment plan that includes educational and psychosocial interventions for children with behavior characterized by:

- moderate-to-severe distractibility
- short attention span
- hyperactivity
- emotional lability
- impulsivity

The widespread use of Ritalin in children is not without controversy. Some experts are vehemently opposed to medicating children who are deemed too inattentive or active for a "normal" classroom. However, there is no specific evidence that clearly establishes the mechanism by which Ritalin produces its mental and behavioral effects in children. Because a diagnosis of ADHD itself is not always straightforward, critics argue that far too many children who are simply extremely energetic are given a diagnosis of ADHD and medicated.

A doctor should prescribe Ritalin only after medical, psychological, behavioral, and educational assessments. The doctor or therapist should talk to the parents and the child and get information from teachers before prescribing stimulants.

It may take up to one month for the medication to achieve its maximum effect in children. Medications like Ritalin are usually taken for as long as is helpful or necessary. While there has been an increase in the number of stimulant prescriptions for children under age five, there is no evidence that these drugs are safe or effective when used on young children. Because of its stimulant properties, however, there have been reports of Ritalin abuse by adults who turn to the drug for its stimulant effects: appetite suppression, wakefulness, increased focus and attentiveness, and euphoria. When abused, the tablets are either taken orally or crushed and snorted. Some abusers dissolve the tablets in water and inject the mixture, although this can cause problems if insoluble fillers in the tablets block small blood vessels.

Because stimulant medicines such as Ritalin have the potential for abuse, the U.S. Drug Enforcement Agency (DEA) has placed stringent Schedule II controls on their manufacture, distribution, and prescription. For example, the DEA requires special licenses for these activities, and prescription refills are not allowed. States may impose further regulations, such as limiting the number of dosage units per prescription.

Side Effects
Common side effects include decrease in or loss of appetite, nervousness, sleep problems, weight loss, or dizziness. Ritalin should not be used in children with anxiety, tension, agitation, irregular heart rhythms, severe angina pectoris, or glaucoma, or in anyone with motor tics or a family history or diagnosis of TOURETTE SYNDROME. Although a rela-

tionship has not been established, suppression of growth has been reported with the long-term use of stimulants in children.

microcephaly A rare neurological disorder in which the circumference of the head is smaller than the average for the age and gender of the infant or child. Microcephaly may be present at birth or it may develop in the first few years of life. The term is used when the head size is less than that of 97 percent to 99 percent of the population.

Symptoms and Diagnostic Path
The signs of microcephaly may vary considerably, causing delay in a child's development that may range from very mild to profound. Severely affected children often have CEREBRAL PALSY, EPILEPSY, visual problems, or feeding difficulties. In other cases, there is only minor intellectual impairment. In some children, microcephaly occurs together with other defects or another syndrome.

Infants with microcephaly are born with either a normal or reduced head size. Subsequently, the head fails to grow while the face continues to develop at a normal rate, producing a child with a small head, a large face, a receding forehead, and a loose, often wrinkled scalp. As the child grows older, the smallness of the skull becomes more obvious, although the entire body also is often underweight and dwarfed. Development of motor functions and speech may be delayed. Hyperactivity and mental retardation are common occurrences, although the degree of each varies. Convulsions may also occur. Motor ability varies, ranging from clumsiness to spastic quadriplegia.

The disorder may be caused by a wide variety of conditions leading to abnormal growth of the brain, and is often a symptom of syndromes associated with chromosomal abnormalities. The great variation in the severity of microcephaly may be explained by the fact that it is caused by so many different abnormalities, both genetic and nongenetic.

Treatment Options and Outlook
There is no specific treatment for microcephaly, other than to treat symptoms. A serious attempt should be made to identify a specific cause of the

disorder. In general, life expectancy for individuals with microcephaly is low and the prognosis for normal brain function is poor. The prognosis varies, depending on the presence of other problems.

Autosomal recessive microcephaly occurs when two healthy parents each carry a faulty gene and they both pass on one copy of this gene to the affected child. Although the chances of both parents carrying the faulty gene are usually rare, the chances are much higher if the parents are closely related. If both parents carry a faulty recessive gene, the chance of conceiving an affected child is one in four.

Autosomal dominant microcephaly occurs when only one of the parents has a faulty gene. If it is passed to the child, it overrides the normal copy from the other parent and is said to be dominant. A parent with a dominant microcephaly gene has a 50 percent chance of passing on that gene (1 in 2).

X chromosome linked microcephaly is caused by a faulty gene located on the X chromosome; this type of genetic disorder is usually diagnosed when a healthy female carrier of the faulty gene has an affected son and another affected close male blood relative. The chance of passing on this gene is one in four when the mother is known to be a carrier.

Humans normally have 46 chromosomes grouped in 23 pairs that carry the genetic code. In some cases, a genetic fault may occur at the chromosomal level. For example, individuals with Down syndrome have an extra copy of chromosome 21. In these cases of chromosome problems, microcephaly is often present along with other problems.

Microcephaly can be caused by a prenatal infection with certain viruses and parasites which are able to cross the placenta. Often the symptoms of these infections may be very mild or even totally absent as far as the mother is concerned. Infections known to cause microcephaly include rubella (German measles), toxoplasmosis (a parasitic infection), and cytomegalovirus (CMV).

External factors such as exposure to radiation or severe substance abuse by the mother can lead to microcephaly.

Examples of microcephaly caused by maternal illness during pregnancy are rare, but maternal PHENYLKETONURIA is one example.

Meningitis (inflammation of the membranes that line the brain and spinal cord) and genital herpes are possible cause of neonatal microcephaly if the infection is active at the time of birth. Other possible causes can include fetal stroke or oxygen starvation at birth.

midbrain Also known as the MESENCEPHALON, this is one of the three divisions of the BRAIN STEM. Found in the upper part of the brain stem situated above the PONS, the midbrain serves as a connecting link between the HINDBRAIN and the FOREBRAIN. The midbrain is the origin of the cranial nerves that control five of the six muscles that move the eye and the muscle that controls the size and reactions of the pupils; it helps maintain balance and receives information about positioning of muscles around eyes and jaw.

The mesencephalon is made up of three main parts: the tectum (containing auditory and visual relay stations, called the inferior and superior colliculi), the tegmentum (containing the midbrain RETICULAR FORMATION that controls attention), the SUBSTANTIA NIGRA and the red nucleus, both of which are involved in motor control.

migraine A severe HEADACHE with accompanying symptoms of nausea, diarrhea, visual disturbances, and depression that attacks about 8 million Americans—75 percent of them women. The symptoms of migraine can occur at any age, although it is common to see the first headache during the teenage years. Most patients have had the first attack by the time they are 40 years old; attacks often recur, but tend to get less severe as a patient ages. Most people with migraine have family members who also have the disorder.

For many patients, specific environmental or internal factors can trigger headache severity or frequency, such as drinking alcohol, sleep deprivation, artificial food additives such as MSG, menstruation, stress, and medication. Sexual activity and heavy exercise may trigger a migraine in some patients. Pregnancy may either cause the headaches to increase in frequency, or result in temporary improvement.

Many studies have confirmed that the initial aura of migraine is explained by a reduction in blood flow to specific areas of the CEREBRAL CORTEX to the OCCIPITAL LOBES, the part of the brain involved in vision. Theories regarding the actual headache and pain in migraine are based on an understanding of the complex pain-sensitive structures in the head. While the brain itself has no pain receptors, the MENINGES (the ultrathin membranes that surround the brain), blood vessels, and bony anatomy of the head have an intricate system of small nerve branches that are sensitive to pain. The TRIGEMINAL NERVE in particular has been found to widen blood vessels and subsequently increase blood flow. When the trigeminal system is activated, neurochemicals are released into different parts of the brain that may in turn activate specific blood cells and cause them to release substances that cause inflammation.

An important substance within the brain called SEROTONIN is thought to be a key chemical compound in antimigraine activity. This accounts for the fact that many of the drugs successfully used to treat migraine are related to the serotonin molecule and may mimic some of its actions.

Symptoms and Diagnostic Path

What characterizes a migraine and differentiates it from other types of headache is its specific symptoms. Of course, not all migraine sufferers experience the same symptoms, and different symptoms can occur at different times. These include:

- **Throbbing or pounding pain**—Unlike other types of head pain, migraine pain is a relentless throbbing or pounding as though the pulse is beating severely in the head. The pain usually begins on one side of the head, at the temple, and can spread downward to the eye, face, and even the neck.

- **Nausea and vomiting**—While nausea and vomiting can be caused by a number of factors, it may also accompany migraines in some sufferers.

- **Aura**—Some people experience visual disturbances, known as aura, immediately before a migraine begins. The aura may look like a shimmer or colored lights, or may involve partial vision loss for 10 to 20 minutes.

- **One-sided head pain**—Migraine sufferers almost always complain of throbbing pain on only one side of the head, usually around the temple, but sometimes a migraine causes pain all over the head.

- **Pain aggravated by activity**—The simple act of moving may be difficult, and pain may be aggravated or worsened by activity.

- **Sensitivity to light, sounds, and smells**—During (and sometimes prior to) a migraine attack, many sufferers experience strong, painful reactions to light, loud noises, and certain odors.

Treatment Options and Outlook

Many new drugs have recently been developed to treat migraines. The use of medication can be divided into two categories: It can treat the patient with an acute migraine, or it can help prevent migraine or decrease its frequency or severity.

It is important for the migraine sufferer to take medication as soon as possible in an attack, to return to normal activity as soon as possible. This form of nonpreventive therapy is useful in patients with relatively infrequent migraines—at most, a few per month. It also is often necessary to use some symptomatic treatment in patients who still have breakthrough headaches despite using prophylactic drugs. Any of the following medications when used often can lead to rebound headaches, a syndrome caused by overusing medication. Analgesic rebound headaches sometimes become worse after a previous dose of medication begins to wear off, requiring more medication to be taken. They usually are seen in patients who take medication for pain more than four days a week. This overuse also can interfere with the effectiveness of prophylactic headache treatment.

- Acetaminophen and aspirin may help a few patients with mild migraine symptoms.

- Nonsteroidal anti-inflammatory drugs (NSAIDs) include naproxen, indomethacin, and ibuprofen.

- Compounds of butalbital, acetaminophen, and caffeine can be helpful for patients with occasional headaches, but compounds with butalbital can become addicting. They may also make people drowsy and interfere with usual activities.
- Ultram (tramadol), a relatively new medication, can be quite effective in both acute and chronic pain syndromes, and be helpful in some patients with migraine. It does not cause the gastrointestinal upset that many medications can.
- Compound of acetaminophen, dichloraiphenazone, isometheptene (Midrin): This medication relieves migraine, tension, and vascular headaches by constricting blood vessels in the brain.
- Opiates (codeine, hydrocodone, oxycodone, propoxyphene), a potent class of medication, may be needed in some patients but can lead to drug addiction. These should only be used when other treatments fail.
- Serotonin receptor medications treat migraine by acting on cerebral blood vessels and inflammation.
- Triptans act rapidly to relieve the pain of the headache and associated symptoms and can be taken at any point in time during the headache, for migraine both with and without aura. They are usually well tolerated and not associated with the sedation that some other drugs can cause. They should be used only for symptomatic treatment, not on a frequent, chronic basis. Some of the more common choices available include sumatriptan (Imitrex), zolmitriptan (Zomig), and rizatriptan (Maxalt).
- Ergots are a class of medications used for many years to treat migraines. They work much like triptans, by blocking blood vessel dilation, preventing inflammation, and acting on serotonin systems. Ergots include DHE (dihydroergotamine, Migranal) or ergotamine tartrate (Cafergot). Ergots can produce side effects similar to those of triptans, including tingling, numbness, flushing, chest tightness, and dizziness. Triptans and ergots should be prescribed with great caution for anyone with risk factors for heart attack or other vascular disease. This includes men over 40, women who have completed menopause, persons with high blood pressure, diabetes, high cholesterol, or who have a history of heart disease.
- Antiemetics (antinausea medications) can help control the nausea and vomiting that may accompany migraine and also can treat the migraine itself in some cases. One commonly prescribed agent is prochlorperazine (Compazine) and can be very effective when used intravenously to treat acute migraine.

There are other types of alternative treatments that some patients explore in their efforts to control migraines, such as biofeedback, TENS units, acupuncture, and so on.

In biofeedback therapy, patients can learn how to reduce pain with a relaxation response that is as effective as Inderol without the side effects. Using a TENS unit can stimulate nerves and reduce muscle spasm in patients with tension and migraine headaches. A health care practitioner's prescription is needed for insurance coverage of these units, which are usually available through medical supply companies. Some chiropractors and physical therapists loan these devices out to patients for a small deposit.

Acupuncture has been effective for some patients in controlling their migraines. Patients should choose a practitioner who holds a full doctorate degree in Chinese medicine, an O.M.D. (Oriental Medicine Doctor), or Lic.Ac (licensed acupuncturist). These practitioners are required to complete several years of training and often have completed internships in China, Japan, or Korea. The letters *TCM* (Traditional Chinese Medicine) after the name mean that the doctor has additional training in prescribing Chinese herbs. The more knowledge practitioners have about Chinese medicine and its supporting philosophy, the better able they are to diagnose and treat symptoms.

Risk Factors and Preventive Measures

The goal behind daily preventive treatment is to decrease the frequency and severity of migraine. These drugs are usually reserved for patients who have fairly frequent headaches and headaches that do not respond to symptomatic treatment. These medications often help make the situation more tolerable, without completely eliminating migraines. Some patients may require treatment with more than one preventive agent, but this should be tried only after treatment with one agent. If the headaches become well controlled, most clinicians recommend tapering the dosages, or discontinuing the medication, if possible.

Beta blockers These drugs likely work on the central nervous system, as well as on serotonin systems. (They have been used for high blood pressure, heart disease, and heart arrhythmias for many years.) They must be taken daily and should be started at the lowest possible dosage. They should not be used in patients with asthma, and in some patients with specific abnormalities within the heart, and should be used with caution in diabetics. Side effects include drowsiness and lightheadedness. Commonly used beta blockers include propranolol (Inderal) and atenolol (Tenormin).

Antidepressants Antidepressants can treat migraine through their action on serotonin systems. The more commonly used agents are the tricyclics, which are usually taken once a day at bedtime, as they can produce drowsiness. They should be started at the lowest possible dosage to avoid side effects such as drowsiness, dry mouth, and dizziness. Commonly used drugs include amitriptyline (Elavil), nortriptyline (Pamelor) and desipramine (Norpramin). Some patients may respond to the newer antidepressants called SSRIs (selective serotonin reuptake inhibitors), such as Prozac. Although they are usually better tolerated than the tricyclic antidepressants, they tend not to be as effective in treatment of migraine. Examples include paroxetine (Paxil), sertraline (Zoloft), and fluoxetine (Prozac).

Valproate (Depakote) This drug has been used to treat seizures for many years, and has also been approved to treat migraine. It is an oral medication which should be taken daily, usually in two divided doses. Laboratory tests, including the blood level of the drug, liver function testing, and a complete blood count, should be monitored. Side effects noted are nausea, diarrhea, hair loss, and weight gain.

Calcium channel blockers (verapamil, Norvasc) These medications are taken orally, either once a day or in divided doses. (They are also used to treat high blood pressure and heart disease.) No blood monitoring is necessary, but side effects can include lightheadedness, drowsiness, and constipation.

mild cognitive impairment A type of memory loss more serious than that associated with normal aging, but less severe than the memory loss of ALZHEIMER'S DISEASE.

Symptoms and Diagnostic Path

People with MCI perform worse on memory tests than healthy people, but they are just as healthy in other cognitive areas—they are not disoriented, generally confused, or unable to perform activities of daily living that are characteristic of Alzheimer's disease.

Over time, the mental and functional abilities of people with MCI decline more quickly than they do in healthy people, but less rapidly than with those diagnosed with mild Alzheimer's disease.

Research also suggests that people with MCI appeared to be at increased risk of developing Alzheimer's disease at a rate of 10 percent to 15 percent per year. In one study at the Mayo Clinic, about half the patients with MCI developed Alzheimer's disease within four years. In the control group, only 1 to 2 percent progressed to Alzheimer's.

MCI cannot be diagnosed by one test; instead, a doctor must assess both physical and neurological assessments to reveal memory problems that are abnormal for age and education—together with normal ability to carry out everyday activities, normal cognitive function, and the absence of dementia.

Treatment Options and Outlook

Scientists hope that with the ability to identify those with MCI, research can focus on finding a treatment that will slow the subsequent development of Alzheimer's disease.

Unfortunately, there is still quite a bit of uncertainty about mild cognitive impairment and how it will progress in any one patient. Some critics object to the idea of MCI as a separate condition instead of simply a very early form of Alzheimer's disease.

While there is currently no approved treatment for MCI, the National Institute on Aging is conducting studies at medical research institutions in the United States and Canada to assess the effectiveness of large doses of vitamin E or DONEPEZIL (Aricept) in slowing the progression from mild cognitive impairment to Alzheimer's disease.

mild head injury   Even the mildest bump on the head is still capable of doing damage to the brain; in fact, research suggests that 60 percent of patients who sustain a mild brain injury are still having symptoms after three months.

Symptoms and Diagnostic Path

Mild head-injury symptoms can result in a puzzling interplay of behavioral, cognitive, and emotional complaints that make it difficult to diagnose. Although research is still limited, studies have found that symptoms following even the mildest head injury can linger, causing ongoing discomfort and interfering with personal lives.

Symptoms include HEADACHE, dizziness, confusion, and memory loss, that may continue for months. Typically, CAT SCANS have yielded negative results for this group of patients. But studies involving MAGNETIC RESONANCE IMAGING (MRI) and brain electrophysiology indicate that contusions and diffuse axonal injuries associated with mild head injury are likely to affect those parts of the brain that relate to functions such as memory, concentration, information processing, and problem solving.

Until recently, diagnostic tools were not sensitive enough to detect the subtle structural changes that can occur and sometimes persist after mild head injury.

CAT scans   While CAT scans are widely available in emergency rooms to assist in the diagnosis of brain HEMATOMAS, many experts believe these scans may not pick up the subtle damage following a mild head injury.

MRI   Many researchers believe MRI is more sensitive in diagnosing many brain lesions beyond a basic hematoma. For example, MRI is more sensitive in detecting the diffuse axonal or shearing injury and contusions often seen in mild head injury.

Quantitative EEG (qEEG)   In many patients, neither CAT nor MRI can detect the microscopic damage to white matter that occurs when fibers

are stretched in a mild, diffuse axonal injury. In this type of mild injury, the AXONS lose some of their covering and become less efficient, but MRI only detects more severe injury and actual axonal degeneration. Mild injury to the WHITE MATTER reduces the quality of communication between neurons in any part of the brain. A quantitative EEG is an enhanced form of an EEG in that the signals from the brain are played into a computer, digitized, and stored. This type of EEG can measure the time delay between two regions of the CORTEX, and the amount of time it takes for information to be transmitted from one region to another.

Evoked potentials   This electrophysical technique is not generally useful in patients with less-serious mild head injury. EPs are not sensitive enough to document any physiologic abnormalities, although the patient may be having symptoms. If testing is done within a day or two of injury, the EP may pick up some abnormalities in BRAIN STEM auditory-evoked potentials.

Neuropsychological testing   These tests may show positive results when imaging tests and neurologic exams are negative. In some patients with persistent symptoms following mild head injury, neuropsychological tests are part of a comprehensive assessment. The tests can also provide information when litigation is an issue.

Future tests   PET (POSITRON EMISSION TOMOGRAPHY), which evaluates cerebral blood flow and brain metabolism, may provide useful information on functional pathology. SINGLE PHOTO EMISSION COMPUTED TOMOGRAPHY (SPECT) is less expensive than PET and might provide data on cerebral blood flow after mild head injury.

Patients who do experience symptoms should seek out the care of a specialist; unless a family physician is thoroughly familiar with medical literature in this newly emerging area, there is a great chance patient complaints will be ignored. Instead, patients with continuing symptoms following a mild head injury are advised to call a local head-injury foundation, which can then refer patients to the best local practitioner.

Treatment Options and Outlook

A 1981 study of 424 patients diagnosed with mild head injury showed that many had recurrent problems with deviant behavior, headaches, dizziness, and cognitive problems; only 17 percent of these patients were symptom-free three months after the accident. A separate 1987 study found that 47 percent of these subjects still had symptoms three months after the accident. A third study in 1989 reached similar conclusions.

Only 12 percent of patients with mild head injury are hospitalized overnight, and instructions they receive upon leaving the emergency room do not address behavioral, cognitive, and emotional symptoms that can occur after such an injury.

minimal brain dysfunction (MBD) A general term used to describe a person who shows behavioral or cognitive signs of brain injury. The term is usually used for cases in which the pattern of thought and action would typically be caused by a disease, but in which none is apparent.

Historically, MBD was the term used to define and classify learning and behavioral difficulties now classified under the category of ATTENTION DEFICIT HYPERACTIVITY DISORDER. It generally includes HYPERACTIVITY, impulsivity, various neurological soft signs and any of a number of learning and language disabilities such as DYSLEXIA and dyscalculia.

The term is often used as though there were an identifiable minimal brain dysfunction syndrome—a collection of fairly specific disorders that could be taken as hallmarks of some underlying neurological cause. Although the issue is far from settled, the evidence to support a single MBD syndrome is unconvincing.

mini-mental state examination (MMSE) A standard brief mental status exam routinely used as a quick way to measure a person's basic cognitive skills, such as short-term memory, long-term memory, orientation, writing, and language. It is often used to screen for dementia or monitor its progression, and provides a brief but relatively thorough measure of cognition.

It doesn't measure mood, perception, or the form and content of thought, and therefore isn't a substitute for a full mental status examination. It is also not a substitute for neuropsychological evalua-

tion, but may well indicate when and what kind of such evaluation is appropriate. It's most suitable for detecting the cognitive deficits seen in syndromes of dementia and delirium and for measuring these cognitive changes over time.

Questions might include today's date, "where are you?" the ability to name three objects slowly and clearly, the ability to count backward from 100 by 7, the ability to spell a common word backward, and the ability to follow a command such as "take this piece of paper with your left hand, fold it in thirds and put it on the table."

mixed receptive-expressive language disorder A LANGUAGE disability causing problems in both understanding and expressing language formerly called developmental receptive language disorder. It is generally understood that receptive language deficit does not occur in isolation, but appears together with problems in expressing language. Between 3 percent and 5 percent of all children have both a receptive and expressive language disorder. Difficulty understanding and using language can cause problems with social interaction and make it difficult to function independently as an adult.

Symptoms Options and Outlook

There are a number of symptoms that indicate this condition, including problems in

- language comprehension
- language expression
- articulation
- recalling early visual or auditory memories

Parents who are concerned about their child's acquisition of language should have the child tested, since early intervention offers the best possible outcome. Standardized receptive and expressive language tests can be given to any child suspected of having problems in this area. An audiogram should also be given to rule out the possibility of deafness.

Treatment Options and Outlook

Speech and language therapy are the best way to treat this type of language disorder. Psychotherapy is also recommended for children because of the possibility of emotional or behavioral problems.

See also LANGUAGE PROCESSING DISABILITIES.

mnesic syndromes   A mixed group of disorders in which memory disturbances are the dominant clinical problem. The disturbances may be of different kinds (AMNESIA, dysmnesia, or HYPERMNESIA) due to organic damage that is specific rather than generalized and usually involves lesions in the HIPPOCAMPUS or the MAMMILLARY BODIES. People with a variety of mnesic syndromes show intellectual impairment as well; there may be clouding consciousness, loss of abstract reasoning, or mental confusion. The best known of the mnesic syndromes is KORSAKOFF SYNDROME.

See also AGNOSIA; AGRAPHIA; ALEXIA; ALZHEIMER'S DISEASE; ANOSOGNOSIA; APHASIA; APRAXIA; BROCA'S APHASIA; cryptomnesia; diencephalic amnesia; dissociative disorders; dysmnesia/dysmnesic syndrome; DYSPHASIA; HYSTERICAL AMNESIA; ischemic amnesia; mixed amnesia; ORGANIC AMNESIA; retrograde amnesia; selective amnesia; TRANSIENT GLOBAL AMNESIA.

molecular neurobiology   The study of genes, proteins, and other microscopic elements of NEURONS and other cells making up the brain and NERVOUS SYSTEM.

Mongolism   See DOWN SYNDROME.

monoamine oxidase (MAO)   An enzyme found in most tissues of the body that triggers the oxidation and breakdown of a large number of monoamines such as EPINEPHRINE, NOREPINEPHRINE, and SEROTONIN.

Antidepressants known as MONOAMINE OXIDASE inhibitors work by blocking the breakdown of monoamines (serotonin, norepinephrine, and DOPAMINE) by an enzyme in the brain called monoamine oxidase.

When NEUROTRANSMITTERS are not broken down, they accumulate in the brain—and because DEPRESSION is associated with low levels of these monoamines, increasing the monoamines eases depressive symptoms.

Unfortunately, monoamine oxidase does not just break down those neurotransmitters; it is also responsible for mopping up another amine called tyramine, a molecule that affects blood pressure. When monoamine oxidase becomes blocked and the monoamine levels rise, levels of tyramine begin to rise too. While a hike in neurotransmitters may be beneficial, an increase in tyramine can be disastrous. Excess tyramine can cause a sudden, sometimes fatal, increase in blood pressure so severe that it can burst blood vessels in the brain.

Every time a person eats chicken liver, aged cheese, broad-bean pods, or pickled herring, tyramine levels rise in the brain. Normally, MAO enzymes take care of this potentially harmful tyramine excess. But if a person is taking an MAO inhibitor, the MAO enzyme cannot stop tyramine from building up. This is exactly what happened when the drugs were first introduced in the 1960s. Because no one knew about the tyramine connection, a wave of deaths from brain hemorrhages swept the country. Other patients taking MAO inhibitors experienced severe HEADACHES caused by the rise in blood pressure. These early side effects were particularly disturbing because nobody knew why they were happening.

The mystery was solved when a British pharmacist noticed that his wife, who was taking MAO inhibitors, had headaches when she ate cheese. But the early MAOIs were considered so dangerous (they also can damage liver, brain, and cardiovascular systems) that even when the MAO-tyramine connection was finally understood, these drugs were taken off the American market for a time. (A related European antidepressant drug, Deprenyl, is marketed in this country as an anti-Parkinson medication; it requires less stringent dietary precautions.)

Eventually the MAOIs were reintroduced in this country despite the tyramine risk because some depressed people do not respond to any other medication. Nevertheless, MAO inhibitors are usually the antidepressant of last resort.

See also SELECTIVE SEROTONIN REUPTAKE INHIBITORS.

mood See EMOTIONS AND THE BRAIN; LIMBIC SYSTEM.

morphine The main component of opium first isolated in 1805 by a German chemist who named it after Morpheus, the Greek god of dreams. Since then, chemists have been able to make other types of OPIATES by slightly altering the morphine molecule. For example, heroin is made by adding two acetyl groups to the morphine molecule, which enables the heroin to enter quickly into the brain, causing the much-desired "rush."

Scientists discovered that the brain contains special opiate RECEPTORS that allow opiate molecules to act on human BRAIN CELLS. Morphine and other opiates resemble molecules produced by the brain itself, called ENDORPHINS or ENKEPHALINS (Greek for "in the head"). Scientists found a high concentration of opiate receptors in the SUBSTANTIA GELATINOSA, which is where pain nerves first connect with the SPINAL CORD. There were also clusters of opiate receptors in the THALAMUS, which is partly involved with deep, lasting pain—the kind that the opiates work best in controlling. There were more opiate receptors in the MIDBRAIN, where pain signals are processed.

Opiates relieve pain, not by eliminating it, but by making the patient indifferent to it. Morphine acts not on the nerves that transmit pain sensations to the brain, but on the brain and spinal cord centers that integrate incoming pain information.

The location of the opiate receptors also explains some of the other effects of morphine and its derivatives. For example, heroin addicts typically exhibit tiny pinpoint pupils; this is because there are many opiate receptors in the pretectal nuclei, located in the brain area that controls pupil size. Opiates can kill by interfering with breathing because there are many opiate receptors in the medulla, pons, and the nucleus of the solitary tract, areas of the brain that control breathing.

Addiction/Tolerance

While a drug addiction does have psychological factors, there are also physiological reasons behind these side effects. When an addict constantly supplies morphine to the NERVE CELLS, they bind to opiate receptors in the brain, triggering a cutback in the body's own production of endorphins. Tolerance occurs because the normal production of endorphins stops and the body then needs more and more outside opiates to meet its needs.

When the drug is stopped, withdrawal symptoms occur because the body needs some time to start to produce its own opiates to replace those supplied from the drug. The brain cannot function normally because some of its neuromodulators are missing, and the addict will experience the side effects of withdrawal (agitation, sleeplessness, DEPRESSION, unusual pain sensitivity, stomach cramps, and diarrhea) until the body's endorphin production returns to normal.

motor aphasia See BROCA'S APHASIA.

motor area See MOTOR CORTEX.

motor association The oldest form of memory, this type of memory is responsible for the fact that once a human learns a physical skill, the motor memory of the experience is never forgotten.

Birds and mammals can remember both sensory and motor associations, but animals farther down the evolutionary ladder (such as fruit flies, cockroaches, and flatworms) can form only motor associations.

Research with cabbage butterflies in 1986 revealed that motor associations enhance survival; while individual butterflies visit flowers of one species, the motor memories of experienced butterflies enable them to work more quickly and obtain more nectar from flowers. Because each flower requires a different method to obtain nectar from it, cabbage butterflies who can select one single species are more productive. Scientists know that recognition depends on memory and not on instinct because different cabbage butterflies favor different species; experiments have shown that if necessary, cabbage butterflies will obtain nectar from a new species and become faithful to those flowers.

motor cortex Part of the CEREBRAL CORTEX that extends from ear to ear across the roof of the brain, concerned with movement and coordination. It lies just in front of the SENSORY CORTEX. Each hemisphere's motor cortex controls the muscles on the opposite side of the body so that if the function of the right motor cortex is impaired, muscles on the left side of the body will be paralyzed.

A variety of regions in the CENTRAL NERVOUS SYSTEM send input to the motor cortex: the sensory cortex, the premotor and supplementary motor areas, the BASAL GANGLIA, and the CEREBELLUM.

The corticospinal tract connects the motor cortex to the motor neurons in the SPINAL CORD and BRAIN STEM; this descending tract also branches out to other structures important in motor activity. Damage to this tract can cause a loss of voluntary movement below the damaged area, although reflex activity will persist because reflex resides segmentally in the spinal cord.

motor homunculus   The term for the brain map representing the body parts and their relative size according to how much of the MOTOR CORTEX is devoted to each. Electrically stimulating areas in the motor cortex, different parts of the body respond. Drawing a map of these activated body areas as they are represented in each region of the motor cortex will reveal a distorted image of a man. (*Homunculus* is Latin for "little men.")

motor nerves   Nerves devoted to carrying impulses outward from the CENTRAL NERVOUS SYSTEM to activate a muscle or gland. Motor nerves cause muscle contractions and stimulate glands to secrete hormones.

motor neuron disease   A progressive degenerative disease of the nerves that control muscles. The condition usually begins in middle age, causing muscle weakness and wasting. Speech or swallowing may deteriorate, with wasting and weakness in muscles of the tongue, hands, and other parts of the body.

It primarily affects the motor cells of the SPINAL CORD, the motor nuclei in the BRAIN STEM, and the corticospinal fibers.

Symptoms and Diagnostic Path

The three distinct forms of motor neuron disease include AMYOTROPHIC LATERAL SCLEROSIS (ALS), progressive muscular atrophy, and progressive bulbar palsy. Though the latter two conditions start with patterns of muscle weakness different from ALS, they usually develop into that disease.

Two types of motor neuron disease (usually inherited) affect much younger patients: infantile progressive spinal muscular atrophy (Werdnig-Hoffmann paralysis) affects infants at birth or shortly after with weakness progressing to death in several months to several years, with rare exceptions. A milder form, chronic spinal muscular dystrophy, begins at any time in childhood through adolescence and causes progressive weakness that may never cause serious problems. The cause is unknown.

Treatment Options and Outlook

Weakness usually spreads to the muscles needed for breathing within four years, but exceptions do occur. Some people have lived more than 20 years after the initial diagnosis. While scientists have no way to slow the degeneration of the nerves, they may be able to lessen disability. Care is usually aimed at lessening discomfort.

See also DEGENERATIVE DISEASES.

motor neurons   The final neuron in the brain-to-muscle pathway that carries nerve impulses to muscles, controlling muscular activity.

See also DEGENERATIVE DISEASES AND THE BRAIN; MOTOR NEURON DISEASE.

motor system disease   See MOTOR NEURON DISEASE.

movement disorders   A group of neurological disorders that involve the motor and movement systems. Some of the more commonly known movement disorders include PARKINSON'S DISEASE, TREMOR, dystonias, HUNTINGTON'S DISEASE, and TOURETTE SYNDROME. These disorders are all caused by problems in the BASAL GANGLIA, deep in the hemispheres of the brain. The movement disorders are characterized by problems that include the inability to move or by severe, constant, and excessive movements.

Most movement disorders, among them Parkinson's disease, affect the speed, quality, and ease of movement. Others, such as tremors, dystonias, tics, progressive supranuclear palsy, Huntington's disease, and Wilson's disease, result in excess movements of varying type, slow movements, or abnormal movements that are not under voluntary control.

Tremors

Tremors are disorders that involve abnormal involuntary movement. They can involve the arms, legs, head, or body. They may be most evident when a person is resting or trying to make fine, coordinated movements. Physiological tremor can affect anyone and may occur with too much caffeine intake or during periods of anxiety.

Essential tremor is most severe when a body part is being used; for example, when trying to write or using fine, coordinated hand movements. It is less obvious when the person is at rest. Essential tremor can occur at any age, although its likelihood increases with age. Some people may have a family history of tremor. If the tremor is disabling, medications can be useful, such as propranolol (Inderal) which acts on the sympathetic nervous system. Side effects include low blood pressure and low heart rate. If it is not tolerated, the antiseizure medication mysoline (Primidone) can be effective.

Resting tremor is the type seen in Parkinson's disease. It is most obvious when arms and legs are at rest, and often subsides when a patient attempts fine movement, such as reaching for an object. If resting tremor interferes with activities, anticholinergic medications or medications to treat Parkinson's disease may be effective.

Dystonia

Dystonia is an involuntary movement disorder characterized by continued muscular contractions that can result in twisted postures of the body or arms and legs. Movements are usually slow and may seem exaggerated. There are many causes of this movement disorder, which can include bio-chemical abnormalities, degenerative disorders, psychiatric dysfunction, toxins, and drugs. Many forms of dystonia are not well understood.

Spasmodic Torticollis

Spasmodic torticollis is a syndrome that usually affects adults, and is characterized by an involuntary turning of the neck to one side. At first, some people may not notice that the head and neck are turned, but eventually the continued turning in one direction can be painful. Treatment may include medications or an injection of Botox, a medication derived from botulinum toxin that can ease the condition by temporarily interfering with the nerve/muscle interaction.

Blepharospasm

An involuntary problem in which the eyelids close intermittently. It may occur so often it interferes with vision. The preferred treatment is Botox injections.

Tic Disorders

Tic disorders usually involve brief, very rapid repeated movements. The more common tics affect the motor systems or the voice. Motor tics often involve the eyelids, eyebrows, or other facial muscles, as well as the upper limbs. Vocal tics may involve grunting, throat clearing, coughing, or cursing. Individuals with tic disorders often describe a strong urge to perform the particular tic. The best-known tic disorder is Tourette syndrome, a condition of multiple motor and vocal tics that usually begins in childhood and is much more common in boys than in girls. The disease often gets better and worse intermittently, with periods of little activity alternating with times when some patients have trouble functioning at all. Medications that lower the amount of dopamine in the brain are effective in these cases, although they carry the risk of side effects.

Progressive Supranuclear Palsy

This condition mimics Parkinson's disease in some ways. Symptoms include eye movement problems, dementia, rigidity, and slow movements, but not usually tremor. Most of the affected people develop this disorder later in life. MRI studies may show that there is evidence of atrophy in the midbrain.

Unfortunately, there is no effective treatment for the disorder.

Huntington's Disease

An inherited disorder with both neurological and psychiatric features that develops when people are in their forties or fifties, characterized by dancelike, jerky, brief movements, clumsiness, jumpiness, facial movements, walking and posture problems, paranoia, confusion, or personality changes. As the disease progresses, a significant dementia develops. MRI brain imaging may show shrinkage of a portion of the basal ganglia known as the CAUDATE NUCLEUS. Unfortunately, there is no cure or effective treatment.

Wilson's Disease

A genetic disorder that involves the nervous system and liver function, causing problems metabolizing copper. As copper builds up in the liver and in specific places in the nervous system, it causes tremors, uncoordination, falling, slurred speech, stiffness, and seizures. Psychiatric problems also can occur, together with severe liver damage. Treatment includes medications that bind copper.

MRI See MAGNETIC RESONANCE IMAGING.

multi-infarct dementia One of the two most common incurable forms of mental impairment in old age, caused by a series of small STROKES that result in widespread death of brain tissue. Multi-infarct dementia causes a step-by-step degeneration in mental ability, with each step occurring after a stroke; memory (especially of recent events) is affected first.

Multi-infarct dementia accounts for about 20 percent of the irreversible cases of mental impairment. In the early stages before severe damage has been done, the person usually is aware of impaired ability, which can lead to frustration and DEPRESSION. CADASIL (cerebral autosomal dominant arteriopathy with subcortical infarcts and leukoencephalopathy) is an inherited type of multi-infarct dementia.

Multi-infarct dementia usually develops more quickly than ALZHEIMER'S DISEASE, and is usually linked to stroke-related physical problems such as paralysis or slurred speech, which aren't symptoms of Alzheimer's disease. Nonetheless, it may be hard to tell the difference between the two dementing conditions. It's also possible for someone to have both Alzheimer's disease and multi-infarct dementia. About one in five of those with senile dementia show signs of both conditions.

Multi-infarct dementia (and the strokes that cause it) are usually the result of an underlying medical condition, such as high blood pressure and artery damage.

Symptoms and Diagnostic Path

Symptoms include confusion, memory problems, wandering, incontinence, laughing or crying inappropriately, problems following instructions, or problems with money. The condition typically begins between age 60 and 75 and affects men more often than women.

Those who are suspected to have multi-infarct dementia should have thorough physical, neurological, and psychiatric evaluations, including a complete medical exam and tests of mental state together with a BRAIN SCAN. The brain scan can rule out curable diseases and may also show signs of normal age-related changes in the brain, such as shrinkage.

Treatment Options and Outlook

Prevention is really the only effective treatment for multi-infarct dementia; patients with high blood pressure, TRANSIENT ISCHEMIC ATTACKS, or earlier strokes should continue treatment for these diseases to minimize the chance of developing DEMENTIA.

While there is no cure for multi-infarct dementia, careful use of drugs can lessen agitation, anxiety, and depression and improve sleep. Proper nutrition is especially important, and the patient should be encouraged to maintain normal daily routines, physical activities, and contact with friends. The patient should be stimulated by providing information about time of day, place of residence, and what is going on in the home and the world; this can help prevent brain activity from failing at a faster rate. Memory aids, such as a visible calendar, lists of daily activities, safety guidelines, and directions to commonly used items, also may help people in their day-to-day living.

multiple intelligences The theory that each person's INTELLIGENCE is actually made up of a number of different abilities that can work individually or together. The idea was first developed by Harvard professor Howard Gardner, who described eight types of intelligences

- body/kinesthetic
- interpersonal
- intrapersonal
- logical/mathematic
- musical/rhythmic
- naturalistic
- verbal/linguistic
- visual/spatial

Each of these eight types represents abilities within a specific area of human function. Gardner believes that intelligence, as it was traditionally measured by most intelligence tests, corresponds to only three types of intelligence as he describes it: verbal/ linguistic, logical/mathematic, and visual/spatial intelligences. This means that traditional measures of intelligence fail to recognize abilities and gifts in other areas, including body/kinesthetic, inter- and intrapersonal, musical, and naturalistic.

Although not validated by research, Gardner's theories have become increasingly accepted by other scientists, yet standard intelligence tests have not changed their basic orientation since the late 1940s; they continue to focus on reasoning measures that depend heavily on linguistic, logical, and visual-spatial abilities. Moreover, the common understanding of intelligence continues to be primarily linked to verbal ability.

At the same time, many schools continue to emphasize linguistic and mathematical intelligence. Often, individuals with learning disabilities have talents that are not valued in academic settings. The theory of multiple intelligences emphasizes the need to acknowledge and cultivate different kinds of thinking and different abilities.

Musical/rhythmic Each individual has a different musical ability. Although musical intelligence may not seem as obvious a form of intellect as mathematical or logical ability, from a neurological point of view the ability to perform and comprehend music appears to work independently from other forms of intelligence.

Bodily/kinesthetic One of the most controversial of Gardner's intelligences is the idea of bodily/ kinesthetic intelligence. In Gardner's theory, each person possesses a certain control of movement, balance, agility, and grace. In some extraordinary athletes, strong bodily/kinesthetic intelligence appears even before formal training begins. These "superathletes" all seem to have a natural sense of how their body should act and react in a demanding physical situation.

Some people argue that physical control should not be included as a form of intelligence, but Gardner and other researchers believe that bodily/kinesthetic ability does deserve such a recognition.

Logical/mathematic Logical/mathematical intelligence is the ability to mentally process logical problems and equations, the type most often found on multiple-choice standardized tests. Logical/ mathematical intelligence often does not require verbal articulation. Individuals who have good logical/mathematical abilities are able to process logical questions at an unusually rapid rate.

Before the advent of the theory of multiple intelligences, logical/mathematical intelligence was considered to be intelligence itself, the "raw intellect" which Western culture revered. Although the theory of multiple intelligences agrees that logical/ mathematical intelligence is indeed a key part of the intellect, it is by no means the only one.

Verbal/linguistic Everyone possesses the ability to use language; although some can master only basic levels of communication, others speak many languages with ease. For years researchers have recognized the connection between language and the brain. Damage to one portion of the brain (BROCA'S AREA) will affect the ability to express clear grammatical sentences, although a person's understanding of vocabulary and syntax remains intact. As Howard Gardner notes, even young children and deaf individuals will begin to develop their own unique language if they are not offered an alternative. A person's ability to construct and comprehend language may vary, but as a cognitive trait it is still universal.

Visual/spatial   Spatial intelligence involves the ability to understand shapes and images in three dimensions. Whether trying to put together a puzzle or create a sculpture, spatial intelligence allows a person to interpret what may or may not be physically seen. Advances in neuroscience have now provided researchers with clear-cut proof of the role of spatial intelligence in the right hemisphere of the brain.

In rare instances, for example, certain brain injuries can cause people to lose the ability to recognize their closest relatives. Though they may see the other person perfectly well, they are unable to comprehend who they see.

And yet a blind person may feel a shape and identify it with ease, although it cannot be seen. Because most people use spatial intelligence in conjunction with sight, its existence as an autonomous cognitive attribute may not seem obvious, but recent research suggests that it is an independent portion of the intellect.

Interpersonal   Humans are social animals who thrive when involved with others. This ability to interact with others, understand them, and interpret their behavior is called interpersonal intelligence. According to Gardner, a person's interpersonal intelligence allows for the awareness of the moods, temperaments, motivations, and intentions of others. Interpersonal intelligence allows an individual to affect others by understanding others; without it, an individual loses the ability to exist socially.

Intrapersonal   Intrapersonal intelligence is the ability to understand and sense the self. Intrapersonal intelligence allows individuals to tap into internal feelings and thoughts. A strong intrapersonal intelligence can lead to self-esteem, self-enhancement, and a strength of character that can be used to solve internal problems.

On the other hand, a weak intrapersonal intelligence (such as with autistic children) prevents a person from recognizing the self as separate from the surrounding environment.

Intrapersonal intelligence often is not recognized from the outside unless it is expressed in some form, such as rage or joy.

Naturalistic   Recently added to the original list of seven multiple intelligences, naturalistic intelligence is a person's ability to identify and classify patterns in nature and relate to one's surroundings. People who are sensitive to changes in weather patterns or are adept at distinguishing nuances between large numbers of similar objects may be expressing naturalistic intelligence abilities.

multiple sclerosis (MS)   A degenerative disease of the CENTRAL NERVOUS SYSTEM believed to involve the immune system, which attacks the MYELIN (protective covering of nerve fibers), disrupting function and causing paralysis. In some patients it also causes memory loss as a result of dysfunctioning FRONTAL and TEMPORAL LOBES. The severity of the disease varies considerably among patients.

The disease usually appears in early adult life in women more than in men and among Caucasians more often than among African Americans or Asians. Some people have a single attack with no recurrence; others have periods when the disease is active (called exacerbations) and times when they are symptom-free (remissions). Finally, some have a chronic, progressive form of the disease that becomes increasingly severe. About 400,000 Americans have MS. About 2.5 million people in the world have MS.

The cause of MS is unknown, but it is thought to be an autoimmune disease in which the body's own defense system treats myelin as an invader, gradually destroying it. Myelin is replaced by scars of hardened patches of tissue called plaques.

While MS is not considered to be a genetic disorder, there seems to be a genetic factor because relatives of affected people are eight times more likely than others to contract the disease. It is believed that the environment may also play a part; the area in which a child spends the first 15 years of life affects future risk of contracting the disease. (MS is five times more common in temperate-zone continents such as the United States and Europe.) It is believed by some that this environmental relationship may involve a slow virus, picked up during a susceptible time of early life, that later triggers an autoimmune disorder.

Recent research suggests that some kinds of antibodies in the immune system may help repair myelin, which may explain the disease's remissions. These antibodies may promise a treatment or even a cure in the future if the antibody level can be increased.

Symptoms and Diagnostic Path

Symptoms vary widely depending on the part of the brain that is affected. They can include tingling, numbness, muscle weakness, muscle cramps, lack of coordination, paralysis, blurry or double vision, abnormal fatigue, confusion, forgetfulness, incontinence, and impaired sexual function; memory loss does not often appear immediately but may occur years later. MS is not fatal; patients can live a normal life span.

Symptoms that wax and wane make diagnosis a challenge. No single test can reveal MS. Confirmation of the disease usually comes only after other diseases have been ruled out; a NEUROLOGIST may perform tests to help confirm the diagnosis, including LUMBAR PUNCTURE (removal of a fluid from the spinal canal for lab analysis) or testing electrical activity in the brain via BRAIN SCANS. MAGNETIC RESONANCE IMAGING has greatly helped in diagnosing MS.

Treatment Options and Outlook

At present there is no cure for MS. However, four medications (Betaseron, Copaxone, Rebif, and Avonex) have been approved by the U.S. Food and Drug Administration (FDA) for relapsing forms of MS. They have helped to lessen the frequency and severity of MS attacks, reduce the accumulation of lesions in the brain, and one has also been shown to slow the progression of disability. In addition to these medications, there is a wide range of treatments that can ease symptoms of spasticity, pain, fatigue, and weakness.

MS does not shorten life span, and most people with the disease can lead fairly normal lives. Recent studies have found that, contrary to earlier beliefs, pregnancy does not worsen symptoms and does not affect the long-term course of the disease. However, some experts caution that a parent with MS may not have the physical stamina to care for a baby or an active child and may need some child care help.

myasthenia gravis (MG) A chronic brain disease in which the voluntary muscles experience marked fatigue and muscle weakness. The fatigue is so profound that muscles are temporarily paralyzed.

It primarily affects teenagers, young adults, and adults over age 40. Women are more often affected, in a 3–2 ratio. The disease affects 5 to 14 per 100,000 Americans each year.

The body's immune system attacks and destroys certain RECEPTORS in muscles. These receptors bind ACETYLCHOLINE, the neurotransmitter released from motor neurons. As a result, nerve impulses are normal but the muscle cannot respond.

Symptoms and Diagnostic Path

This disease affects different people differently and the same person at different times. The affected muscles become worse with use, but they may recover completely with rest. Patients typically experience remissions interspersed with relapses of the condition. In addition to fatigue and weakness, symptoms include drooping of the upper eyelid, double vision, and speech problems. Patients with this disease tire even during slight exertions such as combing the hair, chewing, or talking. Between 15 and 20 percent of patients complain of arm and hand muscle weakness; leg muscle weakness is less common. Progressive weakness of the diaphragm and nearby muscles may produce breathing problems or myasthenic crisis, which is an acute emergency.

Myasthenic crisis is the sudden onset of muscular weakness in myasthenia gravis patients and is usually the result of undermedication or lack of medication. It also may result from progression of the disease, emotional upset, systemic infection, some drugs, surgery, or trauma. Symptoms of such a crisis include sudden breathing problems and an inability to swallow or speak. Weakness of respiratory and laryngeal muscles can depress breathing and obstruct the patient's airway if not treated promptly.

In mild cases, the patient can lead a comparatively normal life. In a few patients, however, the disease progression cannot be stopped; paralysis of the throat and respiratory muscles may be fatal.

Unfortunately, diagnostic delays are common, and a diagnosis is often missed in people with a mild case. The first step to diagnosing the condition is to review the person's medical history and physical and neurological exams. If the doctor suspects MG, several tests are available to confirm the diagnosis:

Blood tests These can detect the antibodies that occur in abnormally high levels in people with MG, but still about 10 percent of sufferers test negative for antibodies. Antibodies also may not be discovered if only eye muscles are affected.

Edrophonium test When this drug is injected, the weak eye muscles of people with MG will briefly get stronger.

Nerve conduction test/repetitive stimulation This test checks for specific muscle fatigue by repetitive nerve stimulation.

Single fiber electromyography (EMG) This test electrically stimulates pairs of single muscle fibers, detecting impaired nerve-to-muscle transmission.

Treatment Options and Outlook

In some patients with mild conditions, regular medication helps transmit nerve impulses to muscles and often suffices to restore the patient's condition to near normal. Anticholinesterase drugs increase the concentration of available acetylcholine, helping to activate the receptors that are left; this improves the response of the muscles to nerve impulses, thereby improving strength. These drugs do not cure the disease, but do improve symptoms. Drugs in current use include pyridostigmine bromide (Mestinon), ambenonium chloride (Mytelase), and neostigmine bromide (Prostigmin). Most patients prefer Mestinon because it causes fewer side effects, such as abdominal cramps, nausea and vomiting, and diarrhea.

Other treatment includes immunosuppressive therapy to remove circulating antibodies, including the administration of corticosteroids, blood plasma exchange, and surgical removal of the thymus. Because the thymus appears to be involved in the production of harmful antibodies, in severe cases its removal causes substantial remission of the disease and sometimes appears to cure the problem. While blood plasma exchange temporarily reduces circulating harmful antibodies and can markedly improve some patients' condition, it cannot treat the underlying disorder.

myelin The white cells (fatty material composed of lipids and proteins) that form a protective sheath around some types of nerve fibers and help facilitate electrical impulse transmission. Myelin also acts as an electrical insulator, increasing the efficiency of nerve conduction. It is myelin that gives the white color to the WHITE MATTER of the brain, composed primarily of myelinated nerve fibers.

The abnormal breakdown of myelin, such as in MULTIPLE SCLEROSIS, is called demyelination, and seriously disrupts normal impulse conduction.

myelin sheath The protein covering that surrounds nerve fibers.

See also MULTIPLE SCLEROSIS; MYELIN.

myelogram An X-RAY examination of the brain and SPINAL CORD to look for tumors or spinal cord injury.

See also MYELOGRAPHY.

myelography A specialized method of X-RAY examination of the spinal canal that involves injection of a radiopaque contrast medium into the SUBARACHNOID SPACE. The X-rays that result are called MYELOGRAMS. This technique is used to recognize tumors of the SPINAL CORD and other conditions that compress the nerve roots.

While noninvasive tests such as CAT SCANS or MAGNETIC RESONANCE IMAGING provide good resolution for diagnosis of spinal problems, myelography may be preferred because of its sharp resolution; fluid obtained during the procedure may provide additional information about cancer, inflammation, and evidence of infection.

Procedure

Before the test, most patients are hospitalized, and no food or drink is given for several hours beforehand. A sedative may be given; the procedure usually takes between 45 and 90 minutes.

In the procedure, a needle is inserted between two of the lower vertebrae and a small amount of cerebrospinal fluid is withdrawn. Contrast media is injected slowly through the LUMBAR-PUNCTURE needle, and a series of X-rays are taken to show the configuration of the space around the spinal cord and whether it is distorted by a protruding disc or bony spur. The table is tilted to move the medium to the location of the suspected disorder in the spine. Most contrast dyes are absorbed by the blood and excreted in the urine and do not usually have to be removed when the procedure is over.

Risks and Complications

The procedure may cause feelings of pressure or nausea, although these effects should be minimized. Afterward, patients may experience a HEADACHE because of changes in the pressure of the CEREBROSPINAL FLUID (CSF); lying down will help alleviate this headache, which is usually brief.

Some conditions (tumors or herniated discs) may be made worse by the change in CSF pressure, requiring an emergency operation. Significant complications are rare.

myelomeningocele A severe and common form of SPINA BIFIDA in which the spine and spinal canal do not close before birth. At delivery, the spinal cord and the covering membranes protrude out of the child's back.

Myelomeningocele is one of the most common birth defects of the brain and spinal cord. Because the bones of the spine do not completely form, the incomplete spinal canal and meninges (the membranes covering the spinal cord) protrude. Myelomeningocele is the most common form of spina bifida, accounting for about 75 percent of all cases. It may affect as many as one of every 800 infants. The other forms of spina bifida are

- spina bifida occulta (in which the bones of the spine do not close, the spinal cord and meninges remain in place, and skin usually covers the defect)
- meningoceles (where the meninges protrude through the vertebral defect but the spinal cord remains in place).

The cause is unknown, but folic acid deficiency is thought to play a part in NEURAL TUBE DEFECTS, including myelomeningocele. The disorder appears to be more common in families; if a child is born with myelomeningocele, siblings are at higher risk than the general population. A viral cause has been implicated, since there is a higher incidence of the defect in children born in the early winter months. Research also indicates possible environmental factors such as radiation.

Symptoms and Diagnostic Path

Symptoms include a saclike protrusion on a newborn's mid to lower back, and weakness of the hips, legs, or feet of a newborn. Because a protruding spinal cord and meninges damages the spinal cord and nerve roots, the function of body areas controlled at or below the defect are impaired. Most defects occur in the lowest areas of the back because this area is normally the last part of the spine to close. Symptoms include partial or complete paralysis and lack of sensation in the legs, and may include loss of bladder or bowel control. The exposed spinal cord is susceptible to infection. Other congenital disorders also may occur, usually involving the spinal cord or the musculoskeletal system such as HYDROCEPHALUS, syringomyelia, hip dislocation, or similar disorders.

Before birth, the condition can be diagnosed with an amniocentesis to reveal high levels of alpha-fetoprotein, indicating problems with the spinal cord. A pregnancy ultrasound may reveal some cases of myelomeningocele.

Treatment Options and Outlook

Treatment is designed to reduce the amount of brain damage caused by the defect and to minimize complications. With treatment, length of life is not severely affected, but brain damage is often irreversible. Early surgical repair of the defect is usually recommended, although surgical repair may be performed later to allow the infant to better tolerate the procedure. Before surgery, the infant must be handled carefully to reduce damage to the exposed spinal cord. Antibiotics may be used aggressively to treat or prevent meningitis, urinary tract infections, or other infections. Gentle downward pressure over the bladder may help drain the bladder; in severe cases, bladder drainage catheters may be needed. A diet high in fiber together with bowel training programs may improve bowel function.

Orthopedic intervention or physical therapy may be needed to treat musculoskeletal symptoms. Other neurologic problems are treated according to the type and extent of the loss of function. The goal of these interventions is to minimize future disability and maximize functioning. Occasionally, surgical shunting to correct hydrocephalus causes the myelomeningocele to spontaneously reduce, and normal growth of the child may cover the defect.

Risk Factors and Preventive Measures

Folic acid supplements may help reduce the risk of neural tube defects such as myelomeningocele. Folic acid (folate) deficiencies must be corrected before a woman becomes pregnant, since the defect develops very early.

naloxone A chemical which can bind to the opiate receptor sites in the brain instead of ENDORPHINS but which has no pain-controlling ability. Considered to be an opiate antagonist, naloxone binds to an opiate receptor without activating it. By binding, it blocks true endorphins from binding and activating.

narcolepsy An often-inherited neurological sleep disorder characterized by irresistible daytime sleep attacks. Other symptoms involve abnormalities of dreaming sleep, such as dreamlike hallucinations and brief feelings of weakness or paralysis. It often becomes noticeable during the teens or early twenties, although it can also appear later in life. It is believed to affect approximately one of every 1,000 people of both sexes and all races.

Narcolepsy is related to the dreaming portion of sleep called REM (rapid eye movement) sleep. During normal REM sleep, the muscles become immobile or "paralyzed" as a protection against acting out dreams. The normal sleep period begins with about 90 minutes of non-REM sleep before REM sleep begins. But for a person with narcolepsy, sleep begins almost immediately with REM sleep. Since the brain may not be totally asleep when dreaming begins, the dream is sometimes experienced far more vividly and is thought of as an hallucination. After waking, REM periods occur inappropriately throughout the day. This explains excessive daytime sleepiness.

Cataplexy is related to the muscle "paralysis" of REM. When automatic behavior occurs, sleep has partially overtaken the brain, but the body continues to perform familiar tasks.

Recent studies have shown that narcolepsy with cataplexy is usually caused by the lack of two related brain chemicals called hypocretin-1 and hypocretin-2 that are essential to the human sleep-wake cycle. Medical researchers have recently identified the cause as the absence of neurotransmitter cells which produce the hypocretin peptide essential to the human sleep-wake cycle. The most likely explanation for the missing brain cells could be that they are destroyed by an autoimmune attack.

Currently, sleep scientists are focusing on genetics, neurotransmitters, and the autoimmune system as possible causes of narcolepsy. Researchers also believe that other factors, such as viruses or bacteria, abrupt changes in wake-sleep cycles, illness, accidents, stress, drug usage, and even hormonal changes may act as triggers, determining whether or not someone with a genetic predisposition to narcolepsy will develop the disorder.

Symptoms and Diagnostic Path

Excessive daytime sleepiness (EDS) includes daytime sleep attacks, which may occur with or without warning (and for many are irresistible); persistent drowsiness, which may continue for prolonged periods of time; and "microsleeps," or fleeting moments of sleep intruding into the waking state.

Cataplexy (the other hallmark symptom of narcolepsy) is a sudden loss of voluntary muscle control, usually triggered by emotions such as laughter, surprise, fear, or anger. It occurs more frequently during times of stress or fatigue. The cataplectic attack may involve only a slight feeling of weakness and limp muscles (such as sagging facial muscles, a nodding head, buckling knees, loss of arm strength, garbled speech); but it may also result in immediate total body collapse, during which the person may appear unconscious, but remains awake and alert. These attacks may last from a few seconds up to 30 minutes.

The two other symptoms are hypnagogic hallucinations (vivid, realistic, often frightening dreams while dozing or falling asleep) and sleep paralysis, a temporary inability to move for a few minutes. Either one of these can occur during the process of going to sleep or waking up, while the brain is partially asleep and partially awake.

The secondary or auxiliary symptoms may include

- automatic behavior: the performance of a routine task, without conscious awareness of doing it, and often without later memory of it
- disrupted nighttime sleep, involving multiple arousals
- intense fatigue and continual lack of energy
- depression
- concentration and memory problems
- vision (focusing) problems
- eating binges
- weak limbs
- trouble handling alcohol

In many cases, a diagnosis is not made until many years after the onset of symptoms. This is often due to the fact that patients do not consult a doctor until many years of excessive sleepiness have passed, on the assumption that sleepiness is not a disease. In one recent study, the average number of years between the onset of symptoms and correct diagnosis was 14 years. Since the symptoms of narcolepsy usually appear during adolescence, this means that most narcoleptic patients are diagnosed too late to prevent the dramatic impact of the disease on their personal and professional development.

Excessive daytime sleepiness (EDS) is often the first symptom to appear; and is the only symptom of narcolepsy for some patients. However, EDS is also a symptom of other medical problems. On the other hand, cataplexy is almost unique to narcolepsy. The combination of EDS and cataplexy would lead to a clinical diagnosis of narcolepsy.

Laboratory tests are needed both to confirm diagnosis and plan treatment. The usual procedure is an overnight polysomnogram (PSG) to determine the presence of excessive daytime sleepiness and perhaps other underlying causes of this symptom. This is followed by the Multiple Sleep Latency Test (MSLT) which measures sleep onset and how quickly REM sleep occurs. The MSLT is the most widely accepted diagnostic test for narcolepsy. Finally, a genetic blood test has been developed which measures certain antigens often found in people who have a predisposition to narcolepsy. Positive results suggest, but do not prove, the existence of narcolepsy. This test is sometimes used when the diagnosis is in question.

Treatment Options and Outlook

Patients with narcolepsy can be substantially helped, but not cured, by medical treatment. The goal of treatment is to use the minimum amount of medication needed to keep the patient as alert as possible during the day and to minimize recurring episodes of cataplexy. In 1999, modafinil was approved for treatment of EDS, and in July 2002, the FDA approved Xyrem (sodium oxybate or gamma hydroxybutyrate, also known as GHB) for treating people with narcolepsy who experience episodes of cataplexy. Due to safety concerns associated with the use of this drug, the distribution of Xyrem is tightly restricted.

In addition, two classes of antidepressant drugs are effective in controlling cataplexy in many patients: tricyclics (including imipramine, desipramine, clomipramine, and protriptyline) and selective serotonin reuptake inhibitors (including fluoxetine and sertraline).

Drug therapy should be supplemented by other strategies, such as taking short, regularly scheduled naps during sleepiest times. Improving the quality of nighttime sleep can help relieve persistent feelings of fatigue. It is also important to maintain a regular sleep schedule, avoid alcohol, and not drink any caffeine-containing beverages before bedtime.

narcotics and the brain Narcotics (drugs that induce stupor and relieve pain) primarily include MORPHINE and other derivatives of opium, although the term also applies to other drugs that depress brain function, such as general anesthetics and hypnotics. In legal terms, a narcotic is any addictive drug that can be illegally abused. OPIATES, which are derived from poppies, contain substances that activate the brain's own ENDORPHIN receptors to produce pain relief, euphoria, and slowed breathing.

Morphine and morphine-like narcotics have been largely replaced as sleeping drugs because of their ability to cause dependence and tolerance, but they are still used for relief of severe pain.

natural opiates   See ENDORPHINS; LIMBIC SYSTEM.

neocortex   The part of the brain that occupies most of the cerebral hemispheres and processes reason, logic, language, mathematics, and speculation about the future. It also influences those behavior patterns set in motion by the more primitive parts of the brain. The neocortex is the brain structure that differentiates mammals from other vertebrates. Scientists assume it is the neocortex that is responsible for the evolution of intelligence.

neostriatum   See STRIATUM.

nerve cells   See NEURONS.

nerve conduction velocity study   A diagnostic technique in which the motor or sensory nerves are stimulated at different points, and the speed of the resulting impulse is measured. This test measures the velocity of the fastest conducting nerve fibers (the large myelinated AXONS). There is normal velocity if the MYELIN is intact; slowed conduction can be caused by demyelination or destruction of large myelinated fibers.

This test is particularly useful in diagnosing GUILLAIN-BARRÉ SYNDROME or conditions such as carpal tunnel syndrome, or to diagnose nerve damage.

Procedure
During the test, sticky pads are placed on the skin over the nerve to record the electrical activity of a patient's nerves, and a computer is used to display, record, analyze, and store the data. One electrode stimulates the nerve with a very mild electrical impulse. The resulting electrical activity is recorded by the other electrodes. The distance between electrodes and the time it takes for electrical impulses to travel between electrodes are used to calculate the nerve conduction velocity.

The test can be used to diagnose some of the following conditions:

- carpal tunnel syndrome
- pinched or trapped nerves
- sciatic nerve problems
- spinal cord dysfunction
- tarsal tunnel syndrome
- spinal disc conditions
- neuromuscular disorders

Risks and Complications
The impulses are completely harmless.

nerve-growth factor (NGF)   A naturally occurring hormone that stimulates the growth of NEURITES (tiny projections of a growing nerve cell that carry information between cells). Nerve-growth factor is one of the human-growth factors currently being studied for its medical potential to restore function in the aging. Human-growth hormone, another growth factor, is also being investigated for its potential to strengthen the elderly.

Growth factors (there are at least eight different varieties currently being studied) each have a different target cell in the body, and each has a possible role in protecting the body's nerve cells against damage from diseases such as ALZHEIMER'S, PARKINSON'S, and LOU GEHRIG'S.

In addition, scientists at the University of California at San Diego found that in a variety of learning and memory tests, infusions of nerve-growth factor into the brain could improve learning capacity and increased the size of brain cells that had previously shrunk. In Sweden, a human Alzheimer's patient reportedly was treated with a similar approach.

TYPES OF USAGE FOR GROWTH-FACTOR HORMONE

Nerve-Growth Factor: Alzheimer's disease

Basic fibroblast-growth factor: Wound healing and Parkinson's disease, stroke

Brain-derived neurotrophic factor: Parkinson's disease

Neurotrophin-3: Nerve damage following trauma, chemotherapy, or diabetes, and in the treatment of Alzheimer's disease.

Neurotrophin-4/5: Alzheimer's and Parkinson's diseases

Ciliary-neurotrophic factor: Lou Gehrig's disease

Glial-growth factor: Peripheral neuropathy

Glial-maturation factor: Nerve injuries

Some scientists are now developing a class of drugs called K252 compounds, which are designed to boost the body's production of nerve-growth factor. Other studies are investigating a possible treatment for Parkinson's disease, amyotrophic lateral sclerosis (Lou Gehrig's disease), and STROKE patients.

The problem with using the different growth factors is that most of these protein molecules are large and difficult to handle and must be pumped directly into the brain because they will not cross the blood/brain barrier. Researchers hope that new kinds of drug delivery systems, such as patches and nasal sprays, may simplify transport problems with these growth factors.

nerve impulse   The electrical message carried by the nerve cells (neurons).

nerve signal   See NERVE IMPULSE.

nervous system   A vast network of cells that carry information coded as NERVE IMPULSES to and from all parts of the body. The system is divided into the CENTRAL NERVOUS SYSTEM (the brain and SPINAL CORD) and the PERIPHERAL NERVOUS SYSTEM (PNS) (the nervous tissue outside the cranium and vertebral column).

In the average adult human, the brain weighs about three pounds and contains about 100 billion nerve cells (neurons) and trillons of "support cells" called glia. The spinal cord is about 43 centimeters long in adult women and 45 centimeters long in adult men and weighs about 35 to 40 grams. The vertebral column, the collection of bones that houses the spinal cord, is about 70 centimeters long. The spinal cord is much shorter than the vertebral column.

The PNS includes the AUTONOMIC NERVOUS SYSTEM, which is further divided into the sympathetic and PARASYMPATHETIC NERVOUS SYSTEMS. The basic functional unit of the nervous system is the nerve cell, or NEURON.

neural graft   A transplant of brain tissue from a healthy brain to a damaged area of the brain or spinal cord.

neural plate   Substance lying along the central axis of the early embryo that forms the NEURAL TUBE and, eventually, the CENTRAL NERVOUS SYSTEM.

neural tube defects   A group of defects occurring at birth caused by a failure of the neural tube to close properly. Between the 17th and 30th day after conception, a ridge of neural-like tissue develops along the embryo's back. As the fetus develops, this material changes into the SPINAL CORD and peripheral nerves at the lower end and the brain at the upper end.

About 2,500 babies are born each year with neural tube defects in the United States—about six of every 10,000 live births. This is a decline from 1970, when there were neural tube defects in about 13 in every 10,000 live births. Most babies with this defect are stillborn or miscarried; only 25 percent of these infants are born alive.

Symptoms and Diagnostic Path

A developmental problem during this time can cause a neural tube defect, leading to abnormalities. The two most common are a total lack of brain (ANENCEPHALY) and SPINA BIFIDA (when the bony arches of the spine do not close, leading to leaks of cerebrospinal fluid). More severe defects of these bones lead to more serious neurological conditions.

A MENINGOCELE refers to the protrusion of the MENINGES through the opening in the spine, with a constant risk of damage and infection to the meninges. In a MENINGOMYELOCELE, the nerve roots and the spinal cord are exposed, and there is a constant risk of infection; this condition is accompanied by paralysis and numbness in the legs and urinary incontinence. There is also usually HYDROCEPHALUS (fluid in the brain) and ARNOLD-CHIARI MALFORMATION as well. If the neural tube fails to fuse at the cranial end (called cranium bifidum), the child will be born with severe mental and physical disorders.

The maternal serum alpha-fetoprotein blood test is given during pregnancy, to detect neural tube defects. This blood test is now available for all women at 16 weeks of pregnancy. Alpha-fetoprotein (AFP) is a chemical made by the fetus that enters the mother's blood; high levels of AFP may mean the fetus has a neural tube defect. While this blood test detects up to 90 percent of NTDs, it is only a screening test. There are other tests also available that can be used to diagnose NTDs during pregnancy.

Both genetic and environmental factors are believed to cause neural tube defects. Studies have shown that the following people are at an increased risk of having an NTD-affected pregnancy:

- women who have low folic acid levels before they become pregnant and through the earliest weeks of pregnancy.
- Caucasians with English/Irish ancestry
- women who do not eat well-balanced diets
- couples who have already had other children with NTDs

Risk Factors and Preventive Measures

It is not possible to predict which women will have a pregnancy affected by a neural tube defect, since 95 percent of cases occur in women with no personal or family history. However, there are some risk factors:

- one NTD-affected pregnancy increases a woman's chance of another by about 20 times
- maternal insulin-dependent diabetes

- anti-seizure medication
- medically diagnosed obesity
- high temperatures in early pregnancy (such as prolonged fever or hot tub use)

In addition, neural tube defects are more common among Caucasians than African Americans, and more common among Hispanic women than non-Hispanic women.

The Centers for Disease Control and Prevention recommends that all women able to have a baby take a multivitamin pill containing 400 micrograms (0.4 mg) of folic acid in addition to eating foods high in folate. Since overcooking can destroy folate and the amount of folate absorbed from food varies, a daily multivitamin pill can guarantee that a woman is receiving the right amount of folic acid.

Women who plan to become pregnant should consult a health care provider about the desirability of using 4 milligrams (4,000 micrograms) of folic acid daily, beginning one month before trying to get pregnant and continuing through the first three months of pregnancy. Although it appears that a lower dose (such as 0.4 milligrams) may have as great a beneficial effect as 4 milligrams, many health care providers recommend the higher dose. This recommendation is based on information from a rigorous scientific study involving women who had previous pregnancies affected by NTDs. This dosage should be prescribed and monitored by a health care provider. Typically, a health care provider will prescribe one prenatal vitamin plus three 1 mg tablets of folic acid a day to get this dosage, because women should not take more than one multivitamin a day since excess vitamin A can hurt the baby.

Folic acid has no known toxic level, even in very high amounts. Nevertheless, experts recommend that women consume no more than 1,000 micrograms of synthetic folic acid a day, since large amounts of folic acid may make it difficult to quickly diagnose a rare vitamin B_{12} deficiency. This condition primarily affects the elderly and, in some cases, can lead to neurological damage. Today, doctors can use a simple test to check for B_{12} deficiency.

While experts do not understand all the causes of neural tube defects, scientists do know that between 50 percent and 70 percent can be prevented by getting sufficient amounts of folic acid.

Recent studies have shown that women who take folic acid before pregnancy and during the first two months of pregnancy can reduce the risk of serious birth defects of the brain and spinal cord. By taking a safe and readily available multivitamin pill with folic acid every day, a woman can cut the risk of NTDs by 50 percent or more. Folic acid is a B vitamin (also known as folate or folacin) that is needed to make new cells in the body. It can be found in most multivitamins and also in certain foods, including peas, corn and dried beans, dark green leafy vegetables, white and whole wheat breads, beef liver and lean beef, bananas, fortified breakfast cereals, or orange juice.

Some personal habits may cause people to have lower levels of folic acid in their bodies. It has been found that people with poor diets or eating disorders, bulimics, cigarette smokers, substance abusers, and users of hormonal birth control have lower amounts of folic acid and should take a multivitamin pill containing folic acid every day.

NTDs also may be caused by a number of environmental agents and genetic factors. Other nutritional factors other than folate have also been suggested as causes of NTDs, including deficiencies of vitamin B_{12} and pantothenic acid. Poor mental health and exposure to environmental pollutants have been implicated as increasing the risk of NTDs in certain areas of the country. The U.S. Public Health Service recommends that pregnant women who use folic acid supplements still be offered prenatal screening for neural tube defects.

neurapraxia   A temporary loss of nerve function characterized by tingling, numbness, and weakness. It is caused by compression of a nerve. Since there is no structural damage, the nerve and the patient should recover completely.

neurasthenia   An outdated term meaning "nervous exhaustion." It was used to describe a group of physical and psychological symptoms including irritability, fatigue, HEADACHE, dizziness, ANXIETY, insomnia, DEPRESSION, and sensitivity to noise that can be caused by organic damage (such as HEAD INJURY), or by neurosis.

neurinoma   Alternate name for ACOUSTIC NEUROMA.

neurite   Tiny projections that sprout from a growing neuron; these neurites may become DENDRITES or axons. If the developing neurite is to become an axon, it may release transmitters from its terminals *before* making synaptic contact. Researchers have shown how this helps shape dendrite arrangement of neurons that the cell in question will eventually contact.

neuroanatomy   One of the oldest of the neurosciences, this is the study of the physical structure of the nervous system from gross anatomy of the brain to the microscopic study of NEURONS.

neurobiology   The study of the biology of the brain.

neuroblastoma   A malignant tumor that develops from the tissues that form the sympathetic nervous system. It may begin in nerve tissue in the neck, chest, abdomen, or pelvis, but usually originates in the abdomen in the tissues of the adrenal gland. It is an aggressive type of cancer that tends to spread rapidly to other areas of the body (most commonly to the lymph nodes, liver, lungs, bones, and bone marrow).

This type of tumor belongs to a group of neuroblastic tumors, which include ganglioneuroblastoma (a malignant tumor comprised of mature ganglion cells and nerve fibers) and ganglioneuroma (a benign tumor composed of Schwann and ganglion cells). Ganglioneuroblastoma is a cancerous neural tumor, but most will act benign; it may look much like a neuroblastoma on imaging, but the prognosis is better for children with these tumors. A ganglioneuroma is a noncancerous tumor composed of mature ganglion cells and nerve fibers. Ganglioneuromas do not spread to other areas like cancerous tumors.

Symptoms and Diagnostic Path

The most common symptoms are the result of pressure by the tumor, or bone pain from cancer that has spread to the bone. Protruding eyes and dark circles around the eyes are common and are caused by cancer that has spread to the area behind the eye. Neuroblastomas may compress the spinal cord, causing paralysis. Fever, anemia, and high blood pressure are found occasionally. Rarely, children may have severe watery diarrhea, uncoordinated or jerky muscle movements, or uncontrollable eye movement.

Neuroblastoma is predominantly a childhood malignancy that is diagnosed only very rarely in adults. Two-thirds of children with neuroblastoma are diagnosed when they are younger than age five. The tumor is often present at birth but usually is not detected until later; in rare cases, neuroblastoma can be detected before birth by fetal ultrasound. Less than 10 percent of all neuroblastomas occur in patients older than age 10.

A careful examination, lab tests, and special X-rays can reveal this type of tumor. Scans may include a CT scan or magnetic resonance imaging (MRI) scan. Often, removal of tissue from the tumor or bone marrow is required to determine whether neuroblastoma exists. A small sample of the tissue may be surgically removed and examined under a microscope.

Once neuroblastoma is found, more tests will be done to find out if the cancer has spread from where it started to surrounding tissues or other parts of the body (staging). Knowing the stage of the disease is important so doctors can plan treatment. For the purposes of treatment the disease is categorized in the following stages

- **Localized resectable**—The cancer is confined to the site of origin, there is no evidence of spread, and the cancer can be surgically removed.

- **Localized unresectable**—The cancer is confined to the site of origin, but the cancer cannot be completely removed surgically.

- **Regional**—The cancer has extended beyond the site of origin to regional lymph nodes and/or surrounding organs or tissues, but has not spread to distant parts of the body.

- **Disseminated**—The cancer has spread from the site of origin to distant lymph nodes, bone, liver, skin, bone marrow, and/or other organs (except as defined for stage IVS).

- **Stage IVS**—Also called "special" neuroblastoma because it is treated differently. The cancer is localized, with dissemination (spread) limited to liver, skin, and/or, to a very limited extent, bone marrow.

- **Recurrent**—This means the cancer has come back or continued to spread after it has been treated. It may come back in the original site or in another part of the body.

Treatment Options and Outlook

There are three main types of treatment for neuroblastoma; surgery, chemotherapy, and radiation. The primary treatment has been chemotherapy, except in situations where the tumor is completely removed surgically.

Chemotherapy is the use of drugs to kill cancer cells and shrink tumors. The drugs may be taken by mouth or injected into a vein or muscle, where the drug enters the bloodstream, travels through the body, and kills cancer cells. Chemotherapy may be given after a tumor has been surgically removed to kill any remaining cancer cells (adjuvant chemotherapy). Chemotherapy can also be given before surgery to shrink the cancer so that it can be removed during surgery (neoadjuvant chemotherapy). Several different chemotherapy drugs are used (usually in combination), including cyclophosphamide, cisplatin, doxorubicin, teniposide, and etoposide. Other drugs, such as ifosfamide, carboplatin, iproplatin, epirubicin, and vincristine are also used.

Surgery is useful in both diagnosing and treating neuroblastoma. The decision to remove a tumor is based on its location, how it affects major blood vessels, and the child's prognosis.

Radiation therapy uses high-energy rays to damage or kill cancer cells and shrink tumors. This type of tumor is considered to be sensitive to radiation, which is often combined with chemotherapy.

Several institutions are now using bone marrow and peripheral blood stem cell transplantation as the treatment of choice for high-risk neuroblastoma. Bone marrow transplantation is a procedure in which healthy bone marrow is given to replace bone marrow destroyed by treatment with high doses of anticancer drugs or radiation. Transplantation may be autologous (the patient's own marrow saved earlier and possibly treated with drugs to kill any cancer cells), allogeneic (marrow from a healthy "matched" donor, usually a brother or sister), or syngeneic (marrow from an identical twin).

Monoclonal antibodies are currently in use by some experts; others are investigating immunotherapy, such as interleukin-2, as a method of treatment. Other agents, such as 13-cis-retinoic acid, have demonstrated good results. Deferoxamine, an iron chelator, also is being studied.

Progress made in the past few decades has improved survival rates for infants and older children with localized disease, but long-term survival for older children whose cancer has already spread at diagnosis remains poor.

Neuroblastoma in adults generally grows at a slower rate than in children, but adult tumors tend to be more resistant to chemotherapy and this group has a worse long-term prognosis regardless of stage or site.

neurochemistry The study of the biochemical processes in the brain.

neurocranium A rare term for the part of the skull that houses the brain.

neurodevelopmental treatment A form of therapy for those who suffer from CENTRAL NERVOUS SYSTEM disorders that cause abnormal movement. The technique attempts to initiate or refine normal stages and processes in the development of movement.

neurofibrillary tangles Normally, every brain cell or neuron contains long fibers made of protein (called tau) that help hold the neuron in its proper shape and help transport nutrients within the neuron. If the structure of tau protein becomes abnormal, it collapses and the fibers begin to twist and tangle. When this happens, the neuron loses its shape and becomes unable to transport nutrients properly; eventually, the neuron dies. The fiber tangles remain in the brain long after the dead neuron has been cleared away.

The development of abnormalities in tau protein appears to be at least a two-step process. First, damaged tau gathers in diffuse tangles and then later forms denser tangles. The diffuse tangles are found more often in the brains of people with the earlier stages of ALZHEIMER'S DISEASE. The denser, fibrillary tangles are found in those whose disease is more advanced.

Neurofibrillary tangles are one of the two findings that define Alzheimer's disease (the other is plaques in the brain). A person who displays all of the behavioral and cognitive symptoms of Alzheimer's disease cannot technically be diagnosed with the disease on autopsy without the presence of tangles and plaques in the brain. In Alzheimer's disease, neurofibrillary tangles are generally found in the neurons of the cerebral cortex and are most common in the TEMPORAL LOBE structures, such as the HIPPOCAMPUS and AMYGDALA.

Whether tau and the tangles develop before or after plaques has been a source of controversy. Recent evidence seems to suggest that the tangles arise after the plaques have done their damage, which implies that preventing the formation of plaques should also prevent the formation of neurofibrillary tangles. This conclusion, however, has not yet been proven.

The tangles were first described by German neuropathologist ALOIS ALZHEIMER in 1906.

neurofibromatosis A group of genetic disorders that trigger the growth of tumors along various types of nerves. The disease also can affect the development of bones and skin, and also can lead to developmental abnormalities, such as LEARNING DISABILITIES. The condition was first described by Dr. Friedrich von Recklinghausen in 1882, when it was called von Recklinghausen's disease. Today, the condition has been classified into two distinct types: NF1 and NF2.

Neurofibromatosis 1 (NF1), also known as von Recklinghausen NF or peripheral NF, occurs in one of every 4,000 births and is characterized by multiple cafe-au-lait spots and neurofibromas on or under the skin. Enlargement and deformities of bones and curvature of the spine also may occur. Occasionally, tumors may develop in the brain, on cranial nerves, or on the spinal cord. About half of patients with NF also have learning disabilities.

Neurofibromatosis 2 (NF2), also known as bilateral acoustic NF (BAN), is much rarer, occurring in one of every 40,000 births. NF2 is characterized by multiple tumors on the cranial and spinal nerves, and by other lesions of the brain and spinal cord. Tumors often affect both auditory nerves, which is why hearing loss beginning in the teens or early twenties is generally the first symptom.

NF in either form is an autosomal dominant genetic disorder; it may be inherited from a parent who has the disease, or it can be caused by a new or spontaneous mutation in the sperm or egg cell. Each child of a parent with NF has a 50 percent chance of inheriting the gene and developing NF. The type of NF inherited by the child is always the same as that of the affected parent, although the severity and the symptoms may differ from person to person within a family.

NF2 is caused by a single mutant gene on chromosome 22, causing the development of acoustic neuromas in almost all people who carry the gene. About 90 percent of those with the NF2 gene develop bilateral acoustic neuromas, and about half have other nervous system tumors. Hormones and growth factors may play a role in the initiation and subsequent growth pattern of acoustic neuromas. Pregnancy is often associated with the onset of symptoms or worsening of existing symptoms, and women are thought to have more problems in general as well as larger and more vascular tumors.

When the gene is transmitted by the mother, the onset of the disorder tends to be earlier. Tumors that develop in the central nervous system involve the sensory nerves, known to be the attachment sites for the female hormone estrogen. So far it has not been possible to document a specific role for estrogen or other hormones in people with NF2.

Symptoms and Diagnostic Path

Patients with NF2 are at a high risk for developing brain tumors, and almost all affected individuals develop tumors on both nerves to the ears (the eighth cranial nerve). The early symptoms of NF2 are the result of dysfunction of the hearing nerve, which carries information about sound to the brain, and the vestibular nerve, which carries balance information to the brain. The first symptoms include hearing loss, ringing in the ears (tinnitus), and problems with balance, beginning in the teens or early twenties. Although tumors on the eighth cranial nerve are most common, persons with NF2 can develop tumors on other nerves as well. These tumors are called Schwannomas because they arise from "Schwann cells," which protect and insulate nerve cells. The symptoms of a Schwannoma depend on its location—those that begin on cranial nerves affect the head and neck unless they grow large enough to push on the base of the brain and affect the body. Those that grow on the nerves as they exit the spinal cord may cause numbness of a part of the body; some tumors may grow large enough to press on the spinal cord and cause weakness and numbness in the legs. Those that grow in the bundles of nerves gathered in the armpits and groin area may cause weakness in one arm or leg. Schwannomas may even grow in tiny nerves in the skin where they can be seen. These peripheral Schwannomas rarely cause neurological symptoms, but they may rub on clothing or be cosmetically disfiguring.

Other symptoms of NF2 may include facial weakness, headache, vision changes, and swelling under the skin caused by the development of a neurofibroma.

In a family member at risk for NF2, the condition is suspected if mild symptoms of NF are found, such as a small lump under the scalp or skin. For NF2, improved diagnostic technologies such as MAGNETIC RESONANCE IMAGING (MRI) scans can reveal tumors as small as a few millimeters in diameter, thus allowing early treatment. Once someone has been diagnosed with NF2, a number of tests may be helpful to define its nature and progression. The two most common tests are MRI and a hearing test. MRI scans are used most often to visualize the brain, although they may also be used to show the spine or nerves in the arms and legs. Although MRI scans can show what a person's body looks like, they cannot show how well the body is working. Hearing tests can reveal how well the hearing portion of the eighth cranial nerve is working. Repeated hearing tests can determine if the functional aspects of a tumor are changing.

Treatment Options and Outlook

Surgery can help some NF1 bone malformations and remove painful or disfiguring tumors, but the tumors may grow back in even greater numbers. In the rare case of a malignancy (3 to 5 percent), treatment may include surgery, radiation, or chemotherapy.

Since the tumors of NF2 lie on nerves near the brain and spinal cord, surgical removal can be risky. Surgery in these small and delicate areas may further injure nerves and cause other neurological problems.

For NF2, better diagnostic technologies (such as MRI scanning) can reveal even tiny tumors, allowing earlier treatment. Other options include surgery to remove tumors completely (which may cause hearing loss), partial removal of tumors, and radiation. If the tumors are not growing fast, some doctors prefer the conservative approach of watchful waiting.

When surgery is no longer an option for a particular person because of medical problems or the size or location of a tumor, radiation may be considered, but it too has both risks and benefits.

In some cases of NF2, the damage to nearby vital structures (such as other cranial nerves and the brain stem) can be life threatening.

Risk Factors and Preventive Measures

Genetic testing is available for families with documented cases of NF1 and NF2; spontaneous mutations cannot be confirmed genetically. A prenatal diagnosis of familial NF1 or NF2 is also possible using amniocentesis or chorionic villus sampling procedures.

neuroglial cells Special cells that are packed around and between the NEURONS, helping to support the delicate nervous tissue. The neuroglial ("nerve glue") cells make up about half the volume of the brain; in addition to support for neurons, they regulate the ionic environment outside neurons. Ionic balance is critical to electrical function.

neurohormone A hormone that acts as a NEUROTRANSMITTER, such as adrenaline (epinephrine).

neuroleptic malignant syndrome (NMS) An uncommon, extremely dangerous reaction to antipsychotic drugs.

Symptoms and Diagnostic Path

It is characterized by sudden high fever with sweating, high blood pressure, delirium, muscle rigidity, racing heart, breathing problems, and feelings of impending doom.

Its exact cause is still unknown, but scientists do know that the main problem comes from high doses of antipsychotic drugs—especially when the drugs are given quickly or injected.

The exact incidence of neuroleptic malignant syndrome is unknown, but several large studies suggest that the incidence rate is about one in 500 to 1,000 patients treated with antipsychotics.

Certain factors may be linked to the risk of NMS, including

- dehydration
- agitation
- catatonia
- mood disorders
- organic brain syndrome
- withdrawal
- the use of rapid dose escalation

Antipsychotic medication can be given again to most patients despite one episode of NMS; usually, the drugs are given at least two weeks after recovery, beginning with a low dose that is gradually increased. Vital signs should be monitored daily and levels of creatine phosphokinase measured once or twice in the first two weeks.

Treatment Options and Outlook

Once neuroleptic symptoms appear, antipsychotic drug administration should be stopped, and symptoms treated. Untreated, the condition has a mortality rate of nearly 30 percent. Early diagnosis can reduce the death rate.

Risk Factors and Preventive Measures

Health care workers should monitor the patient's fluid intake, blood levels of iron, lithium, blood urea nitrogen (BUN), and creatinine. The room should be kept cool and high doses of antipsychotics should be avoided.

neurolinguistics The study of how information is received through the senses, processed in the NEU-RONS and neural pathways of the brain (especially the language areas), and expressed in language and behaviors.

neurological exam A simple systematic assessment of the function of various parts of the NERVOUS SYSTEM that can be performed in a neurologist's office and causes no pain.

Procedure

The most important part of a neurological exam is the description of symptoms and how they developed. Some of the routine tests for nervous system function include tendon REFLEXES, Babinski reflexes, muscle strength, muscle tone, sensory function, and mental status.

Tendon reflexes can be tested by tapping the knee with a rubber-tipped hammer. This test evaluates motor-nerve function, spinal cord connections, and peripheral-nerve conditions. Light stroking of the underside of the foot may produce an involuntary movement of the big toe, called the Babinski reflex; this can suggest an abnormality in the nerve tracts that originate in the brain. Because muscle weakness can be a manifestation of neurological disorder, tests of muscle strength may be part of a neurological exam. To test muscle tone, the physician moves the arm or leg and assesses ease and range of movement. Both legs may be tested, for example, to check for differences between the two sides of the body. Spas-

ticity, rigidity, or flaccidity may suggest problems in the nerves controlling different muscle groups.

Because sensations of pain, heat, and touch travel through the sensory nerves to the central nervous system, sensory tests are an important part of a neurological exam. The sensory functions can be tested by asking patients what they feel when the skin is touched by a pinprick, a hot or cold object, or a tuning fork. Because nervous system disorders can affect the eyes and the senses of taste, hearing, and smell, tests of these senses can be important. Eye testing is especially useful; pupil size and difference in size, range of eye movement, gaze, and field of vision can help diagnose disturbances in nerves affecting vision.

Physicians will also evaluate gait, posture, coordination, and sense of balance by assessing a patient's ability to stand, walk, or move the body in a particular way.

Finally, a patient's mental status may be evaluated by asking questions to determine orientation in place and time and to determine whether judgment or memory are disturbed.

Risks and Complications

There are no risks to the exam.

neurological manifestations of AIDS Acquired immunodeficiency syndrome (AIDS) is caused by infection with the HIV virus that attacks selected cells, and which may cause damage to the brain and spinal cord. This may lead to ENCEPHALITIS (inflammation of the brain), MENINGITIS (inflammation of the membranes surrounding the brain), nerve damage, difficulties in thinking (AIDS DEMENTIA COMPLEX), behavioral changes, poor circulation, headache, and STROKE. AIDS-related cancers such as lymphoma and opportunistic infections may also affect the nervous system.

Symptoms and Diagnostic Path

Neurological symptoms may be mild in the early stages of AIDS, but may become severe in the final stages. Complications vary widely from one patient to another. Cerebral toxoplasmosis, a common problem in AIDS patients, causes such symptoms as headache, confusion, lethargy, and low-grade fever. Other symptoms may include weakness, speech disturbance, seizures, and sensory loss. Progressive multifocal leukoencephalopathy (PML), a disorder that can also occur in AIDS patients, causes weakness and vision loss. Some patients with PML may also develop problems with memory and cognition.

Treatment Options and Outlook

There is no cure for AIDS, but new experimental treatments appear promising. Some symptoms and complications may improve with treatment. For example, antidementia drugs may relieve confusion and slow mental decline, and infections may be treated with antibiotics. Radiation therapy may be needed to treat AIDS-related cancers present in the brain or spinal cord. Neurological complications of AIDS are often underrecognized by AIDS clinicians, so patients who suspect they are having neurological complications should discuss these with their doctor.

The prognosis for individuals with AIDS in recent years has improved significantly because of new drugs and treatments, and educational and preventive efforts.

neurologist A specialist in the diagnosis and treatment of diseases and disorders of the nervous system, including diseases of the brain, spinal cord, nerves, and muscles. Neurologists conduct examinations (such as ELECTROENCEPHALOGRAPHY or LUMBAR PUNCTURE) of patients' nerves, reflexes, motor and sensory functions, and muscles to determine the cause and extent of a problem.

A neurologist can perform detailed examinations of all the neurological structures in the body, including the nerves of the head and neck, muscular strength and movement, sensation, balance, and reflexes. In some cases, detailed questions about memory, speech, and language and other cognitive functions are part of the examination.

Neurologists also use other common tests, including CAT SCANS (computerized axial tomography) and MAGNETIC RESONANCE IMAGING (MRI) scans to provide detailed pictures of the brain, spinal structures, and blood vessels. A neurologist can also perform a lumbar puncture (spinal tap) to obtain

a patient's cerebrospinal fluid for analysis. Some neurologists interpret EEG (electroencephalography) used in the evaluation of seizure disorders, or perform the EMG/NCV (electromyography/nerve conduction velocity tests) to diagnose nerve and muscle problems.

In addition, neurologists use many types of drugs to treat problems involving the nervous system. A neurologist may send a patient for a surgical evaluation, but does not perform surgery.

A neurologist must complete a four-year premedical university degree and four years of medical school. This is followed by at least three years of specialty training in an accredited neurology residency program. After residency training, neurologists may choose to enroll in a one- or two-year fellowship which offers the opportunity to focus on a subspecialty of neurology, such as stroke, dementia, or movement disorders.

After completing the educational requirements, neurologists may seek certification from the American Board of Psychiatry and Neurology (ABPN). To be eligible for certification, an applicant must be a licensed physician with the required years of residency who has passed both a written and oral exam administered by the ABPN.

neurology A medical specialty concerned with the diagnosis and treatment of functional or organic disorders of the BRAIN, SPINAL CORD, and nerves. The science of neurology has developed over the past 200 years, beginning with the study of nerve function in animals during the 18th century by Stephen Hales and Robert Whytt. However, it was not until the mid-19th century that clinical neurology was first studied. During this period, new information was learned about the causes of APHASIA, EPILEPSY, and motor problems caused by BRAIN DAMAGE.

When the ELECTROENCEPHALOGRAPH was invented in the 1920s by Hans Berger, the ability to record electrical brain activity improved the diagnosis of neurological disease. Together with the analysis of CEREBROSPINAL FLUID and the development of cerebral angiography, neurologists were able to more precisely diagnose and treat brain problems.

In the early 1970s, the development of CAT SCANS and of MAGNETIC RESONANCE IMAGING (MRI) in the 1980s yielded detailed views of the inside of the brain, which further improved the diagnosis of brain disease.

neuroma   A benign tumor of nerve tissue that may affect any nerve in the body, usually from an unknown cause. Occasionally, a neuroma develops after a nerve injury.

See also ACOUSTIC NEUROMA.

neurometrics   A method for diagnosing brain disorders by comparing AUDITORY EVOKED POTENTIALS (AEP) from several different regions of the brain with tracings taken from normal, healthy human brains.

neuron   Another name for *nerve cell,* a neuron is the basic functional unit of the NERVOUS SYSTEM. In the brain, neurons are responsible for information processing, converting chemical signals to electrical signals and then back to chemical signals again.

There are about 50 million neurons in the CERE-BRAL CORTEX, 40 billion more in the CEREBELLUM, and another 10 billion in the rest of the brain and SPINAL CORD—about the same as there are stars in the galaxy.

The average number of neurons varies dramatically from one person to the next and seems to have nothing to do with general intelligence (some animals have more neurons than humans do). Apparently, quantity is less important than the quality of the connections between them.

There are two kinds of neurons—motor and sensory. Motor neurons are concerned with movement, and sensory neurons receive impulses from receptors in the eyes, skin, muscles, joints, and organs.

A neuron consists of a compact cell body made up of the nucleus, many long branched extensions (DENDRITES), and a long fiber (the AXON) with twig-like extensions at its end. Neurons are the major type of cell that makes up the brain and nervous system, carrying signals to and from the brain and performing all of the brain's work. Each neuron receives electrical impulses through dendrites, which lie adjacent to one another in a gigantic web whose tiny branches direct signals toward the body of the nerve cell.

If enough arriving signals stimulate the neuron, the neuron fires, sending this electrical pulse down its axon, which connects through synapses into the dendrites of other cells.

Information is carried inside a neuron by electrical pulses, but once the signal reaches the end of the axon it must be carried across the synaptic gap by chemicals called NEUROTRANSMITTERS. On the other side of the synapse is another dendrite, containing RECEPTORS that recognize these transmitting molecules. In a series of complicated steps, the receptor biochemically opens an ionic channel. Charged ions pass through this open channel; the movement of ions generates an electrical current which changes the voltage of the post-synaptic neuron. If the shift is positive enough, this neuron will fire an action potential of its own.

At the same time, the first neuron emits enzymes into the cleft that terminate the transmission and reabsorb any excess transmitter chemicals left in the synapse.

A single neuron can receive signals from thousands of other neurons, and its axon can branch repeatedly, sending signals to thousands more. While researchers have long understood the mechanism of neurons, it is only recently that they have begun to understand how these cells might be able to store memories.

Most researchers agree that when a person experiences a new event, a unique pattern of neurons is activated in some way and within the entire configuration of brain cells, certain cells "light up." Unlike the wiring in the home, however, the brain's circuits are not permanent; as knowledge is acquired, circuits break apart and reform, constantly rewriting themselves and influencing our representations in the world.

The amazing ability of brain cells to make just the right connections may have been gained at the expense of their ability to reproduce; almost all other cells in the body can regenerate, and when these cells die they are replaced by others. Only in the brain are cells irreplaceable. Humans are born with almost all of the brain cells they will ever have, and those that die (about 18 million a year between ages 20 and 70) are lost forever.

By about age 12, through a process called "pruning," children will lose many of the synapses with which they were born. Pruning is the brain's way of getting rid of unneeded synapses and strengthening those that are needed. For example, in a Japanese child, the synapses necessary to make an *R* sound would be pruned, because *R* is not used in the Japanese language.

At the same time, as a child responds to the environment, useful synaptic connections increase. The more connections, the more myelination, and therefore the stronger the brain structure becomes—and the stronger the brain structure, the better the child can learn new skills.

neuronal migration disorders (NMDs) A group of birth defects caused by the abnormal movement of neurons in the developing brain and nervous system from areas where they arise to the areas where they should settle into their proper neural circuits. This occurs as early as the second month of gestation, controlled by a complex group of chemical signals. However, if these signals are incorrect, neurons do not go to the right place, which can result in structurally abnormal or missing areas of the brain in the cerebral hemispheres, cerebellum, brain stem, or hippocampus.

The structural problems found in NMDs include SCHIZENCEPHALY, PORENCEPHALY, lissencephaly, agyria, macrogyria, pachygyria, microgyria, micropolygyria, neuronal heterotopias (including band heterotopia), agenesis of the CORPUS CALLOSUM, and agenesis of the CRANIAL NERVES.

Symptoms and Diagnostic Path

Symptoms vary according to the abnormality, but often feature poor muscle tone and motor function, seizures, developmental delays, mental retardation, failure to grow and thrive, difficulties with feeding, swelling in the extremities, and a smaller than normal head. Most infants with an NMD appear normal, but some disorders have characteristic facial or skull features that can be recognized by a neurologist.

Treatment Options and Outlook

There is no cure, but symptoms can be treated, and may include antiseizure medication and special or supplemental education with physical, occupational, and speech therapies. The prognosis for children with NMDs varies depending on the specific disorder and the degree of brain abnormality and subsequent neurological losses.

Risk Factors and Preventive Measures

Several genetic abnormalities in children with NMDs have been identified. Defects in genes that are involved in neuronal migration have been associated with NMDs, but the role they play in the development of these disorders is not yet well understood. Of the more than 25 syndromes linked to abnormal neuronal migration that have been described, among them are syndromes with several different patterns of inheritance. Genetic counseling thus differs greatly among syndromes.

neuropathology A neurology specialty concerned with the causes and effects of neurological conditions instead of their diagnosis and treatment, which is usually handled by a NEUROLOGIST or a NEUROSURGEON.

neuropathy Any disease of the peripheral nerves. Also called neuritis, it refers to a disease or damage to the peripheral nerves which connect to the BRAIN and SPINAL CORD, to the sense organs, muscles, glands, and internal organs.

Most neuropathies occur from damage or irritation to the AXONS (the conducting fibers that make up nerves) or to the fatty substance called MYELIN that insulates the axons. An axon's myelin sheath may suffer damage ranging from thinning to total loss, which may either slow or completely block the passage of electric signals.

Some cases of neuropathy may have no obvious cause; other instances may be triggered by dietary deficiencies, diabetes, alcoholism, surgery, and so on. Nerves may also become acutely inflamed after a viral infection, such as in GUILLAIN-BARRÉ SYNDROME, or they may result from autoimmune disorders like systemic lupus erythematosus. They may also be found secondary to cancerous tumors such as lung cancer or lymphomas. A group of neuropathies may also be inherited.

Symptoms and Diagnostic Path

It is characterized by numbness and weakness, pain or tingling, depending on which nerves are affected. Precise symptoms depend on whether the affected nerve fibers are sensory or MOTOR NERVES. Sensory nerve damage may cause sensations of cold, numbness, and tingling, whereas motor damage may lead to muscle wasting and weakness. AUTONOMIC NERVOUS SYSTEM damage may cause blurred vision, sweating problems, faintness, and problems with stomach, bladder, intestinal, or sexual functions.

Treatment Options and Outlook

Treating the underlying disorder will help symptoms. If treatment is successful and the damaged nerve cells contain intact cell bodies, a full recovery from neuropathy is possible.

neuropeptides Connected sequences of proteins. First discovered in 1975 by John Hughes and Hans Kosterlitz, two Scottish drug addiction researchers. The two were looking for an internally produced chemical similar to opiate drugs that would plug into existing opiate receptors and trigger the body's own built-in pain-relief system.

The existence of such receptors had been suggested in 1972 by Stanford University psychopharmacologist Avram Goldstein, and was verified in 1973 by Johns Hopkins University researchers Solomon Snyder and Candace Pert. Goldstein suggested that the brain must contain receptors for opiate narcotics since the drugs were able to affect the brain and central nervous system.

Kosterlitz and Hughes discovered an unknown substance they called enkephalin, from the Greek words for "in the head," where it was produced. After analyzing ENKEPHALIN's structure, they discovered that the substance was actually two substances—amino acid chains known as PEPTIDES. Enkephalins were often included under the generic term *endorphins* after the 1975 discovery of the beta-endorphin molecule.

Very quickly, researchers found that the neuropeptides were involved in many activities, from aging to painkilling. Scientists today believe that neuropeptides can be divided into three main categories: enkephalin (two of which, leu-enkephalin and met-enkephalin, were discovered by Hughes and Kosterlitz); beta-endorphin (a large 31-acid molecule that long served as a basic prototype for understanding the neuropeptides); and dynorphin, a substance discovered in 1979 that has much more powerful effects than either enkephalin or simple endorphin.

Although similar to neurotransmitters in a number of ways, neuropeptides are different in that they are made up exclusively of amino acids, rather than inorganic chemical compounds. And while neurotransmitters seem to be a transmission medium for brain messages, neuropeptides seem to be the message itself.

The neuropeptides are found in great numbers in the brain, especially in the LIMBIC SYSTEM, which is the emotional center of the brain. Although more than 20 separate peptides have been identified, most researchers believe hundreds more will be identified in the future.

neuropharmacology See PSYCHOPHARMACOLOGY.

neuropsychiatry The branch of medicine that involves the study, diagnosis, and treatment of disorders caused by organic or physical defects in the brain. In addition, neuropsychiatry is concerned with subtle forms of BRAIN DAMAGE that may underlie psychotic illness. This could include conditions such as TRAUMATIC BRAIN INJURY, cerebral vascular disease, seizure disorders, neurodegenerative diseases (such as ALZHEIMER'S DISEASE or PARKINSON'S DISEASE), brain tumors, infectious and inflammatory diseases of the central nervous system (CNS), alcohol-induced mental disorders, and developmental disorders involving the brain.

Generally, neuropsychiatrists use medication to treat neuropsychiatric disorders and use very specialized equipment to determine the degree of physical defects in the brain. To a greater degree than most psychiatrists, neuropsychiatrists are able to determine specifically what medications should be used and what their effects might be, as opposed to trying various medications on an experimental basis.

Technically speaking, all psychiatrists can present themselves as "neuropsychiatrists" because board certification for psychiatrists includes a joint certification in both psychiatry and neurology. However, the American Board of Psychiatry and Neurology issues certificates based on two different tests. Most practicing psychiatrists pass board exams which ask two-thirds of their questions on psychiatry and one-third on neurology. A neuropsychiatrist has passed the test version which devotes two-thirds of its questions to neurology.

neuropsychological assessment Tests that can evaluate the extent of BRAIN DAMAGE and MEMORY deficits, including assessment of language, memory, perception, reasoning, emotion, self-control, and planning. This kind of testing was first used as a way to distinguish between those whose abnormal behavior was caused by brain dysfunction and those whose problems were caused by psychological factors. Disorders caused by brain dysfunction are called organic; psychological disorders are referred to as functional or psychogenic.

Early tests were based on the assumption that there were common characteristics in all organic impairments and gave a general assessment of "organicity" instead of details about the status of different mental functions.

Although the idea of brain damage as a single concept persists, in fact there is not one simple test that can uncover the often-diffuse problems experienced by those who have brain problems. Because brain damage may cover lesions of different sizes and shapes, different causes in different areas of the brain, uncovering the evidence requires a more sophisticated, comprehensive assessment. In order to properly rehabilitate a patient with brain deficits, it is imperative to have a clear picture of the patient's cognitive strengths and weaknesses to help choose the treatment technique and to measure response to treatment.

neuropsychologist A clinical psychologist with special training in NEUROLOGY as well as intensive training in psychological assessment. The relationship of NEUROPSYCHOLOGY to other neurosciences is an evolving one and may include not only identifying patients who are BRAIN injured, but may also define the nature and extent of brain damage, assess treatment programs and patients' progress, and may plan rehabilitation programs.

A clinical neuropsychologist may enter private practice and offer various forms of psychotherapy and cognitive rehabilitation to individuals, families, or groups, and can administer standardized psychological and neuropsychological tests and interpret and report on their results. Neuropsychologists may furnish legally recognized clinical and diagnostic opinions and conduct diagnostic interviews about the presence, scope, and treatment of cognitive/neuropsychological disorders, behavioral disorders, and mental illness.

A neuropsychologist and a neurologist differ in several ways. A neurologist is a physician (M.D.) who deals with the structural and physiological consequences of brain injury and organic brain disease, while a neuropsychologist (Ph.D) investigates the cognitive and behavioral impact of these conditions.

For example, for a person who suffers serious BRAIN DAMAGE after a bike accident, a neurologist would assess the physical impact of injuries—can the patient walk, move muscles, and maintain hand/eye coordination? The neuropsychologist would test the person's ability to think and reason clearly and check for memory loss or reading, learning, and comprehension problems.

neuropsychology The clinical and experimental discipline within the field of psychology devoted to the study, understanding, assessment, and treatment of behavior directly related to the function of the brain. While NEUROPSYCHOLOGISTS work most often with those whose brains are abnormal, they also investigate individual differences within normal people due to different brain functions or organization.

Neuropsychology is a field somewhere between psychology and NEUROLOGY, closely related to behavioral neurology. Many experts in the field are trained by neurologists in medical settings instead of receiving primary training in psychology.

Experimental neuropsychology deals with both human and animal models and tries to identify the relationship between the brain and behavior. While the fields of clinical and experimental neuropsychology may seem to be similar, the goals of the two are significantly different. While clinical neuropsychology tries to find rules and procedures effective with large numbers of patients with poorly defined disorders, experimental neuropsychology works with patients who have precisely determined disorders as a way of exploring brain-behavior relationships.

neurosurgeon A physician who specializes in surgery involving the brain and nerves, using laser-powered scalpels, operating microscopes, and a range of other technological aids.

Neurosurgeons diagnose, evaluate, treat, and rehabilitate patients with neurological disorders. Because they have extensive training in the diagnosis of all neurological diseases, they are often called upon by emergency room doctors, neurologists, internists, and family doctors for consultations.

Neurosurgeons are more than brain surgeons; they are trained to help patients with head and spine trauma, cerebrovascular disorders, such as brain aneurysms and clogged arteries in the neck that can lead to stroke, chronic low back pain, birth defects, brain and spinal tumors, and abnormalities of the peripheral nerves. Disorders of the brain, spine, and nerves that neurosurgeons often treat range from carpal tunnel syndrome, chronic pain, EPILEPSY, HEAD INJURY, HYDROCEPHALUS, PARKINSON'S DISEASE, SPINA BIFIDA, SPINAL CORD INJURY, STROKE, and tumors.

After four years of medical school and an internship program, the doctor who wants to be a neurosurgeon enters a neurosurgical residency program lasting from five to seven years. While in the program, neurosurgical residents are trained in all aspects of neurosurgery, including cerebrovascular, pediatrics, spine, trauma, and tumor. Some neurosurgeons choose an additional fellowship in a particular area of study after their residency. After residency training and several years in practice, the neurosurgeon may take the American Board of Neurological Surgery examination to become board certified.

neurosurgery The diagnosis and surgical treatment of disorders of the brain, spine, or peripheral nerves. While neurosurgery is ineffective against many generalized NERVOUS SYSTEM disorders (such as MULTIPLE SCLEROSIS), it can be effective against nerve failure due to specific structural changes.

Conditions that may respond to neurosurgery include HEAD INJURY, brain ABSCESSES, tumors, abnormalities of the blood vessels supplying the brain, bleeding inside the skull, some birth defects (such as HYDROCEPHALUS), intracranial pressure, SPINAL CORD compression, intracranial hemorrhage, and nerve damage caused by illness or accidents. NEUROSURGEONS also are involved in the surgical treatment of intractable pain.

The development of neurosurgery has been aided by improvements in anesthesia, scanning techniques, radiology, and antiseptics.

neurosyphilis Infection of the brain or SPINAL CORD that occurs in untreated SYPHILIS many years after first infection. Spinal cord damage from this disorder may cause poor coordination, urinary incontinence, and abdominal and limb pain. Infection in the brain may lead to DEMENTIA, muscle weakness and, sometimes, extensive neurological damage (called "general paralysis of the insane").

neurotensin A painkilling NEUROTRANSMITTER.

neurotoxic drugs Any drug that causes damage to the nervous system. (See also NEUROTOXIN.)

neurotoxin A poisonous or destructive compound that damages nervous tissue. While hundreds of substances have neurotoxic properties, the most common are heavy metals, solvents, pesticides, and drugs (such as alcohol, street drugs, and prescription drugs). Neurotoxins also can be found in the venom of some snakes, and they are released by some types of bacteria, such as those that cause tetanus.

Metals recognized as neurotoxins include lead, mercury, and manganese; industrial settings are common sites for metal neurotoxic poisoning. Fungicides containing mercury have caused mass poisonings; mercuric chloride wastes, which appear as methyl mercury in fish and shellfish, led to serious outbreaks in Japan. Manganese intoxication in the United States has been recognized among those who work in mining, ore crushing, and ferromanganese alloy industries, primarily from inhaling dust particles or fumes. Toxicity may appear four months to 15 years after exposure.

Solvents found in some industries may cause characteristic nerve damage; some harmful solvents include n-hexane, methyl-n-butyl ketone, and toluene.

The actual numbers of neurotoxins in the environment vary widely. Of the 65,000 industrial chemicals registered with the Environmental Protection Agency, for example, estimates range from a low of 2,000 (between 3 and 5 percent) to 18,000 (28 percent). The March of Dimes estimates that between 5 and 10 percent of birth defects are caused by environmental effects, but they have no estimates on the number of neurological birth defects caused by neurotoxins.

Gases including carbon monoxide and methyl chloride have neurotoxic effects, and as many as 39 separate insecticide compounds account for a large number of poisonings among farm workers.

Most commercial products have not been tested for neurotoxicity, which means that permissible exposure limits (PEL) have not even been set.

The hallmarks of neurotoxicity are mood and personality changes, but other symptoms may vary depending on what control centers in the brain are damaged. Symptoms may include memory problems, emotional changes, or physical damage (such as brain swelling). Other symptoms of neurotoxic nerve damage are weakness, numbness, or paralysis of a part of the body served by the affected nerve.

Lead, the most significant environmental hazard, according to the Environmental Protection Agency (EPA) causes a range of symptoms including LEARNING DISABILITIES. Solvents may cause symptoms within two months of exposure and include muscle weakness, sensitivity to touch, slowed MOTOR and SENSORY NERVE function, impaired mental functions, toxic mood disorders, and severe manic depression. Exposure to mercury (a metal that damages a variety of brain areas) may cause cerebellar disorders, irritability, visual problems, deafness, mental

disturbances, ANXIETY, and HALLUCINATIONS or delirium. Manganese toxicity causes apathy, memory problems, progressive problems with walking and motor control, and speech disturbances. Chronic disorders may remain indefinitely.

Neurotoxins interfere with the performance of the NERVOUS SYSTEM—that delicate network of cells that process information transmitted from sensory organs. The nervous system also controls all the body's major functions, including personality, mood, and thought; even a minor interference with the system can have significant effects on everyday performance. Neurotoxins can be inhaled, ingested, or absorbed through the skin, mucous membranes, and the conjunctiva of the eyes. Once ingested, the effects depend on the type of neurotoxin involved, the amount ingested, frequency of exposure, and whether exposure is chronic or acute.

Neurotoxins damage the nervous system by disrupting the NEURONS, their MYELIN nerve sheath that covers the neuron, or the NEUROTRANSMITTERS (chemical messengers in the brain). The nervous system is especially vulnerable to damage because neurons cannot regenerate once they are lost. In addition, certain brain regions and nerves in the brain are directly exposed to chemicals in the blood, and many neurotoxic substances readily cross the BLOOD-BRAIN BARRIER. Finally, because the nervous system depends on a delicate electrochemical balance, it is not hard for neurotoxic substances to interfere with function.

Neurotoxicity is extremely hard to diagnose because the brain feels no pain and because the brain is responsible for such a wide variety of functions that low-level toxicity may go unnoticed. Mental, behavioral, or nervous systems may be attributed not to neurotoxicity but to aging or psychological causes, and the public is often not aware that commercial products can in fact affect brain function.

There are specific blood and urine tests for neurotoxins. Testing for most substances with hair samples is considered inconclusive and experimental. While hair sample tests have been proven unreliable, some physicians and commercial labs still use this test.

The developing fetus is particularly sensitive to neurotoxins because its nervous system is in the process of growing, dividing, and making important connections and because the blood-brain barrier is not yet fully formed. In later stages of fetal development and after birth, exposure to alcohol or lead, for example, can lead to lowered intelligence levels, motor or sensory problems, learning disabilities, and behavior problems. During childhood, the nervous system is still in a state of rapid development, and young children are still vulnerable to neurotoxin damage.

The elderly are also at risk for damage from neurotoxins because of structural and chemical changes in the body beginning at about age 60. Aging leads to a natural decrease in nerve cells, and exposure to neurotoxins can speed up this process of attrition. Aging also alters the way the body metabolizes drugs and chemicals, and a neurotoxin that may have only a slight impact on a younger adult can have a far more serious effect on an elderly person.

In addition, employees of neurotoxic chemical companies are particularly vulnerable to neurological diseases if they do not take proper precautions. Because of this, federal regulations require that protective measures (such as ventilation systems or protective clothing) be used. Unfortunately, some companies ignore the law, some employees may ignore the rules, and some protective systems fail. In addition, the neurotoxic properties of many substances have not yet been adequately studied. For these reasons, neurological disturbances are one of the 10 major forms of occupational hazards, according to the National Institute of Occupational Safety and Health.

While the National Institute of Occupational Safety and Health (NIOSH) recognizes that neurotoxicity is a major cause of occupational disease, it has established safety standards for only 72 substances specifically related to neurotoxicity. Moreover, the EPA tends to concentrate on cancer-causing substances and has issued only a few regulations specifically limiting the use of chemicals for their neurotoxic potential. This lack of regulatory control may be due in part to the fact that the field of neurotoxicity is fairly new; it did not exist as a formal area of study until the early 1970s.

Workers who experience risk of neurotoxic chemical exposure include agricultural employees, degreasers, dentists, dry cleaners, electronics workers, hospital workers, lab workers, painters, plastics workers, printers, rayon workers, steelworkers, transportation workers, and hobbyists.

See also ALZHEIMER'S DISEASE; DEMENTIA; HEADACHES; NEUROTOXIC DRUGS; PARKINSON'S DISEASE; PERIPHERAL NEUROPATHY; TOXIC ENCEPHALOPATHY; TOXIC MOOD DISORDERS.

neurotransmitter A chemical released at the SYNAPSE (space between neurons) that relays a signal from one NERVE CELL to another. When a neurotransmitter is released into the synapse, it moves across the space and attaches to a RECEPTOR in the membrane of a neighboring NEURON. Some neurotransmitters stimulate the release of neurotransmitters from other neurons, while others inhibit the release of neurotransmitters.

Neurons responsible for the same functions contain the same kinds of neurotransmitters; for example, neurons responsible for moving muscles all contain ACETYLCHOLINE, whereas all those in charge of hunger contain NOREPINEPHRINE. In addition, there are both *excitatory* and INHIBITORY neurotransmitters in the brain. Excitatory neurotransmitters include acetylcholine, EPINEPHRINE, norepinephrine, and SEROTONIN; inhibitory neurotransmitters include ENDORPHINS and ENKEPHALINS, gamma-aminobutyric acid (GABA), SUBSTANCE P, and gylcine.

NEUROTRANSMITTER	ACTION
acetylcholine	Affects: short-term memory, thirst, body temperature, motor function
epinephrine (adrenaline)	Affects: fight-or-flight response
norepinephrine	Affects: long-term memory, hunger, sleep/wake cycle
serotonin	Affects: emotions, sleep, satiety
endorphins/enkephalins	Affects: emotions, pain, pleasure, appetite
GABA	Affects: everything
substance P	Affects: pain

Neurotransmitters are made from the protein in food; this protein is first broken down in the stomach and intestines into smaller substances called AMINO ACIDS. These amino acids enter the blood, where they are absorbed by the brain, which uses the amino acids to make neurotransmitters. It is the correct balance of the neurotransmitters in the brain that is responsible for proper function. Any deficiencies in nutrients will upset the level of certain neurotransmitters and interfere with the behaviors or actions for which they are responsible. On the other hand, a problem (such as DEPRESSION) can be corrected by altering the balance of the neurotransmitters; this is precisely what antidepressant medication is designed to do. Different neurotransmitters are manufactured by different nutrients in the diet; therefore, too much or too little of any one nutrient may lead to an abnormal level of neurotransmitters in the brain.

The most common neurotransmitters include acetylcholine, norepinephrine, dopamine, GABA, and serotonin.

New Adult Reading Test (NART) A list of 50 words of increasing difficulty that can establish pre-brain damage intelligence in those of high-average or superior intelligence. Psychologists trying to assess brain damage must somehow quantify loss without knowing how well the person performed before problems began. For example, a person with an IQ of 140 before BRAIN DAMAGE occurred could lose 20 or 30 points and still test as "average." If the person's previous intellectual ability was known, subsequent IQ testing would reveal a significant loss of intellectual ability.

NART was developed to take advantage of the fact that language tends to persist despite brain damage. The test was devised on the basis of research showing that patients with DEMENTIA were able to pronounce unusually spelled words (such as *ache*) despite gradual deterioration in other intellectual spheres.

Scores on this test are considered to be a good predictor of intelligence before deterioration took place in those with high-average or superior intelligence.

nicotine A stimulant drug in tobacco that causes dependence and can affect the brain; while this drug has no medical use, some of its derivatives are used as potent insecticides.

Nicotine activates a range of brain mechanisms by attaching to specific receptors found on the surface of nerve cells in many areas of the central nervous system. It can exert dramatically different actions depending on the location and type of receptor to which it attaches. Nicotine reaches the brain about eight seconds after cigarette smoke is inhaled, but it takes longer (about three to five minutes) to reach the brain when tobacco is chewed rather than smoked. However it is ingested, nicotine increases blood pressure and heart rate, speeds up breathing, constricts arteries, and stimulates the central nervous system.

Although nicotine is one of the most addictive substances known, exactly how it produces addiction and dependence is not clear. Some experts believe that nicotine affects a person's limbic pathways and that it may be responsible for at least part of the addiction.

Nicotine simultaneously activates cholinergic neurons in many different regions throughout the brain, triggering a burst of acetylcholine that causes increased activity in cholinergic pathways throughout the brain, stimulating the body and brain. Through these pathways, nicotine improves reaction time and the ability to pay attention. Stimulation of cholinergic neurons also promotes the release of the neurotransmitter dopamine in the reward pathways of the brain, triggering happy feelings. When drugs like cocaine or nicotine activate the reward pathways, the desire to use these substances is reinforced because the drug makes a person feel happy. Moreover, when a person uses nicotine, it boosts the level of glutamate (a neurotransmitter involved in learning and memory), which may create a memory of good feelings and further increase the desire to use nicotine. Nicotine also raises the level of other neurotransmitters and chemicals that modulate how the brain works. For example, the brain makes more endorphins, the body's own painkiller, in response to nicotine.

Because nicotine's effects last only 40 minutes to a few hours, users must smoke or chew tobacco periodically throughout the day to get more nicotine. In addition, people can also become tolerant of nicotine's effects, so that they need to use more and more to reach the same degree of stimulation or relaxation. As smokers use nicotine-containing products, the body begins to compensate for the effects of the nicotine. Brain cells might increase or decrease the number of receptors or the amount of different neurotransmitters affected by the presence of nicotine. When a smoker quits smoking and there is no longer any nicotine in the body, these physiological adaptations for nicotine remain. As a result, the body cannot function the same way it did before. People trying to quit nicotine experience this process as irritability, anxiety, depression, and craving for nicotine. After about a month, these symptoms and the physiological changes subside, but for many smokers, even a day without nicotine is excruciating. Every year, millions of people try to break the nicotine habit, but only 10 percent succeed.

nimodipine (Nimotop) A drug used successfully to treat symptoms of STROKE patients, which increases blood flow to injured brain tissue. It is being studied for the treatment of ALZHEIMER'S DISEASE and age-associated memory impairment. The drug prevents the constriction of muscle tissue surrounding blood vessels (especially arteries in the brain). This helps keep the arteries open, maintaining blood supply to the brain. Nimodipine also seems to increase ACETYLCHOLINE levels.

It was approved by the U.S. Food and Drug Administration in 1989 to treat hemorrhagic stroke, as it improves blood flow in the brain and lessens oxygen deprivation.

Nimodipine, a calcium channel blocker, is believed to prolong nerve cell survival in Alzheimer's disease by protecting against calcium overload.

NMDA receptor A receptor for the AMINO ACID called GLUTAMATE, which is found in every cell in the body and that plays a central role in brain function. Recent research suggests that glutamate may also be responsible for brain damage as a result of oxygen deprivation following a STROKE. NMDA is named after a synthetic form of glutamate (N-methyl-D-aspartate) used in research. NMDA receptors play heavily in learning and memory systems of the brain, and in mice helped them learn faster and remember longer.

NMR The abbreviation for nuclear magnetic resonance.

See MAGNETIC RESONANCE IMAGING.

nondominant hemisphere The brain hemisphere that is not dominant for speech.

nonverbal learning disabilities (NLD) A form of LEARNING DISABILITY that primarily affects social functioning in areas such as interpersonal skills, social perception, and interaction. Also called right-hemisphere learning disorders, this problem often goes unrecognized for a large part of a child's schooling in part because federal law does not recognize or fund special education for them. Since abnormalities of the right brain hemisphere interfere with understanding and adaptive learning, experts believe that nonverbal learning disabilities are more debilitating than verbal disabilities.

Experts suspect that nonverbal learning disabilities are caused by a problem in the right hemisphere of the brain, either from brain injury or damage before birth. The damage primarily affects visual-spatial perception, processing, and reasoning. Individuals with NLD often display significant strengths in verbal areas and may develop reading and speaking skills earlier than their peers; consequently, their nonverbal learning difficulties may be overlooked.

Nonverbal learning disorders remain predominantly misunderstood and largely unrecognized. Although NLD syndrome was discovered in the early 1970s, even today education professionals are largely unfamiliar with it. Rarely are concerns accepted until the child reaches a point in school where he or she is no longer able to function. These children are often labeled "behavior problems" or "emotionally disturbed" because of their frequent inappropriate and unexpected conduct, despite the fact that NLD has a neurological rather than an emotional origin.

It is especially important to identify children with nonverbal learning disorders because overestimates of the child's abilities and unrealistic demands made by parents and teachers can lead to ongoing emotional problems. Unfortunately, there are few resources available for the child with NLD syndrome through schools or private agencies, and it is hard to find a professional who understands nonverbal learning disabilities.

Nonverbal learning disorders are much less common than language-based learning disorders, affecting only .1 percent to 1 percent of the general population. Unlike language-based learning disabilities, NLD syndrome affects girls as often as boys. Although NLD is rare, experts suspect that as school assessment procedures improve, a higher proportion of children with NLD will be identified.

Symptoms and Diagnostic Path

Individuals with NLD may experience significant difficulties in perceiving and understanding the subtle visual cues important to nonverbal communication which form the basis of social interaction and interpersonal relations. They may misread overt signals of impatience, annoyance, or the desire to end an interaction, and consequently may respond in ways that are perceived by others as inappropriate.

A person with NLD syndrome may have trouble adapting to new situations or accurately reading nonverbal signals and cues. Although these students make progress in school, they have trouble in situations where speed and adaptability are required.

There are three categories of dysfunction

- lack of coordination, severe balance problems, or difficulties with fine motor skills
- lack of image, poor visual recall, faulty spatial perceptions, or difficulties with spatial relations
- lack of ability to understand nonverbal communication, trouble adjusting to new situations, or significant problems with social judgment and social interaction

Children with nonverbal learning disorders often appear awkward and uncoordinated in both fine and gross motor skills. They may have extreme difficulty in learning to ride a bike or kick a soccer ball. Fine motor skills, such as cutting with scissors or tying shoelaces, seem to be impossible for them. Young children with NLD are less likely to explore their environment because they cannot rely on their own perceptions. These children do not learn much from experience or repetition and cannot generalize information.

In the early years, children may often appear confused despite a high intelligence and high scores on receptive and expressive language measures. Closer observation will reveal social ineptness due to misinterpretations of body language and tone of voice. These children do not perceive subtle cues in their environment, such as the idea of personal space, the facial expressions of others, or nonverbal displays of pleasure or displeasure. These are all social skills that are normally grasped intuitively through observation, not directly taught.

Instead, these children cope by relying on language as their principal means of social relating, information gathering, and relief from anxiety, and often develop an exceptional memory for rote material. Since the nonverbal processing areas of the brain are not giving automatic feedback, they rely solely on memory of past experiences, each of which they labeled verbally to guide them in future situations. This, of course, is less effective and less reliable than being able to sense and interpret another person's social cues. Normal conversational "give and take" seems impossible for these children.

It is hard for these children to change from one activity to another or to move from one place to another. A child with NLD needs to concentrate merely to get through a room. Owing to the inability to handle such information-processing demands, these children will instinctively avoid any kind of novelty.

Problems with NLD grow more apparent and more profound during the latter stages of childhood development and into adolescence and adulthood, as pressures on social interaction increase and the requirements for appropriate social performance become more subtle and complex.

Language-based learning disorders are believed to be inherited, but a specific genetic problem has not yet been discovered. Nonverbal learning disabilities involve the performance processes that originate in the right cerebral hemisphere of the brain, which specializes in nonverbal processing.

Brain scans of individuals with NLD often reveal mild abnormalities of the right cerebral hemisphere. A number of children suffering from NLD have at some time early in their development

- sustained a moderate to severe head injury
- received repeated radiation treatments on or near their heads over a prolonged period of time
- shown congenital absence of the corpus callosum
- been treated for hydrocephalus
- had brain tissue removed from the right hemisphere.

All of the damage listed above would involve significant destruction of white matter connections in the right hemisphere. Current evidence suggests that a contributing cause of the NLD syndrome involves early damage of the right cerebral hemisphere or white matter disease that forces the left hemisphere system to function on its own.

Whereas language-based disabilities are usually obvious to parents and educators, nonverbal learning disorders routinely go unrecognized. Many of the early symptoms of nonverbal learning disabilities—the language-based accomplishments—make parents and teachers proud.

This child may speak like an adult at two or three years of age, and during early childhood, he or she is usually considered "gifted" by parents and teachers. Sometimes the NLD child has a history of rote reading at a very young age. This child is generally an eager, enthusiastic learner who quickly memorizes rote material.

Extraordinary early speech and vocabulary development are not often suspected to be a coping strategy used by a child with problems in the right-hemisphere brain system and limited access to nonverbal processing abilities. The NLD child is also likely to acquire an unusual aptitude for spelling, but few adults will consider this to be a reflection of the overdependence on auditory perceptions.

Likewise, remarkable rote memory skills, attention to detail, and a natural facility for decoding, encoding, and early reading development are not generally cause for alarm. Yet these are some of the important early indicators that a child is having trouble relating to and functioning in the nonverbal world.

Dysfunctions associated with NLD are less apparent at the age of seven to eight years than at 10 to 14 years, and they become progressively more apparent and more debilitating with each year. During late elementary school, the child will begin to not complete or turn in written assignments. The child produces limited written output, and the process is always slow and laborious. By the time the problem is revealed, the child may have already shut down in response to impossible academic pressures and performance demands.

Treatment Options and Outlook

Parents and the school should not underestimate the gravity of this disability. The main problem in the painstaking approach to teaching the child is the caregiver's faulty impression that the child is much more adept than he or she is. Everyone tends to overestimate the intelligence of NLD adolescents. The child should be shielded from teasing, persecution, and other sources of anxiety.

Independence should be introduced gradually, in controlled, nonthreatening situations. The more completely the strengths and weaknesses of the child are understood, the better prepared the care providers will be to promote the child's independence. These children should never be left to their own devices in new activities or situations that lack sufficient structure. Goals and expectations must be attainable.

Occupational therapy is a good idea for the younger child. Use of a computer word processor can help, since the spatial and fine motor skills needed for typing are less complicated than those involved in handwriting. Tasks requiring folding, cutting with scissors, or arranging material (maps, graphs, mobiles) will require considerable help. Timed assignments will need to be modified or eliminated.

Adults need to check often that the child understands, and that information is presented clearly. All expectations must be direct and explicit, and the student's schedule must be as predictable as possible. The child should be prepared in advance for any changes in routine such as assemblies, field trips, vacation days, finals, and so on.

A child with NLD should be assigned to one case manager at school who will oversee progress and can make sure all of the school staff are making the necessary accommodations and modifications. In-service training and orientation for all school staff that promotes tolerance and acceptance is a vital part of the overall plan for success, as everyone must be familiar with and supportive of the child's academic and social needs.

An affected child should be in a learning environment that provides daily, nonthreatening contact with nondisabled peers—not a "special" or alternative program—in order to boost social development. This child will benefit from cooperative learning situations when grouped with good role models.

Transitions will always be difficult for these children, so they will need time during the school day to collect their thoughts before "switching gears."

Teachers will need to present strategies for conversation skills, how and when to change the subject, tone and expression of voice, and nonverbal body language (facial expressions, correct social distance).

Isolation, deprivation, and punishment are not effective methods to change the behavior of a child who is already trying hard to conform, but who misinterprets nonverbal cues. If inappropriate behavior causes problems at school, a behavioral intervention plan detailing a course of action may need to be a part of this child's individualized education program or 504 plan.

How well these children progress seems to depend on early identification and accommodation. Typically, children with NLD are regularly punished for circumstances beyond their control, without ever really understanding why, and are often left with little hope that the situation will ever improve. As a result, these children tend to have serious forms of depression, withdrawal, anxiety, and in some cases, suicide.

nonverbal memory Memory for figures, spatial relationships, and so on. Nonverbal memory is assumed to be based in the deep structures of the right temporal lobe.

nootropics A class of drugs designed to improve learning and memory without other CENTRAL NERVOUS SYSTEM effects. The name *nootropic* was taken from the Greek *noos* (mind) and *tropein* (toward).

There is some disagreement about which drugs are to be considered nootropics, but experts usually agree that they include the PYRROLIDONE DERIVATIVES (piracetam and oxiracetam, pramiracetam, and aniracetam).

The mechanism by which these drugs seem to work is not known, although some studies suggest they affect the part of the nervous system that uses ACETYLCHOLINE as a NEUROTRANSMITTER. There also appears to be some involvement with adrenal steroid production in the adrenal CORTEX.

No nootropic drug has been approved by the U.S. Food and Drug Administration; however, nootropic drugs are available to patients outside the United States.

noradrenaline Another name for NOREPINEPHRINE.

norepinephrine A NEUROTRANSMITTER secreted by the adrenal gland and found in the AUTONOMIC NERVOUS SYSTEM (part of the nervous system concerned with control of involuntary bodily functions). Chemically, norepinephrine is a CATECHOLAMINE (a class of compounds that affect the nervous and cardiovascular systems, metabolic rate, and body temperature) and is closely related to EPINEPHRINE. It is also released as a neurotransmitter by sympathetic nerve endings located in the area of the MIDBRAIN called the LOCUS CERULEUS. Isolated in the 1930s, norepinephrine was the second neurotransmitter to be discovered.

Norepinephrine's primary function is to help maintain a constant blood pressure by constricting certain blood vessels when blood pressure drops. This action explains its use as an emergency injection in the treatment of shock or severe bleeding. Among its many other actions, it is responsible for the FIGHT-OR-FLIGHT RESPONSE to danger or stress and is responsible for constricting small blood vessels and increasing blood pressure, increasing blood flow through the arteries of the heart, increasing the rate and depth of breathing, and relaxing the smooth muscle in intestinal walls. It also helps to control emotion and mood.

normal pressure hydrocephalus (NPH) Also known as "water on the brain," this uncommon disorder involves an obstruction in the normal flow of CEREBROSPINAL FLUID, which causes a buildup of cerebrospinal fluid on the brain. It is called "normal pressure" hydrocephalus because the pressure in the spinal fluid is normal, unlike most cases of water on the brain.

NPH may be caused by any of several factors including MENINGITIS, ENCEPHALITIS, and HEAD INJURIES. In addition to treatment of the underlying cause, the condition may be corrected by a neurosurgical procedure (inserting a shunt) to divert the fluid from the brain.

Symptoms and Diagnostic Path

NPH can present with all of the symptoms of classic ALZHEIMER'S DISEASE, especially the DEMENTIA. A CAT SCAN will show the ventricles of the brain are enlarged from an excessive amount of fluid on the brain. Other symptoms include urinary incontinence and difficulty in walking. Presently, the most useful diagnostic tools include the imaging techniques, such as MRI (MAGNETIC RESONANCE IMAGING).

Treatment Options and Outlook

NPH is treated with a surgical procedure called a ventricular-atrial shunt to eliminate the fluid. About 50 percent of cases are cured with this treatment. While its cause is unknown, it is believed to result from an interference of the circulation of fluid in the brain. The condition may also be caused by a brain hemorrhage or inflammation that blocks the fluid; in these cases, shunting does not provide relief.

nuclear magnetic resonance (NMR) See MAGNETIC RESONANCE IMAGING (MRI).

nucleus accumbens A region in the LIMBIC SYSTEM where there are a large number of DOPAMINE NEUROTRANSMITTERS, which are involved in various brain functions, including movement and emotion. Much of the effects of cocaine and amphetamines occur in this part of the brain, which may be permanently damaged by abuse of these drugs.

Chronic administration of these drugs in animals has produced such permanent damage; at its worst, the result may be a psychotic condition much like SCHIZOPHRENIA, which experts also believe is related to dopamine.

nucleus basalis of Meynert An area near where the optic nerves cross that enters into the CEREBRAL CORTEX. When this area is destroyed, it causes a drop in ACETYLCHOLINE activity in the cortex similar to ALZHEIMER'S DISEASE. Scientists suspect that the beginning of Alzheimer's disease may be related to a slow death of cells in the nucleus basalis, which may lead to the formation of the plaques also seen in the disease.

nutrition and the brain What a person eats may have an effect on the brain's performance; when and how much a person eats may have almost as much effect. Research suggests that foods low in protein and high in carbohydrates boost alertness and performance by raising the level of TRYPTOPHAN in the brain.

Researchers believe that certain foods can directly affect brain function in a variety of ways.

Dementia and Memory Problems

In a study of more than 1,000 older people, those with high blood levels of an omega-3 fat called DHA were more than 40 percent less likely to develop DEMENTIA. For this reason, experts suggest people might eat a weekly serving of fish rich in omega-3s, such as salmon.

Other research suggests that sugar may keep memory sharp. In one study, after an overnight fast, healthy people over age 60 drank lemonade sweetened either with sugar or sugar substitute. Those who consumed the real sugar did much better at retelling a short story they read, both a few minutes later and even the next day, after their blood sugar returned to baseline. This may mean that the proper level of blood sugar enhances memory storage, especially for older people.

Research also found that people with high levels of an omega-3 fat called DHA were more than 40 percent less likely to develop dementia (including Alzheirner's disease) over the next nine years than people with low DHA levels. One theory is that since the brain uses DHA to help build membranes around nerve cells, it could be that the more DHA available, the easier the brain finds it can transmit messages.

Depression

Studies have found that the more severe the depression, the lower the level of omega-3 fats. Scientists do not know whether depression causes lower omega-3 levels, or whether lower levels trigger depression. But one theory suggests that a diet deficient in omega-3s could make a person vulnerable to depression, especially if the patient has other risk factors for depression.

Other studies have found that eating several small meals or snacks might temporarily sharpen the mind. In one British study, subjects who ate a light lunch of balanced protein and carbohydrates made fewer errors, and those who ate a heavy lunch made more errors on a task requiring close attention. All light snacks are not equal, however; in one Tufts University study, subjects who ate a nutritionally empty snack did worse on tests of memory and attention than did those who ate a caloric snack.

On the other hand, some studies suggest that a big breakfast does not appear to hamper performance, perhaps because of the body's daily rhythms of alertness and fatigue.

occipital cortex See VISUAL CORTEX.

occipital lobe One of four major pairs of lobes of the CEREBRAL CORTEX in the brain that includes the center of the visual perception system. Although protected from injury because of its location at the back of the brain, any significant trauma here can produce subtle changes to the visual-perceptual system. The occipital lobe is involved in visuospatial processing, discrimination of movement, and color discrimination.

Light reaches the sight centers in the occipital lobe through a complex pathway. After light hits the retina, the information is transmitted to the lateral geniculate nucleus in the thalamus. At this stage the brain interprets the light that the eye receives. From there, the axons then show the image in the visual association cortex that identifies what the eyes are seeing.

Although the occipital lobe is rarely damaged, due to its location, injury may cause changes in sight and perception. When one side of the occipital lobe is damaged, sight is lost in both eyes. Lesions in the occipital lobe can cause unusual side effects, such as "blindsight." A person with blindsight claims to have no vision at all, but when asked, the person can point to or identify objects at a distance unconsciously.

Other lesions in the occipital lobe have been known to cause an inability to identify faces known as prospagnosia. Lesions in the parietal-temporal-occipital association area can also cause writing impairments (AGRAPHIA) and an inability to recognize words (ALEXIA). Disorders of the occipital lobe may cause illusions and visual hallucinations that can cause objects to appear larger or smaller than they really are, or make an object appear to be a different color. Once damaged, the occipital lobe is hard to repair.

occipital neuralgia A chronic pain disorder caused by irritation or injury to the occipital nerve in the back of the scalp, triggering pain originating at the nape of the neck.

Occipital neuralgia can be caused by physical stress, trauma, or repeated contraction of the muscles of the neck.

Symptoms and Diagnostic Path
The pain, often described as throbbing and MIGRAINE-like, spreads up and around the forehead and scalp.

Treatment Options and Outlook
Massage and rest may ease the pain. In some cases, antidepressants may be used when the pain is particularly severe. Other treatments may include local nerve blocks and injections of steroids directly into the affected area.

In most people, the pain is eliminated or reduced with treatment and does not interfere with daily activities.

ocular dominance columns Cells in each of these columns, found in the PRIMARY VISUAL CORTEX, process information from either the right or the left eye; there is no mixing of right-left eye information within columns.

oculomotor nerve Also known as the third cranial nerve, this nerve (together with the fourth and sixth cranial nerves) is responsible for eye movements.

See also CRANIAL NERVES.

Ohtahara syndrome   A neurological disorder characterized by seizures that affects newborns, usually within the first three months of life. The cause of the disorder is unknown.

Symptoms and Diagnostic Path
Babies with Ohtahara syndrome often have MENTAL RETARDATION or other developmental impairments.

Treatment Options and Outlook
There is no cure for Ohtahara syndrome; treatment is symptomatic and supportive. Most drug therapy has limited effect.

Ohtahara syndrome often is fatal; infants who survive suffer from severe mental and physical impairment.

olfactory bulbs   Interior lobes of the brain concerned with the sense of smell. The two olfactory bulbs lie on top of a thin body plate in the roof of the nose and connect to the brain via the OLFACTORY NERVE. Scent particles enter the nose, stimulating smell receptors at the top of the nasal cavity, sending electro-chemical signals through holes in the ethmoid bone to an olfactory bulb; from there, it travels to several brain regions in the lower, more primitive part of the FOREBRAIN.

Connections with the LIMBIC SYSTEM explain the emotional aspects of smell and may explain why some smells can quickly trigger powerful memories. On the other hand, links with the HYPOTHALAMUS can trigger strong physical reactions (such as nausea and vomiting) in response to unpleasant smells. Olfactory connections with the RETICULAR FORMATION explain the stimulating action of smelling salts.

See also SMELL, SENSE OF.

olfactory fatigue   The loss of the ability to detect a certain smell over time. The amount of time that olfactory fatigue remains varies; it is a more extreme version of "smell adaptation," which is the temporary loss of the ability to smell an odor that returns in a few minutes after the cause is removed.

Some scientists believe olfactory fatigue occurs when the brain modifies the sense of smell by transmitting a signal to the nerves, which pick up the "smell" message; the more a person is exposed to these odors, the less he or she notices them.

See also SMELL, SENSE OF.

olfactory nerve   Also known as the first cranial nerve, the olfactory nerve carries the sensation of smell via nerve impulses from the nose to the brain. Smells are detected by hairlike nerve endings (called RECEPTORS) in the mucous membrane lining the top of the nasal cavity. Nerve fibers travel from the receptors through holes in the nasal cavity roof, ultimately forming two structures called the OLFACTORY BULBS. From here, the nerve fibers make their way to the olfactory centers in the brain.

If the olfactory nerves are injured (usually by a HEAD INJURY), the sense of smell may be impaired or completely lost.

See also CRANIAL NERVES; SMELL, SENSE OF.

oligodendroglioma   A rare type of slow-growing primary BRAIN TUMOR that affects several hundred Americans a year. Although this type of tumor is more common in adults, it can occur in children; it is also more common in men than women.

The brain is made up of a number of supporting cells called GLIAL CELLS; a tumor of these cells is known as a GLIOMA. Oligodendroglioma is a type of glioma that develops from cells called oligodendrocytes, which produce the fatty covering of nerve cells. This type of tumor is normally found in the CEREBRUM, particularly in the frontal or temporal lobes.

Oligodendrogliomas may be divided into two types, the slow-growing, well-differentiated tumor or the faster-growing anaplastic oligodendroglioma. Like other gliomas, oligodendrogliomas may be graded between I and IV depending on their malignancy and rate of growth, with grade I the least malignant and grade IV the most.

The cause of oligodendroglioma is unknown.

Symptoms and Diagnostic Path
People with slow-growing oligodendrogliomas may have symptoms for several years before the tumor is diagnosed. The first symptoms of any type of

brain tumor are usually caused by increased pressure within the skull, caused either by a blockage in the ventricles of the brain leading to a build-up of cerebrospinal fluid (CSF), or by swelling around the tumor itself. This high pressure can cause headaches, vomiting, and visual problems. Seizures and behavior or personality changes also may occur.

Oligodendrogliomas can grow in different parts of the brain, and symptoms may relate to the area of the brain that is affected. They are usually found in the frontal or temporal lobes of the cerebrum. A tumor of the frontal lobe of the brain may cause gradual changes in mood and personality and one-sided paralysis. A tumor in the temporal lobe of the brain may cause problems with coordination, speech, and memory.

A neurological examination can assess any effect the tumor has had on the nervous system. A CAT SCAN or MAGNETIC RESONANCE IMAGING scan will be done to find the exact position and size of the tumor. To confirm the type of tumor, the tumor is biopsied and examined under a microscope.

Treatment Options and Outlook
The treatment depends on the person's general health, the size and position of the tumor, and whether it has spread. Before treatment is begun, it is important to reduce any excess pressure within the skull. Steroid medications may help reduce swelling around the tumor. A build-up of fluid may require a shunt to drain off the excess fluid.

When possible, surgery is the preferred method of treatment in order to remove as much of the tumor as possible without damaging the surrounding brain tissue. Depending on the tumor's size and position, it may not be possible to remove completely, and further treatment may be required. In some cases surgery is not possible; tumors may be unreachable or the risk of damage to the rest of the brain may be too high.

Radiation is often used after surgery to destroy any remaining malignant cells, or it may be used to treat oligodendroglioma if surgery is not possible. Radiation is usually given as an external treatment but occasionally it may be given in the form of radioactive implants.

Chemotherapy involves the use of anticancer drugs to destroy cancer cells, and is either given as a sole treatment or together with surgery and/or radiation.

opiates The active element in heroin, morphine, and opium, which are similar in structure to the ENDORPHINS found naturally in the brain.

Within the LIMBIC SYSTEM, BRAIN STEM, and SPINAL CORD, there are places on certain nerve cells that recognize opiates. When stimulated by these opiates, these sites (called opiate receptors) trigger responses in the brain and body. Scientists have identified three types of opiate receptors: delta, mu, and kappa. Each of these receptors is involved in different brain functions. For example, mu is responsible for the pain-relieving effects of morphine.

The limbic system controls emotions. Opiates change the limbic system to produce increased feelings of pleasure, relaxation, and contentment. The brain stem controls the automatic processes of the body, such as breathing and heart rate. Opiates can act on the brain stem to interfere with these automatic processes. The spinal cord transmits pain signals from the body. By acting here, opiates block pain messages and allow people to bear even seriously painful injuries.

Opiates can produce a quick, intense feeling of pleasure followed by a sense of well-being and a calm drowsiness. But they can also cause addiction. If someone uses opiates again and again, the person's brain is likely to become dependent on them. This is because long-term opiate use changes the way nerve cells in the brain work. These cells grow so used to having the opiate that they actually need it to work normally. If opiates are suddenly stopped from dependent nerve cells, many of these cells become overactive. Eventually these cells will work normally again, but in the meantime they cause a wide range of symptoms in the brain and body known as withdrawal symptoms.

Opiates also have medical uses. They are powerful painkillers, and can be used to control severe diarrhea or cough. When used properly for medical purposes, opiates do not produce an intense feeling of pleasure, and patients have very little chance of becoming addicted.

The brain produces its own versions of opiates, called endogenous opioids. These chemicals act just like opiates, binding to opiate receptors. Endogenous opioids are the body's way of controlling pain. Many runners report feeling a pleasant "high" after running; this feeling is probably caused by the release of this natural chemical in the brain.

optical aphasia   The inability to name the object that one sees. Recognition survives—a patient with optical aphasia who sees a bowl of soup can indicate recognition of it, such as by a smile, but would not be able to name what is seen. Other recognition survives, too, so that if the patient can taste or smell the soup, the person can name it; it is only the visual recognition that is lacking.

See also APHASIA.

optic chiasm   The point at which the right and left optic nerves cross.

optic nerve   Also known as the second cranial nerve, this nerve carries impulses from the eyes to the brain.

The small nerves of the retina (the inner surface at the back of the eye) sense light and transmit impulses to the optic nerve, which carries them to the brain. If there is a problem anywhere along the optic nerve and its branches or damage to the areas at the back of the brain that sense visual stimuli, visual changes may result.

The optic nerves follow an unusual route from the eyes to the back of the brain: Each nerve splits, and half of its fibers cross over to the other side at the optic chiasm. Because of this arrangement, damage along the optic nerve pathway causes peculiar patterns of vision loss.

If the optic nerve is damaged between the eyeball and the optic chiasm, vision may be lost in that eye. But if the problem lies farther back in the optic nerve pathway, vision may be lost in only half the visual field of both eyes. If both eyes lose peripheral vision, the cause may be damage at the optic chiasm. If both eyes lose half of the visual field on the same side, the cause is usually damage to the optic nerve pathway on the opposite

side of the brain caused by a stroke, hemorrhage, or tumor.

See also CRANIAL NERVES.

optic neuritis   Inflammation of the OPTIC NERVE characterized by sudden blurry vision. As the nerve tissue becomes swollen and red, the nerve fibers stop working properly. If many of the nerve fibers are involved, the vision may be very poor, but if the optic neuritis is mild, vision is nearly normal.

Many diseases and conditions may cause optic neuritis, which may affect the optic nerve of one or both eyes. Some people (especially children) develop optic neuritis after a viral illness such as mumps, measles, or a cold. In others, optic neuritis may occur as a sign of a neurologic disease affecting nerves in various parts of the body, such as MULTIPLE SCLEROSIS (MS). Studies with up to 10 years of follow-up have demonstrated that approximately 50 percent to 75 percent of people with isolated optic neuritis go on to develop MS. More recent studies reported that those persons with optic neuritis who also had abnormalities in their cerebrospinal fluid or on MRI results were more likely to develop MS.

In a rare condition called Leber's optic neuropathy, which may be hereditary, a special kind of optic neuritis may appear in both eyes within a short span of time. Most of the time, however, there is no known cause.

Symptoms and Diagnostic Path

Optic neuritis usually begins abruptly, with blurred, dim vision in one or both eyes. There may be pain in the eye socket, especially when moving the eyes. Vision may continue to get worse over a week or two, and may seem worse after exercising or a hot bath.

Since the optic nerve enters the back of the eye where it appears as a small disc, an ophthalmologist can examine it by looking in the eye with an ophthalmoscope. Swelling of the optic nerve may or may not be visible depending on whether the optic neuritis is affecting the optic nerve near the eyeball. Since optic neuritis can be confused with many other causes of poor vision, an accurate medical diagnosis is important. If a cause can be found and treated, further damage may be prevented.

Tests may include ultrasound, CT scans, or visual brain wave recordings. Other tests may include assessments of color vision, side vision, and pupil reactions to light.

Treatment Options and Outlook

Treatment includes either IV steroids followed by oral steroids, or no treatment at all, since studies have discovered that those treated with IV steroids had fewer repeat attacks of optic neuritis than did those who took only drugs by mouth. In fact, patients treated with oral steroids alone had a higher risk of repeat attacks of optic neuritis than patients treated with a sugar pill. Even more important, patients treated with IV steroids initially had about half the risk of developing MS in two years as did patients treated with oral steroids only or a sugar pill.

optic tectum The roof of the rear part of the CEREBRUM, which controls visual processes.

organic amnesia Amnesia due to brain dysfunction. Organic memory disorders can be either global or specific; that is, they can affect either a large part of memory (global) or only particular memory bits (specific).

organic brain syndrome A disturbance of consciousness, intellect, or mental functioning of physical as opposed to psychiatric origin, without a precise known physical cause. Organic brain syndrome is a common condition among the elderly, but it is not an inevitable part of aging. The syndrome is not a separate disease, but is a general term used to categorize physical conditions that can cause mental changes. Disorders associated with organic brain syndrome include

- ALZHEIMER'S DISEASE
- arrhythmias
- brain hemorrhage
- brain injury

- carbon dioxide excess
- cardiac infections such as endocarditis or myocarditis
- cardiovascular disorders
- concussion
- CREUTZFELDT-JAKOB DISEASE
- degenerative disorders
- ENCEPHALITIS
- HUNTINGTON'S DISEASE
- infections
- KORSAKOFF SYNDROME
- MENINGITIS
- mental conditions (depression, neuroses, psychoses)
- MULTI-INFARCT DEMENTIA
- MULTIPLE SCLEROSIS
- NORMAL PRESSURE HYDROCEPHALUS
- oxygen loss
- PARKINSON'S DISEASE
- PICK'S DISEASE
- respiratory conditions
- septicemia (blood poisoning)
- STROKE
- substance abuse
- TRANSIENT ISCHEMIC ATTACK (TIA)

Symptoms and Diagnostic Path

In the acute phase of the condition, symptoms can range from a slight confusion to stupor or COMA and may include disorientation, memory impairment, HALLUCINATIONS, and delusions. The chronic form of the syndrome causes a progressive decline in intellect, memory, and behavior.

Treatment Options and Outlook

Treatment varies according to the specific underlying disorder. Many of the associated disorders have no cure. Treatment is supportive.

organic mental disorders A group of mental disorders with a known or presumed physical cause, such as BRAIN TUMORS, drug abuse, HEAD INJURY, metabolic disorders, and so on. Physicians generally make a distinction between organic mental disorders (when the cause is known) and ORGANIC BRAIN SYNDROME, when the cause is not known.

A wide variety of problems can be caused by this problem, such as HALLUCINATIONS, DELUSIONS, DELIRIUM, DEMENTIA, and mood disorders.

osmoreceptors   A group of cells in the HYPO-THALAMUS and lower BRAIN STEM that monitor the concentration of salts and proteins in the blood. If the blood concentration increases, the osmoreceptors trigger nerve impulses to the hypothalamus, which increases the release of VASOPRESSIN from the PITUITARY GLAND, instructing the kidneys to restrict the release of urine until the blood concentration returns to normal.

oxytocin   One of two hormones secreted by the PITUITARY GLAND that initiates labor in pregnant women, stimulates uterine contraction, and plays a part in lactation. This neuropeptide also is involved in grooming and social behavior and may play a role in one type of obsessive-compulsive disorder (OCD). According to research, high levels of oxytocin in the brain are found among patients diagnosed with OCD who do not have a family history of TOURETTE SYNDROME.

In recent studies, scientists collected CEREBRO-SPINAL FLUID from 29 people with OCD, 23 people with Tourette syndrome, and 31 healthy controls. Levels of oxytocin was dramatically higher in the group of OCD patients but not in those who had no personal or family history of tic disorders, or in the control group. Moreover, those with the most severe OCD symptoms had the highest levels of oxytocin.

Paget's disease　A common disorder of middle age in which bone formation is disrupted, weakening and thickening bones of the skull, among others. Because the disease is prevalent in some parts of the country more than others, experts suspect the cause may be viral. Paget's disease affects about 3 percent of the population over age 40; the disorder tends to run in families and affects more men than women.

Symptoms and Diagnostic Path

Changes in the skull may lead to a distortion of the facial bones, producing a lionlike appearance, and to inner-ear damage that may cause deafness, ringing in the ear, VERTIGO, or HEADACHE. Enlarged vertebrae may press on the SPINAL CORD, causing pain and sometimes paralysis.

Paget's disease may be diagnosed using X-rays, alkaline phosphatase blood tests, and bone scans, which can determine the extent and activity of the condition. If a bone scan suggests Paget's disease, the affected bones should be X-rayed to confirm the diagnosis.

Treatment Options and Outlook

Treatment can control Paget's disease and ease symptoms, but there is no cure. A type of bone cancer called osteogenic sarcoma is an extremely rare complication that occurs in less than 1 percent of all patients. The outlook is generally good, particularly if treatment is given before major changes in the affected bones have occurred.

The goal of treatment is to control Paget's disease activity for as long as possible. Five types of bisphosphonates are currently available, including Didronel (etidronate disodium), Aredia (pamidronate disodium), Fosamax (alendronate sodium), Skelid (tiludronate disodium), and Actonel (risedronate sodium).

Miacalcin is administered by injection; 50 to 100 units daily or three times per week for 6–18 months.

Complications resulting from enlargement of the skull or spine may injure the nervous system. However, most neurologic symptoms, even those that are moderately severe, can be treated with medication and do not require neurosurgery.

pain　The experience of pain involves almost every part of the brain, the SPINAL CORD, and the PERIPHERAL NERVOUS SYSTEM, the immune system, endocrine glands, and the metabolic system.

Basically, pain is caused when peripheral nerves are activated by a stimulus to the skin or internal organs. When a pain nerve is stimulated, an electrical signal runs down its AXON. The outer wall of a NERVE CELL is a membrane full of fluid that contains salts (including sodium, potassium, and chloride ions). All are electrically charged particles, and the membrane is surrounded by body fluid that also contains charged particles.

When the neuron is stimulated by pain, its membrane allows a large amount of positively charged sodium ions to enter the cell at the point of stimulation, which changes the properties of the neighboring part of the membrane, allowing sodium ions to enter there as well. The result is a wave of electrochemical activity that moves rapidly down the neuron. The pain information is transmitted electrochemically to the spinal cord, where it is processed and sent to numerous brain regions. In the brain, specific relay nuclei transmit the information to the sensory part of the CEREBRAL CORTEX and to nonspecific nuclei that send out the information to other brain regions.

Information about pain reaches brain regions involved in emotion, sensory perception, body movement, and hormonal release. The pain system also involves a wide range of different NEUROTRANSMITTERS and a group of PEPTIDES (including ENDORPHINS) that are similar to morphine.

The intricacy of the pain system can explain how wounded people may not be consciously aware of their pain and how amputees can still feel pain in the amputated part, despite its absence.

Recent research has suggested that the brain mechanisms behind pain in musculoskeletal areas, skin, and internal organs are different.

painkillers Medications that reduce a person's sensitivity to pain, including general and local anesthetics, aspirin, and opiate derivatives.

General anesthetics act on the BRAIN STEM to induce loss of consciousness, whereas local anesthetics deaden pain by affecting nerve membranes, blocking the transmission of impulses to a body area served by a sensory nerve. Other types of mild, general pain-killers—such as aspirin—apparently act on pain centers in the THALAMUS deep inside the brain, traveling through the blood to all parts of the NERVOUS SYSTEM.

Analgesics are drugs that block pain without interfering with consciousness; for intractable pain, physicians may prescribe morphine or another derivative from opium.

Painkillers, anesthetics, and analgesics can be given by injection into the blood, which very quickly distributes the drug throughout the body; by inhalation; through the rectum; via the SPINAL CORD (an epidural), which enters the CEREBROSPINAL FLUID bathing the brain; or by mouth.

paleocortex An evolutionary early region of the CORTEX; it is the olfactory cortex of the cerebrum. It is composed primarily of the piriform cortex and the parahippocampal gyrus.

paradoxical sleep Another word for RAPID EYE MOVEMENT SLEEP (REM), a deep state wherein dreaming takes place.

parasympathetic nervous system (PNS) One of two parts of the AUTONOMIC NERVOUS SYSTEM, the PNS is responsible for slowing and steadying the body's internal activity, such as heart and breathing rates, by releasing ACETYLCHOLINE. These effects are almost the opposite of the efforts of the SYMPATHETIC NERVOUS SYSTEM. Parasympathetic nerves also increase blood flow to the stomach, liver, intestines, and other organs involved in digestion. In addition, these nerves activate other mechanisms of eating and digestion, including increased salivation, the release into the stomach and intestine of digestive juices, and stimulation of muscles in the intestinal wall to promote the movement of food through the digestive system.

Moreover, parasympathetic nerve fibers contract the pupil and allow the eye to focus on close objects.

The parasympathetic nervous system is made up of one chain of nerves passing from the brain and another leaving the lower SPINAL CORD. The parasympathetic nervous system also helps to maintain erection of the penis in sexually aroused men.

parietal cortex Part of the CEREBRAL CORTEX that regulates special perception; it also contains short-term memory for the perception of motion.

parietal lobes One of four major pairs of lobes of the CEREBRAL CORTEX located at the upper middle part of the brain above the temporal lobes. The parietal lobes include the sensory cortex and the association areas involved in processing information about body sensation, touch, and spatial organization. The association areas in the parietal lobes are also involved in secondary language and visual processing.

Lesions in association areas in the parietal lobe can cause difficulties in learning tasks that require an understanding of spatial perception and the body's position in space. Gerstmann's syndrome is associated with damage to these areas; this syndrome may include left to right confusion, difficulty naming fingers when specific fingers are touched (finger AGNOSIA), problems in writing (dysgraphia), and problems with mathematics (dyscalculia).

parkinsonism Any condition that causes any combination of the types of movement abnormalities seen in PARKINSON'S DISEASE, such as a masklike face, rigidity, and slowed movements. It causes a lack of muscle control because nerve cells cannot transmit messages to the muscles. In addition to the loss of muscle control, some people with parkinsonism often become severely depressed. Although loss of mental capacities is uncommon, with severe symptoms of parkinsonism the person may exhibit overall mental deterioration, such as delirium.

The lifetime risk of developing parkinsonism is 7.5 percent. Parkinson's disease is the most common cause of parkinsonism, but researchers found that Parkinson's itself accounts for only 42 percent of all cases. In every age group, men are twice as likely to develop parkinsonism as women.

Parkinsonism may be caused by disorders such as a STROKE or by brain infections such as ENCEPHALITIS or MENINGITIS. The influenza epidemic during the early part of the 20th century caused a number of cases of encephalitis and resulting parkinsonism.

Other diseases of the brain that combine parkinsonism with additional nerve disorders include Wilson's disease, HUNTINGTON'S DISEASE, Shy-Drager syndrome, cortical-basal ganglionic degeneration, PROGRESSIVE SUPRANUCLEAR PALSY, diffuse Lewy body disease, CREUTZFELDT-JAKOB DISEASE, and even ALZHEIMER'S DISEASE. Alzheimer's patients can have movement problems just as Parkinson's patients can have dementia. It is a case of which is first and which is worse.

A few drugs used to treat blood pressure, vomiting, mental disorders, and seizures can cause or worsen parkinsonism. Other drugs causing parkinsonism include tranquilizers (such as haloperidol), metoclopramide, and phenothiazine medications, narcotics, or general anesthesia.

Poisons that can cause parkinsonism include manganese, carbon monoxide, carbon disulfide, the cycad nut, and the illicit drug MPTP (methylphenyl tetrahydropyridine).

Parkinsonism caused by medications is usually reversible. However, symptoms caused by toxins, infections, or disorders may or may not be reversible. When there is no underlying triggering cause, the condition is called Parkinson's disease, and is characterized by the depletion of chemicals that facilitate electrical transmission between nerve cells.

Symptoms and Diagnostic Path

Initial symptoms may be mild and nonspecific, such as a mild tremor, or the feeling that one leg or foot is stiff or dragging. Other symptoms include muscle rigidity, stiffness, difficulty bending arms or legs, posture problems, movement difficulties, loss of balance, shuffling, slow movements, difficulty initiating any voluntary movement, freezing when the movement is stopped, muscle aches and pains, shaking, tremors, finger-thumb rubbing, reduced ability to show facial expressions, masklike appearance, staring, inability to close mouth, slow speaking, low-pitched or monotone voice, difficulty chewing or swallowing, loss of fine motor skills, difficulty writing, difficulty eating, frequent falls, mild decline in intellectual function, depression, confusion, or dementia.

Examination may show increased muscle tone, tremors of the Parkinson's type, and difficulty initiating or completing voluntary movements. Reflexes are usually normal. Tests are not usually specific for parkinsonism but may be used to confirm or rule out other disorders that may cause similar symptoms.

Treatment Options and Outlook

Treatment is aimed at control of symptoms. If the symptoms are mild, no treatment may be required. If the condition is caused by a medication, the benefits of the medication may be weighed against the severity of symptoms. If appropriate, medications may be stopped or changed. Treatment of underlying conditions may reduce symptoms.

When drugs such as levodopa (L-Dopa) are taken orally, many of the worst symptoms are lessened. New drugs such as pramipexole (Mirapex) and ropinirole (Requip) can delay the need for levodopa. Future approaches to treatment include a focus on early detection and slowing progression of the disease. Encouraging results have been reported from certain experimental surgical treatments, such as transplantation of fetal dopamine-producing cells and insertion of a pacemaker-like device deep in the brain to suppress uncontrolled movements. Traditional surgery can alleviate some tremors, and physical therapy may help mobility.

Good general nutrition and health are important. Exercise should continue. Regular rest periods and lack of stress are recommended, because tiredness or stress can make the symptoms worse. Physical therapy, speech therapy, and occupational therapy may help promote function and independence, and may help maintain skills, foster a positive attitude, and minimize depression.

Parkinson's disease A motor system disorder that causes muscle tremor, stiffness, and weakness; there is evidence that motor deficits may be accompanied by cognitive problems including poor memory. The disease was first described by James Parkinson (1755–1824) of London.

In the normal brain, some nerve cells produce the chemical dopamine, which transmits signals within the brain to produce smooth movement of muscles. In Parkinson's patients, 80 percent or more of these dopamine-producing cells are damaged, dead, or otherwise degenerated. This causes the nerve cells to fire wildly, leaving patients unable to control their movements. These damaged cells are primarily located in the substantia nigra of the BASAL GANGLIA of the brain.

About one in 200 people are affected by the disease, with 50,000 new cases diagnosed each year. The incidence of Parkinson's disease is lower among women and people who smoke.

Symptoms and Diagnostic Path
Though full-blown Parkinson's can be crippling, early symptoms of the disease may be so subtle and gradual that patients sometimes ignore them or attribute them to the effects of aging. At first, patients may feel overly tired or a little shaky. Their speech may become soft and they may become irritable for no reason. Movements may be stiff, unsteady, or unusually slow. Parkinson's disease usually begins with a slight tremor, followed by a stiff, shuffling walk, trembling, a rigid stoop, and a fixed expression. The intellect is unaffected until late in the disease, although speech may become slow; DEPRESSION is common.

Symptoms mimic a wide range of other disorders, including adverse drug reactions, carbon-monoxide poisoning, STROKE, HEAD INJURY, and BRAIN TUMOR. While initial symptoms are so mild they may be easily overlooked, as the disease progresses it becomes so clear-cut a physician may be able to diagnose the condition by a simple examination. However, other possible disorders should be excluded via tests (CT or MRI SCANS or blood work).

Treatment Options and Outlook
The first-line treatment for the disease is L-dopa (levodopa), which was approved for the treatment of Parkinson's disease in 1970. Levodopa helps restore muscle control once it is converted to dopamine in the brain. (It is not possible to give dopamine to patients directly, since the chemical cannot penetrate the blood-brain barrier.) Although levodopa can pass through the blood-brain barrier, it changes to dopamine so quickly that only a small amount actually arrives in the brain. As a result, in order to relieve symptoms many patients need to take fairly large doses of levodopa, which can cause side effects such as nausea and dyskinesias (involuntary movements).

To reduce the chance of these side effects, doctors often prescribe a combination of levodopa and carbidopa (Sinemet). Carbidopa delays the conversion of levodopa to dopamine until it reaches the brain, often preventing levodopa's side effects. Carbidopa also decreases the amount of levodopa needed.

Because each Parkinson's patient reacts differently to treatment, doctors must work closely to find a balance between the drug's benefits and side effects. The levodopa-carbidopa combination can be very effective, but the combination does have problems. Doses must be increased over time, and in advanced cases the drug intermittently stops working.

Three drugs were approved in 1997 for the treatment of Parkinson's disease: Mirapex (pramipexole dihydrochloride), Requip (ropinirole hydrochloride), and Tasmar (tolcapone). Mirapex and Requip, which mimic dopamine's role in the brain, allow patients to regain some of their lost muscle control. Both are approved for use alone or with levodopa. Combining Mirapex with levodopa allowed patients to reduce those doses by up to 25 percent. Requip trials showed similar benefits, allowing patients to reduce levodopa doses by an average of 31 percent.

Tolcapone (Tasmar) is a new kind of drug called a COMT inhibitor that also can be used with levodopa drugs. Tasmar blocks a key enzyme responsible for breaking down levodopa before it reaches the brain. In studies, patients who took Tasmar noted significant improvements in talking, writing, walking, and dressing.

Other drugs also used for Parkinson's disease include Parlodel (bromocriptine) and Permax (pergolide), which mimic dopamine's role in the brain. They are sometimes given with levodopa drugs to improve response. Eldepryl (selegiline hydrochloride), also called deprenyl, can enhance and prolong levodopa response by delaying the breakdown of naturally occurring and levodopa-formed dopamine, allowing accumulation in surviving nerve cells.

In August 2000 the U.S. Food and Drug Administration approved a type of implant to control tremors consisting of a wire surgically implanted deep within the brain and connected to a pulse generator similar to a cardiac pacemaker, implanted near the collarbone. Whenever a tremor begins, patients can activate the device by passing a hand-held magnet over the generator. The system delivers a mild electrical stimulation that blocks the dysfunctional brain signals that cause tremor. Effects are often dramatic. With the implant, patients who could not raise a glass of water without spilling it can within hours sip from the glass with no signs of their disability.

Pallidotomy is a type of brain surgery that can help many Parkinson's patients, especially those in late stages of the disease. Doctors are not sure why the procedure works, although they caution that some of the surgery's effects diminish after two years and long-term effectiveness of the procedure is unknown. In pallidotomy, a surgeon makes a tiny hole in the skull and uses a small electric probe to destroy a small portion of the globus pallidus, which experts believe is overactive in Parkinson's patients. Before operating, the surgeon maps the patient's brain to decide where the probe should go. During surgery the patient is awake but sedated, so the surgeon can note responses to stimuli. Although both sides of the brain have a globus pallidus, pallidotomies typically are performed on one side at a time. After the patient has recuperated, a second procedure is done if needed.

In January 2002, the FDA approved deep brain stimulation using two implanted electrodes, one on each side of the brain. More recently, the FDA also approved a technologically advanced electrode apparatus that can be controlled by the patient through use of a remote control device.

Alternatively, thalamotomy may be performed to destroy a specific group of cells in the thalamus, the brain's communications center. This type of surgery is designed for the 5 percent to 10 percent of Parkinson's patients with disabling tremor in the hand or arm. It reduces or eliminates tremor in as many as 90 percent of patients.

Scientists are currently working in several areas of potential Parkinson's treatments. Some experts are studying neurotrophic proteins that seem to protect nerve cells from the premature death that prompts Parkinson's. Others are studying neuroprotective agents—naturally occurring enzymes that appear to deactivate free radicals, which some scientists think may be linked to the damage done to nerve cells in Parkinson's. Still other researchers are studying ways to implant neural tissues from fetal pigs into the brain to restore the degenerate area. Finally, some scientists are modifying the genetic code of individual cells to create dopamine-producing cells from other cells, such as those from the skin.

Without treatment, the disease progresses over 10 to 15 years to severe weakness and incapacity; about one-third of patients eventually go on to develop dementia. Experiments with transplants of dopamine-replacing adrenal tissue are now being conducted.

Penfield, Wilder (1891–1976) Canadian neurosurgeon who discovered that stimulating various areas of the CORTEX produced a range of responses from patients; however, only stimulation of the TEMPORAL LOBES elicited meaningful, integrated experiences, including sound, movement, and color.

Interestingly, some of these memories that popped up during stimulation were unremembered in the normal state. Furthermore, the memories Penfield stimulated appeared to be far more detailed, accurate, and specific than normal recall.

Penfield did not set out to study MEMORY; he wanted to reduce SEIZURES in epileptic patients by removing the damaged tissue in the brain that triggered the seizures. Penfield knew that the seizures always were preceded by a "mental aura" (a warning sensation the patient experiences before a seizure). He planned to open the skulls of fully conscious patients and move a stimulating electrode across the brain. This would deliver a weak electrical shock to various areas to find the site that produced the mental aura. If he found such a site, he reasoned, he could destroy it and end the seizures.

While his technique was often successful, his discovery of the ability to stimulate memories radically altered ideas that were popular at the time about how the brain worked. Stimulating one side of the brain brought back a certain song to one patient, the memory of a moment in a garden listening to a mother calling her child in another. Interestingly, stimulating the same point elicited the same memory every time. It seemed that Penfield had found an ENGRAM—the site in the brain where memory was stored.

As a result of his findings, Penfield believed that the brain makes a permanent record of every item to which a person pays conscious attention, although this record may be forgotten during day-to-day life.

peptides A class of substances made up of chains of AMINO ACIDS joined end to end. Some NEUROTRANSMITTERS are peptides.

perception The process through which sensory information (hearing, sight, touch, movement, taste, smell) is recognized and interpreted. Perception involves both the intake of information through the senses and the processing and making sense of information through cognition. While sensory experience itself is largely automatic for humans, perception also involves learned behavior and intellectual capacity.

perceptual disorder A disorder involving the perception of stimuli from one or more of the senses. Unlike visual or hearing problems, perceptual disorders involve the processing of information received through a sense, either in perception or understanding. A number of distinct brain problems are caused by defects in visual, sensory, and hearing perception that represent fundamental defects in perception rather than complex problems of memory, reasoning, or motor function. They usually involve only parts of the brain.

peripheral nervous system (PNS) All parts of the NERVOUS SYSTEM lying outside of the CENTRAL NERVOUS SYSTEM (the brain and SPINAL CORD). The PNS comprises the nerves extending to every part of the body and includes the cranial nerves and the spinal nerves. The part of the PERIPHERAL NERVOUS SYSTEM that controls involuntary movements and vegetative functions is called the AUTONOMIC NERVOUS SYSTEM, which is divided into the SYMPATHETIC and the PARASYMPATHETIC NERVOUS SYSTEMS. Because the PNS is not protected by the BLOOD-BRAIN BARRIER, as is the central nervous system, the PNS is far more vulnerable to neurotoxic damage.

peripheral neuropathy Damage to the nerves of the PERIPHERAL NERVOUS SYSTEM, caused by a number of diseases and one of the most common results of poisoning with NEUROTOXINS. Damage can occur either to MOTOR NERVES (causing muscle weakness) or to sensory nerves (interfering with sensations of touch to cold, heat, pain, and pressure, or causing pain). Often neurotoxic exposure causes damage to both types of nerves. This condition can develop either quickly, with intense symptoms, or accumulate slowly over a long period of time.

During the 1930s, widespread outbreak of peripheral neuropathy was caused by solvent contamination of Ginger Jake, a popular tonic used as a digestive aid and to treat flu and menstrual problems. Normally, ingredients included ginger, castor oil, and a large amount of alcohol. However, varnish was substituted for the more expensive castor oil by one unscrupulous distributor, and as many as 100,000 people were diagnosed with "Ginger Jake syndrome"—symptoms ranging from numbness to permanent paralysis.

Symptoms and Diagnostic Path

The first signs of peripheral neuropathy are often cramps in the legs, problems in climbing stairs, or problems in grasping heavy objects. Other symptoms include continual numbness and tingling in the feet similar to the "pins-and-needles" feeling when a leg or foot is compressed and "falls asleep." In severe cases, there may be paralysis.

Treatment Options and Outlook

Successful treatment of peripheral neuropathy requires management of the condition causing the pain if possible. Successful treatment of the underlying condition will cause the pain to resolve on its own.

If it is not possible to identify or treat the underlying pathology causing peripheral neuropathy, there are several treatment options. For minor pains, over-the-counter pain medications (aspirin, naproxen sodium, ibuprofen, acetaminophen), heat, ice, rest, bandaging, elevation, or gentle massage may provide sufficient relief. For more severe, unremitting pain, narcotic pain drugs, lidocaine patches, anti-seizure medications, and even antidepressants can provide relief. Long-term, severe pain may require referral to a pain management clinic, physical therapy, or use of a transcutaneous nerve stimulator (TNS) unit. Some chronic peripheral neuropathy patients have claimed to obtain relief through meditation, yoga, tai chi, qi gong, or acupuncture.

The outlook for relief from peripheral neuropathy depends on the cause of the pain. Transient irritations or injuries will generally resolve in due course of time regardless of the treatment. Nerve damage and systemic illnesses may provide intractable pain that resists any treatment and may last for a longer time. Many patients must receive pain management training to be able to live with their pain for long periods. One of the authors (Dr. Harris) has severe, intractable pain from damaged vertebrae in his neck and nerve damage in his shoulder from a head-on collision with an inebriated driver in the 1990s. Since it was not practical (or healthy) for him to take narcotic medication for more than a few days, it was necessary for him to receive pain management therapy with referral to a physical therapist who trained him in the use of a TNS unit.

personality The concept of personality is complex, taking into account a whole range of a person's traits and behaviors. Psychologists define personality as an enduring tendency to act and feel in particular ways.

There is evidence that part of the CEREBRAL CORTEX known as the PREFRONTAL CORTEX in the FRONTAL LOBE plays a role in personality traits such as planning and organizational ability, ethical and moral sense, and overall emotional control.

One of the best examples of the relationship between the PREFRONTAL CORTEX and personality is in the unfortunate example of Phineas A. Gage, who was injured when a three-foot iron rod pierced his skull during an explosion in 1848. Incredibly, he did not die, but his left frontal lobe was destroyed when the bar entered the skull. Before the accident, he had been a well-liked, calm, and steady worker, but afterward his friends noticed extreme personality changes. He became deeply disagreeable, tactless, profane, and restless. It appeared that a sort of civilizing influence over his personality had been lost when his frontal lobe was obliterated. Interestingly, alcohol appears to mimic this type of prefrontal control over behavior because intoxication can lead to similar personality changes such as increased profanity, vulgarity, aggression, and loss of sexual restraint.

Some researchers have begun to study the effect of certain NEUROTRANSMITTER levels on personality. Initial results suggest that the levels of DOPAMINE seem to correlate with the degree of extroversion.

Of course, personality is more than the sum total of a person's neurotransmitters; it is shaped by a variety of factors, including genetic and environmental influences. Family size, income, position within the family (eldest or youngest, for example), nutrition, and body size or shape can all affect personality.

Pervasive Developmental Disorders (PDDs)   PDDs include a wide spectrum of social and communication disorders, including AUTISTIC DISORDER and AUTISM SPECTRUM DISORDERS such as ASPERGER'S DISORDER.

Symptoms and Diagnostic Path

PDDs can be especially difficult to diagnose, given the vagueness of symptoms of these disorders and the young ages of children when symptoms of PDDs begin to emerge. For example, a young child's tendency to be contrary at times may be perfectly normal but may give the incorrect impression there is a PDD present. Most psychologists and physicians observe that PDDs are identifiable by age three.

Parents and physicians of children with PDDs note they first noticed problems in infancy and the toddler period with acquiring language; difficulty relating to people, things, and events; extreme resistance to changes in routine; unusual play with toys and other objects; obsession with certain toys or other objects to the exclusion of other things; and self-stimulation behavior such as head-banging, scratching themselves, or staring into lights as they switch them on and off.

Children with PDDs vary widely in ability: Although some test in the deficient range of intelligence, others have been extremely intelligent. Some never speak, and others develop language to some extent.

Treatment Options and Outlook

There is no one treatment for PDDs. Speech and language therapists provide extensive therapies with those who are able to acquire language and enhance their ability to communicate. Physical and occupational therapists work to assist individuals with PDDs in strengthening their muscles and developing coordination. Psychologists may offer assistance with behavior management and help parents and teachers develop specific behavior modification programs to help these individuals develop socially appropriate behavior. Physicians may prescribe medications to help lessen behavioral symptoms. Some children with PDDs will require highly specialized special education and related services in segregated classrooms with small student-to-teacher ratios, while others will be able to integrate into the mainstream effectively.

Early identification and treatment of children with PDDs significantly improves these individuals' long-term outcomes. Many will require 24-hour cooperation between home and school over their entire school career to maximize the benefits of special education and related services. Parents, for example, may have specific roles in reinforcing the activities of the speech and language therapist by participating in "homework" assigned by the clinician or enhance the child's physical therapy by having them play games that enhance their fine- and gross-motor coordination.

Although many individuals with PDDs have life-long disabilities in social, behavioral, and language functioning, many achieve sufficient gains through appropriate treatment to be able to pursue productive adult employment and function independently.

pesticides and the brain   One of many NEUROTOXINS that can adversely affect the NERVOUS SYSTEM, damaging and inhibiting the enzyme acetylcholinesterase, which is essential for proper neuromuscular function.

Of the many different types of pesticides commercially available, the organophosphates (originally developed as nerve gas during World War II) are the most commonly used; they include malathion, disulfotan, and dementon. Even a tiny amount of exposure to organophosphate may cause toxic mood disorders and NEUROPATHY; concentrated exposure can kill. Most neurological damage is reversible, once exposure has ended.

The most common way for a person to become poisoned with pesticides is by skin absorption—especially farm workers and those who work in pesticide manufacturing plants. Many people may be exposed at home by spraying in gardens or to prevent bug infestations. Pesticides can also contaminate groundwater or food.

petit mal seizure   A temporary disturbance of brain function caused by abnormal electrical activity in the brain that occurs during childhood and adolescence, but rarely in adulthood. These seizures are characterized by a momentary loss of awareness resembling a daydream. This type of seizure may last up to 30 seconds at a time and may occur hundreds of times daily.

Petit mal seizures are also known as absence seizures, which cause a loss of consciousness that is usually brief and barely noticeable. The neurons in a normal brain communicate by firing tiny electric signals. During a seizure, the firing pattern of the brain's electric signals becomes abnormal and unusually intense, affecting an isolated area of the brain or the entire brain.

Petit mal seizures occur in two of every 1,000 people, usually in children between the ages of six to 12; they rarely begin after age 20. Typically, girls suffer from absence epilepsy more often than boys, and in most cases the underlying reason for the seizures is unknown. Research suggests that genetic factors play some role in the development of absence epilepsy.

Symptoms and Diagnostic Path
During a seizure, the individual simply stops moving or speaking, stares blankly, and does not answer questions. While the seizure is happening, the child's eyelids may blink or flicker rapidly or an arm or leg may twitch or jerk. When the seizure ends, the child resumes normal activities without realizing that anything has happened, and with no memory of the seizure. A child with repeated absence seizures is said to have childhood absence EPILEPSY or petit mal epilepsy.

Seizures may occur for weeks or months before they are noticed because symptoms commonly occur during quiet rest periods rather than periods of activity. Petit mal seizures can be infrequent, or they may occur many times an hour. The more often a child has these seizures, the more likely they will interfere with school function and learning. All too often, teachers may interpret these seizures as lack of attention or other misbehavior.

A review of the child's medical history, especially any history of birth trauma, serious HEAD INJURY or infections involving the brain, and family history, is the first step in reaching a diagnosis. This is followed by a physical and neurological examination and routine blood tests to rule out common medical illnesses that can mimic epilepsy

or trigger seizures. An ELECTROENCEPHALOGRAM (EEG) can detect the electrical activity in the brain. Petit mal seizures generally present a very characteristic appearance on the EEG, with a specific combination of spike and wave patterns that confirms the diagnosis. In some cases, the doctor also may order an MRI (magnetic resonance imaging) or CT (computed tomography) scan of the child's brain to look for a tumor or other abnormality.

Treatment Options and Outlook
The goal of treatment is to prevent progression to more serious types of seizures. Antiseizure medications may prevent or minimize the number of seizures. Reevaluation should occur at least yearly. Monitoring of blood drug levels is important for continued control of seizures and reduction of medication side effects.

Petit mal seizures usually respond to valproic acid, ethosuximide, or clonazepam. Multiple, frequently repeated seizures are treated by intravenous diazepam (Valium).

Almost all children who have petit mal seizures have significantly fewer (or no) seizures with the use of medications. Petit mal seizures may stop spontaneously after the child reaches adulthood, or they may continue indefinitely. In some cases, the person may begin having grand mal seizures. Most people with petit mal seizures live a fairly normal life. As adulthood approaches, restrictions may be placed on driving or operating dangerous machinery if seizures continue.

See also GRAND MAL SEIZURE

PET scan Positron emission tomography is an imaging technique used to record and create images of the chemical activity in regions of the brain that are used primarily as a research tool.

Procedure
This type of scan creates computerized images of the distribution of radioactively labeled GLUCOSE in the brain in order to show brain activity. The more active a part of the brain is, the more glucose it uses. PET sensors are arrayed around the head of a patient, who sits with the head behind black felt to keep out

distractions. The scan can pinpoint the source of the radioactivity (and heightened activity). These data are sent to computers that produce two-dimensional drawings showing the neural "hot spots." While PET accurately tracks brain function, it can resolve brain structures less than a half-inch apart.

PET scans are especially helpful for investigating the brain, where they can be used to detect tumors, to pinpoint the location of epileptic activity, and to investigate brain function in mental illness.

PET scans of labeled drugs that attach to specific RECEPTORS can show the distribution and number of those receptors.

Risks and Complications

There are no known risks to the procedure.

See also BRAIN SCANS; CAT SCAN; NUCLEAR MAGNETIC IMAGING; SPECT; SQUID.

phenylalanine An AMINO ACID from which the brain manufactures norepinephrine, which plays a major role in learning and MEMORY. It is converted into TYROSINE in the body; in the inherited disease PHENYLKETONURIA, the enzyme that converts phenylalanine into tyrosine is defective. Unless phenylalanine (a natural constituent of most protein foods) is eliminated from the diet, it builds up in the brain and causes severe MENTAL RETARDATION.

phenylketonuria (PKU) An inherited metabolic disease (also called an inborn error of metabolism) that leads to MENTAL RETARDATION and other developmental disabilities if untreated in infancy. In this condition, an amino acid called PHENYLALANINE builds up in the bloodstream, causing brain damage.

PKU is inherited as an autosomal recessive disorder, which means that each parent of a child with PKU carries one defective gene for the disorder and one normal gene. In a recessive condition, an individual must inherit two defective genes in order to have the disorder. Individuals with only one copy of a defective gene are called carriers, show no symptoms of having the disease, and usually remain unaware of their status until they have an affected child. In order for a child to inherit PKU, both parents must be PKU carriers. When this occurs, there

is a one in four chance of the parents producing an affected child with each pregnancy. Boys and girls are equally at risk of inheriting this disorder.

The disease affects at least one of every 16,000 babies, mostly those of northern European background. Jews, Asians, and Africans are less commonly affected.

Untreated, the condition can lead to MENTAL RETARDATION by age one, in addition to behavior problems or a LEARNING DISABILITY.

Symptoms and Diagnostic Path

Before the 1960s, most infants born with PKU developed mental retardation and CEREBRAL PALSY. Infants with untreated PKU appear to develop typically for the first few months of life, but by 12 months of age most babies with PKU will have a significant developmental delay and will be diagnosed with mental retardation.

Although treatment for PKU using a low-phenylalanine diet was first described in the 1950s, the inability to detect PKU early in the child's life limited effective treatment. The first newborn screening test was developed by Dr. Robert Guthrie in 1959 specifically to test for PKU. This simple yet effective and economical test was developed to screen newborn infants for PKU before leaving the hospital.

Today, all states routinely screen newborns for PKU. The American Academy of Pediatrics recommends that infants receiving the test during the first 24 hours of life be retested at two to three weeks of age during their first postnatal pediatric visit.

To test for PKU, a few drops of blood are taken from the infant's heel and tested in a state laboratory for abnormal amounts of phenylalanine. The normal phenylalanine level is less than 2 milligrams per deciliter (mg/dl). Those with phenylalanine levels of 20 mg/dl or higher are considered likely to have "classical" PKU. Infants with these high levels are further tested to confirm the diagnosis before treatment is started.

Treatment Options and Outlook

Although PKU is not preventable, its symptoms can often be treated successfully through the use of a carefully regimented diet with a restricted phenylalanine content. Babies are given a special formula that contains very low phenylalanine levels; they gradually progress to eating certain vegetables and other foods that are low in phenylalanine. Affected children must have their blood tested regularly to ensure the presence of the correct level of phenylalanine. Foods recommended for those affected by PKU contain small amounts of protein, such as fruits and vegetables, limited amounts of cereal and grain products, and special low-protein products.

High-protein foods such as meat, fish, eggs, poultry, dairy products, nuts, peanut butter, legumes, and soy products, as well as products containing Nutrasweet, should be avoided. The food program used to treat those with PKU is quite expensive, typically costing up to $10,000 a year or more. Although health departments may pay for the formula in some states and mandated insurance coverage may cover the cost in other states, most insurance companies do not cover the cost of treatment for those with PKU because it is considered nutritional rather than medical therapy.

While phenylalanine restricted diets have proven to be highly effective in preventing mental retardation, it is now recognized that there may still be subtle cognitive deficits. Usually the individual has a normal IQ, but the incidence of ATTENTION DEFICIT HYPERACTIVITY DISORDER (ADHD) and learning disabilities is higher compared to those children who do not have PKU.

Recent studies have found that children with PKU who stopped the diet in early childhood did not develop as rapidly as children who remained on the diet, and had more learning disabilities, behavioral problems, and other neurological problems. Thus, until research provides alternative treatments, everyone with PKU should remain on a restricted diet indefinitely in order to maintain a safe level of phenylalanine (believed to be in the range of 2–6 mg/dl).

Some infants with slightly higher levels of phenylalanine have mild hyperphenylalanemia. Today many clinicians believe that any child with a phenylalanine level greater than six or eight mg/dl should be treated with a modified phenylalanine-restricted diet.

Pregnancy and PKU

Pregnant women with PKU who do not receive dietary therapy have high levels of phenylalanine that can damage their unborn child, causing mental retardation and other congenital defects. High levels of phenylalanine are extremely toxic to the brain of a fetus. Although the child may not have PKU, there will be brain damage from the toxic effects of phenylalanine in the womb. This is known as maternal PKU.

More than 90 percent of infants born to women with PKU who are not on a specialized diet will have mental retardation, and may also have small head size, heart defects, and low birth weight. These infants cannot be treated with a special diet since they do not have PKU. Therefore, women who have PKU should be on a phenylalanine-restricted diet at least one year before pregnancy and should stay on the diet while breast-feeding to increase the chance of having a healthy child.

phenytoin (Dilantin) This well-known treatment for EPILEPSY may also improve intelligence, concentration, and learning, according to some studies. In the United States, the only approved use for this drug is to control various types of SEIZURES, which it does by stabilizing electrical activity in cell membranes. It is a cerebral vasodilator.

Excess amounts of the drug have the opposite effect on MEMORY, intelligence, and reaction time. Many patients are allergic to the drug.

phrenology The belief that there is a relationship between the structure of the skull and the science of a person's character. The term *phrenology* is derived from the Greek roots *phren* ("mind") and *logos* ("study of"). The theory was developed by idiosyncratic Viennese physician Franz Joseph Gall (1758–1828), who believed that the brain is composed of distinct, innate faculties and that because they are distinct, each faculty must have a distinct seat in the brain. Gall also believed that the size of the different areas in the brain was a measure of their power, and that the shape of the brain was determined by the development of the various areas.

As the skull takes its shape from the brain, Gall believed, the surface of the skull could therefore be read as an accurate index of psychological aptitudes and tendencies. Gall himself never approved of the term *phrenology*, but called his system *organology* or simply "the physiology of the brain."

Gall and the phrenologists never conducted independent rigorous research, but tried only to confirm their preconceived ideas. Any evidence that supported their theory was readily accepted as proof, whereas any contradictory findings (such as a selfish person with a well-developed "organ of benevolence") were always explained away.

The first phrenological society was founded in Edinburgh in 1820, and many more followed. During the theory's popular crest in the 1820s and 1830s, many employers could demand a character reference from a local phrenologist to ensure that the employee was honest and hardworking. This belief that the protuberances on the skull provided an accurate index of talents and abilities was especially important in education and criminal reform of the time. Phrenologists thought they could determine the best careers for their subjects—and even find a good marital match—with great accuracy. During the heyday of phrenology, visiting a phrenologist was much like seeking the advice of a psychic or astrologer today. At the time, phrenology was popular not just among some scientists but also with political and social reformers, as well as with devout evangelicals who saw evidence for the design of a creator.

However, most phrenologists were not religious, but saw the theory as more of a self-help method. From Britain, the practice of phrenology spread to America and France in the 1830s.

By the mid-1850s it had become far less popular in Britain, as a new, less scientific and more entrepreneurial movement was introduced to Britain by the American "phrenological Fowlers" in the 1860s and 1870s. The Fowlers had begun lecturing and reading heads in New York in the 1840s, and swept through Britain on a successful lecture tour before establishing various phrenological institutions, societies, and publishing businesses.

Phrenologizing involved mostly head reading and character delineations as well as speculation on the relationships between the phrenological faculties. Most phrenologists would run their bare fingertips or palms over a person's head to distinguish any elevations or indentations, although some experts would use calipers, measuring tapes,

and other instruments. A skilled phrenologist knew not just the map of the head according to the latest phrenological chart, but also the pros and cons of each of the 35 organs.

Phrenology has been almost universally discredited as a science since the mid-19th century; even during the peak of its popularity between the 1820s and 1840s, phrenology was always controversial and never achieved the status of an accredited science. Phrenology eventually became deeply unfashionable amongst the well-to-do who had previously espoused it, degenerating into a sect of extremists. (Even so, the British Phrenological Society founded by L. N. Fowler in 1887 was disbanded only in 1967.)

The history of phrenology is now of interest to historians and those seeking the early roots of modern cerebral localization and neuroscience. Phrenology was the first system to attribute psychological behavior to localized regions of the CEREBRAL CORTEX, an approach that has become increasingly well accepted after the work of PIERRE-PAUL BROCA and others in France and CARL WERNICKE in Germany in the 1870s.

physiological causes of memory loss Because the brain is susceptible to fluctuating levels of fluids, oxygen, and nutrients, anything that affects the physiological health of the body may affect memory systems as well.

Fluid Imbalances Too much or too little water in the body can disturb brain function, because water contains electrolytes (potassium, sodium, chloride, calcium, and magnesium) that are crucial to the function of cells that make up the memory system.

Hypoglycemia Because brain cells require an adequate amount of sugar (glucose) to maintain metabolic activity, a drop in the body's blood sugar level can lead to a host of memory problems.

Malnutrition Dementing brain disease can be produced by a diet that lacks enough of the B-complex vitamins (especially NIACIN, thiamine, and B_{12}). This is one reason behind the memory problems of serious alcohol abusers, who typically lack thiamine because they do not eat properly. Vegetarians who do not get enough vitamin B_{12} also may experience symptoms of memory deficits; recent research suggests that those with low-normal levels of B_{12} in their blood tend to experience depression with memory problems. A more serious lack of this vitamin can lead to spinal cord degeneration and associated brain diseases, including memory loss.

physostigmine   A drug used as eyedrops in the treatment of glaucoma that also may produce mild memory improvement among ALZHEIMER'S DISEASE patients. Physostigmine also reverses memory loss following the administration of SCOPOLAMINE in normal subjects.

Physostigmine is believed to improve memory by enhancing levels of ACETYLCHOLINE, which is important in a range of memory processes.

The drug improves efficiency and reduces the effort needed to perform working memory tasks while altering the activity of some of the brain regions activated by this memory task, according to a study by the National Institute on Aging. The drug may enhance efficiency during the processing of information by focusing attention on the task at hand, or it may help minimize the effects of distracting stimuli. Either way, a more efficient working memory could be a great advantage for patients with ALZHEIMER'S DISEASE and other memory impairments.

TACRINE, the first approved drug for treatment against Alzheimer's disease, acts on the acetylcholine system in a way similar to physostigmine. Some scientists believe that since physostigmine improves the brain's response to memory tasks, similar drugs that enhance the cholinergic system might help relieve symptoms in Alzheimer's disease patients.

pia mater   The innermost layer of the membranes surrounding and protecting the brain that dips into all the furrows of the brain. Made up of fine tissue, it also contains many blood vessels that supply the brain. Sometimes, the pia mater and the ARACHNOID are regarded as one membrane, which is then called the pia-arachnoid.

Pick's disease   A form of DEMENTIA characterized by a slowly progressive deterioration of social skills and changes in personality leading to impairment of intellect, memory, and language. The condition is almost impossible to distinguish from ALZHEIMER'S DISEASE except on autopsy, although it is much less common. Alzheimer's disease causes 50 percent to 60 percent of dementia cases, whereas Pick's disease accounts for about 5 percent of cognitive deterioration.

On average, patients contract this disease at about 55 years of age, with death following within about seven years. After the midfifties, the likelihood of developing Pick's disease decreases; there have been only three cases of Pick's disease diagnosed in patients over age 70.

The disease is characterized by "Pick's bodies" in the brain cells—miscellaneous bits of the normal cell. Although the parts are recognizable, their normal relationships have been disrupted. The cause is unknown.

Pick's disease was first identified in 1892 by Dr. Arnold Pick, who described the progressive mental deterioration in a 71-year-old man. On autopsy, his brain showed an unusually shrunken frontal cortex—the region involved in reasoning and other higher mental functions. This shrinkage is different from the brain changes associated with Alzheimer's disease.

Symptoms and Diagnostic Path

The disorder begins in the frontal lobes, triggering changes in personality and social behavior. Memory problems later appear, until eventually patients become mute, incontinent, and immobile. Although the disease varies greatly in the way it affects individuals, there is a common core of symptoms among patients which may be present at different stages of the disease. These symptoms include loss of memory, lack of spontaneity, difficulty in thinking or concentrating, and disturbances of speech. Other symptoms include gradual emotional dullness, loss of moral judgment, and progressive dementia. Although the disease usually affects individuals between the ages of 40 and 60, the age of onset may range from 20 to 80. The condition is more common in women than men.

Pick's disease is diagnosed in a process similar to that involved in diagnosing Alzheimer's disease. Often a patient is diagnosed with "probable

Alzheimer's," and later the diagnosis is changed to Pick's.

Treatment Options and Outlook

There is no cure or specific treatment for Pick's disease, and its progress cannot be slowed down. However, some of the symptoms of the disease may be treated effectively.

The course of Pick's disease is an inevitable progressive deterioration that may take anywhere from less than two years to more than 10 years. Death is usually caused by infection.

pineal gland   A tiny structure within the brain responsible for secreting the hormone MELATONIN, which induces sleep and regulates CIRCADIAN RHYTHM, affecting mood and mental quickness. The amount of this hormone varies over a 24-hour period and is greatest at night. It is believed that the secretion of this hormone is controlled by nerve pathways from the retina; light affects the secretion.

Because the pineal gland is not duplicated in each hemisphere, philosopher RENÉ DESCARTES chose this site as the place where the body and soul are integrated.

The gland is located deep within the brain, just below the back part of the CORPUS CALLOSUM, the band of fibers that connects the two halves of the CEREBELLUM. Several tumors may occur rarely in the pineal gland.

pineal gland tumors   There are a number of types of tumors that may be found in the PINEAL GLAND, located at the back of the third ventricle of the brain. The most common type of tumor found in this part of the brain is called a germinoma. Other tumors include ASTROCYTOMAS, teratomas, MENINGIOMAS, pineocytomas, and pineoblastomas. Germinomas, which develop from germ cells, are malignant tumors that grow quite quickly, often spreading to other parts of the brain.

Pineal region tumors are very rare and make up a very small percentage of primary brain tumors. They occur more often in children than adults, and are most common in teenagers. They are also more common in boys than girls.

Symptoms and Diagnostic Path

Tumors in the pineal region usually produce symptoms related to increased pressure within the skull that may be caused by a block in the ventricles of the brain which leads to a buildup of cerebrospinal fluid, or by swelling from the tumor itself.

The first sign of this type of tumor in children is often water on the brain (HYDROCEPHALUS), which can cause an enlarged skull. Other symptoms include headaches, vomiting, visual problems, lethargy, and irritability. Some symptoms may be caused by the tumor pressing on surrounding areas of the brain, which could lead to problems with coordination and balance. People with this condition often have trouble walking and may appear to stumble. Tumors in the pineal region may extend to the pituitary gland and result in delayed puberty or other hormonal problems.

A neurological examination can assess any effect the tumor has had on the nervous system. A CT or MRI scan can pinpoint the precise location of the tumor. A biopsy can confirm the type of tumor, and blood tests for hormone levels will probably be taken, particularly if there are signs that the pituitary gland is affected. A lumbar puncture (spinal tap) may be done to obtain a sample of cerebrospinal fluid, since some germinomas contain distinctive cells that can be detected under a microscope. (This test cannot be done if intracranial pressure is too high.)

Treatment Options and Outlook

The treatment for tumors in the pineal region depends on the size and position of the growth. Before any treatment, any excess pressure in the skull must be reduced. Steroid medications may be given to reduce swelling around the tumor, or a shunt may be inserted to drain off the excess cerebrospinal fluid.

The position of the pineal region in the center of the brain often makes surgical removal of these tumors very difficult. However, when possible, surgery is the preferred treatment for pineal tumors in order to remove as much of the tumor as possible without damaging the surrounding brain tissue.

Radiation is often used to treat tumors in the pineal region; germinomas in particular respond well to radiotherapy. Radiation is often given after surgery to destroy any remaining cancer cells. If there are signs that the cancer has spread to the spine, radiation will be given to both the brain and the spinal cord. When surgery is not possible, radiation may be given alone or combined with chemotherapy.

Chemotherapy to destroy cancer cells is often used in combination with radiation to treat germinomas. It is rarely used for other pineal tumors.

pituitary adenoma A tumor of the PITUITARY GLAND, which lies behind a bone at the base of the skull. Almost all adenomas are benign, which means that they are relatively slow-growing and are slow to invade surrounding tissues. They rarely spread to other areas of the body. Typically, they appear in young or middle-aged adults, affecting men and women equally.

Symptoms and Diagnostic Path
A pituitary adenoma causes symptoms either from compression of nearby brain structures or from abnormal hormone production. Secondary effects of tumor growth can lead to compression of the optic chiasm, which has a position slightly above and in front of the pituitary gland. Such damage leads to visual problems.

Treatment Options and Outlook
Surgical therapy, medicinal therapy, or radiotherapy are the three treatment options for pituitary adenomas.

Surgery is indicated if there is evidence of tumor enlargement, especially when growth is accompanied by compression of the optic chiasm, sinus invasion, or the development of pituitary hormone deficiencies. Visual improvement following treatment is often dramatic, with the greatest degree of improvement occurring within the first few months.

The surgical removal of a pituitary adenoma can usually be performed by a method called a transsphenoidal operation. The surgeon approaches the pituitary gland by making an incision beneath the upper lip to expose the nasal passage. Using a microscope and specialized instruments, the surgeon enters the sphenoid bone, and eventually an

opening is made in the wall of the bone to expose the pituitary gland. When the tumor is removed, the cavity is sealed and the surgeon then applies a "glue" made from the patient's own blood donated before surgery. Vaseline gauze is then packed into the nasal cavities and the procedure is completed. Conventional radiation may be added after surgery to prevent tumor regrowth.

See also PITUITARY TUMORS.

pituitary gland Located just below the HYPOTHALAMUS, this gland produces many hormones as well as ENDORPHINS. In conjunction with the hypothalamus, the two essentially run the endocrine system. This "master gland" secretes hormones that control hormone secretion by other endocrine glands. It affects the growth of bones, muscles, the thyroid, adrenal cortex, secretion of testosterone and estrogen, development of follicles, ovulation, water balance, blood pressure, and uterine contraction.

pituitary tumors About 10 percent of brain tumors are pituitary tumors, almost all of which are benign. They are most often found in young or middle-aged adults. Pituitary tumors are considered either "secreting" or "nonsecreting." Secreting tumors release excess amounts of one of the pituitary hormones and are named after that hormone—for example, "prolactin-secreting tumor."

Symptoms and Diagnostic Path
Symptoms of pituitary tumors are either caused by direct pressure from the tumor itself or by a disruption in normal hormone levels. As the tumor grows, it puts pressure on the optic nerve, causing headaches and visual problems. Symptoms caused by a disruption in hormone levels usually take a long time to develop. Prolactin-secreting tumors are the most common type of secreting tumor. Women with this type of tumor may notice that their menstrual periods stop; they also may produce small amounts of breast milk. Symptoms in men may include impotence. Infertility is common in both men and women with this type of tumor, which may be diagnosed during routine tests for

infertility. Symptoms of other secreting tumors are related to the hormones they release.

Excess secretion of growth hormones can cause a condition called gigantism which leads to abnormal growth, causing enlargement of the hands and feet and leading to high blood pressure and diabetes. A very rare tumor that releases too much TSH causes a disruption in the body's normal metabolism. Overproduction of ACTH can produce a number of symptoms, including Cushing's syndrome, which is characterized by a round face, weight gain, increased facial hair in women, and mental changes, such as depression.

Tumors that secrete FSH or LSH are very rare and are likely to cause infertility.

Tumors in the posterior pituitary are also very rare; disturbances in this area are more likely to be caused by pressure from the surrounding tissues. The most common symptom of this type of tumor is a condition called diabetes insipidus (as opposed to diabetes mellitus), the main symptom of which is the production of large quantities of very weak urine.

Pituitary tumors are often discovered during when a blood test reveals excess amounts of pituitary hormones. This may be followed by a CT or MRI scan to confirm the diagnosis of a pituitary tumor. Eye tests can reveal pressure on the optic nerve that may indicate a tumor.

Treatment Options and Outlook

Surgery is the most common treatment for most pituitary tumors; it will remove the tumor but leave at least some of the normal pituitary gland behind. This is not always possible, and in certain cases the entire gland must be removed. Surgery is usually done by approaching the pituitary from the nose or by a small opening under the lip. This makes recovery after surgery much quicker than in other operations for brain tumors.

Some prolactin-secreting tumors can be treated with a drug called bromocriptine, which reduces the production of prolactin. If the entire pituitary gland is removed, medications must be taken to replace the missing hormones.

Radiation treatment is often used after pituitary surgery for all types of tumors. Treatment of pituitary tumors is usually very successful.

PKU See PHENYLKETONURIA.

planum temporale Part of the brain that is involved in understanding speech; in most healthy people, it is much larger in the left hemisphere.

plasticity A neuron's ability to change its structure or function. The brain is not a computer that is wired forever at birth. Instead, it remodels itself constantly in response to experience, aging, hormones, illness, injury and learning. It is plastic— that is, it can be molded. It is this plasticity that helps the brain quickly learn new things, such as memorizing a phone number or practicing the piano. In fact, something as simple as remembering a name or address can't be performed until something changes in the brain.

The new understanding of how much the brain is constantly changing is partly due to advances in brain scan techniques that allow scientists to see inside the living, thinking brain. Images from positron emission tomography (PET) and FUNCTIONAL MAGNETIC RESONANCE IMAGING (fMRI) let scientists track changes in the brain as they happen. Activated areas of the brain "light up" on these scans, revealing increased blood flow and electrical energy.

It all takes place on the level of the connections between individual brain cells. The human brain has up to 100 billion nerve cells; about 10 billion are in the NEOCORTEX, the outer layer of gray matter responsible for conscious experience. All the action in the brain occurs at the cells' connection points, called the SYNAPSES, where electrical pulses that carry messages leap across gaps between cells. Each neuron can form thousands of links, giving a typical brain about 100 trillion synapses.

As a person learns, behaves, and experiences the world and stores memories, changes occur at the synapses, and more and more connections in the brain are created. The brain organizes and reorganizes itself in response to experience and sensory stimulation, and these changes are reinforced with use. As a person learns and practices new information, intricate circuits of knowledge and memory are laid down.

The interconnections between neurons are not fixed, but change all the time. Researchers at Rockefeller University have discovered that neurons don't act alone, but work together in a network, organizing themselves into groups and specializing in different kinds of information processing. For example, if one neuron sends many signals to another neuron, the synapse between the two gets stronger. The more active the two neurons are, the stronger the connection between them grows. Thus, with every new experience, your brain slightly rewires its physical structure. In fact, how a person uses his brain helps determine how the brain is organized. It is this flexibility, this "plasticity," that helps the brain rewire itself once it has been damaged, helping a person recover lost or damaged functions in the wake of stroke, for example.

Periods of Plasticity

Periods of rapid change occur in the brain under four main conditions:

- developmental: when the immature brain first begins to process sensory information
- activity-dependent: when changes in the body alter the balance of sensory activity received by the brain
- learning and memory: when we alter our behavior based on new sensory information
- injury-induced: after damage to the brain

Brain Repair

In the past, scientists thought that the nervous system could not repair itself, and that brain cells, once lost, could never be replaced. But today scientists know that the brain can reorganize itself to an astonishing degree. Some very new research with rats even suggests that new brain cells can be created.

Unfortunately, the brain's ability to adapt is not limitless. Normal plasticity can't fully compensate for severe damage from tumors or trauma, for example. It is also possible for the brain to become *too* plastic, and overreact. This is what happens when an amputee feels a "phantom pain" in a missing limb.

At Any Age

This plasticity means the human brain has the capacity to remodel itself at any age. It is experience—both good and bad—that is behind the brain's continual remodeling. Even illness or trauma is a kind of "learning" for the brain. This could mean that one day, the best treatment for a degenerative disease like Parkinson's might be not a drug but an intense relearning process that could help the patient unlearn the illness.

Twenty years ago, experts thought that the structure of the brain develops during childhood and, once organized, it left very little room for changes. Today we know that this isn't true—adult brains remain plastic to some degree. It is true, however, that while humans never stop learning, this remodeling is harder for adults than for children. Studies of children learning to play the violin showed that their brain plasticity, as evidenced by changes in their brains in response to practicing, is greatest in those under age 13. Scientists believe this is because the younger a person is, the more room in the brain's hemisphere for new connections to be made.

Scientists believe a person loses about 1,000 neurons each day after age 40. However, this loss can be offset by regular stimulation. If a neuron is being used, it secretes substances that affect nearby cells responsible for the neuron's nourishment. These cells, in turn, produce a chemical that appears to keep the neuron from being destroyed. If the neuron doesn't get that substance, it dies. So as long as a person is actively using his brain and learning new things, research suggests it's possible to offset the death of neurons.

No matter how plastic the brain, however, it is still true that memory does deteriorate with aging. Yet while there is some physical breakdown and memory loss as adults age, the biggest obstacle to continued learning is the patterns the brain has already learned. Neurons are shaped much like trees, with branches going off in all directions. Each time a nerve cell branches out, it allows for more subtle connections with other neurons far away, not just those close by that do similar things. Scientists believe this means that an adult's mind may lose details but gain more depth and richness, much like seeing the majesty of the forest instead of the details of an individual oak.

In the Future
Once scientists fully understand how the brain makes its new connections, it would be possible to create more effective drugs or physical exercises to enhance the natural plastic processes.

pleasure centers Deep within the HYPOTHALAMUS is a structure which appears to be associated with pleasure. The existence of this structure has been proven primarily through animal research; rats with electrodes connected to this region would incessantly press a lever to stimulate the region and experience pleasure. A similar area in the hypothalamus in humans has been found during NEUROSURGERY.

These pleasure centers involve certain NEU-ROTRANSMITTERS of the LIMBIC SYSTEM, and it is the action of these chemicals that is mimicked by psychoactive drugs. DOPAMINE and NOREPINEPHRINE (two neurotransmitters found in NEURONS of the limbic system) are released by the use of cocaine and AMPHETAMINES. Opiate receptors are also found throughout the limbic system, and these are also stimulated by morphine, heroin, and other narcotics. Scientists believe that these drugs cause a sense of euphoria by stimulating one or more of these pleasure centers in the brain.

pneumococcal vaccine See MENINGITIS, PNEUMOCOCCAL

pneumoencephalography A technique used in the X-RAY diagnosis of diseases inside the skull, in which air is introduced into the VENTRICLES of the brain to displace the CEREBROSPINAL FLUID. X-ray photos can show the size and condition of the ventricles and the SUBARACHNOID SPACES.

polioencephalitis A type of viral brain INFEC-TION that attacks the GRAY MATTER of the CEREBRAL HEMISPHERES and the BRAIN STEM. The term is now

usually restricted to infections of the brain by the POLIOMYELITIS virus.

polioencephalomyelitis Any viral infection of the CENTRAL NERVOUS SYSTEM, such as RABIES, that affects the GRAY MATTER of the brain and the SPINAL CORD.

poliomyelitis (polio) An infectious viral brain INFECTION once known as infantile paralysis that kills motor NEURONS in the SPINAL CORD and BRAIN STEM. The virus is excreted in the feces of an infected person, from where it may be spread directly or indirectly. Air-borne transmission also occurs.

While the disease is most common where sanitation is poor, epidemics may occur even in hygienic conditions where individuals have not acquired immunity to the disease during infancy or through vaccination.

However, since the development of effective vaccines in the 1950s in the United States, polio has virtually been eliminated from the United States and Europe. Cases do occur in people who have not been fully vaccinated, and polio remains a serious risk for unvaccinated travelers visiting southern Europe, Africa, or Asia. No wild polio has been reported in the United States in 20 years.

Of those who have been paralyzed with polio, more than half eventually make a full recovery. Another quarter suffer minor permanent muscle weakness, and less than a quarter are left with a severe disability. Fewer than one in 10 patients dies; those who do are primarily adults and those with a severely infected brain stem.

In some cases, years after extensive paralysis with some recovery, there is a "postpolio" degeneration with new weakness and pain in some of the recovered muscles.

Symptoms and Diagnostic Path
This viral infection causes problems ranging from slight disability to total paralysis. About 85 percent of children infected with the virus have no symptoms at all; the rest have a short illness with a slight fever, sore throat, HEADACHE, and vomiting

that lasts for a few days, after which most children recover completely.

In abortive poliomyelitis, only the throat and intestines are infected, and the symptoms resemble stomach ache or flu. In nonparalytic poliomyelitis, the symptoms are accompanied by muscle stiffness (especially in neck and back). Paralytic poliomyelitis is much less common and includes weakness and eventual paralysis of the muscles. After a short period of apparent health, there is a major illness with symptoms of MENINGITIS, with fever, severe headache, stiff neck and back, and aching muscles. This progresses (often in just a few hours) to extensive paralysis of muscles. If infection spreads to the brain stem, there are problems in swallowing and breathing. In bulbar polio, the muscles of the respiratory system are involved, and breathing is affected.

Treatment Options and Outlook
There is no specific drug treatment for polio other than to treat symptoms. Bulbar polio may require the use of a respirator. In cases of paralysis, physical therapy is required to prevent muscle damage while the virus is active; later, it may retain muscle function.

Risk Factors and Preventive Measures
The American Academy of Pediatrics recommends the IVP (inactivated polio vaccine) be given during infancy at two, four, and 18 months, with an optional extra dose at six months and a booster at four to six years. The vaccine contains all three types of poliovirus, and immunity develops against each in turn. There are two alternative types of vaccine: IVP, which contains dead viruses and is given by injection, and OPV (oral poliovirus vaccine), which contains live but harmless strains of virus and is given by mouth. IVP is the vaccine of choice in the United States, because of a small risk (about one in 5 million) of the live vaccine causing polio in the vaccinated person or in a close contact.

Most adults do not need a polio vaccine because they were already vaccinated as children, according to the CDC, but three groups of adults at higher risk *should* consider polio vaccination: people traveling to areas of the world where polio is common, laboratory workers who might handle polio virus, and health care workers treating patients who could have polio.

Adults in these three groups who have never been vaccinated against polio should get three doses of IPV—the first dose at any time, followed by a second dose one or two months later, followed by a third dose six to 12 months after the second. Adults in these three groups who have had one or two doses of polio vaccine in the past should get the remaining one or two doses, no matter how long it has been since the earlier doses.

pons One of the three divisions of the BRAIN STEM, the pons receives sensations from facial skin and from the eyes, nose, mouth, and teeth. The pons tells the jaw muscles to chew, controls the outer eye muscle that moves the eye to the side, receives taste sensations from the front of the tongue, works the muscles that control facial expressions, receives nerve impulses from sounds that enter the ear, receives signals from the cochlea, and causes secretion of saliva and tears.

porencephaly An extremely rare disorder of the central nervous system involving cysts or cavities in a cerebral hemisphere that are the remnants of destructive lesions, but are sometimes the result of abnormal development. The disorder can occur before or after birth; most affected infants show symptoms of the disorder shortly after birth.

Symptoms and Diagnostic Path
Delayed growth and development, slight or incomplete paralysis, poor muscle tone, seizures, and abnormally large or small head. Individuals with porencephaly may have poor or absent speech development, EPILEPSY, HYDROCEPHALUS, shrinkage or shortening of a muscle, and MENTAL RETARDATION.

Treatment Options and Outlook
Treatments include physical therapy, medication for seizure disorders, and a shunt for hydrocephalus.

The prognosis varies according to the location and extent of the lesions. Some patients with this disorder may develop only minor neurological problems and have normal intelligence, while others may be severely disabled. Still others may die before the second decade of life.

positron emission transaxial tomography (PETT) scan   See PET SCAN.

postcentral gyrus   A part of the brain where touch and pressure sensation is perceived; also known as somatosensory cortex.

postconcussion syndrome   A syndrome of symptoms following even a mild bump on the head that can include dizziness and memory loss for six months or longer. Research suggests that 60 percent of patients who sustain a mild BRAIN INJURY are still having symptoms after three months.

The fact that a head injury can produce symptoms throughout the body has been known for at least the past 3,000 years; the Edwin Smith Surgical Papyrus, written between 2,500 and 3,000 years ago, contains information about 48 cases; eight describe head injuries that affect other parts of the body.

Symptoms and Diagnostic Path

Mild head injury symptoms can result in a puzzling interplay of behavioral, cognitive, and emotional complaints that make it difficult to diagnose. Although research is still limited, studies that do exist have found that symptoms following even the mildest head injury can linger, causing ongoing discomfort and disrupting lives.

Symptoms following a head injury may be due both from the direct physical damage to the brain and also to secondary factors such as lack of oxygen, swelling, and vascular disturbances. An injury that pierces the skull may also cause a brain INFECTION.

The kind of injury the brain receives during a closed head injury depends on the type of accident; whether or not the head was unrestrained on impact, and the direction, force, and velocity of the blow. If the head is resting on impact, the maximum damage will be found at the impact site;

a moving head will cause a "contrecoup" injury, where the damage will occur on the side opposite the point of impact.

Both kinds of injuries cause swirling movements throughout the brain, tearing nerve fibers and causing widespread vascular damage. There may be bleeding in the CEREBRUM or SUBARACHNOID SPACE leading to HEMATOMAS, or else brain swelling may raise pressure inside the cranium, cutting off oxygen to the brain.

After a head injury, there may be a period of impaired consciousness followed by a period of confusion known as post-traumatic amnesia. For some reason, the physical and emotional shock of an accident can interrupt the transfer of all information that happened to be in the short-term memory just before the accident; this is why some people can remember information several days before and after an accident but not information right before the accident occurred. Both the length of time of unconsciousness and post-traumatic amnesia have been linked to how well a person recovers after a head injury.

Until recently, diagnostic tools were not sensitive enough to detect the subtle structural changes that can occur and sometimes persist after mild head injury. Typically, CAT SCANS have not been able to reveal damage with this group of patients. But studies involving MAGNETIC RESONANCE IMAGING (MRI) and brain electrophysiology indicate that contusions and diffuse axonal injuries associated with mild head injury are likely to affect those parts of the brain that relate to functions such as memory, concentration, information processing, and problem solving.

In fact, a study of 424 patients diagnosed with mild head injury showed that many had recurrent problems with deviant behavior, HEADACHES, dizziness, and cognitive problems; only 17 percent were symptom-free three months after the accident.

Only about 12 percent of patients with mild head injury are hospitalized overnight, and instructions given upon release from the emergency room usually do not address behavioral, cognitive, and emotional symptoms that may occur after such an injury.

While CAT scans are widely available in emergency rooms to help in the diagnosis of neural hematomas, many experts believe these scans may not pick up the subtle damage following a mild head injury.

Many researchers believe that MRI is more sensitive in diagnosing many brain lesions beyond a basic hematoma. For example, an MRI is more sensitive in detecting the diffuse axonal or shearing injury and contusions often seen in this type of brain accident.

In many patients, neither CT nor MRI can detect the microscopic damage to WHITE MATTER that occurs when fibers are stretched in a mild, diffuse axonal injury. In this type of mild injury, the AXONS lose some of their covering and become less efficient, but MRI only detects more severe injury and actual axonal degeneration. Mild injury to the white matter reduces the quality of community between different parts of the CEREBRAL CORTEX. In these cases, a quantitative EEG may be used. This type of assessment is different from an EEG in that the signals from the brain are played into a computer, digitized, and stored. This type of EEG can measure the time delay between two regions of the CORTEX and the amount of time it takes for information to be transmitted from one region to another.

The study of evoked potentials is an electrophysical technique not generally useful in patients with less serious head injury. Evoked potentials are not sensitive enough to document most physiologic abnormalities, although the patient may be having symptoms. If testing is done within a day or two of the injury, the EP may pick up some abnormalities in brain stem auditory-evoked potentials.

Neuropsychological tests may show positive results when imaging tests and neurologic exams are negative. In some patients with persistent symptoms following mild head injury, neuropsychological tests are part of a comprehensive assessment. The tests can also provide information when litigation is an issue.

POSITRON EMISSION TOMOGRAPHY (PET SCAN), which evaluates cerebral blood flow and brain metabolism, may provide useful information on functional pathology following mild head injury. SINGLE PHOTO EMISSION COMPUTED TOMOGRAPHY (SPECT) is less expensive than PET and might provide data on cerebral blood flow.

Treatment Options and Outlook

Patients who do experience symptoms should seek out the care of a specialist; unless a family physician is thoroughly familiar with medical literature in this newly emerging area, experts caution that there is a great chance that patient complaints will be ignored. Patients with continuing symptoms after a mild head injury are advised to call a local head-injury foundation, which can refer patients to the best local practitioner.

postpolio syndrome (PPS) A condition that can strike polio survivors 10 to 40 years after their recovery from polio. The syndrome is caused by the death of individual nerve terminals that remain after the initial polio attack. Doctors estimate that PPS affects about 25 percent of polio survivors.

Symptoms and Diagnostic Path

Symptoms include fatigue, slowly progressive muscle weakness, muscle and joint pain, and muscular atrophy. The severity of PPS depends upon how seriously patients were affected by the first polio attack.

The only way to be sure a person has PPS is through a neurological examination together with other lab studies such as MAGNETIC RESONANCE IMAGING (MRI), neuroimaging, electrophysiological studies, and muscle biopsies or spinal fluid analysis.

Treatment Options and Outlook

At present, no treatment can cure or prevent PPS. Some experimental drug treatments, including pyridostigmine and selegiline, show promise in treating symptoms of the disorder. Doctors recommend that polio survivors follow a healthy lifestyle, with good diet, moderate exercise, and regular checkups. PPS is a very slowly progressing condition that is marked by long periods of stability. PPS patients, compared with control populations, do not show any increase in antibodies against the polio virus, and since PPS affects only certain muscle groups, doctors question whether the polio virus can cause a persistent infection in humans. Except in people with severe respiratory impairment, PPS is not usually life threatening.

Scientists are studying a number of possible treatments for postpolio syndrome, including insulin-like growth factor (IGF-1) and other growth factors. Other researchers are looking at the mechanisms behind fatigue. Scientists are also trying to determine if there is an immunological link in this disorder.

potassium The most important ion in the brain. Potassium ions allow brain cells to discharge, sending messages to other neurons.

Prader-Willi syndrome (PWS) A complex genetic disorder that causes short stature, MENTAL RETARDATION or a LEARNING DISABILITY, incomplete sexual development, characteristic behavior problems, low muscle tone, and an involuntary urge to eat constantly. This, coupled with a reduced need for calories, leads to obesity.

PWS is found in people of both sexes and all races, and in about one in 14,000 people in the United States. It is one of the 10 most common conditions seen in genetics clinics and is the most common known genetic cause of obesity.

Although PWS is associated with an abnormality of chromosome 15, it is generally considered not to be an inherited condition, but rather a spontaneous genetic birth defect that occurs at or near the time of conception. The faulty chromosome affects functioning of the hypothalamus.

Symptoms and Diagnostic Path

Newborns with PWS have poor muscle tone, and cannot suck well enough to get sufficient nutrients. Often they must be fed through a tube for several months after birth until their muscle control improves. By preschool age, children with PWS develop an increased interest in food and quickly gain excessive weight if calories are not restricted.

In addition to sometimes extreme attempts to obtain food, people with PWS are prone to temper outbursts, stubbornness, rigidity, argumentativeness, and repetitive thoughts and behaviors. Strategies to deal with these problems usually include structuring the environment, implementing behavioral management techniques, and occasionally prescribing drug therapy.

Early diagnosis of Prader-Willi syndrome gives parents an opportunity to manage their child's diet and avoid obesity and its related problems from the start. Since infants and young children with PWS typically have developmental delays in all areas, early diagnosis may help a family take advantage of early intervention services and help identify areas of need or risk. Diagnosis also makes it possible for families to get information and support from professionals and other families who are dealing with the syndrome.

Many doctors will refer a suspected patient to a medical geneticist who specializes in diagnosing and testing for genetic conditions such as PWS. After taking a history and doing a physical examination, the diagnostician will arrange for specialized genetic testing to be done on a blood sample to evaluate for the genetic abnormality found in people with PWS.

Treatment Options and Outlook

People with PWS can attend school, enjoy community activities, get jobs, and even move away from home, although they need a lot of support. Students with PWS are likely to need special education and related services, such as speech and occupational therapy. In community, work, and residential settings, adolescents and adults often need special assistance to learn and carry out responsibilities and to get along with others. People with PWS always need around-the-clock food supervision. As adults, most affected individuals do best in a special group home for people with PWS, where food access can be restricted. Although in the past many patients died in adolescence or young adulthood, preventing obesity will allow a person with PWS to have a normal lifespan.

praxia The ability to know or recognize objects; it is dependent on an intact parietal lobe.

prefrontal cortex Located in the telencephalon, this brain structure is important in judgment, planning, tact, impulse control, and abstract thinking. In addition, the prefrontal cortex is intimately connected with the LIMBIC SYSTEM. Moreover, input to the prefrontal cortex from the THALAMUS, HYPOTHALAMUS, and MIDBRAIN seems to provide information about the internal emotional and motivational states; these influences, together with other information synthesized by the prefrontal cortex from incoming sensory information, help to give meaning and significance to external events.

Researchers suspect that the prefrontal cortex plays a role in structuring behavior by helping prepare sensory and motor systems for action, by holding some information in a flexible memory. Relatively more developed in humans than any other species, there is an enormously complex interaction between this area and other parts of the brain. When this area is damaged, doctors cannot point to any one particular skill or function that is lost; rather, it appears as if an essential quality of "being human" is lost.

In recent research, scientists tested chess players who answered increasingly complex questions designed to identify parts of the brain used for a particular type of thinking. Results of the study suggested that the prefrontal cortex is where the brain plans and processes events or thoughts that are considered as a unit.

pregnancy and memory

pregnancy and memory   Many women say they experience memory lapses during pregnancy, probably because of emotional and hormonal conditions—although, because of a lack of studies, scientists do not really know why.

The physical symptoms that occur during pregnancy (such as nausea and fatigue) can be emotionally disruptive and could cause forgetfulness. Also, the powerful hormonal changes that take place during pregnancy alter the brain's chemistry, which could reduce the capacity for remembering.

The situation is not permanent, however; women who experience memory loss during pregnancy usually report that the problem fades away a few weeks after delivery at the latest.

pregnenolone   A simple steroid that, in recent research trials, seems to enhance MEMORY in rats and restore normal levels of neurotransmitters (such as ACETYLCHOLINE) which decline during aging. The drug has been tested in humans as a treatment for arthritis and was found to produce no side effects. The hormone was used during the 1940s to treat rheumatoid arthritis but had been abandoned when physicians discovered that cortisone was far more effective.

Pregnenolone is one of several steroid drugs researchers are investigating for possible memory enhancement properties. While several rat and mice studies have seemed to suggest a link between memory improvement and the steroid, the mechanism by which steroids influence memory and learning remains little understood. Scientists suggest pregnenolone might enhance memory because it serves as a raw material for the production of all steroid hormones used in storing information in memory. Concentrations of many of these steroids decline with age; by restoring these levels, pregnenolone may bring back memory abilities that had begun to erode.

premotor cortex   A part of the brain found in the FRONTAL LOBE closely associated with the MOTOR CORTEX that is connected to the RETICULAR FORMATION of the BRAIN STEM. The premotor cortex is responsible for identifying objects in space, choosing strategies of action, and programming movement; it also sends output fibers to those reticular NEURONS that influence the muscles of the back, hips, shoulders, and thighs and appears to help regulate POSTURE and stabilize the trunk and limbs during complex movements.

primary lateral sclerosis (PLS)   A rare neuromuscular disease characterized by progressive muscle weakness in the voluntary muscles that typically begins after age 50. PLS belongs to a group of disorders known as motor neuron diseases that occur when specific nerve cells in the CEREBRAL CORTEX that control voluntary movement gradually degenerate, causing the muscles under their control to weaken. The disease, which scientists believe is not hereditary, progresses gradually over a number of years, or even decades, leading to stiffness and weakening of the affected muscles.

There is no evidence in PLS of the degeneration of spinal motor neurons or muscle wasting that occurs in a similar disorder called AMYOTROPHIC LATERAL SCLEROSIS (ALS, or Lou Gehrig's disease).

Symptoms and Diagnostic Path

Difficulty with balance; weakness and stiffness in the legs; clumsiness, together with possible stiffness in the hands, feet, or legs which produces slowness and awkward movement; dragging of the feet; and facial involvement resulting in poorly articulated speech. The disorder usually begins in the legs, but it may also begin in the tongue or the hands.

For the first few years after symptoms begin, there is a possibility that the true diagnosis is ALS, which can have some of the same symptoms as PLS. For this reason, most neurologists follow a patient for a few years before making a diagnosis of PLS.

Treatment Options and Outlook

There is no cure, but symptoms can be treated. Baclofen and tizanidine may reduce spasticity; quinine or phenytoin may decrease cramps. Physical therapy may help prevent joint immobility, and speech therapy may be useful for patients with speech problems. The disorder is not fatal.

primary visual cortex   Signals from the eyes are fed into this region of the brain from the lateral geniculate bodies. This is where information from both eyes is first combined.

prions   Common term for "proteinaceous infectious particle," a kind of infectious protein that is unlike bacteria or viruses.

Although experts understand very well the identity and general properties of prions, exactly how they infect and grow remains a mystery. It is often assumed that the diseased form directly interacts with the normal form to make it rearrange its structure.

Prions are believed to cause a range of brain diseases in animals and humans. In animals, they cause scrapie in sheep, BOVINE SPONGIFORM ENCEPHALOPATHY (BSE) in cows, transmissible mink encephalopathy (TME) in mink, chronic wasting disease (CWD) in elk and mule deer, feline spongiform encephalopathy in cats, and exotic ungulate encephalopathy (EUE) in nyala, oryx, and greater kudu.

In humans, they cause several varieties of CREUTZFELDT-JAKOB DISEASE (CJD), such as iatrogenic Creutzfeldt-Jakob disease, variant-Creutzfeldt-Jakob disease, familial Creutzfeldt-Jakob disease, and sporadic Creutzfeldt-Jakob disease, Gerstmann-Sträussler-Scheinker syndrome (GSS), FATAL FAMILIAL INSOMNIA (FFI), KURU, and ALPERS DISEASE.

The term was invented in 1982 by Stanley B. Prusiner, a researcher at the University of California, San Francisco School of Medicine.

About 60 years ago scientists discovered that sheep were catching a disease (scrapie) that transformed their brains into pitted sponges, but researchers could never zero in on the virus. Then neurobiologists discovered a strange movement disorder among New Guinea tribesmen. Both, it turned out, were caused by prions.

Physicians have traced about 40 cases of a prion disease in adults to injections of infected growth hormone administered during childhood. A few others have caught prion diseases after receiving transplanted brain tissue or corneas from infected donors.

Called the prion protein molecule (PrP) this protein arises from cells it may one day destroy. Normally, it can be found harmlessly on the surfaces of NERVE CELLS until something induces it to infect a new cell and replicate by transforming the cell's normal PrP into another version of the mutant PrP.

About 10 percent of prion diseases are hereditary; that is, the gene for PrP mutates, which leads to substitutions or alterations among the 253 AMINO ACIDS that make up PrP. Somehow, these slight differences induce the protein to switch its shape. Different diseases will result depending on the makeup of the rest of the gene.

Some scientists think that accumulation of toxic forms of PrP causes cellular destruction; others believe that imbalances in normal PrP concentrations can hurt cells.

Some scientists suspect that the loss of functional PrP can lead to the disintegration of the brain. They also believe that normal PrP helps produce SYNAPSES, without which nerve cells cannot communicate.

progressive multifocal leukoencephalopathy (PML)

An uncommon disorder of the nervous system that primarily affects individuals with suppressed immune systems such as transplant patients, cancer patients, and nearly 10 percent of patients with AIDS. The disorder is characterized by destruction of the fatty myelin sheath that covers and insulates nerve cells in the brain.

The disease is caused by a common human polyomavirus known as JC virus.

Symptoms and Diagnostic Path

Mental deterioration, vision loss, speech disturbances, inability to coordinate movements, and paralysis. Eventually, the patient experiences coma as the brain lesions spread. In rare cases, seizures may occur.

Treatment Options and Outlook

There is no cure for PML, nor is there currently an effective treatment for the disorder. Treatment is symptomatic and supportive. The course of PML is relentless and progressive. Death usually occurs between one and four months after symptoms appear; but there have been a number of reported cases with survival for months to years.

progressive supranuclear palsy (PSP)

A rare brain disorder that causes serious and permanent problems with control of gait and balance. The most obvious sign of the disease is an inability to aim the eyes properly, caused by lesions in the area of the brain that coordinates eye movements.

Symptoms and Diagnostic Path

The symptoms of PSP are caused by a gradual deterioration of brain cells in a few tiny, important places in the brain stem.

In addition to the blurry vision caused by problems in aiming the eyes, PSP patients often exhibit changes in mood and behavior, including depression and apathy, in addition to mild DEMEN-TIA. However, the pattern of symptoms can vary considerably from one person to the next. PSP is a progressive disease but is not itself directly life threatening. Patients do tend to have serious complications, as a result of swallowing problems. The most common complications are choking, pneumonia, head injury, and fractures from falls. The most common cause of death is pneumonia. With good attention to medical and nutritional needs, however, most PSP patients live well into their seventies and beyond.

PSP is often misdiagnosed because some of its symptoms are so much like those of PARKINSON'S DISEASE, ALZHEIMER'S DISEASE, and rarer neurodegenerative disorders, such as CREUTZFELDT-JAKOB DISEASE. The key to establishing a diagnosis is to identify early gait instability and problems moving the eyes, as well as ruling out other similar disorders.

Treatment Options and Outlook

There is currently no effective treatment, although scientists are searching for better ways to manage the disease. In some patients the slowness, stiffness, and balance problems may respond to antiparkinsonian drugs such as levodopa, or levodopa combined with anticholinergic agents, but the effect is usually temporary. The speech, vision, and swallowing difficulties usually do not respond to any drug treatment. Antidepressants such as fluoxetine (Prozac), amitriptyline (Elavil), or imipramine (Tofranil) may be of some modest help. Nondrug treatment for PSP may include weighted walking aids to offset the tendency to fall backward, and bifocals or special prism glasses to ease the problem of looking down. Physical therapy has not been proven to help, but certain exercises can help keep the joints limber. The surgical procedure known as gastrostomy may be necessary to improve swallowing problems. This surgery involves placing a tube through the skin of the abdomen into the intestine to avoid having to eat by mouth.

Scientists are studying the use of free radical scavengers (drugs that can get rid of potentially harmful free radicals). In addition, better understanding of the related diseases of Parkinson's and Alzheimer's will help solve the problem of PSP.

prosopagnosia A form of AGNOSIA in which patients have special difficulty recognizing human faces. However, this definition may be too narrow, since these patients also may have problems in recognizing certain other classes of objects, such as species of birds.

protein kinase C (PKC) A molecule found on the surface membrane of NERVE CELLS existing in all animal cells, where it plays a role in growth, blood clotting, and the action of hormones. It was first discovered in the early 1970s by a Japanese scientist.

PKC acts by attaching a phosphate group onto specific sites on the other molecules, changing the function of those molecules, increasing or decreasing their level of activity.

Scientists first realized the potential of PKC in 1986 when Princeton University researchers noted that the protein mimicked cellular changes that occur during learning. Scientists already knew that the electrochemical action in NEURONS changes as an animal learns, and that a protein requiring calcium is involved.

When researchers realized that a single molecule was responsible for learning and memory, they reasoned that its appearance should coincide with learning, and its disappearance with forgetting. Research suggests that PKC orchestrates neuronal functions necessary for learning and memory.

Researchers have also discovered that chemicals that block PKC prevent short-term (but not long-term) memory in snails, suggesting that other mechanisms might be responsible for memories that last more than a few minutes.

Scientists are also investigating the role of PKC in memory disorders such as ALZHEIMER'S DISEASE. One recent study at the University of California, San Diego found that the brains of 11 Alzheimer's victims contained only half as much PKC as the brains of seven people who had died of natural causes.

pseudodementia A disorder that mimics DEMENTIA but that includes no evidence of brain dysfunction; nearly one out of 10 of those thought to be suffering from true dementia in fact have a depressive illness. Unlike dementia, DEPRESSION is treatable; many people respond well to antidepressant drugs. Not surprisingly, pseudodementia is found most often in elderly patients.

Pseudodementia is believed to be a way of avoiding depression or asking for help; when it occurs after a minor BRAIN INJURY it is often linked to the patient's desire to avoid an unpleasant experience. Pseudodementia can also be found among those who have experienced a minor organic brain injury, which after recovery appears to produce a degree of impairment in excess of what would be expected.

pseudotumor cerebri A condition (also called benign intracranial hypertension) in which there is increased pressure in the brain. The term literally means "false brain tumor," since many of its symptoms resemble that condition. It is most common in women between the ages of 20 and 50.

Symptoms and Diagnostic Path

Symptoms include headache, nausea, vomiting, and pulsating intracranial noises, all of which closely mimic symptoms of brain tumors. Symptoms may appear as a result of the abnormal buildup of pressure within the brain.

Treatment Options and Outlook

Pressure within the skull may be controlled by removing excess fluid with repeated spinal taps or by shunting. Steroids may be prescribed to reduce swelling of brain tissue. Drugs to reduce cerebrospinal fluid production may be used. Once the disorder is treated, pseudotumor cerebri generally has no serious consequences. However, any visual loss may be permanent regardless of treatment. In some cases, pseudotumor cerebri recurs.

psychedelic drugs A term for HALLUCINOGENS that was coined by psychiatrist Humphrey Osmond in the 1960s from the Greek word for "mind-manifesting."

psychic blindness The inability to recognize objects despite normal vision.

psychopharmacology A branch of pharmacology concerned with the effects of drugs on mental processes and behavior. Drugs have been used for hundreds of years to induce sleep and lessen pain, but it was not until the mid-20th century that psychotropic and neuroleptic drugs were introduced.

The term *psychotropic* (from the Greek *psyche* for "mind" and *tropikos* for "turning") describes drugs that affect mood, including antidepressants, sedatives, stimulants, and tranquilizers. *Neuroleptic* (from the Greek *neuro* for "nerve" and *lepsis* for "taking hold") refers to one of a group of drugs used to modify the manifestation of psychosis. They are also known as major tranquilizers or antipsychotics.

Psychopharmacologic drugs include the following drug classes: antipsychotics, anti-neurotics (or antianxiety drugs), and antidepressants.

psychosurgery Any brain operation performed to treat mental symptoms as a last resort in cases which have not responded to any other treatment. While psychosurgery was first practiced as long ago as 2,000 B.C., the first widespread use of this treatment was not until the 1930s; it reached its peak in the 1960s and began to decline in the 1970s.

In the first half of the 20th century, prefrontal LOBOTOMY was the most common type of psychosurgery, but it has been replaced by other safer operations because of its harmful side effects.

The most effective targets for this type of surgery were the FRONTAL LOBES; other regions included the cingulum, the AMYGDALA, several areas in the THALAMUS, and the HYPOTHALAMUS.

The most common type of psychosurgery today is stereotaxic surgery in which a scalpel or probe is inserted into a small drilled hole in the skull above one temple. Under X-RAY control, the probe is guided to a specific brain area where the surgeon makes small cuts in nerve fibers. This type of surgery is used to treat severe DEPRESSION, ANXIETY, or severe OBSESSIVE-COMPULSIVE DISORDER.

Other psychosurgical techniques include more complex operations in which the brain is exposed by cutting away a portion of the skull; parts of the brain are then removed. Temporal lobe EPILEPSY is treated this way by removing parts of the temporal lobe; rarely, complete lobes are removed to treat violent or aggressive behavior.

Psychosurgery remains a controversial treatment because, while benefiting some subjects, it involves destroying perfectly healthy brain tissue, it may have unpredictable results and may cause negative changes in intellect or personality. Critics of the procedure liken it to the abuses of human subjects during biomedical experiments in Germany during World War II. Proponents argue that prohibiting psychosurgery deprive patients of their right to effective medical treatment.

punch drunk syndrome A problem resulting from multiple repeated blows to the head (such as those experienced by boxers or football players) that can result in a short-term MEMORY problem and abnormal findings on neuropsychological tests.

The condition was first described in 1928 when it was noted that the punch drunk brain viewed under a microscope showed signs in common with ALZHEIMER'S DISEASE: widespread NEUROFIBRILLARY TANGLES and neural scarring. It is believed that the BRAIN DAMAGE and resulting memory loss is caused by rapid movements of the head, causing HEMORRHAGES and damaged BRAIN CELLS. In particular, the brains of boxers often exhibit nerve degeneration and loss of nerve fibers in the HIPPOCAMPUS to a degree far exceeding those in the brains of patients with Alzheimer's disease.

Purkinje, Jan Evangelista (1787–1869) This pioneer Czech experimental histologist and physiologist helped create a modern understanding of the brain and heart function, vision, mammalian reproduction, embryology, and the composition of cells. He is best known for the discovery of large nerve cells in the CORTEX of the CEREBELLUM (named Purkinje cells in 1837).

A graduate of the University of Prague, he published his doctoral dissertation on vision and was later appointed as professor of physiology at the university. It was here that he discovered the phenomenon known as the Purkinje effect (as light intensity decreases, red objects are perceived to fade faster than blue objects of the same brightness). He also republished his doctoral dissertation in two volumes, *Observations and Experiments Investigating the Physiology of Senses.*

Purkinje created the world's first department of physiology at the University of Breslau, Prussia, in 1839 and the first official physiological laboratory in 1842. The experimental method he used to explore the sensory experience helped lay the foundation for future research. He is best known for his discovery in 1837 of what came to be known as Purkinje cells—large nerve cells with many branching dendrites found in the cortex of the cerebellum, and for his 1839 discovery of Purkinje fibers, the unusual tissue that conducts the pacemaker stimulus along the inside walls of the ventricles to all parts of the heart. Purkinje introduced the terms *plasma* to describe the clear liquid remaining after blood has been cleared of its various corpuscle components, and *protoplasm,* used to describe young animal embryos.

Purkinje described the effects of camphor, opium, belladonna, and turpentine on humans in 1829. An early user of the improved compound microscope, he also discovered the sweat glands of the skin (1833) and the germinal vesicles (1825). He recognized fingerprints as a means of identification in 1823, and noted the protein-digesting power of pancreatic extracts in 1836. Purkinje died at the age of 82 on July 28, 1869.

pyramidal cells   Cortical cell type involved in motor activity; the neurons are named for their pyramidal shape.

pyroglutamate (2-oxo-pyrrolidone carboxylic acid, or PCA)   This AMINO ACID is an important flavor enhancer found naturally in a wide variety of fruits and vegetables, dairy products, and meat; it is found in large amounts in the brain, CEREBROSPINAL FLUID, and blood. It is also a suspected enhancer of cognitive ability.

PCA is able to penetrate the BLOOD-BRAIN BARRIER, where some researchers believe it stimulates cognitive function, improving memory and learning in rats. At least one study has shown it is effective in alcohol-induced memory deficits in humans and in patients suffering from MULTI-INFARCT DEMENTIA. Administration of this amino acid increased attention and improved short- and long-term retrieval and long-term memory storage.

When compared with a placebo in studies of memory deficits in 40 aged patients, results indicated that PCA improved verbal memory functions in those who were already affected by an age-related memory decline.

One form of the substance has been used in Italy to treat SENILITY, MENTAL RETARDATION, and alcoholism, where it is found in health food and vitamin stores in a variety of preparations under several names.

pyrrolidone derivatives   A class of NOOTROPIC drugs including piracetam and its analogues oxiracetam, pramiracetam, aniracetam, and others. The mechanism behind their memory-enhancing properties seems to be the increase in transmissions at all synapses; most research suggests that the drugs affect the cholinergic system and the adrenal cortex in the brain.

Pythagoras (c. 580 B.C.–c. 500 B.C.)   Greek philosopher who suggested that the mind was located in the brain and that the brain was the home of the soul.

rabies Known medically as hydrophobia, this acute viral disease of the CENTRAL NERVOUS SYSTEM can cause fatal BRAIN STEM ENCEPHALITIS. It is usually transmitted to humans by the bite of an infected animal.

While the usual incubation period is between one and two months for bites on the extremities, incubation periods ranging from 10 days to more than a year have been reported. Bites on the face or neck can have an incubation period as short as two weeks.

Symptoms and Diagnostic Path

Symptoms usually begin with personality changes and periods of excitement. This is followed by malaise, fever, breathing problems, salivation, and painful throat-muscle spasms induced by swallowing. Eventually, merely seeing water can induce convulsions and paralysis; death occurs after this stage within four to five days from respiratory failure or heart arrhythmia. This disease is nearly 100 percent fatal during the acute stage.

Treatment Options and Outlook

Rabies vaccine and antiserum should be administered to anyone with an animal bite sustained in an unprovoked attack. If a person is bitten by an infected animal, daily injections of rabies vaccine, together with an injection of rabies antiserum, may prevent the disease from developing. Foxes, bats, raccoons, and skunks are the major animal reservoirs in the United States, and a rabies epidemic in the 1990s among wild animals has been reported among certain areas in the Northeast.

Risk Factors and Preventive Measures

A pre-exposure series for all human rabies vaccines is given in three shots on the first day, day 7, and day 21, or 28. How often boosters are given depends on how good a person is at producing antibodies. People who have received the pre-exposure series only need two boosters if they are later exposed to rabies.

People in high-risk jobs are encouraged to have their blood tested at regular intervals so boosters can be given if antibody levels fall below a safe range. The average high-risk worker needs boosters only about once every two years.

rapid eye movement (REM) sleep Also known as paradoxical sleep, this is one of two types of sleep characterized by an increase in electrical activity within the brain. (The other type of sleep is known as NREM, or nonrapid eye movement sleep.)

During REM sleep, the temperature and blood flow to the brain increases, and brain waves begin to resemble the active pattern of an awake person. Eyes move rapidly and dreaming occurs.

REM sleep usually begins about 90 to 100 minutes after a person first falls asleep. The first REM period lasts only about 10 minutes, but each period lasts longer and longer throughout the night; the last of a night's four or five REM periods may last as long as an hour. Babies spend about half of their sleeping time in REM sleep because REM is related to brain growth during development; adults spend about one-fifth of their time asleep in REM. When REM sleep intrudes into wakefulness, this is known as NARCOLEPSY.

See also SLEEP AND THE BRAIN; SLEEP APNEA; SLEEP DISORDERS.

reading The ability to read is a complex process handled by an elaborate network of brain regions that utilize visual information and make sense of words. While scientists do not agree on the precise process, some researchers suggest that the ability to read depends on specific brain structures. Critics of this view believe that reading is the result of more general brain activities, such as those responsible for sorting objects into meaningful groups.

Recent research has lent credence to the specific structure theory, finding that the FUSIFORM GYRUS showed distinctive electrical responses to patterns of letters. Researchers suspect that this activity takes place in a portion of the brain's visual system that specializes in word recognition.

While electrical activity during this process typically occurs on both the sides of the brain, other parts of the visual system on the side more heavily involved in language (usually the left) probably also contribute to word recognition. For example, recent BRAIN SCANS have found that reading both real and nonsense words increases blood flow in a visual area on the left side of the brain.

rebound headaches   See HEADACHES.

recall   A term used to denote the ability to retrieve information from long-term memory. Recall is involved in a broad range of tasks and specific tests, from remembering a phone number to calling up information for a school exam. While useful as a descriptive term, it does not refer to a specific area of cognitive function.

Difficulty recalling information may be caused by a number of different learning problems. This may include problems imprinting information during processing because of poor attention or short-term memory, as well as difficulty with rapid retrieval tasks that are typically found in expressive-language disorders.

receptive language   The forms of language that are received as input from listening and reading. Listening and reading are receptive skills that involve feeding information into the brain, as opposed to speaking and writing, which are the expressive forms of language. Most individuals maintain a fairly similar set of receptive and

expressive, oral and written language function, but those with learning problems may have specific deficits in one or more of these areas.

Individuals with DYSLEXIA or specific reading disabilities have problems with receptive language, involving deficits in both oral language and processing sounds (phonological processing), and significant problems in decoding and understanding texts. Some individuals with these problems still have relatively strong oral expression, although most will have problems with written expression due to problems with reading written language.

Experts assess receptive language in several ways. One informal assessment involves giving an individual a multistep instruction, such as "Here is a penny. Put the penny on the floor beside you, open the door, and turn off the light."

More formally, tests such as the Peabody Picture Vocabulary Test-Fourth Edition (PPVT-IV) evaluate receptive language by presenting a series of pictures and instructing the child to choose one based on a verbal description (such as "Choose the one that shows 'swimming'").

receptors   Bits of protein embedded in the wall of nerve cells that bind neurotransmitters. Each receptor binds a specific neurotransmitter, turning a particular biochemical or cellular mechanism on or off. Receptors are generally found in the dendrites and cell body of NEURONS. In order to record a memory, the recording agent must be able to respond within a fraction of a second to a stimulus and then keep the information indefinitely.

Some scientists believe that some older people lose their memory abilities because their bodies have stopped producing the enzymes that keep their receptors healthy.

reflex   An automatic, predictable action that occurs in response to a particular stimulus over which the person has no voluntary control. While the brain controls most of the body's actions at any one moment, there are times when the body must react as quickly as possible without waiting for a response to reach the brain, which might be preoccupied elsewhere. These "emergency reactions" of reflexes take place without any conscious instruction from the brain.

The simplest sort of reflex involves a sensory NERVE CELL at the skin surface that reacts to a stimulus (such as touching a finger to a hot pan). The cell sends a signal along its nerve fiber to the SPINAL CORD; messages are conveyed to neurons in the central GRAY MATTER of the cord, where they split up and follow two paths. One path follows a short reflex loop through the spinal cord via relay NEURONS and back out along MOTOR NEURONS. Almost immediately muscles contract to pull the finger away. Some other messages travel the second path up the spinal cord to the brain; once in the brain, awareness of the stimulus dawns, but by this time the finger has already been pulled away.

The neurons involved in this circuit, encompassing the original sensation to the final action, are called a reflex arc.

One of the best-known reflexes is the simple knee-jerk reflex. When a rubber hammer taps the knee just below the knee cap, it stretches a tendon of one of the thigh muscles; a signal passes via a sensory neuron to the spinal cord, which activates a pool of motor neurons; these neurons cause the muscle to contract, jerking the lower leg.

Many reflexes are present at birth, including those that control basic body functions, such as shivering in response to cold or breathing faster when the level of carbon dioxide rises in the blood. The part of the NERVOUS SYSTEM concerned with these processes is the AUTONOMIC NERVOUS SYSTEM, and parts of the BRAIN STEM and the HYPOTHALAMUS help process information for this system. Some automatic system reflexes can be controlled to a degree—it is possible to stop emptying the bladder voluntarily—but ultimately, reflex is stronger than voluntary will.

On the other hand, some inborn reflexes are found only among infants, and disappear later in life; these include the grasp reflex that causes an infant to grasp a finger that is placed in its palm. NEUROLOGICAL EXAMINATIONS typically include testing of some simple inborn reflexes, such as the knee jerk, pupil constriction in the presence of light, and the plantar reflex (curling toes when the sole of the foot is irritated). Abnormal reflex reactions may be a symptom of a malfunctioning nervous system. The examination of vital reflexes

controlled by the brain stem is the basis for diagnosing BRAIN DEATH.

Reflexes that are not inborn but that are learned as a result of experience are called conditioned reflexes. They occur as a result of conditioning—when new pathways and connections within the nervous system are formed as a result of learning. Operant conditioning is an especially important part of learning; once an acceptable response to a new situation has been discovered and repeated several times, it is then automatically elicited by that stimulus and becomes a reflex. For example, a person who drives to work every day can make the same drive without consciously making the effort to follow the route.

Primitive reflexes, as opposed to inborn reflexes, are automatic movements present at birth that occur in response to a stimulus but that disappear during the first few months of life. They are believed to represent actions that might have been an important survival tactic during earlier stages of evolution.

Examples of these primitive reflexes include:

- **Grasp reflex**—For the first four months of life, an infant will firmly grasp any object placed in its palm.

- **Moro's reflex**—If a baby's head is momentarily unsupported, arms will be swung outward and brought together in an embracing movement while legs are extended and the baby cries. This reflex lasts for the first three or four months of life.

- **Tonic neck reflex**—During the first week of life when a baby turns its head to one side, the arm and leg on that side are stretched out, while the arm and leg on the opposite side flex.

- **Walking or stepping reflex**—When a baby is held upright with the feet touching the ground, a forward-stepping movement is made by each leg as the weight is placed on the other foot. This reflex is present for the first two months of life and then returns at about the age of six months.

- **Rooting reflex**—Touching a baby's cheek with the fingertip near the corner of the mouth will cause the head to turn so that the finger enters the mouth; this reflex enables the baby to find the nipple.

REM See RAPID EYE MOVEMENT SLEEP.

reptilian brain Another name for the "primitive BRAIN," this most basic part of the neurological components is responsible for instinctive behavior, such as reproduction, self-preservation, and fighting to establish territory. In evolutionary terms, it is the oldest part of the brain, and is also called the reptilian complex.

reticular activating system (RASY) A system of nerve pathways in the brain concerned with the level of consciousness (from states of sleep, drowsiness, and relaxation to full attention). It filters out extraneous stimuli and helps a person stay focused. The system combines information from all of the senses and from the CEREBRUM and CEREBELLUM and determines the activity of the brain and the AUTONOMIC NERVOUS SYSTEM.

The diffuse pathways extend from the caudal medulla to the MIDBRAIN. The ascending and descending long tracts of the BRAIN STEM pass through and around the RETICULAR FORMATION. Because its NEURONS tend to have long AXONS, the system can have profound effects on overall brain and SPINAL CORD activity.

A network of nerve fibers (also known as the reticular formation) located in the brain stem moderates the level of central nervous system activity, controlling arousal, consciousness, and attention. It is also involved in breathing and cardiac functions, movement, awareness, and sleep.

reticular core A network of neurons in the brain stem that receives impulses from all sensory systems. The reticular core is the center for arousal and calming.

reticular formation A network of nerves deep in the brain from the MEDULLA OBLONGATA to the MIDBRAIN. This structure (*reticular* is derived from the Latin word for "net") receives information from all over the body, sending it to cells in the HYPOTHALAMUS, CEREBRAL CORTEX, CEREBELLUM, and SPINAL CORD. In this way, the reticular formation controls the activity level of the entire nervous system and plays a role in movements that do not call for conscious attention; it is also involved in sending or inhibiting sensations of pain, temperature, and touch.

The reticular formation, in conjunction with neurons in the THALAMUS and others from various sensory systems of the brain, make up the RETICULAR ACTIVATING SYSTEM—the basic process that allows people to maintain consciousness.

It is the reticular activating system that allows a person to focus, excluding background information and distractions. It also serves as an effective filter for the continuous stimuli bombarding a person's nervous system; it is this filtering that allows a person to nap while riding in the car but to suddenly snap to attention when the sound of the car's engine changes as it slows down to a stop.

retinoblastoma A rare malignant tumor of the retina (the thin nerve tissue, responsible for sensing light and forming images, that lines the back of the eye). Although retinoblastoma may occur at any age, it most often occurs in younger children, usually before the age of five, affecting one in every 20,000 births. Retinoblastoma is usually confined to the eye (either one or both) and does not spread to nearby tissue or other parts of the body. A child's chance of recovery and retaining sight depend on the extent of the disease.

Symptoms and Diagnostic Path
Once retinoblastoma is found, tests can determine the size of the tumor and whether it has spread to surrounding tissue or to other parts of the body.

For the purposes of treatment, retinoblastoma is categorized into intraocular, extraocular, and recurrent types. In intraocular retinoblastoma, tumors are found in one or both eyes, but the cancer has not spread into the tissues around the eye or to other parts of the body. In extraocular retinoblastoma, cancer has spread beyond the eye and may be confined to the tissues around the eye, or it may spread to other parts of the body. Recurrent retinoblastoma refers to cancer that has returned or continued to grow after it has been treated. It may recur in the eye, in the tissues around the eye, or elsewhere in the body.

Treatments Options and Outlook

Most children can be cured of this type of tumor. The type of treatment given depends on the extent of the disease within the eye, whether the disease is in one or both eyes, and whether the disease has spread. Treatment includes

- enucleation: surgery to remove the eye
- radiation therapy: high-energy radiation to kill cancer cells and shrink tumors. Radiation may be external or internal (placing radioactive material into or near the tumor).
- cryotherapy: the use of extreme cold to destroy cancer cells
- photocoagulation: the use of laser light to destroy blood vessels that supply nutrients to the tumor
- thermotherapy: the use of heat to destroy cancer cells
- chemotherapy: drugs to kill cancer cells. In children with retinoblastoma, chemotherapy is under investigation

For intraocular retinoblastoma, treatment depends on whether the cancer is in one or both eyes. If the cancer is in one eye, treatment may include surgery to remove the eye (enucleation) for large tumors when useful vision cannot be preserved. External radiation therapy, photocoagulation, cryotherapy, thermotherapy, or radiation may be used with smaller tumors when sight may be preserved. For cancer in both eyes, treatment may include surgery to remove the eye with the most cancer, and/or radiation therapy to the other eye. Radiation therapy to both eyes may be considered if there is potential for vision in both eyes.

In patients with extraocular retinoblastoma, treatment may include radiation or chemotherapy. Clinical trials are testing new combinations of chemotherapy drugs, with or without peripheral stem cell transplantation, and different ways of administering chemotherapy drugs.

Risk Factors and Preventive Measures

A hereditary form of retinoblastoma may occur in one or both eyes, and generally affects younger children. Most retinoblastoma occurring in only one eye is not genetic, and is more often found in older children. When the disease occurs in both eyes, it is always hereditary. Because of the hereditary factor, the patient's siblings should have periodic examinations to determine their risk for developing the disease.

Children with hereditary retinoblastoma may also be at risk of developing a tumor in the brain (atrilateral retinoblastoma) while they are being treated for the eye tumor. Patients should be periodically monitored for the possible development of this rare condition during and after treatment. A child with retinoblastoma (especially the hereditary type) also is at higher risk for developing other types of cancer later.

For patients with recurrent retinoblastoma, treatment depends on the site and extent of the recurrence or progression. If the cancer comes back only in the eye and is small, the child may have surgery or radiation therapy. If the cancer returns outside of the eye, treatment depends on many factors.

retrieval The searching-and-finding process that leads to recognition and recall to bring information out of long-term MEMORY.

retrograde amnesia (RA) A type of AMNESIA that is principally a deficit of recall and recognition of information in which the patient has a gap in memory extending back for some time from the moment of damage to the brain. The memory gap usually shrinks over time.

Retrograde amnesia appears to be most pronounced for the period immediately before the trauma, with less disruption of more remote memories. This means that older patients with retrograde amnesia can probably describe their college graduation but would have trouble talking about what happened the day before the trauma.

Retrograde amnesia may occur following STROKE, HEAD INJURY, administration of electroconvulsive therapy, or in cases of psychogenic amnesia.

Symptoms and Diagnostic Path

RA usually causes an inability to remember personal and public events instead of loss of language, conceptual knowledge, or basic cognitive skills.

Psychologists have developed tests for RA that can measure a patient's memory for events. By compiling a life history of the patient from relatives and friends, the tester can compile a series of questions about each period of a patient's life with which to test the patient. Examiners can also use an autobiographical cueing procedure involving the recall of personal events in response to specific words. This test can uncover retrograde amnesia if the patient can recall events only from certain periods of his or her life. However, this procedure may be unreliable because it is hard to determine whether the patient's memories are accurate. Retrograde amnesia may also be tested by measuring a patient's ability to remember public events because it is assumed that memory for public and personal events have a common basis.

The most extensive test for retrograde amnesia is the Boston remote memory battery, which has three parts with easy and difficult questions. The easy questions may be answered on the basis of general knowledge, while the difficult questions reflect information requiring a particular time period. Unfortunately, this test is culture specific and cannot be used effectively outside the United States without being reformatted.

Treatment Options and Outlook

Treatment depends on the root cause. If there is an underlying cause that continues to be active, such as pressure on the brain, then it should be treated. Otherwise, there is varying benefit of general cognitive rehabilitation. Prognosis also varies according to the root cause. If there is permanent brain damage, such as from a stroke or traumatic brain injury, the amount of improvement expected from treatment is less than that expected if the root cause is a more reversible condition, such as pressure on the brain or pseudodementia brought on by, for example, toxicity or drug interactions.

Generally, retrograde amnesia is less of a problem for patients with memory deficits than is ANTEROGRADE AMNESIA (problems acquiring new information after trauma or an illness).

See also SHRINKING RETROGRADE AMNESIA; TEMPORAL LOBECTOMY.

Rett syndrome A progressive neurological disorder in which individuals exhibit a LEARNING DISABILITY, poor muscle tone, autistic-like behavior, useless hand movements, lessened ability to express feelings, avoidance of eye contact, a lag in brain and head growth, walking abnormalities, and seizures. Loss of muscle tone is usually the first symptom.

The syndrome occurs in about one of every 10,000 to 15,000 live female births, with symptoms usually appearing in early childhood, between the ages of six months and 18 months. Experts believe that while boys can get Rett syndrome, in boys the condition is fatal and they do not survive long past birth. The gender difference is caused by the difference in sex chromosomes. Females have two X chromosomes, but only one is active in any particular cell. That means that only about half the cells in a girl's nervous system will actually be using the defective gene. Because boys have a single X chromosome, all of their cells are obliged to use the faulty version of the gene, which presumably is what results in fatal defects.

Rett syndrome follows a tragic and irreversible course. Although the child develops normally for the first six to 18 months of life, she begins to gradually deteriorate mentally and physically. As the damage to the nervous system worsens, she loses the ability to speak, begins to have trouble walking or crawling, and experiences seizures. One of the most striking symptoms is loss of conscious control of the hands, leading to continual, compulsive hand-wringing. Though rarely fatal, Rett syndrome nevertheless leaves its victims permanently impaired.

Predicting the severity of Rett syndrome in any individual is difficult, but in spite of the significant impairments that characterize this disorder, most people with Rett syndrome survive at least into their forties. Girls and women with Rett can continue to function and enjoy life well into middle age and beyond. They experience a full range of emotions and show engaging personalities as they take part in social, educational, and recreational activities at home and in the community. However, the risk of death increases with age, and sudden, unexplained death often occurs, possibly from brain stem problems that interfere with breathing.

First described by Dr. Andreas Rett, the condition received worldwide recognition after research by Bengt Hagberg and colleagues was published in 1983. In October 1999, Huda Zoghbi and colleagues discovered a mutation on the MeCP2 gene on the X chromosome that has been linked to Rett syndrome. MeCP2 is a protein that controls gene function, but scientists do not yet understand its role in Rett syndrome. This mutation has been found in up to 75 percent of typical and atypical cases of Rett. Continued research will focus on other still-unidentified genetic factors which contribute to the condition. Researchers agree that its severity is probably not linked to the exact location of individual mutations on the gene, but to the X inactivation patterns in each affected girl.

The gene produces part of a switch that shuts off production of as-yet-unidentified proteins. Experts suspect that overproduction of some proteins might cause the nervous system deterioration characteristic of the disease. Discovery of the gene will enable scientists to unravel the disease process and could eventually lead to the development of drugs to lessen the damage.

Symptoms and Diagnostic Path

Rett syndrome is essentially a neurological disorder with reduced brain weight, a drop in volume of the frontal cortex and CAUDATE NUCLEUS, with reduced melanin in the SUBSTANTIA NIGRA. Brain cells are smaller than normal, and many of the body functions controlled by the brain, such as breathing and language, are affected by the condition.

The child with Rett syndrome usually shows an early period of apparently normal or near-normal development until six to 18 months old. A period of temporary stagnation or regression follows, during which the child loses communication skills and purposeful use of the hands. Soon, stereotyped hand movements, gait disturbances, and slowing of the rate of head growth become apparent.

Most girls with Rett do not crawl typically, but may "bottom scoot" without using their hands. Many begin independent walking within the normal age range, while others show significant delay or inability to walk independently. Some begin walking and then lose this skill, while others continue to walk throughout life. Still others do not walk until late childhood or adolescence.

Problems may include seizures, which can be severe, but tend to lessen in their intensity in later adolescence. Disorganized breathing patterns also may occur and tend to decrease with age. Scoliosis is a prominent feature of Rett, and it can range from mild to severe.

Apraxia (dyspraxia), the inability to program the body to perform motor movements, is the most fundamental and severely handicapping aspect of the condition. It can interfere with every body movement, including eye gaze and speech, making it difficult for the child to do what she wants to do. Due to apraxia and lack of verbal communication skills, an accurate assessment of intelligence is difficult. Most traditional testing methods require use of the hands or speech, which may be impossible for the girl with Rett. Some children start to use single words and word combinations before they lose this ability.

Diagnosing the disorder before the child is four or five years old is often difficult. However, the discovery of the genetic mutation means that a blood test can reveal the genetic pattern and improve the accuracy of early diagnosis. If combined with an effective therapy, the test might allow doctors to forestall the drastic consequences of the disease.

The condition is most often misdiagnosed as AUTISM, CEREBRAL PALSY, or nonspecific developmental delay. While many health professionals may not be familiar with Rett syndrome, it is a relatively frequent cause of neurological dysfunction in females.

Treatment Options and Outlook

There is no cure for Rett syndrome; however, there are several treatment options, including treatments for the learning disabilities and seizures that may occur. Some children may require special nutritional programs to maintain adequate weight.

Most girls who have been diagnosed are under 18 years of age, and little is known about life expectancy for these children. A girl with Rett syndrome has about a 95 percent chance of living until age 25. Death may be caused by seizures or swallowing problems.

Reye's syndrome   A rare condition nearly exclusive to children under age 15, characterized by BRAIN DAMAGE following chicken pox, influenza, or an upper respiratory infection. Because it has been associated with the administration of aspirin, physicians recommend that children never be given aspirin for viral infections or fever of unknown cause.

Symptoms and Diagnostic Path

About a week into the viral illness, signs of Reye's syndrome begin with vomiting, confusion, lethargy, disorientation, and jaundice. As the brain swells, it may trigger seizures, coma, heart disturbances, and breathing problems.

Treatment Options and Outlook

There is no specific treatment; corticosteroid drugs and mannitol infusions control brain swelling; dialysis or blood transfusions may correct blood chemistry changes; a ventilator may assist breathing. This type of supportive care has reduced the death rate to 10 or 20 percent.

Reye's syndrome is a leading cause of death among children beyond infancy. The death rate from this condition has dropped dramatically from 60 percent to 10 percent as scientists begin to understand the disorder. The chances for recovery are not as good for those who experience SEIZURES or deep COMA. Severe attacks carry the risk of lasting brain damage.

right brain   The right CEREBRAL HEMISPHERE, linked with spatial skill.

See also HANDEDNESS; SPLIT-BRAIN RESEARCH.

rivastigmine (Exelon)   Drug that was approved as a treatment for mild to moderate ALZHEIMER'S DISEASE in 2000, which works by blocking enzymes that break down ACETYLCHOLINE, a brain chemical that carries messages between brain cells. Patients with Alzheimer's appear to produce smaller amounts of acetylcholine in their brains. According to some studies, patients who took this drug showed greater improvement in thinking and remembering, in the ability to carry on activities of daily living, and in overall functioning.

Normally, the human brain produces acetylcholine to carry messages, and then it is broken down by a special enzyme called acetylcholinesterase. Like other drugs designed to treat Alzheimer's, rivastigmine prevents the last part of the cycle so that acetylcholine is not broken down. As a result, there is more acetylcholine available to carry messages in the brain.

According to the manufacturer (Novartis), studies show that between 25 and 30 percent of people who take the medication score better on tests of memory, understanding, and activities of daily living after six months than they did before starting therapy. However, between 10 percent and 20 percent of patients taking the placebo also scored better on the same tests at the end of six months. Another 20 percent of patients who took the drug were more or less the same after six months on the drug as when they started, whereas about another 10 percent of those on the placebo were no worse. (Normally most people with Alzheimer's disease would decline noticeably over this period of time.) The drug had no clear effect on the remaining patients.

Rivastigmine has received approval for use against Alzheimer's in 60 countries around the world. It is normally taken twice a day with food, beginning with a low dose of 1.5 mg twice a day, building to a total of 6 to 12 mg a day.

Side Effects

The drug causes side effects including nausea, vomiting, loss of appetite, fatigue, and weight loss. In most cases, these side effects are temporary and decline with continuing treatment, but sometimes the nausea and vomiting are severe enough that patients lose weight. In clinical trials, 26 percent of women and 18 percent of men who took high-dose rivastigmine lost at least 7 percent of their initial body weight due to nausea and vomiting and because of this, the drug should be taken with meals.

Side effects are more common when treatment first starts or when the dose is increased. It is not possible to tell who will have side effects and who will not.

Sandhoff disease A rare genetic lipid storage disorder causing a progressive deterioration of the central nervous system. Although Sandhoff disease is a severe form of TAY-SACHS DISEASE prevalent in people of European Jewish descent, it is not limited to any ethnic group. Onset of the disorder usually occurs at 6 months of age.

The condition is caused by a deficiency of the enzyme hexosaminidase which results in the buildup of certain fats in the brain and other organs of the body.

Symptoms and Diagnostic Path

Symptoms include progressive weakness, startle reaction to sound, early blindness, progressive mental deterioration, frequent respiratory infections, an abnormally enlarged head and doll-like facial appearance, cherry-red spots in the back of the eyes, seizures, and muscle contractions.

Treatment Options and Outlook

There is no specific treatment for Sandhoff disease: treatment is symptomatic and supportive. The prognosis for patients with Sandhoff disease is poor; death usually occurs by age three and is generally caused by respiratory infections.

Schilder's disease A rare, progressive demyelinating disorder which usually begins in childhood, featuring widespread destruction of the myelin sheath of the NEURONS in the CEREBRAL HEMISPHERES of the brain. The disorder is a variant of MULTIPLE SCLEROSIS.

Symptoms and Diagnostic Path

DEMENTIA, APHASIA, seizures, personality changes, poor attention, tremors, balance instability, incontinence, muscle weakness, headache, vomiting, and vision and speech impairment.

Treatment Options and Outlook

Treatment for the disorder is similar to that for standard multiple sclerosis therapy, and includes corticosteroids, beta-interferon or immunosuppressive therapy, and symptomatic treatment. Like multiple sclerosis, Schilder's disease is unpredictable. For some patients, the disorder progresses with a steady, unremitting course; others may experience significant improvement and remission. In some cases, Schilder's disease is fatal.

schizencephaly An extremely rare developmental disorder characterized by abnormal clefts in the brain's cerebral hemispheres. Schizencephaly is a form of PORENCEPHALY in which there is a cavity in the cerebral hemispheres.

Symptoms and Diagnostic Path

Individuals with clefts in both hemispheres are often developmentally delayed, with delayed speech and language skills. Individuals with smaller clefts in only one hemisphere are often paralyzed on one side of the body, but may have normal intelligence. Patients with schizencephaly may also have varying degrees of abnormally small head, MENTAL RETARDATION, partial or complete paralysis, and reduced muscle tone. Most patients have seizures, and some may have HYDROCEPHALUS.

Treatment Options and Outlook

Typically, treatment includes physical therapy, treatment for seizures, and, in cases that are complicated by hydrocephalus, a shunt to divert fluid. The prognosis for individuals with schizencephaly

317

varies depending on the size of the clefts and the degree of neurological deficit.

schizophrenia The most common form of psychosis, affecting about one percent of the population, schizophrenia (or "fragmented mind") results in a break from reality involving bizarre delusions, illogical thinking, incoherence, and HALLUCINATIONS.

Originally termed *dementia praecox* by German psychiatrist Emil Kraepelin, the cause of schizophrenia has eluded researchers who have spent a great deal of time searching for evidence of physical dysfunction in the brains of schizophrenia patients.

It appears that schizophrenia may be caused by a malfunctioning DOPAMINE system, and new research suggests that the roots of schizophrenia appear much earlier in brain development. In fact, considerable evidence suggests that malfunctioning fetal brain development may set the stage for later appearance of the disorder. It may be that aberrant organization of fetal BRAIN CELLS during development may combine intact and impaired NEURONS together in dysfunctional circuits. Some researchers suggest that viral infections during pregnancy (together with other prenatal or birth problems) may play a role in the development not just of schizophrenia, but also of AUTISM and DYSLEXIA. As evidence, researchers cite a Finnish study that found a higher rate of schizophrenia among children of women exposed to a flu epidemic during the second trimester of pregnancy. Schizophrenia has also been linked to birth in the winter when viral infections are common.

Twin studies have also shown that some type of genetic mechanism strongly influences about half of all cases of schizophrenia.

Some researchers believe that many schizophrenia patients' brain development begins to break down in midpregnancy when many large neurons arrive at their final destination. In parts of the CORTEX (the brain's outer layer) and within deeper regions associated with emotion and memory, researchers have found disorganized ensembles of neurons.

By staining schizophrenics' brains after autopsy, scientists have also found missing or abnormally sized neurons and abnormal myelination of nerve fibers.

People with both a family history of schizophrenia and a second trimester exposure to viral infection may experience the greatest chance of developing schizophrenia themselves. Minor complications at birth or shortly thereafter may boost these odds even further, scientists suggest. Other scientists suggest that families with high percentages of schizophrenia may lack the genetic instructions that guide cortical neurons during development to their final destination in circuit formation.

More recent research suggests that the root of schizophrenia may lie in abnormalities in the THALAMUS and related structures; scientists have already suspected that the thalamus helps focus attention and process sensory information. When comparing brains of normal and schizophrenic patients, researchers at the University of Iowa Hospitals and Clinics in Iowa City found that the area of greatest difference in strength of signal during MAGNETIC RESONANCE IMAGING (MRI) was found in the thalamus and nearby tissue leading to the front of the cortex. Schizophrenic men also had a much smaller thalamus than normal men.

Malfunctions in the underlying function of the thalamus, which develops before or shortly after birth, may be the root of the problem that underlies the various symptoms of schizophrenia.

Symptoms and Diagnostic Path
Schizophrenia interferes with the ability to concentrate on and think about incoming information, but it is unclear to what extent this depends on the subtype of the disorder and to what extent it reflects the patient's problems with paying attention to outside events.

Treatment Options and Outlook
Since the 1950s, doctors have used the phenothiazines (especially CHLORPROMAZINE) to tame the symptoms of schizophrenia. More recently, haloperidol has also been helpful in controlling some of the most problematic symptoms; neither drug offers a complete cure.

Recent Swiss research suggests that training to improve attention, memory, and basic reasoning skills may play a role in treating many cases of the disease. Their approach of cognitive rehabilitation differs from other more traditional programs, which focus on teaching social skills. In studies at the University of Bern, researchers emphasize thinking abilities by having patients sort cards containing geometric shapes, colors, and days of the week. Training then advances to word problems and interpreting the meaning of social interactions and other complete social skills. As many as 18 months after the program, participants showed substantial improvement on tests measuring attention and overall mental condition. However, these patients are still not capable of complex thought and social interaction.

scopolamine   An antispasmodic drug that blocks neurotransmission of certain chemicals in the brain, including ACETYLCHOLINE, important in the normal function of memory. If given to normal subjects, the drug causes a severe memory loss which is reversed by the administration of PHYSOSTIGMINE. Under the influence of scopolamine, retention remains intact, but effortful retrieval is impaired. Scopolamine appears to disrupt efficient encoding processes leading to a deficiency in effective retrieval of information. It has a more potent effect than sedatives or tranquilizers on human cognitive abilities, but the strength of the AMNESIA following scopolamine administration depends on the memory task used to define it.

seasonal affective disorder (SAD)   A syndrome of winter DEPRESSION, SAD is specifically related to changes in the length of daylight across the seasons. While its exact cause is not known, the disorder has been linked to a malfunction in the brain's biological clock that controls temperature and hormone production.

As many as 12 million Americans may suffer from this disorder, and up to 35 million others may experience milder forms. It is at least four times as common among women, usually beginning in the twenties and thirties (although it has been reported in some children and teenagers). Other estimates suggest that as many as half of all women in northern states experience pronounced winter depression, but very few receive the necessary treatment because their doctors do not differentiate between typical depressive symptoms and SAD.

The PINEAL GLAND appears to be particularly important in the development of SAD. Nestling near the center of the brain, the pineal gland processes information about light through special nerve pathways and releases the sleep-inducing hormone MELATONIN, also responsible for regulating CIRCADIAN RHYTHMS. Melatonin is produced in the dark and peaks during the winter. Experts believe it may suppress mood and mental quickness. Interestingly, people with bipolar disorder are extremely sensitive to light, and their melatonin levels plummet when exposed to light.

Symptoms and Diagnostic Path

The body is regulated by some sort of biological clock that sets the pace for everyday rhythms of sleep, activity, temperature, and cortisol and melatonin release. Most people maintain a certain flexibility in this system, allowing them to synchronize this biological clock to environmental changes. But experts suspect that some people—perhaps those prone to depression—do not synchronize their clocks so easily. It could be that their internal clock is out of step with the world's 24-hour rhythm so that melatonin is released too early (causing evening sleepiness and early morning awakening) or too late (causing insomnia and problems awakening).

Treatment Options and Outlook

While some cases eventually disappear, others persist for a lifetime. The best treatment for this disorder is phototherapy—exposure to additional special types of light during the winter—which will reverse this type of depression in most people.

Treatment is effective and inexpensive; patients must only be sure to get an accurate diagnosis and the right kind of light box to provide enough high-intensity light for a certain time each day. After a few days spent sitting for a few hours under special, bright fluorescent lights, symptoms subside; symptoms reappear if treatment stops. In general, patients must sit about three feet away from a bank of special lights of between six and eight fluorescent bulbs about three hours daily. Ordinary room light is not bright enough to affect SAD.

While researchers are still studying this treatment, many physicians recommend it for this type of depression. *Treatment should only be given under the supervision of an expert.* Experts believe that the treatment works by increasing the secretion of the hormonal chemical melatonin in the brain, helping to regulate the natural circadian rhythm.

Because light therapy may be only partly successful in eradicating symptoms, treatment may be bolstered by the use of antidepressants. Antidepressants alone may be used instead of light therapy for people with SAD, but often the two treatments are used together, since giving two treatments together often means that lower doses of antidepressants can be used. Many physicians adjust the dose of antidepressants with the changing seasons—increasing the dose as the days become shorter, decreasing it as the days lengthen.

More doctors are considering SELECTIVE SEROTONIN REUPTAKE INHIBITORS (SSRIs) to be the drug of choice for SAD, primarily because the SEROTONIN system is believed to be part of the problem in this disorder. Desyrel has also been used successfully with SAD patients. Other antidepressants also may be beneficial, such as the tricyclics desipramine or imipramine. (Doctors often avoid prescribing the more sedating tricyclics, such as amitriptyline and doxepin, because people with SAD tend to sleep too much as it is.)

seasonal rhythm   See CIRCADIAN RHYTHM.

sedatives   Drugs that relieve anxiety and tension, including BARBITURATES, administered at lower doses than those needed for sleep. They have been generally replaced by tranquilizers, which are less likely to cause dependence.

See also CENTRAL NERVOUS SYSTEM DEPRESSANTS.

seizure   A sudden burst of abnormal electrical activity from some area in the brain caused by one of a number of different conditions. While all seizures used to be called epilepsy, today the more modern term is *seizure disorder.* Seizures that occur on a regular basis, however, are still termed epileptic.

Seizures may be caused by a wide variety of neurological or medical problems, including STROKE, heart disease, kidney problems, sinus infection, middle-ear disorders, injury, high fever, chemical abnormalities in the blood, acute alcoholic toxicity, drug poisoning, or old scar tissue from an injury. When a clear-cut cause cannot be found, doctors usually assume that a seizure is caused by a metabolic disorder or a birth injury.

Symptoms and Diagnostic Path

A seizure that arises in only a small portion of the brain may set off a simple case of tingling in a small area of the body. Other symptoms may include HALLUCINATIONS, intense feelings of fear, or DÉJÀ VU. If the abnormal electrical activity spreads across the brain, the patient loses consciousness and experiences a GRAND MAL SEIZURE.

In order to determine the cause of seizures, doctors need to have an accurate description of the seizure, complete physical exam, blood tests, and ELECTROENCEPHALOGRAM (EEG), CAT SCAN, or MAGNETIC RESONANCE IMAGING (MRI).

Treatment Options and Outlook

Seizures can be prevented in more than 90 percent of cases, especially if the cause has been identified. The most common antiseizure medication is valproic acid. Alternatively, other antiseizure medications include PHENYTOIN (Dilantin), carbamazepine (Tegretol), or phenobarbital. Medication that works the best with the fewest side effects should be continued for at least five years after the last seizure.

See also SEIZURE, FEBRILE.

seizure, febrile   A common type of childhood SEIZURE triggered by a rapidly escalating fever and characterized by twitching limbs and loss of consciousness. About one in 20 children will have one or more febrile seizures, which tend to run in families and are not considered serious. They usually appear in children between six months and five years.

Most children who experience febrile seizures are completely normal; about 30 to 40 percent will experience another such seizure within the following six months.

The fever that triggers the seizure usually develops with an acute infectious illness such as an ear infection or tonsilitis. The seizures themselves are caused by a disturbance in the normal electrical activity of the brain.

Symptoms and Diagnostic Path
Loss of consciousness followed by uncontrollable twitching of arms or legs for several minutes.

Treatment Options and Outlook
During the seizure, the mouth should never be wedged open to prevent biting of the tongue, which rarely occurs anyway. If the child has not had previous seizures, a physician should be contacted. Any seizure that lasts longer than five minutes should be treated as an emergency. No other treatment is necessary for the seizure other than treatment of the underlying illness.

Risk Factors and Preventive Measures
The chances of recurrent febrile seizures are increased if there are mental problems or a family history of EPILEPSY, or if the first seizure was prolonged. Children with all three risk factors have a 10 percent chance of developing epilepsy. However, in healthy children, the risk of developing epilepsy is small.

Seizures may be prevented by lowering the child's temperature by using acetaminophen at the first sign of fever. Bedclothes should be removed, and a fan pointed toward the child. While sponging the child with lukewarm water may be comforting, it will most likely not help in reducing the temperature.

selective serotonin reuptake inhibitors (SSRIs)   A class of antidepressants that prevents brain cells from reabsorbing SEROTONIN, thus effectively raising the levels of this NEUROTRANSMITTER. A malfunctioning serotonin system has been implicated in the development of DEPRESSION. The SSRIs include citalopram (Celexa, Cipramil, Emocal,

Sepram, Seropram), escitalopram oxalate (Lexapro, Cipralex, Esertia), fluoxetine (Prozac, Fontex, Seromex, Seronil, Sarafem), fluvoxamine maleate (Luvox, Faverin), paroxetine (Paxil, Seroxat, Aropax, Deroxat, Paroxat), sertraline (Zoloft, Lustral, Serlain), and dapoxetine (no known trade name).

In addition to depression, these antidepressants appear to be effective in treating a wide range of other mood disorders such as ANXIETY or panic disorders, post-traumatic stress, eating disorders, or obsessive-compulsive disorder.

These SSRIs have moved to the forefront of modern psychiatric treatment because they work as well as any of the older antidepressants while causing far less serious side effects. This lack of side effects is primarily due to the fact that they work so selectively in the brain, affecting just one neurotransmitter system (serotonin) instead of other neurotransmitter systems and RECEPTOR sites throughout the brain. This is quite different than the shotgun approach of older antidepressants such as the MONOAMINE OXIDASE (MAO) INHIBITORS or TRICYCLIC ANTIDEPRESSANTS, which interfere with neurotransmitters and receptor sites all over the brain.

When a drug blocks a specific neurotransmitter, it causes side effects; the more neurotransmitters that are blocked, the more variety of side effects will result. For example, blocking the reuptake of NOREPINEPHRINE can produce tremors, sexual dysfunction, and tachycardia. Blocking the reuptake of DOPAMINE can produce movement disorders and changes in the endocrine system. By specifically blocking serotonin alone, scientists can sidestep those problems (although patients may still experience stomach upset, insomnia, and anxiety).

The more receptors and neurotransmitters that are affected, the more side effects are produced. This is why a tricyclic antidepressant, which blocks the reuptake of norepinephrine and serotonin plus four different types of receptors, is associated with many more side effects than the SSRIs, which affect only one neurotransmitter and barely disturb receptors at all.

Interestingly, it now appears that the serotonin neurotransmitter system may be far more complex than anyone had realized, linking areas throughout the brain in an interwoven tapestry of serotonin-producing connections. Not surprisingly, serotonin receptors are especially plentiful in the areas of the brain controlling emotion. What is more, there are at least six different receptor types in the serotonin system, each responsible for sending different signals to different parts of the brain. The next step is to find a drug that can affect just one of these receptor types and to develop a simple lab test that can identify specific serotonin malfunctions. While it is apparent that serotonin is of vital importance in the development of depression, scientists are not so sure that it is a simple cause-and-effect relationship; the brain's biochemical pathways for emotion and mood are just too complex. While it may be true that scientists can directly relieve depression by increasing serotonin, it is also true that altering serotonin levels causes slight effects in other neurotransmitter systems and that those changes affect depression.

self-hypnosis   See HYPNOSIS.

semantic memory   Memory for facts, such as the information that would be contained in a dictionary or encyclopedia with no connection to time or place. People do not remember when or where they learn this type of information. Semantic MEMORY registers and stores knowledge about the world in the broadest sense; it allows people to represent and mentally operate on situations, objects, and relations in the world that are not present to the senses. A person with an intact semantic memory system can think about things that are not here now.

Because semantic memory develops first in childhood—before episodic memory—children are able to learn facts before they can remember their own experiences.

The seat of semantic memory is believed to be located in the medial temporal lobe and diencephalic structures of the brain.

senile dementia   In the past, DEMENTIA was divided into two forms: presenile (affecting people under

age 65) and senile (over age 65). These designations are no longer used today.

Senile dementia (or SENILITY) is a catchword that has been used for many years to label almost any eccentric behavior in the elderly. It has sometimes been equated with chronic brain failure, CHRONIC BRAIN SYNDROME, ORGANIC BRAIN SYNDROME, or ALZHEIMER'S DISEASE.

Fifty percent to 60 percent of older people with impaired memories have Alzheimer's; approximately 20 to 25 percent of brain impairment is caused by STROKE, and the remainder is the result of other causes, including normal aging.

There are a number of reasons for confusion, forgetfulness, and disorientation besides Alzheimer's disease. It could be caused by overmedication or medication interaction, chemical imbalances, DEPRESSION, sudden illness, malnutrition and dehydration, or social isolation.

senility   A term that once referred to changes in mental ability caused by old age. However, the term *senile* simply means "old" and therefore, senility does not really describe a disease. In addition it is considered by many people to be a derogatory or prejudicial term.

Most people over age 70 suffer from some amount of impaired memory and reduced ability to concentrate. The risk of DEMENTIA rises to affect about one of five people over age 80. Depressive illness and confusion due to physical disease are also common.

The terms *chronic ORGANIC BRAIN SYNDROME* and *acute* or *reversible organic brain syndrome* have been used respectively to refer to those dementias that cannot be treated (chronic) and to those that respond to treatment (acute).

See also AGING AND MEMORY; ALZHEIMER'S DISEASE.

senses and the brain   One of the chief responsibilities of the brain is the processing and interpretation of information picked up by the body's five senses: sight, smell, touch, sound, and taste. The primary receiving centers for the major sensory nerves are the THALAMUS, located in the MIDBRAIN next to the third ventricle, and the BASAL GANGLIA. The thalamus integrates all the various sensory impulses (such as recognizing pain) and, like some giant traffic manager, sends all sensory stimuli to the CEREBRAL CORTEX, where the messages are received and translated into a response. The thalamus is also responsible for the sense of movement and position and the ability to identify sizes and shapes of objects.

Sensory impulses travel on three major pathways depending on the type of sensation and typically involve three NEURON relays. Information about these paths is of crucial importance when making a neurological diagnosis.

AXONS, which are responsible for carrying messages of heat, cold, and pain, make connections with the cells of secondary neurons in the SPINAL CORD. Temperature and pain fibers pass immediately to the opposite side of the spinal cord and travel upward to the thalamus.

Sensations of touch, light pressure, and limb localization travel for some distance before entering the gray column of the spinal cord, completing the connection.

Stimuli from muscles, joints, and bones (including the sense of position in space and vibration) travel uncrossed to the BRAIN STEM via the axon of the primary neuron.

In the MEDULLA, connections are made with secondary neuron cells whose axons then cross to the opposite side and travel to the thalamus.

Cutting a sensory nerve will cause the total loss of sensation in the area of the body it serves. Severing the spinal cord will therefore permanently anesthetize the area below the injury.

Assessment of the health of this system involves testing (with eyes closed) tactile sensation, superficial pain (such as a pinprick), vibration, and proprioception (subjective sense of joint position). Tactile sensation is tested by lightly touching a cotton ball to the same areas on each side of the body; the sensitivity of different areas of the body is compared.

Because pain and temperature sensations are transmitted together, it is not usually necessary to test separately for temperature sensation. A patient's sensitivity to superficial pain can be evaluated by asking the person to differentiate between the sharp and blunt ends of a broken wooden cotton swab stick or tongue depressor applied with equal intensity to both sides of the body. A safety pin should not be used because it can break the skin.

Vibration and proprioception are transmitted together, and the strength of these senses are often lost together. A person's sense of vibration is evaluated by having the patient report when a low-frequency tuning fork stops vibrating when placed against a bony prominence of the body. Side-to-side comparisons are made.

A person's ability to sense body position in space can be tested by having the patient close both eyes and describe the direction in which the toes have been moved.

After all these peripheral sensations have been tested, it is also important to determine if the brain is correctly integrating these sensations. This can be tested by evaluating whether a patient can perceive how many objects have been touched when touching two sharp objects at the same time. Similarly, a person should be able to tell when he or she is touched in two places on the body at the same time (with eyes closed).

sensory area   Part of the CEREBRAL CORTEX that receives tactile sensory information from the skin, including pressure receptors, thermo-receptors, and so on.

sensory cortex   A part of the CEREBRAL CORTEX parallel to the MOTOR CORTEX that is responsible for awareness of body sensations such as hot or cold.

sensory deprivation   The removal of a person's normal sights, sounds, and physical feelings. Studies have shown that sensory deprivation can produce a variety of mental changes and a slowing of brain activity. Volunteers who lay immobile in a darkened environment, wearing masks and gloves in a sound-proof room, reported feelings of unreality, concentration problems, and HALLUCINATIONS.

sensory integration   The process of absorbing sensory information, organizing this information in the CENTRAL NERVOUS SYSTEM, and using the information to function smoothly in daily life. Sensory experiences include touch, movement, body awareness, sight, sound, and the pull of gravity; as the brain organizes and interprets this information, it provides a crucial foundation for later, more complex learning and behavior. This critical function of the brain is responsible for producing a composite picture of a person's existence, so that the person can understand who he or she is physically, where he or she is, and what is going on in the environment. Sensory integration is a continual process: As children gain competence, their sensory integration improves, so that the more children do, the more they can do.

For most people, effective sensory integration occurs automatically and unconsciously, without effort. For others, the process is inefficient, demanding effort and attention with no guarantee of accuracy. Children develop sensory integration in the course of ordinary childhood activities. But for some children, sensory integration does not develop efficiently. When the process breaks down, a number of problems in learning, development, or behavior may develop.

The concept of sensory integration comes from a body of work developed by occupational therapist A. Jean Ayres, Ph.D., who was interested in the way in which sensory processing and motor planning disorders interfere with daily life and learning. This theory has been developed and refined by other occupational and physical therapists.

sensory integration dysfunction (DSI) A somewhat controversial theory about the inefficient brain processing of information received through the senses. A child with DSI has trouble detecting, discriminating, or integrating sensations. Children with sensory integration problems may be bright, but they may have trouble using a pencil, playing with toys, or taking care of personal tasks such as getting dressed. Some children with this problem are so afraid of movement that ordinary swings, slides, or jungle gyms trigger fear and insecurity. On the other hand, some children whose problems lie at the opposite extreme are uninhibited and overly active, often falling and blundering into dangerous situations. In each of these cases, a sensory integrative problem may be an underlying factor. Its far-reaching effects can interfere with academic learning, social skills, even self-esteem.

Research clearly identifies sensory integrative problems in children with developmental or learning difficulties, and independent research shows that a sensory integrative problem can be found in some children who are considered learning disabled by schools. However, sensory integrative problems are not limited to children with learning disabilities; they can affect all ages, intellectual levels and socioeconomic groups.

A number of situations can trigger sensory integration problems:

Prematurity As more premature infants survive today, they enter the world with easily overstimulated nervous systems and multiple medical problems. Parents need to learn how to give their premature infant the sensory nourishment their child requires for optimal development, and how to avoid harmful overstimulation.

Developmental disorders Severe problems with sensory processing are a hallmark of AUTISM. Autistic children seek out unusual amounts of certain types of sensations, but are extremely hypersensitive to others. Similar traits are often seen in other children with developmental disorders. Improving sensory processing will help these children develop more productive contacts with people and environments.

Learning disabilities As many as 30 percent of school-age children may have learning disabilities. While most of these children have normal intelligence, many are likely to have sensory integrative problems. These children are also more likely than their peers to have been born prematurely, to have had early developmental problems, and to have poor motor coordination. Early intervention can improve sensory integration in these children, minimizing the possibility of school failure before it occurs.

Brain injury Trauma to the brain as a result of accidents and strokes can have profound effects on sensory functioning.

This complex neurological problem leads to either sensory-seeking or sensory-avoiding patterns, or a motor planning problem called dyspraxia.

Symptoms and Diagnostic Path

Sensory seekers have nervous systems that do not always process sensory input that is sent to the brain. As a result, they respond too strongly to sensations. Children who are underresponsive to sensation seek out sensory experiences that are more intense or of longer duration. They may

- be hyperactive as they seek more and more movement input
- be unaware of touch or pain, or touching others too often or too hard (may seem aggressive)
- engage in unsafe behaviors, such as climbing too high
- enjoy sounds that others perceive as too loud, such as TV or radio volume

At the other end of the spectrum of this disorder are sensory avoiders, who have nervous systems that feel sensation too easily or too much, making them overly responsive to sensation. As a result, they may have "fight or flight" responses to sensation, a condition called sensory defensiveness. They may

- respond to being touched with aggression or withdrawal
- be afraid of, or become sick with, movement and heights
- be very cautious and unwilling to take risks or try new things
- be uncomfortable in loud or busy environments such as sports events or malls
- be very picky eaters or overly sensitive to food smells

Treatment Options and Outlook

Sensory integration dysfunction is believed to be a neurological problem that affects behavior and learning. Medicine cannot cure the problem, but occupational therapy can address the child's underlying problems in processing sensations. A good sensory treatment plan may be a major component in treating the child with DSI. Taking a conservative approach often helps the inattentive child whose problem is not ADD, but developmentally delayed sensory processing.

If a child is suspected of having a sensory integrative disorder, a qualified occupational or physical therapist can conduct an evaluation consisting of both standardized testing and structured observations of responses to sensory stimulation, posture, balance, coordination, and eye movements. After carefully analyzing test results and other assessment data, along with information from other professionals and parents, the therapist will recommend appropriate treatment.

If therapy is recommended, the child will be guided through activities that challenge the child's ability to respond appropriately to sensory input by making a successful, organized response. Training of specific skills is not usually the focus of this kind of therapy. Instead, adaptive physical education, movement education, and gymnastics are examples of services that typically focus on specific motor skills training. Such services are important, but they are not the same as therapy using a sensory integrative approach.

The motivation of the child plays a crucial role in the selection of the activities in a sensory integrative approach. The most important step in promoting sensory integration in children is to recognize that it exists and that it plays an important role in the development of a child. The goal of occupational therapy is to enable children to take part in the normal "jobs" of childhood, such as playing, eating, dressing, and sleeping.

septo-optic dysplasia (SOD) A rare disorder characterized by abnormal development of the optic disk, pituitary deficiencies, and often absence of the part of the brain that separates the lateral ventricles.

Symptoms and Diagnostic Path

Symptoms may include blindness in one or both eyes, pupil dilation in response to light, nystagmus (a rapid, involuntary back-and-forth movement of the eyes), inward and outward deviation of the eyes, low muscle tone, seizures, and hormone problems, and sometimes jaundice at birth.

Intellectual problems vary in severity among individuals. Some children have normal intelligence but others have a LEARNING DISABILITY and

MENTAL RETARDATION; most are developmentally delayed due to vision impairment or neurological problems.

Some people with this condition have near normal vision in one eye, while others have decreased vision in both eyes, and others are severely affected and nearly blind. An eye doctor can diagnose this problem by looking inside the eye with an ophthalmoscope.

Treatment Options and Outlook

Hormone deficiencies may be treated with hormone replacement therapy, but visual problems are generally not treatable. Vision, physical, and occupational therapies may be required.

serotonin A chemical that is found in many tissues of the body. In the brain, serotonin acts as a NEUROTRANSMITTER (a chemical involved in transmitting nerve signals between NERVE CELLS) that is believed to be involved in mood states (especially DEPRESSION) and consciousness.

Antidepressant drugs called SELECTIVE SEROTONIN REUPTAKE INHIBITORS (SSRIS) (including Prozac, Zoloft, and Paxil) are used to treat depression by inhibiting the absorption of serotonin in the brain, effectively boosting the levels of the neurotransmitter.

sex differences in the brain See GENDER DIFFERENCES IN THE BRAIN.

sexuality and the brain While sexual activity appears to be a physical activity, it is the brain that is of profound importance in sexuality itself. Sexual activity is moderated by the LIMBIC SYSTEM structures in the TEMPORAL LOBE; damage in this area has been linked to hypersexuality, an abnormal condition characterized by an increased sex drive and an indiscriminate choice of partners. In both men and women, the sex drive and sexual response appear to be triggered by the sense organs or HYPOTHALAMUS. Instinctual sexual behavior is genetically programmed in the hypothalamus and the limbic system and is triggered by sex hormones in these areas.

In most mammals, sexual arousal is linked to chemicals (pheromones) with distinctive odors that the female releases when she is in heat (the period of time when her eggs are ready to be fertilized). These pheromones stimulate males of the same species to try to mate with the female.

However, in humans there is no period when the female is in heat, although some women do feel more interested in sex after ovulation. Moreover, in humans, males seem fairly uninterested by pheromones, even though such chemicals do exist to stimulate the human male sex drive.

sexual orientation and the brain The process that makes a person male or female in orientation is quite complex. A child's outward sexual characteristics—his or her gender—is determined at conception by the X or Y chromosome present in the fertilizing sperm. This sets off a series of hormonal events culminating in the development of characteristically male or female genitals and gonads.

While the bodies of both boys and girls in early childhood (other than genitals) appear to be identical, by the teenage years hormonal activity begins to influence the development of adult sex differences. However, hormonal activity appears to be most important in infancy because research has suggested this affects the physiological makeup of the infant's brain, affecting personality traits.

Research has shown that natural or artificially induced hormone imbalances can produce "male" changes in female brains and vice versa, together with related personality changes—girls exhibit more aggression, and boys become gentler. These results suggest that sex roles may be as much a result of brain development as social conditioning. Research suggests that the brain's exposure to sex hormones at a specific critical phase in very early life determines sexual behavior for the rest of life, no matter what a person's outward sexual characteristics. In rat experiments, females given male hormones for a few days just after birth fail to mate as females should and cannot ovulate. In addition, the preoptic part of their hypothalami shows a more characteristic male, not female, brain-cell pattern.

Moreover, in 1991 researchers discovered that the brains of homosexual men were anatomically different from those of heterosexual men. In homosexual men, a tiny node in the front of the HYPOTHALAMUS (an area of the brain concerned with sexual behavior) was only about a third of the size of the node in heterosexual men; this node was roughly the same size as in heterosexual women. Researcher Simon LeVay of the Salk Institute in San Diego emphasized that his findings did not prove that the brain variation caused homosexuality, nor did he know when the brain abnormality appeared. LeVay's study was based on autopsies of 19 homosexual men, and 16 men and six women believed to be heterosexual. (The researchers could not obtain the brains of lesbian women because these women rarely die of sexually transmitted diseases and, therefore, their sexual orientation was not often noted on medical charts.) While the brains of all subjects were fairly young (about age 40), more than half had died from AIDS. This prompted critics to attribute the differences in the brains to the disease and not to sexual preference.

Other researchers have found a second difference between the brains of homosexual and heterosexual men. A pair of researchers at the University of California at Los Angeles discovered a difference in the ANTERIOR COMMISSURE, a pencil-sized bundle of nerves that may carry sensory information between the lobes of the brain. The brain structure in gay men was 34 percent larger than in heterosexual men and 18 percent larger than in heterosexual women. Researchers concluded that the difference could mean homosexual men may process information differently.

shaken baby syndrome A type of brain damage caused by forceful shaking of an infant or young child by the arms, legs, chest, or shoulders that can lead to hemorrhages and swelling of the brain.

A baby's head and neck are especially vulnerable to injury because the head is so large and the neck muscles are still weak. In addition, the baby's brain and blood vessels are very fragile and are easily damaged by whiplash motions such as shaking, jerking, and jolting.

About 50,000 cases of shaken baby syndrome occur each year in the United States; one shaken baby in four dies as a result of this abuse. Head trauma is the most frequent cause of permanent damage or death among abused infants and children, and shaking accounts for a significant number of those cases. Some studies estimate that 15 percent of children's deaths are due to battering or shaking and an additional 15 percent are possible cases of shaking. The victims of shaken baby syndrome range in age from a few days to five years, with an average age of six to eight months.

While shaken baby abuse is not limited to any special group of people, 65 percent to 90 percent of shakers are men. In the United States, adult males in their early twenties who are the baby's father or the mother's boyfriend are typically the shaker. Females who injure babies by shaking them are more likely to be baby-sitters or child care providers than mothers.

Severe shaking often begins in response to frustration over a baby's crying or toileting problems. The adult shaker also may be jealous of the attention that the child receives from a partner.

Shaken baby syndrome is also known as abusive head trauma, shaken brain trauma, pediatric traumatic brain injury, whiplash shaken infant syndrome, and shaken impact syndrome.

Symptoms and Diagnostic Path

Shaken baby syndrome can cause MENTAL RETARDATION, speech and LEARNING DISABILITY, paralysis, seizures, blindness, hearing loss, and death. It is difficult to diagnose unless someone accurately describes what happened. Physicians often report that a child with possible shaken baby syndrome is brought for medical attention due to falls, difficulty breathing, seizures, vomiting, altered consciousness, or choking. The caregiver may report that the child was shaken to try to resuscitate it. Babies with severe or lethal shaken baby syndrome are typically brought to the hospital unconscious with a closed head injury.

To diagnose shaken baby syndrome, physicians look for bleeding in the retina of the eyes, blood in the brain, or increased head size, indicating buildup of fluid in the tissues of the brain. Damage to the spinal cord and broken ribs from grasping the baby too hard are other signs of shaken baby syndrome. Computed tomography (CT) and magnetic resonance imaging (MRI) scans can reveal injuries in the brain, but are not regularly used because of their expense. A milder form of this syndrome may be missed or misdiagnosed. Subtle symptoms which may be the result of shaken baby syndrome are often attributed to mild viral illnesses, feeding dysfunction, or infant colic. These include a history of poor feeding, vomiting, or flulike symptoms with no accompanying fever or diarrhea, lethargy, and irritability over a period of time. Without early medical intervention, the child may be at risk for further damage or even death, depending on the continued occurrences of shaking.

Treatment Options and Outlook

Treatment of survivors falls into three major categories—medical, behavioral, and educational. In addition to medical care, children may need speech and language therapy, vision therapy, physical therapy, occupational therapy, and special education services. Some may need the assistance of feeding experts and behavioral consultants.

Immediate medical attention can help reduce the impact of shaking, but many children are left with permanent damage. Fewer than 10 percent to 15 percent of shaken babies recover completely; the rest have a variety of disabilities, including partial or complete loss of vision, hearing problems, seizure disorders, CEREBRAL PALSY, sucking and swallowing disorders, developmental disabilities, AUTISM, cognitive or behavior problems, or a permanent vegetative state.

short-term memory   Another word for consciousness, short-term memory has a range of other names: Primary memory, immediate memory, working memory. But while some researchers describe a distinct short-term memory system of limited capacity and a long-term system of relatively unlimited capacity, others do not distinguish between the two. Instead, they suggest there is only one system with what appears to be "short-term" memory as only memory with very low levels of learning.

This type of memory storage is necessary in order to perform many tasks; for example, when reading a book, the beginning of the sentence must be kept in mind while reading the last part of the sentence in order for the whole phrase to make sense.

Short-term memory receives information from sensory memory. If not processed further, the information quickly decays; among typical subjects without any memory training, short-term memory seems as if it can deal only with about six or seven items at once for about 15 to 30 seconds at a time. Research suggests that the information in short-term storage is highly vulnerable to distraction or negative interference. (For example, when you lose your train of thought during a conversation after being interrupted.)

Once placed in short-term storage, information can then either be transferred into long-term storage (or "secondary memory") or it can be forgotten.

If a person looks up a number in a phone book, sensory memory registers the number and passes it into short-term memory. As the number is repeated over and over while dialing, it is retained in short-term memory. The limited capacity of short-term memory determines how much information a person can pay attention to at any one time. Going over information keeps it in short-term memory; after a person has looked up an unfamiliar phone number and repeated it over and over, the person could probably make a phone call without having to look up the number again in the book. However, if the person was interrupted while dialing, it is likely that the number would be forgotten when the person tried to redial.

Short-term memory also is limited in capacity to about five or 10 bits of information, which can be enlarged by using MNEMONICS—strategies to help remember information. For example, grouping a phone number into segments of three, three, and four makes it much easier to remember than if the number was remembered as one long continuous line of 10 digits.

If data is to be transferred into long-term store, a permanent memory trace is formed that provides the basis for restoring the information to consciousness. To remember a phone number for a long period of time, it must be "encoded" and moved into LONG-TERM MEMORY—preferably using sight or sound to help remember it. A person could sing the number or think about a picture of the number to help retrieve it from long-term memory.

Short-term memory is an important part of a person's memory in that it serves as a sort of temporary notepad, briefly retaining intermediate results while we think and solve problems. It helps maintain a concept of the world by indicating what objects are in the environment and where they are located, keeping visual perceptions stable.

A person's visual perception darts around a scene taking about five retinal images per second and integrating information from all the snapshots into one sustained model of the immediate scene. New changes are included in an updated model, while old ones are discarded, thanks to short-term memory.

Short-term memory maintains the file of our intentions in "active" mode, guiding behavior toward those goals. It keeps track of topics that have been mentioned in conversations. If two friends are discussing a third acquaintance, they can refer to the person as "she" without using her name, and each will know whom the "she" refers to, because of short-term memory.

However, these early processes are extremely complex, including the necessity of word identification and object recognition. By the time information has reached short-term store, a great deal of processing has already occurred of which people are not consciously aware. What passes into consciousness and short-term store is simply the *result* of those unconscious processes. Researchers suggest that only information that has been consciously perceived is transferred from short- to long-term store.

Many researchers liken a person's short-term memory to a computer's central processing unit (CPU). Almost all computers are designed with a sort of "short-term memory" within the CPU, which receives data, stores it in memory, retrieves it and can display it on a screen or print it out. These functions are strikingly similar to short-term memory.

shrinking retrograde amnesia   The gradual recovery from RETROGRADE AMNESIA, with older memories

returning first. The existence of the phenomenon of shrinking retrograde amnesia is not surprising, considering that earlier memories can be derived from a different source from that needed to recall more recent experiences.

As recovery occurs, more and more of the episodic record becomes available and more recent memories can be recalled. It is believed that older experiences are more broadly distributed than newer events and that a gradual recovery process will restore some component of older memories before it restores more narrowly distributed newer memories.

shunt, brain   A procedure in which a narrow piece of tubing is inserted into the brain to receive excess intracranial pressure. In the technique, the shunt is inserted into the back portion of the lateral ventricle and then threaded under the scalp toward the neck; still under the skin, the tubing is threaded to another body cavity, where the SPINAL FLUID is drained and absorbed.

Shy-Drager syndrome   A progressive disorder of the central and sympathetic nervous systems characterized by a drop in blood pressure when a patient stands up, causing dizziness or momentary blackouts. The syndrome has been classified clinically into three types

- olivopontocerebellar atrophy (OPCA), which primarily affects balance, coordination, and speech
- striatonigral degeneration, which can resemble Parkinson's disease because of slow movement and stiff muscles
- mixed cerebellar and parkinsonian form

Symptoms and Diagnostic Path

All three forms of the disease may cause a drop in blood pressure on standing, together with constipation, impotence, and urinary incontinence. Constipation may be unrelenting and hard to manage. Other symptoms that may develop include impaired speech, difficulties with breathing and swallowing, and inability to sweat.

Shy-Drager syndrome may be hard to diagnose in the early stages. For most patients, blood pressure is low when the patients stand up and high when the patients lie down.

Treatment Options and Outlook

The low blood pressure is treatable, but there is no known effective treatment for the progressive central nervous system degeneration. General treatment is aimed at controlling symptoms. Antiparkinsonian medication may be helpful. To relieve low blood pressure while standing, dietary increases of salt and fluid may help. Medications to raise blood pressure, such as salt-retaining steroids, are often necessary, but they can cause side effects and should be carefully monitored by a physician. Alpha-adrenergic medications, nonsteroidal anti-inflammatory drugs, and sympathomimetic amines are sometimes used.

Sleeping with the head elevated at night reduces problems with low blood pressure on arising. An artificial feeding tube or breathing tube may be surgically inserted for management of swallowing and breathing difficulties.

Shy-Drager syndrome usually ends in death within seven to 10 years after diagnosis. Breathing problems, airway obstruction, or cardiopulmonary arrest are common causes of death.

sight See VISION.

sleep and the brain In order to function with peak skills, it is essential to get enough sleep and rest the brain, which can be taxed by too much work during the day and poor sleeping at night. In fact, sleep is an active process of the nervous system. Most people spend about a third of their lives sleeping, although the amount of sleep needed varies at any one time. Babies sleep for about 16 hours a day in several periods; at age five most children sleep 10 or 11 hours at night. Adults need between seven or eight hours of sleep to stay healthy and alert, although illness, exertion, and pregnancy increase the need for sleep. A few people, known as nonsomniacs, need only one or two hours of sleep each night.

As evening wears on and darkness falls, the eyes register the fading light with the brain's biological clock—the PINEAL GLAND, found deep within the brain. This gland then secretes MELATONIN, a sleep-related hormone that affects BRAIN CELLS that use SEROTONIN. Melatonin is concentrated in the raphe nuclei found along the BRAIN STEM behind the RETICULAR ACTIVATING SYSTEM—the part of the brain responsible for consciousness itself.

During sleep, the sensory input to the reticular activating system drops, and the electrical activity up through the CEREBRAL CORTEX drops. This does not mean that a sleeping brain is completely switched off, however. In sleep, the brain undergoes repeated activity cycles marked by several distinct stages.

Stage I sleep is characterized by relaxation as the person drifts in and out of sleep; heartbeat and breathing slow down, muscles relax, and a slight noise would awaken the sleeper. After a few minutes, sleepers pass into Stage II, a stage of light sleep where the eyes roll slowly from side to side. The ELECTROENCEPHALOGRAM (EEG) will show "sleep spindles," and sleepers will not awaken unless the noise is much louder. As the body grows still more relaxed, the person enters Stage III sleep, wherein the long, slow DELTA WAVES appear. Heartbeat, breathing, body temperature, and blood pressure fall further, and muscles become more relaxed. About 20 to 30 minutes after sleep begins, the person enters Stage IV—deep sleep. At this point, EEG tracings show primarily delta waves; some sleepers may talk or sleepwalk in this stage. Then the cycle slowly reverses itself over the next 30 to 40 minutes, and the person slowly surfaces from Stage III to II. But instead of going on to experience Stage I again, the sleeper enters the first of several phases of REM SLEEP as the eyes suddenly start to flicker back and forth while breathing and heartbeat becomes irregular. Sleepers awakened during this stage report dreams.

During REM, noradrenalin-producing cells in the PONS (the middle section of the brain stem) trigger a burst of signals that spread to nearby cells, eventually affecting the entire cerebral cortex. Some scientists believe that the cortex then draws on its memory banks to construct a pattern of these signals—resulting in a dream. While this is going on, the brain electrically "freezes" motor neurons that control the large muscles; this prevents violent movements of arms and legs that would be harmful during REM sleep.

Periods of REM sleep alternate with NREM (non-REM) sleep in about a 90-minute cycle; the REM portion becomes longer each time as the NREM shortens. The fourth or fifth period of REM sleep may last as long as an hour. Eventually, sleep becomes shallower and the sleeper awakens.

Each sleep cycle lasts about 90 minutes, and there are about four or five cycles per night. During sleep, the brain revises, manipulates, and stores information. Of course, sleep is not a continuous process throughout the night. Instead, according to researchers at France's National Center for Scientific Research, the brain processes, reviews, consolidates, and stores information during "paradoxical sleep," (REM) which lasts for just about 20 minutes and occurs every 90 minutes in humans. During this portion of sleep, all the senses are put on hold, disconnecting the brain from the outside world.

Despite popular ideas to the contrary, it is not possible to learn while asleep, even though some people cannot learn effectively *without* sleep. Because both the conscious and subconscious play a role in the memory process, one cannot work without the other.

The inability to sleep deprives a person not just of valuable memory consolidation during rest but also interferes with learning during waking hours. This problem particularly affects the elderly, who often have more sleep problems and get very little fourth-stage, or "deep," sleep, during which the brain recharges itself. After a while, the person lives in a chronic state of fatigue and finds it difficult to pay attention.

sleep apnea Episodes of failure to breathe during sleep that may last for 10 seconds or longer. It may be caused either by a failure of the brain's regulation of breathing during sleep or by excessive muscular relaxation.

Symptoms and Diagnostic Path

In the less common central sleep apnea, the patient's airway stays open, but the diaphragm and chest muscles do not work because of a disturbance in the brain's regulation of breathing during sleep.

Obstructive sleep apnea, on the other hand, is far more common and is caused by excessive relaxation during sleep of the muscles of the soft palate at the base of the throat. These muscles block the airway, making breathing labored and causing loud snoring. A complete blockage will halt breathing, making the sleeper stop snoring. As the pressure to breathe makes muscles of the diaphragm and chest work harder, the blockage is opened and the patient gasps and briefly wakes. This type of sleep apnea may also be caused by enlarged tonsils and adenoids, a large tongue, or a small airway.

Some people experience both central and obstructive sleep apnea (called mixed apnea), which is characterized by a brief period of central apnea followed by a longer period of obstructive apnea.

The periods of arousal during the night are brief and are not usually remembered; people who experience them will often complain of being sleepy during the day. Severe sleep apnea may lead to high blood pressure, heart failure, heart attack, or STROKE.

Obstructive sleep apnea affects one in every 100 men between the ages of 30 and 50, especially if they snore and are overweight. However, the condition may be found in women as well and in all ages. Some experts suggest that some cases of sudden infant death syndrome (SIDS) may be caused by sleep apnea; it becomes more and more common as a person ages.

Treatment Options and Outlook

Because most people with severe sleep apnea are overweight, the condition is eased with weight loss. In addition, people subject to sleep apnea should not drink alcohol within two hours of going to sleep and should not take sleeping pills. (Both substances slow down the breathing muscle activity and may worsen the condition.)

More and more patients are finding relief with "continuous positive airway pressure" (CPAP)—a mask that is worn over the nose and mouth during sleep, forcing oxygen into both nasal passages and the airway to keep them open.

Protriptyline and supplemental oxygen may help some people; surgery to remove excess tissue at the back of the throat may be helpful in some cases. Some may find relief with a tracheostomy (an opening in the windpipe), which bypasses the obstructed airway, allowing air to flow directly to the lungs during sleep.

sleep disorders One in three adults in the United States suffers from one of the more than 100 disorders of sleeping and waking. The disorders are divided into four main categories: the insomnias (problems in falling or staying asleep), problems staying awake, problems adhering to a consistent sleep/wake schedule, and problems with sleep-disruptive behaviors.

Insomnias are classified as transient (lasting just a few nights, usually due to excitement or minor stress), short-term (lasting up to three weeks due to major stress or illness), and chronic (continued poor sleep that may be caused by physical illness, psychological issues, poor sleeping environment, or lifestyle). While insomnias are not considered a disease, they are a symptom that can benefit from medical treatment.

Problems in staying awake are the usual reasons that drive people to seek help at one of the more than 200 sleep-disorder centers in this country. These problems are usually the result of SLEEP APNEA (a potentially fatal disorder in which breathing stops intermittently during sleep) and NARCOLEPSY (a disorder causing daytime sleep attacks).

Those people who have problems maintaining a consistent sleep/wake cycle usually have disruptions in their internal sleep center in the brain controlling sleeping and waking. A common example of this problem is JET LAG, in which the body's internal clock is upset by rapid travel across time zones (especially west to east). A form of this type of jet lag occurs among employees who must work rotating shifts, constantly changing their hours for waking and sleeping. Those who work night shifts also complain of more problems with poor sleep and daytime drowsiness.

sleeping sickness A serious infectious disease of tropical Africa spread by the bite of the tsetse fly, which transmits the protozoa *Trypanosoma brucei* to humans and animals. The protozoa multiply and spread to the bloodstream and eventually the brain, where it induces the strange lethargy from which the disease gets its name.

There are two forms of the disease: sleeping sickness of western and central Africa is spread primarily from person to person, while the east African version primarily affects wild animals, although it is occasionally transmitted to humans.

While sleeping sickness can be controlled by eradicating the tsetse fly, many thousands of Africans (and some tourists) still contract the disease each year.

Symptoms and Diagnostic Path

First, a painful nodule develops at the bite site; the West African version then slowly proceeds with fever and lymph-gland enlargement until the protozoa migrate to the brain, setting off HEADACHES, confusion, and severe lassitude with eventual complete inactivity, drooping eyelids, and a vacant expression. Untreated, the disease is fatal.

The East African form of the disease runs a faster course, beginning with a high fever a few weeks after infection. If the disease is not at first fatal from attacking the heart, the protozoan will continue to affect the brain.

Treatment Options and Outlook

Drug treatment will cure the disease, although the drugs can cause serious side effects. If the infection has already spread to the brain, it can cause brain damage.

Risk Factors and Preventive Measures

Tourists should protect themselves against the bite of the tsetse fly in order to avoid the disease.

slow viruses of the brain A group of viruses of the CENTRAL NERVOUS SYSTEM (including the brain) that cause symptoms of memory loss and DEMENTIA 10 or 20 years after the initial infection. The diseases take a slow course, the end of which is usually fatal. Included among diseases suspected to be caused by such a slow virus may be at least one type of ALZHEIMER'S DISEASE, KURU, CREUTZFELDT-JAKOB DISEASE, a rare complication of measles called subacute sclerosing panencephalitis, and MULTIPLE SCLEROSIS.

smell, sense of   One of the five senses, it enables a human being to distinguish several thousand different odors, although scientists are not sure of the exact mechanism by which this is possible.

A person is able to smell when odors travel up the nasal cavity to the OLFACTORY NERVES, which send electrical signals to the brain where the interpretation of smell occurs. Any glitch along this path will interfere with a person's ability to detect or identify odors.

The sense of smell is made possible because of the presence of smell RECEPTORS (specialized NERVE-CELL endings) in a small area of mucous membrane lining the roof of the nose. These receptor cells have cilia that reach down to the surface of the mucous membrane, and are stimulated by odor molecules. Odor molecules must dissolve in mucus before they can stimulate receptors, which is why this area must be kept moist.

When the molecule "keys" fit into the receptor "locks," the process triggers nerve impulses in the olfactory nerve that are transmitted to the brain, where they are translated in parts of the LIMBIC SYSTEM and FRONTAL LOBES. The system is exquisitely sensitive; as little as four molecules will give a recognizable smell.

A person may either lose the sense of smell (anosmia) or experience distortions in this sense (dysosmia). Because the senses of smell and taste are so intimately intertwined, problems in smell usually affect the ability to taste as well; this is why elderly people often complain that food has lost its taste. Temporary problems with smell may occur when the mucous membrane in the nose becomes inflamed, such as with a cold, flu, or rhinitis. Cigarette smoking may also inflame the nose and interfere with the sense of smell. Overgrowth of the adenoids or a deviated septum will block airflow and interfere with the sense of smell. In rare cases, a person may lose the ability to smell because of a MENINGIOMA (tumor of the MENINGES,

the membranes surrounding the brain) or a tumor behind the nose.

MEDICATIONS THAT CAN AFFECT SENSE OF SMELL
Antibiotics
Anticoagulants (anti-blood-clotting drugs)
Antihistamines
Blood pressure medicine
Chemotherapy drugs
Dietary supplements
Nose drops
Oil of peppermint
Toothpaste
Vitamin D (high doses)

In addition, the olfactory nerves can be damaged during HEAD INJURY; if both nerves are completely torn, the person will permanently lose the ability to smell. Less severe damage may result in temporary smell distortions as the nerves heal. Between 5 and 10 percent of all major head injuries result in some malfunction in the sense of smell.

Fleeting unpleasant odors (cacosmia) may occur as a result of DEPRESSION or SCHIZOPHRENIA, in some forms of EPILEPSY, and during recovery from severe alcoholism. Sometimes, a person with dysosmia may be convinced that the smell originates in the person's own body and may begin to wash compulsively.

Many diseases, including neurological problems, endocrine diseases, hereditary disease, cirrhosis, or kidney failure, may also interfere with the sense of smell. Damage to brain tissue caused by STROKE or toxic chemicals may alter the sense of smell, as can dietary deficiencies (especially in vitamin A, vitamin B_{12}, or zinc).

Smell may also be altered as a side effect of medications, dietary supplements, and nose drops, or radiation therapy to the head. (See also OLFACTORY FATIGUE.)

Smith, Edwin, surgical papyrus of   An ancient Egyptian medical treatise that describes how a HEAD INJURY can have effects throughout the body. The papyrus, written between 2,500 and 3,000 years ago, contains information about 48 cases, in which eight describe head injuries that affect other parts of the body.

Apparently intended as a textbook on surgery, it begins with the clinical cases of head injuries and works its way down the body, describing in detail the examination, diagnosis, treatment, and prognosis in each case.

The papyrus was acquired in Luxor in 1862 by the American egyptologist Edwin Smith, a pioneer in the study of Egyptian science. After his death in 1906, the papyrus was given to the New-York Historical Society, which turned it over for study to Egyptologist James Henry Breasted in 1920. He published a translation, transliteration, and discussion in two volumes in 1930.

smoking and the brain See ADDICTIONS; NICOTINE; STIMULANTS AND THE BRAIN.

sodium pentothal See TRUTH DRUGS.

somatic nervous system The somatic ("bodily") nervous system features motor and sensory nerves; motor nerves branch from the CENTRAL NERVOUS SYSTEM and trigger muscle action on orders from the brain or SPINAL CORD, whereas sensory nerves bring information from sensory receptors in skin, tongue, eyes, nostrils, joints, and muscles. The information from these two groups of nerves is used by the body to control how we move and hold our body erect. Together, the AUTONOMIC NERVOUS SYSTEMS and the somatic nervous system make up the PERIPHERAL NERVOUS SYSTEM.

source amnesia Loss of memory for when and where particular information was acquired.

spasticity A condition in which certain muscles are continuously contracted, causing stiffness or tightness of the muscles that may interfere with movement and speech. Spasticity is usually caused by damage to the portion of the brain or spinal cord that controls voluntary movement. It may occur together with spinal cord injury, MULTIPLE SCLEROSIS, CEREBRAL PALSY, BRAIN DAMAGE, severe head injury, and some metabolic diseases.

Symptoms and Diagnostic Path
Increased muscle tone, clonus (a series of rapid muscle contractions), exaggerated deep tendon reflexes, muscle spasms, scissoring, and fixed joints. The degree of spasticity varies from mild muscle stiffness to severe, painful, and uncontrollable muscle spasms. The condition can interfere with rehabilitation in patients with certain disorders, and often interferes with daily activities.

Treatment Options and Outlook
Medications such as baclofen, diazepam, or clonazepam can be administered. Muscle stretching, range-of-motion exercises, and other types of physical therapy may help prevent joint shrinkage or muscle shortening.

spatial memory See MEMORY.

SPECT (single-photon emission computerized tomography) A type of brain scan that tracks blood flow and measures brain activity. Less expensive than PET (POSITRON EMISSION TOMOGRAPHY) SCANS, SPECTS may be used to identify the subtle injury following mild head trauma.

Procedure
SPECT is a type of radionuclide scanning, a diagnostic technique based on the detection of radiation emitted by radioactive substances introduced into the body. Different radioactive substances (radionuclides) are taken up in greater concentrations by different types of tissue; this gives a clearer picture of organ function than other systems.

The radioactive substance is swallowed or injected into the bloodstream, where it accumulates in the brain. Gamma radiation (similar but shorter than X-RAYS) is emitted from the brain, detected by a gamma camera, which emits light, and used to produce an image that can be displayed on a screen; using a principle similar to CS scanning, cross-sectional images can be constructed by a computer from radiation detected by a gamma camera that rotates around the patient. It is also possible to create moving images by using a computer to record a series of images right after the administration of the radionuclide.

Risks and Complications

Radionuclide is a safe procedure requiring only tiny doses of radiation. Because the radioactive substance is ingested or injected, it avoids the risks of some X-ray procedures in which a radiopaque dye is inserted through a catheter into the organ (as in ANGIOGRAPHY), and unlike radiopaque dyes, radionuclides carry almost no risk of toxicity or allergy.

speech   The intrinsic ability to speak is hardwired into the brain at birth and usually starts with vocalized vowels at about seven weeks of age. Learning how to speak involves the ability to make and monitor sounds. It occurs when the brain activates MOTOR NERVES, sending signals to operate larynx, vocal cords, pharynx, soft palate, tongue, and lips. Sensory nerves bring the brain signals from speech muscles and from the ears, which pick up sound waves made by the voice. With this type of feedback system, a child can learn how to modify sounds to match words that are heard. This is why children who are deaf will not learn to speak on their own.

Infants learn first how to babble, and the responses of adults around them help them select sounds to reproduce. By the time infants are 16 weeks old, they can make consonant sounds and by 20 weeks can utter some syllables. The first meaningful word usually appears before the first year. By 21 to 24 months, a child is using two-word phrases, and by the age of three, most children speak constantly.

In an English-speaking country, a child will speak the *a* and other vowels, followed by *m, b, g, k,* and *p*. By 32 weeks most children can say *t, d,* and *w*. The sounds of *s, f, h, r,* and *th* come later.

Speech disorders may be due to problems of articulation (anarthria or dysarthria) of LANGUAGE function (aphasia or dysphasia), problems in the production of voice sounds (aphonia or dysphonia), or to mental illness.

speech-language pathologist   An expert who specializes in the assessment and treatment of speech, language, and voice disorders. Also known as a speech pathologist or speech therapist, the speech-language pathologist evaluates and treats individuals with communication problems resulting from LEARNING DISABILITY, hearing loss, brain injury, cleft palate, emotional problems, development delays, or STROKE. They also provide clinical therapy to help those with speech and language disorders, and help them and their families understand the disorder and develop better communication skills.

Speech-language pathologists perform screening tests and make recommendations for the type of speech language treatment required. Treatment could include a specific program of exercises to improve language ability or speech, together with support from the client's family and friends.

They conduct research to develop new and better ways to diagnose and treat speech and language problems, work with children who have language delays and speech problems, and provide treatment to people who stutter and to those with voice and articulation problems.

Educational requirements include a master's degree in speech-language pathology, more than 300 hours of supervised clinical experience, and successful completion of a certifying exam. Those who meet the strict requirements of the American Speech-Language and Hearing Association are awarded the certificate of clinical competence.

spina bifida   A general name for congenital abnormalities caused by the failure to close of an embryo's membrane-and-tissue-covered tube housing the CENTRAL NERVOUS SYSTEM. Literally meaning "spine in two parts," spina bifida is also known medically as a NEURAL TUBE DEFECT.

While defects can be found anywhere on the spine, they are generally found on the lower back.

The precise cause is not clear, but there appear to be both environmental and genetic causes.

Symptoms and Diagnostic Path

There are several types of spina bifida, including spina bifida occulta, MENINGOCELE, MYELOMENINGO-CELE, encephalocele, and ANENCEPHALY.

In *spina bifida occulta,* there is a small, incomplete closure but no obvious damage to the SPINAL CORD. Found in 20 percent or more of the population, the damage is so minor that many people do not know they have it (hence the name *occulta,* or "hidden"). The site may be marked by a dimple, hair tuft, or telangiectasia (red skin caused by expanded blood vessels). It may be associated with urinary or bowel problems, together with weakness or poor circulation in the legs that appears in adulthood.

Meningocele is characterized by the appearance of the MENINGES (the membrane covering the spinal cord) pushing out through an abnormal opening in the vertebrae, forming a sac that looks like a bulge. The spinal cord itself is not damaged, and the sac is covered by skin. This defect can be easily repaired by surgery during the first few days of life.

The most severe form of spina bifida is myelomeningocele, which is what most people think of when they hear the term *spina bifida.* This abnormality is characterized by the protrusion of nerve and tissue from the spinal cord into a sac, which may or may not be covered by skin on the outside. Symptoms include muscle weakness, loss of sensation, paralysis below the defect, and incontinence. In addition, a malformation at the base of the BRAIN STEM can lead to a HYDROCEPHA-LUS (a buildup of CEREBROSPINAL FLUID) which must be relieved via a SHUNT to avoid BRAIN DAMAGE, including blindness, deafness, SEIZURES, and LEARNING DISABILITIES.

Anencephaly is the medical term for the absence of the brain or spinal cord—the skull does not close and only a groove appears where the spine should be. There is no medical treatment that can save these infants, most of whom will die during the first few hours of life.

Genetic screening tests (including alpha fetoprotein, ULTRASOUND, and amniocentesis) can diagnose the condition.

Treatment Options and Outlook

In the past, most children with the most severe cases of spina bifida (myelomeningocele) died soon after birth, but today immediate surgery saves the lives of most of these children. They usually must have a series of operations as they grow and usually need special devices to help them walk. With this treatment, about 80 percent of these children can walk by the time they enter school. Most need special training (such as how to insert catheters) to manage bowels and bladder and prevent serious bladder infections and kidney problems. Special diets and schedules allow many children to achieve bowel continence, especially when started in the preschool years.

These children may also experience lack of feeling, pressure sores, spinal disorders, eye problems, excess weight, MENTAL RETARDATION, or learning disability.

As adults, many can function sexually although some (especially males) may have some problems due to nerve damage. A woman with spina bifida can give birth, but she has a 4 to 5 percent chance of bearing a child with the same problem.

spinal accessory nerve Also known as the 11th cranial nerve, this nerve is responsible for movements of neck and back muscles.

See also CRANIAL NERVES.

spinal cord The very center of the NERVOUS SYSTEM, the spinal cord is a long bundle of nerves extending from the base of the brain running along the inside of the spine (backbone). The spinal cord is the main link between the body and the brain, merging with the base of the brain; the lower end is about two-thirds of the way down the spine. Below this, the spinal cord splits to form several main nerves that continue within the spine, ending up at the legs and feet.

Like the brain, the spinal cord contains both GRAY and WHITE MATTER. The gray matter lies in the center of the cord and consists of thousands of the cell bodies of the MOTOR NEURONS that pass signals to body muscles. A thick layer of white matter surrounds the gray matter; white matter is made up primarily of AXONS (long, thin, wiry extensions of the cells) and contains the nerve fibers that pass signals to and from the brain.

The spinal cord is almost totally enclosed by the spinal bones; 31 pairs of large nerves called spinal nerves branch off the spinal cord at regular intervals and pass through the narrow gaps between the spinal bones. Each spinal nerve contains both sensory and motor neurons. Spinal nerves in the neck handle signals to and from the head, arms, and hands; nerves in the chest lead to the chest muscles, skin, and other organs (such as lungs and heart). Nerves from the lower end of the cord branch out through the stomach area, down into the legs and feet.

Some parts of the nerves carry information to the spinal cord, which relays the messages to the brain; these include nerve messages from the skin detailing touch, temperature, and pain, and messages from internal organs and muscles. Nerves carrying incoming messages are called sensory nerves.

Motor nerves carry outgoing information—signals from the brain traveling down the spinal cord that activate muscles and control the movements of the body.

The spinal cord, like the brain, is wrapped in three layers of MENINGES, and cushioned from shock by the fluid between the arachnoid and PIA MATER layers. It is also possible to have an INFECTION here, called MENINGITIS; in some cases, the inflamed meninges may press on the brain or spinal cord and cause damage or even death.

See also LUMBAR PUNCTURE.

spinal cord tumors Abnormal growths of tissue found inside the bony spinal column, one of the primary components of the central nervous system. Because the spinal column is a rigid, bony structure, any abnormal growth (whether benign or malignant) can place pressure on sensitive tissues and impair function. Tumors that originate in the spinal cord are called primary tumors. Most primary tumors are caused by out-of-control growth among cells that surround neurons. In a small number of individuals, primary tumors may be caused by a specific genetic disease, such as NEUROFIBROMATOSIS or TUBEROUS SCLEROSIS, or from exposure to radiation or cancer-causing chemicals.

The cause of most primary tumors remains a mystery. They are not contagious and, at this time, not preventable.

Symptoms and Diagnostic Path
Spinal cord tumor symptoms include pain, sensory changes, and motor problems. The first test to diagnose spinal column tumors is a neurological examination, followed by CT scans, magnetic resonance imaging, and positron emission tomography. Lab tests include the EEG and the spinal tap. A biopsy helps doctors diagnose the type of tumor.

Treatment Options and Outlook
The three most commonly used treatments are surgery, radiation, and chemotherapy. Doctors also may prescribe steroids to reduce the swelling inside the central nervous system.

Symptoms of spinal cord tumors generally develop slowly and worsen over time unless they are treated. The tumor may be classified as benign or malignant and given a numbered score that reflects how malignant it is. This score can help doctors determine how to treat the tumor and predict the likely outcome, or prognosis, for the patient.

Researchers are studying the effectiveness of using small radioactive pellets implanted directly into the tumor, and advanced drugs and techniques for chemotherapy and radiation therapy. In gene therapy for spinal cord tumors, scientists insert a gene to make the tumor cells sensitive to certain drugs, to program the cells to self-destruct, or to instruct the cells to manufacture substances to slow their growth. Scientists are also investigating why some genes become cancer-causing. Since tumors are more sensitive to heat than normal tissue, research scientists are testing hyperthermia as a treatment. Scientists also are looking for ways to duplicate or enhance the body's immune response to fight against spinal cord cancer.

spinal tap See LUMBAR PUNCTURE.

split-brain research Research that divides a brain surgically into right and left halves so that each half can be trained and tested independently.

While the two CEREBRAL HEMISPHERES may appear almost as two separate brains, in fact they are joined by the CORPUS CALLOSUM—a bundle of 300 million nerve fibers.

The left hemisphere in most people is dominant—it is responsible for writing, computing, speaking, and thinking logically. The right (or secondary) hemisphere handles spatial recognition. The right brain is concerned with creative activities such as art and music, while the left is more analytical and logical. In general, the left hemisphere deals with analysis, while the right hemisphere deals with synthesis.

In the 1950s, scientists successfully treated severe EPILEPSY by severing the nerve fibers connecting the two hemispheres. Despite common fears at the time, the mind did not split in two. While these patients appeared quite normal, a few quirks did exist. For example, a patient with severed hemispheres can describe an unseen object in the right hand but not in the left.

Scientists studying ELECTROENCEPHALOGRAMS have concluded that language dominance is found in the left hemisphere in most people, no matter whether they are right- or left-handed. Speech centers in some people are found in both hemispheres and a few others in the right hemisphere. In young children, the potential for speech can be found in both hemispheres; if the left is damaged, speech will develop in the right. By age 10, speech dominance is usually solidified.

spongiform encephalopathies A group of rare diseases (including KURU and CREUTZFELDT-JAKOB DISEASE) that are characterized by spongy appearance of the CORTEX, diffuse degeneration of NEURONS in the CEREBRUM, BASAL GANGLION, and SPINAL CORD, and the proliferation of GLIAL CELLS.

Symptoms and Diagnostic Path

The diseases cause a rapid, progressive DEMENTIA similar to ALZHEIMER'S DISEASE but also accompanied by striking rigidity, weakness, and muscle spasms. In addition, there is usually a characteristic EEG pattern.

Treatment Options and Outlook

There are no specific treatments; the muscle spasms may respond to benzodiazepine drugs, such as clonazepam and diazepam.

See also MAD COW DISEASE.

SQUID (superconducting quantum interference device) A type of brain-scanning device that senses tiny changes in magnetic fields. When brain cells fire, they create electric current; electric fields induce magnetic fields, so magnetic changes indicate neural activity.

Stanford-Binet Intelligence Scale: Fifth Edition (SB 5) A type of intelligence quotient (IQ) test that can be used to assess intelligence for individuals over age two. First developed in 1910, the test is a standard tool for many school psychologists and yields a mental age (M.A.) and an IQ.

In its revised form, the test provides multiple area IQ scores (called S.A.S.'s) in addition to an overall IQ score. In addition to measuring the verbal and nonverbal areas of a child's development, the Stanford-Binet also provides a quantitative score, measuring the child's mathematical reasoning, and a memory score, measuring the child's short-term memory. (While the Wechsler scales also have subtests which measure these areas, they do not provide IQ scores isolating these abilities.)

The Stanford-Binet test is a good choice for children who are slow at processing information because it contains only one timed subtest. However, this lack of timing can make the testing session extremely long. In addition, test scores may be substantially lower than those resulting from the WAIS-IV for very bright individuals over age 16.

See also WECHSLER INTELLIGENCE SCALE FOR CHILDREN 4TH ED. (WISC-IV).

stars, seeing What appears as random bursts of light when people hit their heads is actually caused by a jolt to the BRAIN CELLS responsible for vision. Normally, these cells respond to the electrical messages sent by the eyes, interpreting the signals as faces, objects, or whatever people are viewing. But a sudden blow to the head can also trigger activity in visual cells unrelated to, or less active during, the given visual scenario. This overactivity of visual processing cells is a burst of electricity that the brain interprets as bursts of light.

Stars most often appear following a blow to the back of the head because that is the location of the visual CORTEX. In fact, stimulating the cells in this part of the brain with a probe can also set off a twinkling-star show. Scientists also believe that the pulsing star-like visual HALLUCINATIONS often seen by MIGRAINE sufferers is caused by spontaneous electrical signaling in the visual cortex.

While "stars" do not normally appear unless the head has received a strong blow, the twinkling lights do not usually signal serious problems. On the other hand, the appearance of twinkling lights after only a slight blow—or none at all—should prompt a visit to the physician. Showers of lights or snake-shaped streams of light may signal a torn retina (nerve cells blanketing the back of the eye).

A torn retina may be repaired with a laser, but if left untreated the retina may completely detach, causing partial or total blindness.

status epilepticus   Repeated or prolonged attacks of epileptic SEIZURES lasting at least five minutes without regaining consciousness between seizures. This medical emergency may be fatal if not treated quickly. This condition is most likely to occur if anticonvulsant drugs are suddenly stopped or taken inconsistently.

stereogram   Two pictures each viewed by one eye, which when combined by the brain give the illusion of a three-dimensional shape.

stereotactic radiosurgery   Also known as gamma knife surgery, this technique of tightly focused radiation is used for patients with an inoperable BRAIN TUMOR. The procedure was pioneered in the late 1960s by Lars Leksell, M.D., a Swedish neurosurgeon at the Karolinska Institute in Stockholm. Since then, thousands of patients around the world have undergone the procedure to destroy tumors or correct life-threatening blood vessel problems, with no reported deaths or complications from the procedure.

Procedure
In the technique, the surgeon uses a small directed beam of radiation to treat areas that may be inaccessible by conventional surgery or for patients who may not be able to withstand an operation. The one-time application is an outpatient procedure that may serve as a substitute for the 20 to 30 radiation treatments normally required. Using the precisely directed beams of radiation, surgeons can focus on and destroy the diseased tissue and spare nearly all of the surrounding healthy tissue.

The key is to locate the diseased tissue and program those coordinates into a linear accelerator—the unit that emits the radiation beam. The accelerator is rotated around the target area in the patient's brain, allowing high doses of radiation to be given directly to the designated site. The procedure usually takes an entire day and is performed with a local anesthetic. A CAT SCAN is used to determine the exact coordinates of the diseased tissue; with that information, doctors then affix a metal ring to the head, which helps the linear accelerator focus on the target area.

At present, this type of radiation is being used for patients with various types of brain tumors, as well as brain tumors that have not responded to conventional radiation therapy. It also can be used to treat malformed blood vessels in the brain that can cause seizures and are usually inoperable under normal situations.

The technique is also used to obtain a brain biopsy, to insert a permanent stimulating wire to control intractable pain, and to destroy areas of the brain to treat disabling neurological disorders.

Risks and Complications
Although the technique often costs less than traditional neurosurgery, it is still not widely practiced, and treatment is not always easy to find.

stimulants and the brain   A class of drugs that increase nerve activity in the brain by triggering the release of NOREPINEPHRINE. These stimulant drugs include NICOTINE, CAFFEINE, AMPHETAMINES, and COCAINE.

There are two main types of stimulant drugs—those that stimulate the nerves of the CENTRAL NERVOUS SYSTEM (including the amphetamines) and those that affect the respiratory system. Central nervous system stimulants reduce drowsiness and increase alertness by their action on the RETICULAR ACTIVATING SYSTEM in the BRAIN STEM. Respiratory stimulants act on the respiratory center in the brain stem. Nerve stimulants include caffeine, dextro-amphetamine, and methylphenidate; respiratory stimulants include doxapram and nikethamide.

Caffeine boosts the brain's flow of thoughts and output of motor signals to the muscles. Too much caffeine can cause heartbeat and respiration to increase and bring on insomnia. Amphetamine is a synthetic product resembling ephedrine available as tablets, powder, or ampules for injection. They are chemically similar to the natural neurotransmitter NORADRENALIN, and enhance the activity of noradrenalin in the brain by releasing quantities of noradrenalin stored in NERVE CELLS and preventing its reabsorption by blocking MAO. Amphetamine also may act on the RECEPTORS of certain cells.

Nerve stimulants can be given to treat NARCO-LEPSY (a disorder characterized by excess sleepiness); they are also effective in the treatment of hyperactivity in children. They also may suppress appetite, but their adverse effects make these drugs a poor choice in the treatment of obesity.

stimulus Any sensory event (such as a flashing light or the touch of a feather) that causes the brain to become active.

stimulus-response memory The type of memory involved when a dinner gong triggers a trained dog to salivate. This type of memory occurs in the brain below the outer CORTEX.

Stokes-Adams syndrome Recurrent, temporary loss of consciousness that occurs as a result of insufficient flow of blood to the brain caused by heart problems. In most cases, when the heart begins beating regularly again, the skin reddens and the person wakes up.

Symptoms and Diagnostic Path
Symptoms include sudden attacks of fainting followed by a bluish tinge to the skin if the person does not regain consciousness quickly. There is a rapid breathing rate and slow pulse. Seizures may occur due to lack of oxygen to the brain.

Treatment Options and Outlook
No treatment is needed if the patient wakes up. If consciousness does not return, prompt cardiopulmonary resuscitation may be needed to prevent brain damage. Most patients with this problem wear a pacemaker to regulate their heart rhythm and prevent future attacks.

stress and the brain The limbic system produces emotional arousal and the CORTEX monitors and modulates that arousal, but if more stressors accumulate, the balance in the brain may be disturbed. ANXIETY may represent tension between limbic and cortical impulses.

Social stress may intensify the damage from STROKE, SEIZURES, or the aging process in key brain structures, according to research.

striate cortex The primary VISUAL CORTEX.

striatum A term used for the combined entity of the CAUDATE NUCLEUS and the putamen; it is one of the four separate nuclei in the BASAL GANGLIA. The area of the striatum (Latin for "striped") receives information, including all forms of sensory information and data about the state of activity in the motor system, from almost all parts of the CERE-BRAL CORTEX. Its so-called stripes are made up of heavily myelinated AXONS of the connections from the motor and sensory cerebral cortices.

Recordings in the striatum show that the neurons' activity starts just before and during a particular movement.

stroke Also called a cerebral vascular accident, this causes interruption of blood supply to the brain or leakage of blood outside of vessel walls.

Any area in the brain damaged by the stroke will affect further brain function, including sensation, movement, and memory. Strokes are fatal in about one-third of cases, and are a leading cause of death in developed countries. In the United States, stroke will occur in about 200 out of every 100,000 people each year; incidence rises quickly with age, and is higher in men than women.

A stroke may be caused by any of three mechanisms: CEREBRAL THROMBOSIS (clot), cerebral embolism, or HEMORRHAGE. *Cerebral thrombosis* is a blockage by a clot that has built up on the wall of a brain artery, depriving the brain of blood; it is responsible for almost half of all strokes.

Cerebral embolism is a blockage by material that is swept into an artery in the brain from somewhere else in the body, depriving the brain of oxygen; it accounts for 30 to 35 percent of strokes.

Less common is *cerebral hemorrhage,* the most serious form of stroke, caused by the rupture of a blood vessel and bleeding within or over the surface of the brain. Hemorrhages account for about a quarter of all strokes. The hemorrhage is usually from a vessel at the base of the brain, where blood leaks into the brain substance itself, often resulting in COMA and paralysis. Death is almost inevitable if the hemorrhage is large.

Symptoms and Diagnostic Path

Ominously, a survey of 71,000 people conducted by the Centers for Disease Control (CDC) in 2005 found that 44 percent of the respondents could name the five warning signs of a stroke. According to the CDC these warning signs include

- sudden numbness or weakness of the face, arm or leg, especially on one side
- sudden confusion or difficulty speaking
- sudden trouble walking, dizziness or loss of balance
- sudden trouble with vision in one eye or both
- severe headache with no known cause

According to the National Stroke Association if you think someone may be having a stroke it is critical to act F.A.S.T. and perform this simple test

- **F**ace: Ask the person to smile. Does one side of the face droop?
- **A**rms: Ask the person to raise both arms. Does arm drift downward?
- **S**peech: Ask the person to repeat a simple sentence. Are the words slurred? Can he or she repeat the sentence correctly?
- **T**ime: If the person shows any of these symptoms, time is important. Call 911 or get the person to a hospital fast.

A stroke that affects the dominant of the two CEREBRAL HEMISPHERES in the brain (usually the left) may cause disturbance of language and speech. Symptoms that last for less than 24 hours followed by full recovery are known as TRANSIENT ISCHEMIC ATTACKS (TIAS); such an attack is a warning that a sufficient supply of blood is not reaching part of the brain. If circulation through smaller vessels is inadequate, brain tissue may die.

Blockage of the anterior cerebral artery on one side of the brain usually causes paralysis and sensory loss in the limb on the opposite side. If the artery of the dominant hemisphere (almost always left) is affected, mental confusion and speech impairment (APHASIA) may also occur.

A blockage of the main branch of the middle cerebral artery on one side produces paralysis and sensory loss on the opposite side, mainly affecting the face and arm. Aphasia also can occur when the area is in the dominant hemisphere. Blockage of smaller vessels of the middle cerebral artery produces one-sided blindness, inability to read (ALEXIA) or to recognize sensory stimuli (agnosia) or to perform skilled movements (apraxia) in combinations or as isolated symptoms.

Blockage of the main part of the posterior cerebral artery on one side causes damage to the THALAMUS and the VISUAL (OCCIPITAL) CORTEX, with occasional muscular weakness and sensory loss accompanied by burning pains, and ataxia.

Blocking the basilar artery on the underside of the brain is serious, often causing paralysis and sensory loss in all extremities and in the muscles supplied by the BRAIN STEM (cranial) nuclei. Blockage of the vertebral artery that runs toward the

SPINAL CORD is not usually fatal, although symptoms can be disabling.

A brain hemorrhage of any size is likely to be fatal, whereas the majority of patients with a clot are likely to recover from the initial damage. A number of patients do die in the first weeks after a stroke from complications, such as pneumonia, heart problems, or kidney malfunction.

Stroke survivors may find that their brain problems gradually improve over months following a stroke.

Treatment Options and Outlook

Unconscious or semiconscious hospital patients require a clear airway, tube feeding, and regular changing of position. Any fluid accumulation in the brain may be treated with corticosteroid drugs or diuretics. A stroke caused by an embolism is treated with anticlotting drugs to help prevent recurrences. Long-term administration of these drugs also has been recommended for those with intermittent symptoms of stroke. Sometimes, aspirin or vascular surgery (cleaning out the vessels in the neck for patients with arteriosclerotic narrowing) has been tried with moderate success.

General care in the first stages following a stroke, such as physiotherapy and speech therapy, are important to a patient's recovery. While about half of patients recover more or less completely from their first stroke, any intellectual impairment and memory loss is usually permanent.

Risk Factors and Preventive Measures

While most stroke victims are elderly, a third of all stroke victims are under age 65. Certain things can increase the risk of stroke: high blood pressure that weakens the walls of arteries or ATHEROSCLEROSIS (thickening of the lining of arterial walls). Stroke can also be caused by conditions that cause blood clots in the heart that may migrate to the brain: irregular heartbeat (atrial fibrillation), damaged heart valves, or heart attack. Conditions that increase the risk of high blood pressure or atherosclerosis can also cause stroke, such as hyperlipidemia (fatty substances in the blood) or polycythemia (high level of red blood cells in the blood). Diabetes mellitus is a risk factor; people with diabetes are five times as likely to have a stroke as nondiabetics. How-

ever, the National Institutes of Health notes that diabetics who monitor their GLUCOSE levels closely and inject insulin have fewer diabetes-related complications, including stroke. In addition, smokers have a higher risk; one study found that those who smoke more than 25 cigarettes a day have three times higher risk of stroke from a clot, and 10 times higher risk of stroke from a burst blood vessel. But those who quit smoking can cut the risk to that of a nonsmoker in just two years.

Oral contraceptives also increase the risk of stroke in women under 50; however, the older high-dose pills were far more dangerous than today's low-dose versions. Several studies have suggested an increased risk for low-dose pills, but others have found a significant risk only in women who smoke as well as take the pill. Women who smoke, use birth control pills, and have MIGRAINES appear to have an even greater chance of having a stroke.

Scientists do not yet understand why, but African Americans and Hispanics have a higher incidence of stroke; one reason could be that African Americans are more prone to high blood pressure.

Pregnancy is yet another risk factor; stroke is 13 times more common during the nine months of pregnancy because of changes in blood consistency. Pregnancy-related high blood pressure may predispose a woman to stroke.

Finally, a history of untreated TIAs is a risk factor of stroke; one third of those who have had a TIA will have a stroke within five years. Small doses of aspirin daily (as little as one-tenth of a tablet) may lessen that risk. The anticlotting drug Ticlid, approved by the U.S. Food and Drug Administration, is slightly more effective but has been associated with potentially serious side effects.

See also CEREBROVASCULAR ACCIDENT.

Sturge-Weber syndrome A rare congenital condition that affects the brain and the skin in which a malformation of blood vessels in the brain may cause weakness on the opposite side of the body, MENTAL RETARDATION, and EPILEPSY. There is usually a large port-wine birthmark covering one side of the face, usually involving an upper eyelid or forehead.

Symptoms and Diagnostic Path

In the brain, excessive blood vessel growth develops on the back region of the brain, on the same side as the port-wine stain. These growths, called angiomas, often lead to SEIZURES that usually begin by age one. The convulsions usually appear on the side of the body opposite the port-wine stain, and vary in severity. A weakening or loss of the use of one side of the body opposite the port-wine stain also may develop.

Developmental delay of movement and cognitive skills also may occur in varying degrees. In about 30 percent of patients, increased pressure within the eye (glaucoma) can occur at birth or develop later. Enlargement of the eye also can occur. The glaucoma and enlargement is usually restricted to the eye affected by the port-wine stain.

Treatment Options and Outlook

Lasers can lighten or remove port-wine stains in children as young as one month of age. Anticonvulsants are used to control the seizures, and surgery and/or eye drops are used to control the glaucoma.

subarachnoid hemorrhage A type of brain hemorrhage in which a blood vessel ruptures, spreading blood over the surface of the brain. This is a fairly unusual type of STROKE that usually affects a younger patient who is less likely to suffer from widespread CEREBROVASCULAR DISEASE.

About 8 percent of all stroke patients have this type of HEMORRHAGE, which is usually caused by the rupture of an intercranial aneurysm bleeding into the SUBARACHNOID SPACE around the brain. Common sites for these ruptures include the ANTERIOR COMMUNICATING ARTERY lying between the FRONTAL LOBES, the middle cerebral artery, and the posterior communicating artery.

Less commonly, the hemorrhage might be caused by a ruptured ANGIOMA (an abnormal proliferation of blood vessels within the brain).

This type of hemorrhage usually occurs spontaneously, and is not usually caused by any type of HEAD INJURY—but it may follow on the heels of unaccustomed physical exertion.

A patient who loses consciousness after such a stroke may regain consciousness, but recurrent strokes are common and may be fatal.

About five to 10 Americans per 100,000 suffer a subarachnoid hemorrhage each year. It is particularly common among patients between 35 and 60. Subarachnoid hemorrhages are slightly less common than an intracerebral hemorrhage (another form of stroke), characterized by bleeding within the brain itself.

Symptoms and Diagnostic Path

Immediate loss of consciousness or a sudden violent HEADACHE are usually the primary symptoms. Typically, the patient will experience symptoms similar to KORSAKOFF SYNDROME shortly after the hemorrhage—disorientation, confabulation, and memory problems. If the person remains awake, other symptoms may follow: photophobia (intolerance of bright light), nausea and vomiting, drowsiness, and neck stiffness.

The diagnosis is confirmed by CAT SCAN and large amounts of blood in the CEREBROSPINAL FLUID. An ANGIOGRAM may pinpoint the site of the burst blood vessel.

About one-third of patients recover; another one-sixth recover partially but have some disability (such as paralysis, mental problems, or epilepsy). Half of all patients die from the initial or subsequent strokes.

Treatment Options and Outlook

Treatment is generally aimed at preventing future strokes, such as control of high blood pressure. A burst ANEURYSM or angioma may be surgically removed or obliterated.

subarachnoid space An area of the brain located between the arachnoid and the PIA MATER. The space has a spongy appearance and is filled with CEREBROSPINAL FLUID. The subarachnoid space is wider in the SPINAL CORD than in the brain, especially in the lower part of the vertebral canal.

subdural hemorrhage A large blood clot (HEMATOMA) that forms within the skull when blood seeps into the space between the DURA MATER, the tough outer layer of the MENINGES (covering of the brain) and the middle meningeal layer. The most common cause of this seeping blood is a torn vein on the inside of the dura mater resulting from a HEAD INJURY. Subdural hemorrhages are most common among the elderly who have fallen.

Symptoms and Diagnostic Path

Because the bleeding is very slow, months may pass before symptoms appear as a result of rising pressure inside the skull from the weight of the blood pressing on the brain. Fluctuating symptoms include HEADACHE, confusion, and drowsiness and the development of weakness and paralysis on one side. Because these symptoms are similar to STROKE, any recent head injury (within the past several months) should be reported.

The presence of such a hemorrhage is diagnosed by ANGIOGRAPHY and CAT SCANS. Following surgical treatment, most patients recover fully.

Treatment Options and Outlook

Treatments include CRANIOTOMY (drilling burr holes in the skull), draining the blood, and repairing damaged blood vessels.

subliminal learning Learning that takes place below the level of consciousness, as contained in messages or information that is presented too quickly for normal awareness. The idea of subliminal learning is related to sleep learning, in which material to be learned is presented when the subject is asleep.

Subliminal advertising first reached public awareness during the 1950s, when some outdoor movie theaters reported huge concession sales following messages saying "eat popcorn" and "drink Coca-Cola" that flashed on the screen during a six-week period. Popcorn business reportedly increased 50 percent, and soda sales rose 18 percent.

There is some research support to the notion that in a laboratory, subjects can process limited sensory information without conscious awareness if they are playing close attention to the task, but studies could not duplicate the subliminal effect reported during the 1950s. Scientists have concluded that it is unlikely anyone could learn or remember information if the person is not aware that it is being presented.

substance abuse Many scientists believe that the key to understanding substance abuse lies in the brain, particularly since the discovery that the brain has many RECEPTORS for many drugs such as NICOTINE, marijuana, HEROIN, and other OPIATES and BENZODIAZEPINES (such as Valium). Because scientists have discovered that drugs have specific actions in certain brain regions, they may be able to discover how to disrupt the effects of these drugs.

The problem is complex, however, because addiction involves not just the physical presence of receptors but also the psychological reality of motivation and pleasure that can lead to addiction. Addiction to harmful substances is related to the involvement of brain systems that control normal pleasurable activities associated with eating, drinking and socialization.

Scientists still do not fully understand either the location, organization, or chemistry of the brain system underlying positive emotions and pleasure, although they have found some interesting clues. They discovered that animals preferred cocaine to food and would ignore food completely in the presence of cocaine; however, this behavior would be completely reversed if the neurotransmitter DOPAMINE is removed from one particular area of the brain (the nucleus accumbens).

substance P A neuropeptide involved with the transmission of pain signals.

substantia gelatinosa The part of the brain where nerves for pain, temperature, and touch make the first contact with the SPINAL CORD.

substantia nigra A black-pigmented band of matter (its name means "black substance") located in the BASAL GANGLIA of the MIDBRAIN that produces the NEUROTRANSMITTER DOPAMINE. The absence of dopamine produces rigidity and tremor.

In patients with PARKINSON'S DISEASE, the neurons in the substantia nigra that transmit dopamine die; the loss of these neurons is directly connected with the onset of symptoms. This loss of dopamine fibers is devastating to motor control, resulting in problems making voluntary movements and with uncontrollable tremors of the head, hands, and arms. However, patients can be successfully treated at first by boosting the stores of dopamine with the drug LEVODOPA. However, eventually, Levodopa stops working.

sulci The valleys on the surface folds of the CEREBRAL CORTEX that become wider in cases of brain atrophy.

sumatriptan (Imitrex) A MIGRAINE medication that appears to cancel pain from migraine and cluster HEADACHES. Although other migraine medications exist, sumatriptan was specifically created to take advantage of particular biochemical features of migraines. Sumatriptan was designed to block receptor binding of SEROTONIN, a NEUROTRANSMITTER whose role in headaches has long been suspected.

Migraine headaches are believed to be caused by dilated blood vessels in the head. Sumatriptan constricts these blood vessels, relieving migraine headache. However, while it is very effective in relieving migraine, it does not prevent or reduce the number of migraine attacks.

Side Effects
Possible side effects may include pain or tightness in the chest or throat, tingling, flushing, weakness, dizziness, abdominal discomfort, and sweating.

Patients with coronary artery disease and those with poorly controlled high blood pressure should avoid sumatriptan. It should be given with caution to patients at risk for coronary artery disease (those with high blood pressure, diabetes, elevated blood cholesterol, obesity, cigarette smoking, or strong family history of heart attacks).

superior colliculus Nuclei within the THALAMUS that is most critical in carrying out the function of vision. This structure got its name by the way it looked to early scientists; the "colliculi" are two "pairs of hills" on top of the midbrain (brain stem), of which the highest (or "superior") two deal with vision.

supplementary motor area Found in the FRONTAL LOBE of the brain, this structure receives input fibers from the BASAL GANGLIA and sends output back to the basal ganglia, the RETICULAR FORMATION, and the MOTOR CORTEX. The supplementary motor area is involved in planning and initiating movement. A malfunction in this area can interfere with voluntary movement and speech.

suprachiasmatic nucleus A pair of small cell clusters that receive and integrate visual information in the brain found in the HYPOTHALAMUS, which uses information about light intensity to coordinate internal rhythms. This brain structure gets its name from the Latin word for "above," because it lies just above the optic chiasm, where the nerve fibers from the eyes cross each other.

Each suprachiasmatic nucleus (there is one on either side of the hypothalamus) is made up of about 10,000 small, tightly packed cell bodies with sparsely branching DENDRITES. Researchers suspect that several different NEUROTRANSMITTERS might be released by NEURONS in these nuclei; however, SEROTONIN is the only neurotransmitter found there in high concentrations.

Sydenham chorea Once called St. Vitus' dance, this childhood movement disorder is characterized by rapid, irregular, aimless, involuntary movements of the muscles of the limbs, face, and trunk. The disorder, which is considered a manifestation of rheumatic fever, typically occurs between the ages of five and 15, more often among girls.

Experts suspect that the movements are caused by an autoimmune problem triggered by the streptococcal infection, which causes the body to make antibodies to specific brain regions.

Symptoms and Diagnostic Path
Symptoms may appear abruptly or gradually, and may include muscle weakness, decreased muscle

tone, and clumsiness. The symptoms vary from mild—involving restlessness, grimacing, and slight lack of coordination—to severe—involving incapacitating involuntary movements. The disorder may strike up to six months after the fever or infection has gone away.

Treatment Options and Outlook

There is no specific treatment for Sydenham chorea, which may include bed rest, sedatives, and the drug diazepam to control movements. Penicillin may treat the fever or infection.

Complete recovery often occurs; the average case lasts three to six weeks, although occasionally it may be longer.

sylvian fissure (fissure of Sylvius)   A major crevice in the cerebrum separating the temporal and PARIETAL LOBES.

Sylvius, Franciscus (1614–1672)   A Dutch professor also known as Franz de la Boe, for whom the fissures of Sylvius are named. (These fissures are deep grooves in each side of the CEREBRAL CORTEX.)

Dr. Sylvius was a very important figure in the 17th century's scientific revolution. He was born in Hanau, Germany, on March 15, 1614, after his family had fled the southern Low Countries during the war against Spain. He studied medicine at several northern European schools, earning a degree at the University of Basel (Switzerland) in 1637 and then settled at the age of 24 at Leiden University (Holland), where he held a position as an unsalaried lecturer. With no prospect of a professorship, however, he moved to Amsterdam and opened a private practice. By the time he began his practice, he had already discovered (1641) the deep cleft separating the brain's temporal, frontal, and parietal lobes, known today as the Sylvian fissure (or the aqueduct of Sylvius).

In 1658, he was offered twice the usual salary to return to Leiden University as its professor of practical medicine. Sylvius accepted, and some nine years later, he was appointed vice chancellor of the university.

That summer a plague struck Leiden, killing nearly half of the university faculty and forcing the university to close temporarily. Despite becoming gravely ill himself, Sylvius attempted to study the disease. He later recovered, and began to concentrate on writing his *New Idea in Medicine*. He had completed only the first volume before his death on November 15, 1672, at the age of 58. It was left to Sylvius's many loyal students to spread his new ideas throughout Europe.

Leiden University's medical laboratory is now named after Sylvius, as is a computer program for studying the brain.

sympathetic nervous system   A division of the AUTONOMIC NERVOUS SYSTEM that controls such activities as hormone secretion and heartbeat. It consists of two chains of nerves passing from the SPINAL CORD throughout the body. Into these organs and other structures, the nerve endings release EPINEPHRINE and NOREPINEPHRINE. During the FIGHT-OR-FLIGHT RESPONSE, the sympathetic nervous system increases the heartbeat, dilates the airways and the blood vessels in muscles, and constricts those in the skin and abdominal organs. This increases blood flow to the muscles and decreases the activity of the digestive system.

See also PARASYMPATHETIC NERVOUS SYSTEM.

synapse   The point at which a nerve impulse passes from the AXON of one NEURON (NERVE CELL) to a DENDRITE of another. To send a signal, one neuron transmits an electrical signal to another by firing across the synapse gap between adjacent dendrites, which triggers the release of chemical messengers (NEUROTRANSMITTERS) that diffuse across the spaces between cells, attaching themselves to RECEPTORS on the neighboring nerve cell. The receiving dendrite has receptors that recognize the chemical transmitter and speed the signal through the neuron.

The human brain contains about 10 billion neurons joined together by about 60 trillion synapses. For a long time, scientists have believed that change in the brain's synapses is the critical event in information storage. But researchers do not agree about how synaptic change actually represents information. One of the most popular ideas is that the specificity of stored information is determined by the location of synaptic changes in the NERVOUS SYSTEM and by the pattern of altered neuronal interaction that these changes produce.

synaptic change and memory The theory that memory occurs as a result of functional changes in the brain's SYNAPSES caused by the effects of external stimuli prompted by training or education. Nerve cells (NEURONS) connect with other cells at junctions called synapses; they transmit electrical signals to each other by firing across this junction, which triggers the release of neurotransmitters (special signaling substances) that diffuse across the spaces between cells, attaching themselves to receptors on the neighboring nerve cell. The human brain contains about 10 billion of these nerve cells, joined together by about 60 trillion synapses.

Researchers generally have agreed that anything that influences behavior leaves a trace (ENGRAM) somewhere in the nervous system. As long as these memory traces last, theoretically they can be restimulated, and the event or experience that established them will be remembered.

See also NEUROTRANSMITTERS AND MEMORY.

syphilis A sexually transmitted or congenital disease which can have devastating effects on the brain. Syphilis of the brain (neurosyphilis) also can cause paralysis in addition to DEMENTIA.

Syphilis is caused by a type of bacterium called *Treponema pallidum*. Usually transmitted by sexual contact, the organism enters the body via minor cuts or abrasions in the skin or mucous membranes. It also could be transmitted by infected blood or from a mother to her unborn child during pregnancy.

Neurosyphilis usually occurs 10 to 20 years after the initial infection, when it is considered to be the end stage of the disease. Rarely seen today, it is occasionally diagnosed in elderly demented patients who were never properly treated for syphilis in their youth.

Symptoms and Diagnostic Path

Symptoms include subtle changes in personality, lack of attention, poor judgment, aggression, bizarre behavior, mood swings, and problems in concentration; some patients experience delusions of grandeur, but about 50 percent have a simple dementia.

Treatment Options and Outlook

Syphilis is not nearly as deadly as it once was, due to the introduction of penicillin; however, treatment at the late stage takes longer. More than half of those treated suffer a severe reaction six to 12 hours later, because the body reacts to the sudden annihilation of large numbers of syphilitic spirochetes (a type of bacteria). Brain damage already caused by the disease, however, cannot be reversed.

Risk Factors and Preventive Measures

Infection can be avoided by maintaining monogamous relationships; condoms offer some measure of protection but are not absolutely foolproof. People infected with syphilis are infectious during the primary and secondary stages, but not the end stage.

tacrine (Cognex) The first drug approved by the U.S. Food and Drug Administration (FDA) to treat some of the symptoms of mild to moderate ALZHEIMER'S DISEASE. However, the effects of this drug are only slight, and there are unfortunate side effects.

It works by preventing the breakdown of ACETYLCHOLINE, a brain chemical important to memory. Acetylcholine deficiency is thought to result in memory loss associated with Alzheimer's disease. The drug has been shown to increase cognition in about a third of patients with mild to moderately demented Alzheimer's disease; unfortunately, the drug does not stop the degeneration of brain tissue, and so it cannot cure the disease.

The FDA approved tacrine largely because a 30-week study showed that high doses improve cognition in people with mild to moderate Alzheimer's. Since its approval, clinical experience has been disappointing. Depending on the study, tacrine helps only 20 to 40 percent of those who take it. Doctors cannot predict who will respond to tacrine, to what extent, and for how long. Tacrine may help somewhat, but only for a minority of people with Alzheimer's.

Side Effects

Side effects are related to the fact that tacrine boosts an enzyme that can lead to liver damage; the long-term effects of this rise remain unclear. About half of patients give up on the drug because of the side effects. Of those who continue, less than half of patients with mild to moderate stages of Alzheimer's notice a slight improvement. Patients taking very high dosages of the drug (more than 160 mg per day) show the most improvement, but they also have the highest risk for liver damage; discontinuing the drug reverses any liver problems.

Other frequent side effects include nausea, vomiting, diarrhea, abdominal pain, indigestion, and skin rash.

Although tacrine can harm liver function during treatment, the risk of permanent damage from long-term treatment is not known. Patients should have their blood tested every other week for at least 16 weeks when first taking tacrine to make sure it is not affecting the liver. If any abnormality in liver function occurs, doctors must adjust the dosage accordingly or discontinue administration of this drug.

tardive dyskinesia A type of movement disorder caused by long-term use of neuroleptic medication. Scientists believe that the disorder appears more often in those who have had acute reactions to neuroleptic drugs (such as chlorpromazine) and who have an underlying affective disorder. Neuroleptic drugs are usually prescribed for psychiatric disorders.

Symptoms and Diagnostic Path

Symptoms may include facial and limb movements, writhing or involuntary movements, and posture disorder with spasm in the muscles of the shoulder, neck, and trunk. The involuntary movements are often restricted to the head and neck, such as chewing or tongue-thrusting. Symptoms may fluctuate, taking months or years to disappear after drug withdrawal. About half of the cases are reversible within five years, but some cases may never improve. The movements do not typically worsen once a plateau has been achieved.

Stopping and starting neuroleptic drugs is not effective and may even be associated with increased risk. Symptoms may remain long after the neuroleptic drugs have been stopped. With careful treatment, some symptoms may improve or even disappear.

Treatment Options and Outlook

Treatment is difficult. Drugs that may help include tetrabenazine and reserpine. Other drugs that have been tried with varying success include baclofen, valproic acid, DIAZEPAM, alpha antagonists, amantadine, clonidine, and carbidopa-L-dopa.

taste   The sense of taste is far less acute than the sense of smell, partly because a person's taste CHEMORECEPTORS are far less sensitive than the olfactory receptors in the nose. A person would need 25,000 times more of a chemical compound to taste it than to smell it.

While a person's ability to taste is fairly crude (differentiating only sweet, sour, salty, and bitter), the sense of smell can enable a person to distinguish the most flavors. In fact, the sense of smell is so important to the sense of taste that losing the ability to smell (such as during a cold) will interfere with a person's ability to taste anything.

The mechanism of taste depends on the translation of a chemical signal into an electrochemical one, and it begins in the taste buds on the tongue, palate, throat, and tonsils. Adults have about 9,000 of these taste buds, each containing groups of taste-sensitive cells with taste-sensitive hairs. (Taste buds for sweetness lie at the tip of the tongue; sour is found on the left and right front sides; salt behind sour and bitter along the back of the tongue).

Substances must first dissolve in water or saliva to allow the molecules to bind to the surface of a taste bud; chemicals in food or drinks dissolve in saliva, flowing into the pores found in the protuberances of the tongue; around these pores are taste buds. The molecules produce an electrochemical change within the taste-bud receptor cell and stimulate hairs projecting from the taste-bud cells, triggering signals sent from the cells along nerves to taste centers in the brain via part of the seventh nerve (GLOSSOPHARYNGEAL NERVE) to centers in the lower BRAIN STEM, on to the thalamus, and then to the CEREBRAL CORTEX. Because olfactory nerves cross over in the MEDULLA, tastes from each side of the tongue are registered in the opposite BRAIN HEMISPHERE.

tau protein   The major protein that makes up neurofibrillary tangles found in degenerating brain cells, especially in ALZHEIMER'S DISEASE. Tau is normally involved in maintaining the internal structure of the nerve cell, but in Alzheimer's disease the tau proteins begin to twist and tangle.

In the late 1980s scientists discovered that in healthy brain cells, the internal structure (called a microtubule) is formed like a parallel set of train tracks with crosspieces holding them together, which carry nutrients from the body of the cell to the ends of the axons. The crosspieces between the parallel microtubules are made of tau protein.

In cells of patients with Alzheimer's, this parallel structure collapses as the tau protein crosspieces twist into paired helical filaments. If tau does not function properly, the microtubules collapse and tangle together, and can no longer shuttle substances throughout the cell.

Scientists know that the development of Alzheimer's involves two normally harmless proteins in the brain, tau and BETA-AMYLOID. Alzheimer's disease develops when something triggers beta-amyloid to fold and twist into a different shape. As it changes, beta-amyloid begins forming abnormal strands that accumulate on brain cells. It also appears to induce tau protein to become a killer as well. Together, the two destroy the brain cells, forming the plaques and tangles that have been the hallmarks of the disease since it was first described in 1907 by ALOIS ALZHEIMER.

Scientists disagree about whether it's the sticky plaques of beta-amyloid in the brain or the tangles of tau protein inside brain nerve fibers that play a more central role in the destruction of brain cells. While tangles of tau have been found in the brains of people with Alzheimer's, many scientists believed that tangles were probably a secondary part of the disease. Instead, most Alzheimer's researchers have focused attention on amyloid as the substance that kills brain cells. Other think the plaques and tangles are really a marker left by nerve cells killed by some other cause.

What is known is that increases of beta-amyloid in brain tissue are associated with increasing severity of mental decline, with the highest levels of beta-amyloid found in the brains of patients with the most dementia.

Tay-Sachs disease An inherited fatal brain disorder, most commonly found among Ashkenazi Jews, in which harmful quantities of a fatty substance build up in the nerve cells in the brain. It is found in one of every 2,500 Ashkenazi Jews, which is about 100 times higher than in any other ethnic group.

The disease is caused by a deficiency of the enzyme hexosaminidase, a protein essential for regulating chemical reactions in the body. This deficiency is what causes the buildup of the fatty substance known as gangliosides. Gangliosides are made and biodegraded rapidly in early life as the brain develops.

Symptoms and Diagnostic Path

Infants with Tay-Sachs disease appear to develop normally for the first few months of life. Then, as nerve cells become distended with fatty material, a relentless deterioration of mental and physical abilities occurs. The child becomes blind, deaf, demented, and unable to swallow. Muscles begin to atrophy and paralysis sets in. An extreme startle response to sound is one of the earliest symptoms. The disease progresses rapidly, and is usually fatal by age three.

A much rarer form of the disorder that occurs in patients in their twenties and early thirties is characterized by unsteadiness of gait and progressive neurological deterioration.

The disease is diagnosed with a physical exam and family history, and confirmed with an enzyme analysis of tissue samples.

Treatment Options and Outlook

There is no treatment for this disease. Prenatal screening may reveal an affected fetus.

Risk Factors and Preventive Measures

Carriers, or those with an affected relative, should receive genetic counseling before planning a pregnancy. The gene for Tay-Sachs is recessive; for example, an Ashkenazi Jew has a one in 25 chance of carrying the gene; if two carriers marry, there is a one in four chance that they will have an affected child.

tectum, midbrain Midbrain "roof," a term referring to the inferior and superior colliculi.

tegmentum The region of the MIDBRAIN below and in front of the cerebral aqueduct that contains the nuclei of several CRANIAL NERVES, the RETICULAR FORMATION, and the pathways that link the FOREBRAIN and the SPINAL CORD.

telencephalon Also known as the endbrain, this is one of two subdivisions of the FOREBRAIN; telencephalic structures account for about 75 percent of the weight of the entire human CENTRAL NERVOUS SYSTEM. These structures include the two CEREBRAL HEMISPHERES that (while separated by a large fissure) are connected by a mass of crossing fiber tracts (corpus callosum).

temperature regulation The control of the body's temperature is of critical importance to proper function of the brain. It is believed to be controlled by the HYPOTHALAMUS, which acts like a type of thermostat that constantly monitors internal temperature, automatically activating mechanisms to compensate for changes.

The need to raise or lower internal temperature is monitored by the body's heat receptors. When the body's temperature falls, blood vessels in the skin constrict, shunting blood away from the skin to deeper vessels to prevent excessive cooling. The hypothalamus also sends nerve impulses to stimulate shivering, which generates heat by making muscles work harder.

Conversely, when the body overheats, the hypothalamus triggers sweating, increases and dilates blood vessels in the skin, boosting blood flow in order to radiate heat away from the body. This is why the skin of an overheated individual appears to be quite red.

A whole variety of factors can disrupt the body's heat-regulating system, causing heat stroke, fever, or hypothermia. These factors could include thyroid disorders, infection, and overexposure to cold or extreme heat.

The average normal body temperature measured in the mouth is 98.6°F. However, normal body temperature by no means remains constant at this level; body temperature varies among individuals and also in the same person depending on exercise, sleep, eating, and drinking. Moreover, temperature fluctuates according to the time of day (lowest at about 3 A.M. and highest about 6 P.M.). It also depends on the stage of the menstrual cycle (lowest during menstruation and highest at ovulation). In most people, temperature varies between 97.8°F and 99°F.

Where the temperature is taken also can have an effect; temperature measurement is highest when taken rectally (rising by about 0.5°F. to 0.7°F.) and is lower when taken in the armpit by about 0.3°F.

temporal artery   A branch of the external CAROTID ARTERY that supplies blood primarily to the temple and the scalp.

temporal cortex   See TEMPORAL LOBE.

temporal lobe   The part of the brain that forms much of the lower side of each half of the CEREBRUM (the main mass of the brain). The temporal lobes are concerned with smell, taste, hearing, visual associations, some aspects of memory, and a person's sense of self. Any interference in the normal function of the temporal lobes may cause peculiarities in any of these functions. A HEAD INJURY may cause direct and diffuse effects in the temporal lobe; there is some evidence that the tips and undersurface of the temporal lobe are particularly vulnerable to trauma.

A great deal of research has centered on the temporal lobe. Some scientists have spent time probing the lobes and recording the resulting effects in patients; others have studied the results of removing part or all of the temporal lobe.

During the 1950s, Canadian surgeon WILDER PENFIELD was the first to stimulate this part of the brain during surgery. He found that while stimulating various areas of the CORTEX produces a range of responses from patients, only stimulation of the temporal lobes elicits meaningful, integrated experiences (including sound, movement, and color) that are far more detailed, accurate, and specific than normal recall. Interestingly, some of the memories that popped up during Penfield's stimulation were unremembered in the normal state, while stimulation of the same spot in the temporal lobe would elicit the exact same memory again and again.

Research also suggests that removing the left temporal lobe (TEMPORAL LOBECTOMY) causes verbal memory deficits, while removal of the right lobe impairs nonverbal memory (such as memory for mazes, patterns, or faces).

Recent studies of gender differences in the brain have found that in cognitively normal men, a tiny region of the temporal lobe behind the eye has about 10 percent fewer NEURONS than it does in women. The neurons in this region are responsible for understanding language as well as melodies and speech tones.

See also LEUCOTOMY.

temporal lobectomy   The surgical removal of both TEMPORAL LOBES is associated with severe AMNESIA, when the HIPPOCAMPUS is also removed. Amnesia does not develop following lesions involving the uncus or AMYGDALA as long as the hippocampus is not removed.

Removing one of the temporal lobes results in a material-specific memory deficit; that is, removing the left temporal lobe causes a verbal memory deficit, while those with right temporal lobectomies have more problems in remembering nonverbal material such as faces, patterns, and mazes. Left temporal lobectomies result in more problems in learning and retaining verbal material (such as paired associates, prose passages, or Hebb's recurring-digit sequences). In addition, stimulation of the left temporal lobe leads to a number of naming errors and impaired recall.

Different areas within the left temporal lobe cause two different kinds of memory problems.

Stimulating the anterior region causes an ANTERO-GRADE AMNESIA; stimulating the posterior section causes a RETROGRADE AMNESIA.

Patients who have undergone removal of the right temporal lobe can usually perform verbal tasks but have problems with learning visual or tactile mazes or in figuring out whether or not they have seen a particular geometric shape before. They also have problems recognizing tonal patterns or faces. But those with right temporal lobectomies are impaired in maze learning only if there was extensive hippocampal lesions. The same is true for recognition of photographs.

In fact, researchers have found that the more extensive the section of hippocampus removed, the greater the memory deficit. Among those whose left temporal lobe was removed, those with extensive hippocampus involvement had more problems with short-term verbal memory than those with no or little involvement.

temporal-lobe epilepsy   See EPILEPSY.

tension headaches   See HEADACHES.

tetrahydroaminoacridine (THA)   See TACRINE.

thalamus   The crucial brain structure that first receives messages from the body about heat and cold, pain and pressure, smell and taste. Named for the Greek word for "chamber" or "inner room," the thalamus is important in the factual memory circuit and serves as the entrance chamber to the perceptual CORTEX.

All sensory organs (except for smell) enter the cortex via the thalamus. It is the part of the brain that automatically responds to extremes in temperature and pain. It is critical to states of awareness and all sensori-motor function.

A bit smaller than the CEREBELLUM, the thalamus is found deep inside the HEMISPHERES of the CEREBRUM, above the HYPOTHALAMUS.

One of the main parts of the DIENCEPHALON, the thalamus is active during memory and is involved in many cases of memory disorder—particularly

in WERNICKE-KORSAKOFF SYNDROME. One of the best-known cases of thalamic damage and memory problems is a patient known as N.A., a man who was stabbed in the thalamic region at age 22 and who suffered significant memory problems. Other cases of memory problems involving the thalamus have been reported, primarily with tumors, which can lead to a rapidly developing DEMENTIA.

The thalamus also seems to regulate cycles of sleep and wakefulness and seems to direct the way a person sometimes feels well or poorly.

theta waves   A type of brain wave commonly seen in children under five and usually in adults suffering from extreme mental illness.

thirst   The urge to drink. Control of the body's fluid intake is one of the most crucial functions of the brain because the proper function of each and every cell depends on a proper fluid environment. Thirst is one way to control the amount of water in the body; the other way is by the volume of urine that is produced by the kidneys. Sufficient fluids are even more important in maintaining life than food.

The HYPOTHALAMUS controls fluid intake, partly by monitoring the amount of dissolved substances in the blood to assess how dilute the blood is and the total blood volume. The concentration of sugar, salt, or other substances in the blood rises when fluid intake drops; as this particle concentration rises, the concentrated blood passes through the hypothalamus in the brain. Here, special nerve RECEPTORS are stimulated, inducing the sensation of thirst.

When the body needs to boost its fluid intake (such as after a large loss of blood or during dehydration in hot weather), thirst increases; at the same time, the PITUITARY GLAND releases antidiuretic hormone (ADH) to retain water and decrease the urine volume.

Thirst is depressed when there is too much water in the blood; when this happens, urination increases and the need to drink disappears.

thought   Mental activity involving problem solving, reasoning, and the formation of judgments.

The hallmarks of thought are the substitution of symbols (words, numbers, or images) for objects, the formation of these symbols into ideas, and the arrangement of ideas in a certain order in the mind. Certain aspects of thought can be tested; these include speech and efficiency, idea content, and logical relationships between ideas.

In recent research, neuroscientists have recorded a visual representation of the chemical and electrical activity that characterize thinking in the brain cells. Using a technique called optical imaging, cameras recorded tiny differences in reflected light flashing across the surface of the brain as thinking occurred. Scientists do not know what causes the changes, which are too subtle to be seen by the naked eye. The procedure was used to help surgeons figure out which part of the brain to preserve during surgery to treat EPILEPSY. Before this technique was tried, information had to be obtained by scattering tiny electrodes across the brain's surface and mapping the trajectories of electrical impulses.

thought disorders Conditions that feature abnormalities in the structure or content of thought as evidenced by a person's speech, writing, or behavior. SCHIZOPHRENIA is one of the most common mental illnesses that is characterized by thought disorders. Patients can lose a logical connection to associations, jumping from one unrelated subject to another, or making indirect associations or "clang associations" (words that sound the same but do not connect logically).

Other thought disorders found in schizophrenia include neologisms (inventing new words), thought blocking (interrupted train of thought), auditory HALLUCINATIONS, and having the feeling that thoughts are being introduced or removed from the mind by an outside entity.

All types of confusion (such as DEMENTIA and DELIRIUM) feature an inability to think clearly; flight of ideas (rapidly switching from one idea to another) is characteristic of mania as a result of loosening of associations.

Recurrent ideas that seem to keep returning to a person's mind are characteristic of obsessive-compulsive disorder, while slowed thinking is a hallmark of clinical DEPRESSION.

Finally, delusions (false beliefs) are a form of distorted thinking and are found in schizophrenia and other psychotic illnesses.

thyroid stimulating hormone (TSH) Also known as thyrotropin, this is a hormone that is synthesized and secreted by the anterior PITUITARY GLAND under the control of thyrotropin-releasing hormone and that stimulates activity of the thyroid gland. Defects in the production of this hormone may lead to an over- or underproduction of thyroid hormones. TSH is also given in an injection to test thyroid-gland function.

TIA See TRANSIENT ISCHEMIC ATTACK.

tic douloureux See TRIGEMINAL NEURALGIA.

Todd's paralysis A neurological condition characterized by a brief period of temporary paralysis after a seizure. The cause of Todd's paralysis is not known, but an episode indicates that a SEIZURE has occurred. It is important to distinguish the condition from a STROKE, which requires treatment.

Symptoms and Diagnostic Path
The paralysis may be partial or complete, but usually occurs on one side of the body and usually fades away completely within two days. Todd's paralysis also may affect speech or vision.

Treatment Options and Outlook
No treatment is necessary, since the paralysis disappears quickly.

tomogram A photograph of a section of skull and brain made by a computer from CAT or PET SCANS.

tomography The process of scanning through a single section of tissue and bone using X-rays or ultrasound. By producing a series of slices at different depths, a three-dimensional image of the body structure can be given.

topectomy A more conservative type of psycho-surgery that destroys parts of the frontal CORTEX itself instead of the white fibers below it, as in LEUCOTOMY. The operation was designed to avoid the problems of HEMORRHAGE, memory loss, and vegetative states that often occurred after other more radical LOBOTOMY.

The procedure was developed by research scientist J. Lawrence Pool at Columbia University in 1947 and was performed on patients at the New Jersey State Hospital in Greystone Park, New Jersey.

TORCH disorders Also known as *TORCH syndrome*, a collection of infectious agents that cause defects in the developing fetus. The acronym TORCH stands for Toxoplasmosis, Other (HIV, AIDS), Rubella, Cytomegalovirus, and Herpes Simplex.

Symptoms and Diagnostic Path

TORCH disorders can cause similar symptoms, including fever, difficulties feeding, subcutaneous bleeding (causing purple spots on the skin), enlargement of the liver and spleen, and yellowing of the skin. The enlargement of the liver and spleen will frequently appear from the physician's feeling the abdominal area and then confirmed by ultrasound. Additional diagnostic procedures, including blood chemistry, urine and stool samples, and sometimes tissue samples attempt to uncover the underlying condition. Additional diagnostic procedures may include blood incompatibility tests and blood pathology tests.

Treatment Options and Outlook

Prevention and treatment of fetal infections with TORCH disorders as a result of increased public health services greatly decreased the incidence of birth defects in the United States but continues to present a challenge in nonindustrialized countries. Advances in providing clean water supplies and sanitation through the Peace Corps and other humanitarian efforts are making significant impact on the occurrence of TORCH disorders in the Third World. In many cases, there will be no treatment for some TORCH disorders, and the infected mother must take care to avoid additional complications such as secondary infections. Appropriate levels of rest, hydration with clean drinking water, adequate nutrition, and sanitary surroundings can minimize the risk of developing additional complications.

Risk Factors and Preventive Measures

The potential of TORCH disorders for causing birth defects, such as congenital deafness, transient cold- and flulike symptoms, skin lesions, and damage to the organs of the developing fetus, has prompted physicians and public health services to educate expecting mothers in general hygiene and the importance of obtaining regular medical care. Pediatricians, especially those working in nonindustrialized countries, are reminded to monitor newborns for signs of congenital infections. Some of the more valuable preventive measures include avoidance of cat feces, drinking water from tested sources, use of condoms, regular hand washing, washing soiled clothing with bleach, and decontamination of food preparation surfaces with antibacterial agents or bleach.

Recently, the ready availability of hand sanitizers and antibacterial and bleach-containing cleaning cloths that people can carry with them make it easier to avoid bacterial and viral infections away from soap and water. Teaching children effective sickness hygiene, such as covering their mouths when coughing, avoiding others' discarded tissues, and not eating or drinking after others can minimize the likelihood pregnant mothers will come into contact with infectious agents.

See also TOXOPLASMOSIS, AIDS, and CYTOMEGALO-VIRUS.

Tourette syndrome A neurological disorder characterized by tics, or rapid, sudden movements that occur involuntarily and repeatedly in a consistent fashion. To be diagnosed with Tourette syndrome, an individual must have multiple motor tics as well as one or more vocal tics over a period of more than one year. These need not all occur simultaneously, but in general the tics may occur many times a day, usually in brief, intense groupings, nearly every day or intermittently.

Many patients with Tourette syndrome also have other conditions, such as ATTENTION DEFICIT HYPERACTIVITY DISORDER (ADHD), obsessive-compulsive disorder, or LEARNING DISABILITY.

Up to 20 percent of children have at least a transient tic disorder at some point. Once believed to be rare, Tourette syndrome is now known to be a more common disorder that represents the most complex and severe manifestation of the spectrum of tic disorders.

Symptoms and Diagnostic Path

Common simple tics include eye blinking, shoulder jerking, picking movements, grunting, sniffing, and barking. Complex tics include facial grimacing, arm flapping, coprolalia (use of obscene words), repeating words (either one's own or another's words or phrases). The type, location, frequency, and severity of tics may vary over time. In some cases, symptoms may disappear for a period of weeks or even months. Although there is an involuntary quality to the tics, most people have some control over their symptoms at least briefly, and even for hours at a time. However, suppressing tics tends simply to postpone more severe outbursts, since the impulse to express tics is ultimately irresistible. Tics often will increase in response to stress and become less frequent with relaxation or intense focus on a task. Symptoms include obsessions, compulsions, impulsive behavior, and mood swings. Tourette is commonly associated with other syndromes, including ADHD, anxiety, mood or panic disorders, obsessive-compulsive disorder, behavior problems, and learning disabilities. Anxiety, stress, and fatigue often intensify tics, which usually diminish during sleep or when the patient is focused on an activity. Psychoactive drugs, particularly cocaine and stimulants, have a tendency to worsen tics.

In most patients, tics peak in severity between ages nine and 11, but between 5 percent and 10 percent of patients continue to have unchanged or worsening symptoms in adolescence and adulthood. In this population, the likelihood of tics continuing for decades is substantial. Patients in their seventh, eighth, and ninth decades of life may have tics that have been present since childhood. In most older patients, the tics tend to become quite stable over time, although occasionally new tics

will be acquired. There is no reliable way to predict which children will have a poorer prognosis.

An accurate diagnosis is the single most important component in managing the condition. Tics occur suddenly during normal activity, unlike other movement disorders. A complete physical examination, with specific attention to the neurologic exam, is important. The thyroid-stimulating hormone (TSH) level should be measured in most patients, since tics often occur together with hyperthyroidism. A throat culture should be checked for group A beta-hemolytic streptococcus, especially if symptoms get worse or better with ear or throat infections. However, the evidence of strep infection with a single occurrence of worsening tics is not enough to make a diagnosis of streptococcus-induced, autoimmune-caused Tourette syndrome.

An electroencephalogram is useful only in patients in whom it is difficult to differentiate tics from EPILEPSY.

Treatment Options and Outlook

Positive reinforcement programs appear to be most helpful in managing tic disorders. The most common drugs used to manage tics are haloperidol (Haldol), pimozide (Orap), risperidone (Risperdal), and clonidine (Catapres). Guanfacine (Tenex) is not labeled for use in children under 12 years of age. Less often, clonazepam (Klonopin) may be prescribed. For tics of mild to moderate severity, or in patients who are wary of drug side effects, an initial trial of clonidine or guanfacine may be tried. These medications are modestly effective in tic control and have a range of less specific benefits.

Most patients with Tourette syndrome require medication for up to one to two years. About 15 percent of patients require long-term medication for tic control. When tics appear to be stable and adequately controlled for a period of four to six months, a slow and gradual reduction in medication should follow. With such a strategy, occasional "drug holidays" may be possible in some patients as tics lessen. If tics increase, incremental increases in medication may be needed.

Sedation, weight gain, poor school performance, social anxiety, and unusual body movements, including TARDIVE DYSKINESIA, a potentially irreversible drug-caused movement disorder that may be difficult to distinguish from tics may result from medications. When pimozide is used, baseline and follow-up electrocardiograms are recommended.

Risk Factors and Preventive Measures
An abnormal metabolism of the neurotransmitters dopamine and serotonin are linked to the disorder, which is genetically transmitted. Parents have a 50 percent chance of passing the gene on to their children. Girls with the gene have a 70 percent chance of displaying symptoms; boys with the gene have a 99 percent chance of displaying symptoms.

toxic encephalopathy A type of ENCEPHALOPATHY (a degenerative disease of the brain) caused by long-term exposure to any of a variety of toxic substances. Symptoms include personality changes, memory problems, and fuzzy thinking, listlessness, convulsions, COMA, and respiratory arrest. Recovery from this condition may take weeks, and some people may never recover.

toxic mood disorders Personality and mood changes caused by exposure to NEUROTOXINS that damage the brain. There are a wide variety of substances that may cause mood or personality changes, but the most common sources are lead and mercury, some solvents and gases, and pesticides. The solvent carbon disulfide, used primarily in industrial uses, can cause a severe manic DEPRESSION.

While regulations today require ventilation in the rayon and cellophane industries, which use this product, even regulated levels may cause toxic mood disorders and symptoms of DEPRESSION, irritability, and insomnia.

Symptoms and Diagnostic Path
The symptoms of a toxic mood disorder may be subtle or wrongly associated with depression; other symptoms may be obvious or subtle. They may include personality changes such as irritability, social withdrawal, and the inability to cope with even minor problems. Mental changes may include short-term MEMORY LOSS, concentration problems, mental slowness, and difficulty in following instruc-

tions. NEUROTOXINS also may interfere with the hormones regulating sleep, causing some people to sleep too much and others to experience insomnia. Chronic fatigue caused by neurotoxic exposure also will have neuropsychiatric impairment that may show up only with specialized tests. Symptoms may also include problems in walking, muscle weakness, or diminished manual dexterity.

To identify whether a particular set of symptoms are toxic in nature, the patient should have a careful history and physical, including a neuropsychological evaluation and standardized testing by a certified neuropsychologist, various lab tests, and specific toxicological assessments.

Treatment Options and Outlook
Once exposure has been eliminated, symptoms can fade away within days, but the symptoms may reappear and worsen if exposure continues.

See also TOXIC ENCEPHALOPATHY.

toxoplasmosis This is one of the TORCH DISORDERS that can cause birth defects. It comes from a one-celled parasite *Toxoplasma gondii.* People contract toxoplasmosis through swallowing cat feces when, for example, they touch their hands to their mouths after cleaning a cat's litter box or working in a garden where an infected cat has defecated. Eating uncooked and undercooked meat, especially pork, eating food prepared with utensils contaminated by uncooked meat, drinking water contaminated by *Toxoplasma gondii,* and receiving blood transfusions from an infected donor can also cause contraction of the parasite.

Symptoms and Diagnostic Path
Most healthy people do not experience symptoms because healthy immune systems suppress illness from it, although some individuals experience flu-like symptoms with swollen glands or body ache for a month or more.

Severe ocular infestations can cause reduced and blurred vision, light sensitivity, eye redness, and tearing. Ophthalmologists may, in acute cases, prescribe medication for symptomatic relief. Although most infants infected at birth do not show symptoms, some develop symptoms later in life or suffer serious eye or brain damage.

Physicians diagnose toxoplasmosis with blood tests.

Treatment Options and Outlook

Most healthy people do not require treatment for toxoplasmosis. However, physicians will sometimes prescribe pyrimethamine (Daraprim), an antimalarial medication, for acute infections. For particularly recalcitrant toxoplasmosis infections, they may prescribe sulfadiazine in combination with pyrimethamine. Physicians may treat pregnant women with previous toxoplasmosis infestations with medications to prevent reactivation of symptoms.

According to the Centers for Disease Control and Prevention, more than 60 percent of individuals in the United States will contract this parasite.

Risk Factors and Preventive Measures

Severe infections can cause damage to the brain, eyes, and other organs. Occasionally, an individual who contracted toxoplasmosis early in life will find it reactivated due to a compromised immune system much later. Infants born to mothers who experience toxoplasmosis infestations shortly before giving birth and individuals with compromised immune systems are especially susceptible to development of severe reactions.

The best prevention is washing hands thoroughly after handling cat litter—or wearing rubber gloves when handling it—avoiding drinking water from sources not known to be clean (such as from streams in the wild), and avoiding cross-contamination from utensils and work surfaces used to prepare uncooked meats.

tranquilizers Tranquilizers are divided into major tranquilizers (antipsychotics) and minor tranquilizers (antianxiety drugs).

Antipsychotic drugs work by blocking the action of DOPAMINE, a NEUROTRANSMITTER acting on the brain. LITHIUM is an antipsychotic drug that is thought to reduce the release of NOREPINEPHRINE, another neurotransmitter. They are used to treat psychoses, particularly SCHIZOPHRENIA and manic DEPRESSION. They are also used to calm or sedate those with other mental disorders, such as DEMENTIA, who have become agitated.

Antipsychotics include the phenothiazines (chlorpromazine, fluphenazine, perphenazine, thioridazine, trifluoperazine) and others, such as haloperidol and lithium.

Antianxiety drugs include benzodiazepines and beta-blockers. Benzodiazepines work by reducing nerve activity in the brain; beta-blockers reduce the physical symptoms of ANXIETY, such as shaking and palpitations. They are used to relieve symptoms of anxiety when it threatens a person's ability to cope in everyday life. They are also sometimes used to calm a person before surgery.

transient global amnesia An abrupt loss of memory lasting from a few seconds to a few hours without loss of consciousness or other impairment.

During the period of amnesia, the subject cannot store new experiences and suffers a permanent memory gap. At the same time, the subject may also lose memory of many years prior to the amnesia attack; this retrograde memory loss gradually disappears, although a permanent gap in memory that usually extends backward no more than an hour before onset of the amnesia attack results.

Attacks of transient global amnesia may occur more than once and are believed to be caused by a temporary reduction in blood supply in areas of the brain concerned with memory, sometimes heralding a stroke, although several toxic substances have been associated with transient global amnesia.

Victims are usually healthy and over age 50; an attack may be precipitated by many things, including sudden changes in temperature, physical stress, eating a large meal and even sexual intercourse. This type of amnesia is not common, and it disappears within a day or two. It was first described in 1964.

See also RETROGRADE AMNESIA.

transient ischemic attack (TIA) A temporary impairment of the brain caused by an insufficient supply of blood, which can result in brief memory or speech problems, weakness, paralysis, dizziness, or nausea. Episodes usually last for a few minutes, but they may occur for up to a few hours. An attack that lasts for more than 24 hours is considered to be a STROKE.

Unlike a stroke, which may have the same symptoms but involve a lasting deficit, TIA symptoms fade without permanent damage. However, they should be regarded as a possible forerunner of stroke and should be reported to a physician. Stroke does occur in from one-fourth to one-third of all patients with TIAs.

TIAs may be caused by a temporary block to an artery supplying the brain (EMBOLISM) or by a narrowed artery thick with fat deposits (ATHEROSCLEROSIS).

Symptoms and Diagnostic Path

A wide variety of symptoms may occur, depending on the site of the block and how long the blood flow is impaired. Symptoms may include weakness or numbness in legs or arms, disturbed speech (APHASIA), dizziness, or partial blindness. A TIA is always followed by complete recovery.

Symptoms of TIA may be confused with a BRAIN TUMOR or SUBDURAL HEMATOMA (blood-filled swelling); diagnosis may include BRAIN SCANS and blood tests; ULTRASOUND, ANGIOGRAPHY, or heart studies may be needed to pinpoint the problem.

Because there is no way to tell whether symptoms are from a TIA or a stroke, patients should assume that all strokelike symptoms are an emergency and should not wait to see if they go away. A prompt evaluation within an hour can identify the cause of the TIA.

Treatment Options and Outlook

Depending on the diagnosis, the doctor may recommend drug therapy or surgery to reduce the risk of stroke in people who have had a TIA. The use of antiplatelet drugs such as aspirin is a standard treatment for patients at risk for stroke. People with atrial fibrillation (irregular beating of the heart) may be prescribed anticoagulants.

transient memory disorders A group of temporary memory disorders in which a person's memory stops functioning normally for a certain period of time. Causes include vascular disorders, closed HEAD INJURY, medications, or aftereffects of electroconvulsive therapy (ECT). Psychogenic disorders also may be of a transient nature. (See also ELECTROCONVULSIVE THERAPY AND MEMORY.)

Transient Global Amnesia A form of sudden-onset ANTEROGRADE AMNESIA, coupled with RETROGRADE AMNESIA for recent events, disorientation in time, and no loss of personal identity. Attacks may last from minutes to days and can be set off by many things, including temperature change, toxins, physical stress, or even sexual intercourse. The underlying dysfunction is believed to be a temporary drop in blood supply to the memory centers of the brain.

Posttraumatic Amnesia Most victims of closed head injury suffer only a temporary memory loss from between a few seconds to several months. It is believed that the injury interferes somehow with the transfer of information from short- to long-term memory.

ECT and Memory Loss Many patients who undergo ECT report a temporary anterograde or retrograde amnesia that gradually fades away.

traumatic brain injury The common general term for brain injuries that impair thinking as a result of physical trauma severe enough to cause loss of consciousness or damage to the brain structure. Each year, about 2 million Americans sustain a brain injury—about one every 15 seconds. More than a million brain injuries are sustained by children, 30,000 of whom will have permanent disabilities.

Males, especially those between the ages of 14 and 24, are twice as likely to be injured as females, followed by infants and then the elderly. Children are more likely to incur traumatic brain injury during the spring and summer. Traffic accidents account for almost half of the injuries; about 34 percent occur at home and the rest in recreation areas.

Traumatic brain injury includes both open and closed head injury. In an open head injury, the force of impact can cause scalp injuries and skull fractures, together with blood clots and bruising. This type of injury usually affects one place in the brain, producing specific problems. A closed head injury can cause more widespread damage, as the force of impact causes the brain to smash against the opposite side of the skull, tearing nerve fibers and blood vessels. This type of injury may affect the brain stem, causing physical, intellectual, emotional, and social problems. The entire personality of the person may be forever changed.

In young children, abuse is the primary cause of this type of injury; 64 percent of babies under age one who are physically abused have brain injuries, usually by shaking. In children under age five, half are related to falls. Car and biking accidents and suicide attempts are the primary causes of traumatic brain injury in school-age children and adolescents.

Symptoms and Diagnostic Path

The symptoms after a traumatic brain injury may be elusive, but it is important to understand that head injuries tend to get worse over time. Obvious warning signs include

- lethargy
- confusion
- irritability
- severe headaches
- changes in speech, vision, or movement
- bleeding
- vomiting
- seizure
- coma

More subtle signs of head injury may also appear, including

- long- and short-term memory problems
- slowed thinking
- distorted perception
- concentration problems
- attention deficits

- communication problems (oral or written)
- poor planning and sequencing
- poor judgment
- changes in mood or personality

Sometimes, certain behaviors may appear long after the traumatic brain injury occurs. These behaviors may include overeating or drinking, excessive talking, restlessness, disorientation, or seizure disorders.

Some patients may experience COMA after a brain injury; the degree of the coma severity is measured by the Glasgow Coma Score, which assigns a number to the degree to which patients can open their eyes, move, or speak. X-rays and brain scans may help if a skull fracture is suspected.

Treatment Options and Outlook

Rehabilitation should begin as soon as possible after the accident, focusing on the problem areas, including physical or occupational therapy, or speech and language therapy. (See also BRAIN DAMAGE.)

tremor An involuntary, rhythmical alternating movement that may affect the muscles of any part of the body, although the hands, feet, jaw, tongue, and head are most often affected. Tremors are caused by the rapid alternating contraction and relaxation of muscles and are a common symptom of neurologic disease. Occasional tremors may be felt by almost everyone (usually during fear or excitement), triggered by the increased production of the stress hormone EPINEPHRINE.

Some tremors are unrelated to disease; these include the slight, persistent tremor common among the elderly. Another common tremor not associated with disease is essential tremor, a mild movement that runs in families and may sometimes be relieved by small doses of alcohol or by taking beta-blockers. Both of these types of tremor increase with movement of the affected part of the body.

More persistent tremors are caused by trauma, tumors, STROKE, or degenerative disease. Coarse tremors (four to five movements per second) that occur during rest, diminishing during movement, are a common sign of PARKINSON'S DISEASE. Intention tremors (tremors that worsen on movement) are a sign of CEREBELLUM disease. Tremors often accompany such diseases as MULTIPLE SCLEROSIS, Wilson's disease, mercury poisoning, thyrotoxicosis, and liver encephalopathy.

In addition, tremors may appear as a side effect of certain drugs (such as AMPHETAMINES, ANTIPSYCHOTICS, ANTIDEPRESSANTS, CAFFEINE, or LITHIUM) or as a sign of withdrawal. Alcohol withdrawal also may trigger tremors, indicating the presence of alcohol dependence. These "morning shakes" occur as the blood alcohol level falls; the tremors disappear when more alcohol is consumed.

trephining The ancient practice of boring and scraping of the skull to release "evil spirits" conducted by prehistoric physicians, a treatment that usually relieved intracranial pressure caused by TUMORS, HEMORRHAGES, and skull fractures. CRANIOTOMY is an extension of trephining in which a flap of skull is entirely removed, exposing the MENINGES (brain covering) that covers the CEREBRAL CORTEX.

tricyclic antidepressants A class of antidepressant drugs named for their three-ring chemical structure that have been used to treat DEPRESSION since the 1950s. Tricyclics include amitriptyline, amoxapine, clomipramine, despiramine, doxepin, imipramine, nortriptyline, and protriptyline. They are sometimes used for other disorders in addition to depression, including obsessive compulsive disorder, panic disorder, and (in the case of imipramine) bedwetting.

The tricyclic antidepressants work by raising the brain's level of the NEUROTRANSMITTERS NOREPINEPHRINE and SEROTONIN—chemicals that are abnormally low in depressed patients. The problem with cyclics is that they do not stop there. They go on to interfere with a range of other neurotransmitter systems and a variety of brain cell receptors, slowing down nerve cell communication all over the brain. The more neurotransmitter systems and receptors that are affected, the more side effects a

patient will have. Still, for some people the cyclics work better than any other drug.

Side Effects

The FDA has proposed black box warnings on the labels for antidepressants for use with individuals ages 18 to 24 due to increased probability of suicide ideation (thoughts), gestures, and attempts. See DEPRESSION for a list of antidepressants with known increased suicidality with this age group.

Among other brain systems, the tricyclics act on histamine receptors, activating the body's FIGHT-OR-FLIGHT RESPONSE, speeding up the heart and shunting blood away from bodily functions, such as waste removal. The result is dry mouth, blurred vision, constipation, and urinary problems. These side effects may be especially annoying with amitriptyline, clomipramine, doxepin, imipramine, or protriptyline. Amoxapine (Asendin) or desipramine have the lowest risk for these side effects. Other side effects include weight gain, nausea, HEADACHES, inability to sweat, increased heart rate, drowsiness, sun sensitivity, decreased blood pressure, sexual function problems, or dizziness when standing up.

Like all antidepressants, tricyclics may be associated with a mild manic high or suicide attempts in some people. In one study of 231 nonsuicidal patients, about 3.5 percent taking the antidepressant drug Prozac became suicidal after beginning treatment, but about 6.5 percent taking both Prozac and a tricyclic became suicidal. In a retrospective study published in the *British Medical Journal* of 3,065 patients with major depression, tricyclics worsened suicidal thinking slightly more than Prozac did (16.3 percent versus 15.3 percent). Actual suicidal acts were reported as 0.3 percent for Prozac and 0.4 percent for tricyclics.

In addition, tricyclics may affect a diabetic patient's blood sugar levels or may cause dry eyes; this dryness may adversely affect contact lenses, coating them with deposits of thick secretions and making them feel gritty, itchy, or painful.

Patients who use clomipramine for too long run the risk of developing a group of symptoms called neuroleptic malignant syndrome, including fever, fast or irregular heartbeat, sweating, weakness, muscle stiffness, SEIZURES, or loss of bladder control.

Amoxapine causes tardive dyskinesia, speech or swallowing problems, lip smacking or puckering, loss of balance, cheek puffing, rapid or wormlike tongue movements, shakiness or trembling, shuffling walk, slow movements, arm or leg stiffness, uncontrolled chewing movements, and uncontrolled movements of hands, arms, or legs).

Some side effects may appear after treatment stops: headache, irritability, lip smacking or puckering, nausea or vomiting, diarrhea, abdominal pain, convulsions, puffing of cheeks or rapid wormlike tongue movements, restlessness, insomnia, vivid dreams, uncontrolled chewing movements, uncontrolled leg or arm movements, or unusual excitement. There may be rebound mild mania or mania in manic-depressive people not taking LITHIUM at the same time.

trigeminal nerve This nerve is responsible for facial sensation and jaw movements and is also known as the fifth cranial nerve. It arises from the PONS (part of the BRAIN STEM) and then branches into three parts, which then subdivide even further into a web of smaller nerves. These nerves supply sensations to the face, scalp, nose, teeth, mouth lining, upper eyelid, sinus, and front part of the tongue. They also control the amount of saliva and tears, and are also involved in chewing.

Damage or disease in one area supplied by the trigeminal nerve may cause pain in a different area (such as tooth pain caused by inflamed sinuses).

See also CRANIAL NERVES; TRIGEMINAL NEURALGIA.

trigeminal neuralgia A disorder of the fifth cranial nerve (TRIGEMINAL NERVE) that causes brief episodes of stabbing pain involving the cheek, lips, chin, or gums on one side. It usually begins in one particular "trigger" point and is often brought on by touching the face, talking, chewing, or swallowing. Its nickname, *tic douloureux* ("painful twitch"), refers to the fact that the intense pain often causes wincing.

Symptoms and Diagnostic Path
Trigeminal neuralgia most often occurs in women over age 50, but it also may be found in younger people with MULTIPLE SCLEROSIS. Attacks recur in clusters of brief episodes that may last for weeks; the recurrences tend to occur closer and closer together with time.

Treatment Options and Outlook
Anticonvulsants such as carbamazepine may suppress the pain in most people, but others develop a resistance to the drug.

Baclofen, clonazepam, gabapentin, and valproic acid may also be effective and may be used in combination to achieve pain relief. If medication fails to relieve pain, surgical treatment may be recommended.

The disorder often waxes and wanes; successive recurrences may be incapacitating. Due to the intensity of the pain, even the fear of an impending attack may interfere with activities of daily life. However, trigeminal neuralgia is not fatal.

trochlear nerve Also known as the fourth cranial nerve, this nerve (together with the third and sixth cranial nerves) is responsible for eye movements. It arises from the MIDBRAIN (part of the BRAIN STEM) and passes through the skull, entering the eye socket via a gap in the skull. It supplies only one muscle of each eye; by contracting this superior oblique muscle, the eye rotates outward. If this nerve is damaged, it may cause double vision.

See also CRANIAL NERVES.

truth drugs A group of drugs including sodium pentothal that are useful in psychiatry to help patients recall experiences and emotions they have tried to suppress. The drugs act on the brain, lowering the inhibitory processes.

tryptophan An AMINO ACID converted by the brain into the NEUROTRANSMITTER SEROTONIN, linked to mood and sleepiness. Scientists have found that depressed patients often have low blood levels of tryptophan; lowering the levels of this amino acid appears to worsen mood in healthy people. Some research appears to suggest that administering tryptophan may help ease DEPRESSION and boost the effectiveness of certain antidepressants.

However, tryptophan is no "happy pill"—giving it to people with normal mood does not make them even happier, most likely because their serotonin levels are not abnormal.

Several years ago the U.S. Food and Drug Administration banned the sale of tryptophan after 38 people died of a muscle-nerve disease associated with tryptophan pills; this disease was eventually traced to one batch of contaminated pills. Whether tryptophan is harmful at all has not been determined, although some scientists suspect that large doses of any amino acid may lead to eventual metabolic disturbances.

tuberous sclerosis A rare congenital inherited disorder characterized by MENTAL RETARDATION, seizures, and skin lesions. Severe cases may be fatal by age 30.

Symptoms and Diagnostic Path

Symptoms include EPILEPSY and mental retardation, although INTELLIGENCE may be normal in mild cases. This multisystem disease affects the brain, kidneys, heart, eyes, lungs, and other organs. Small tumors may grow in the brain.

Treatment Options and Outlook

There is no cure; treatment is aimed at relieving symptoms, such as treating epilepsy and removing tumors, and medication for neurobehavioral problems.

Risk Factors and Preventive Measures

The gene for tuberous sclerosis can now be detected at an early stage of pregnancy. Genetic counseling is recommended for affected families who are considering having children.

tyrosine An AMINO ACID that plays a role in controlling blood pressure and is associated with alertness.

Scientists have found that tyrosine supplements may improve alertness during stress, lessening fatigue and boosting mental agility. Other studies found that giving tyrosine pills improved cognitive performance in the presence of loud, irritating noise.

However, some scientists caution that taking large doses of any amino acid may eventually disrupt the body's metabolic balance.

ultradian rhythms Rhythms that appear more than once per day (*ultra* for "beyond," or more than once a day). For example, the cycle of stages that occurs within the normal six-to-eight-hour period that humans sleep is one example of an ultradian rhythm. Several hormones (luteinizing hormone and follicle-stimulating hormone) are secreting into the bloodstream in an ultradian rhythm.

Some human ultradian rhythms occur without conscious knowledge—occurring about every hour and a half during wakefulness and sleep. Verbal and spatial matching tasks also show that human alertness and cognitive performance also seem to run in 90-minute cycles. The night-time portion of this ultradian rhythm (sleep) has been studied for many years. During sleep, the brain passes through several different states of activity in cycles of about 90 minutes.

See also SLEEP AND THE BRAIN.

ultrasound scan Also known as neurosonography, this diagnostic technique utilizes a computer image produced by analysis of echoes of high frequency sound generated by a device placed on the skin's surface, deflected from interfaces between structures of different density.

This technique is particularly useful in evaluating prenatal, neonatal, and infant-brain problems. Because the baby's skull before birth is poorly mineralized and not completely fused, sound waves can penetrate into the brain. Once the fontanelles close, the cranial bones disperse sound waves and make ultrasounds useless.

unconsciousness Loss of awareness of the self and of the surroundings caused by a drop in the activity of the RETICULAR FORMATION of the BRAIN STEM.

Symptoms and Diagnostic Path

Unconsciousness may either be brief (such as in FAINTING) or more profound (such as in a COMA). A CONCUSSION is a brief state of unconsciousness after a HEAD INJURY.

Sleep is a normal form of altered consciousness.

Treatment Options and Outlook

To treat an unconscious breathing person, the airways should be open and the mouth free from debris. If the person is not breathing but the heart is beating, artificial respiration should be started. Tight clothing should be loosened. An unconscious person should not be left alone.

V

vagus nerve   Also known as the 10th cranial nerve, this nerve is the longest of all cranial nerves and is responsible for breathing, swallowing, taste, circulation, and digestion. It is a primary component of the parasympathetic nervous system, emerging from the MEDULLA OBLONGATA (part of the BRAIN STEM), through the neck and chest to the abdomen, with branches to most of the major organs of the body.

It affects other organs by releasing ACETYLCHOLINE, which is responsible for a wide range of bodily processes (narrows the bronchi, slows heart rate, boosts stomach acid and pancreatic juice production, stimulates gall bladder, and increases peristalsis). It is also involved in coughing, swallowing, sneezing, and speech.

If this nerve becomes too active, it can influence the development of a peptic ulcer by speeding up the production of stomach acid. It can also be damaged by infection, STROKE, or TUMORS. This type of damage could result in problems ranging from the gag reflex, swallowing, or hoarseness.

See also CRANIAL NERVES.

Valium (diazepam)   A BENZODIAZEPINE, antianxiety drug.

See DIAZEPAM.

Varolio, Constanzo (1543–1575)   The Italian surgeon and anatomist, who in 1573 illustrated the PONS, part of the BRAIN STEM overlooked earlier by the Belgian anatomist Andreas Vesalius, who had produced the first anatomy book of the brain.

See also BRAIN IN HISTORY.

vasopressin   Another name for ADH (antidiuretic hormone), this chemical functions as a NEUROTRANS-MITTER in the brain—and it also may be part of the ink with which memories are written.

Vasopressin is released from the PITUITARY GLAND and acts on the kidneys to increase the reabsorption of water into the blood. It reduces the amount of water lost in the urine and helps control the body's overall water balance. Water is continually being taken into the body in food and beverages and is also produced by the chemical reactions in cells. At the same time, water is always being lost in urine, sweat, feces, and breath; vasopressin helps maintain the optimum amount of water in the body.

Its production is controlled by the HYPOTHALAMUS (located in the center of the brain), which detects changes in the concentration and volume of the blood. If the blood concentration loses water, the hypothalamus stimulates the pituitary gland to release more vasopressin, and vice versa.

External vasopressin is approved for treatment of diabetes as a way of preventing the frequent urination common in this disease. It is given via the nose or by injection, since high IV doses cause narrowing of blood vessels. Vasopressin has also been used to treat memory deficits of aging, senile DEMENTIA, ALZHEIMER'S DISEASE, KORSAKOFF SYNDROME, and AMNESIA.

Research has shown that when subjects are given vasopressin, they remember long lists of words better and seem to chunk and encode better. (Chunking, or grouping words together, is a trick that memory experts teach to improve memory.) Vasopressin is also being studied as a possible memory enhancement drug.

Because cocaine, LSD, AMPHETAMINES, RITALIN, and Cylert (pemoline) cause the pituitary to step up the release of natural vasopressin, abuse of these drugs can result in a depleted pool of vasopressin and resulting mental slowness. On the other hand, alcohol and marijuana suppress the release of vasopressin.

Side Effects

Vasopressin is available by doctor's prescription in the United States. It is available in a nasal spray and produces noticeable effects within seconds because it is absorbed by the nasal mucosa. However, it can produce a range of side effects from congestion to HEADACHE and increased bowel movements, abdominal cramps, nausea, drowsiness, and confusion. It has not been proved safe during pregnancy. Because it temporarily constricts small blood vessels, it should not be used by anyone with hypertension, angina, or ATHEROSCLEROSIS and should be used cautiously in the presence of EPILEPSY.

ventricles Four fluid-filled cavities of the brain. The lateral ventricles (paired first and second ventricles) are found one in each cerebral HEMISPHERE and communicate with the third ventricle in the center of the brain. The fourth ventricle is found between the BRAIN STEM and the CEREBELLUM. CEREBROSPINAL FLUID circulates within all the ventricles linked by special ducts and around the brain's outer rim before being reabsorbed by the blood. This fluid effectively reduces the weight of the brain, buffering the brain against trauma. The cerebrospinal fluid is secreted by tufted clusters of blood vessels called the choroid plexus that line the ventricles. As a person ages, the ventricles enlarge.

ventriculitis An inflammation of the VENTRICLES of the brain that is usually caused by an INFECTION. It may be caused by the rupture of a cerebral abscess into the cavity of the ventricle or from the spread of a severe form of MENINGITIS from the SUBARACHNOID SPACE.

ventriculoatriostomy A surgical procedure to relieve excess pressure due to the build-up of CEREBROSPINAL FLUID caused by HYDROCEPHALUS. The fluid is drained via a system of catheters into the jugular vein in the neck.

ventriculography An outdated type of procedure that illuminates the ventricular cavities within the brain to be seen on X-RAY film after air or a contrast medium has been introduced. This technique has largely been replaced by CAT SCANNING and MRI.

ventriculoscopy Examination of the VENTRICLES of the brain using a fiberoptic instrument.

ventriculostomy A surgical procedure to introduce a hollow needle into one of the lateral VENTRICLES of the brain to relieve high intracranial pressure, to obtain CEREBROSPINAL FLUID from a ventricle for testing, or to deliver antibiotics or contrast medium for X-RAY examination.

verbal memory Memory for verbal information. Verbal memory is assumed to reflect functioning of the deep structures of the left temporal lobe.

vertebrobasilar insufficiency Periods of dizziness, weakness, double vision, and speech problems that come and go because of the reduced flow of blood to the BRAIN STEM and CEREBELLUM. Usually, such a drop in blood flow is caused by fat deposits that narrow arteries around the base of the brain.

vertigo A sensation of spinning (of either a person or the person's surroundings) that is a common complaint only rarely caused by disease. It is usually caused by a disturbance of the semicircular canals in the inner ear or the nerve tracts branching from the canals. Healthy people can experience vertigo on amusement park rides, while sailing, or even while watching a movie.

On the other hand, *severe* vertigo (usually occurring with other symptoms) is usually caused by disease, such as inflammation of the semicircular canals (labyrinthitis) or Ménière's disease. Less commonly, it may be caused by a BRAIN TUMOR (on the BRAIN STEM) or by MULTIPLE SCLEROSIS. It may also be caused by psychological problems.

Antihistamines may help prevent recurring attacks.

vestibular nerve   Part of the VESTIBULOCOCHLEAR NERVE, this nerve carries sensory impulses from the semicircular canals in the inner ear to the CEREBELLUM. Combined with information from the eyes and joints, this nerve controls balance.

vestibular system   The system found in the inner ear that helps maintain balance and judge a person's position in space, even with the eyes shut. The three looped semicircular ducts of the system communicate with the saclike saccule and utricle. Hair cells on each structure are linked to nerve fibers; when a person moves the head, fluid flows through the ducts and sacs, moving hair cells that trigger signals from nerve fibers to the brain via the eighth cranial nerve (VESTIBULOCOCHLEAR NERVE).

Since different movements of the head can activate different sets of fibers, the semicircular ducts can register nodding, turning, or tilting of the head. The saccule and utricle relay to the brain the position of the head in relation to gravity. This is how a person is able to stand or walk in the dark.

vestibulocochlear nerve   Another name for the eighth cranial nerve, this nerve controls balance and hearing and carries sensory impulses from the inner ear to the brain. The nerve enters the brain between the PONS and the MEDULLA OBLONGATA (parts of the BRAIN STEM).

The vestibulocochlear nerve really has two parts, the VESTIBULAR NERVE and the ACOUSTIC NERVE (also called the cochlear or auditory nerve). Disorders of this nerve include tumor (ACOUSTIC NEUROMA) or INFECTION (such as MENINGITIS or ENCEPHALITIS).

See also CRANIAL NERVES.

vestibulo-ocular reflex   This visual reflex located in the BRAIN STEM permits continued fixation of the eyes on an object while the head is in motion. With this sophisticated reflex, the neurons of the retina, the oculomotor system, and the vestibular system combine. It can best be understood by a simple test: A person who stares at an index finger while turning the head rapidly from side to side can easily retain focus on the finger; it is far more difficult to focus on the finger when the head is still and the finger is moved rapidly back and forth.

vincamine   An extract of periwinkle, this drug is a vasodilator (widens blood vessels) and increases blood flow and oxygen use in the brain. It has been used to treat memory defects.

In some studies, vincamine has been shown to improve memory in ALZHEIMER'S DISEASE patients and has normalized the brainwave patterns in elderly people with memory problems or with alcohol-induced ORGANIC BRAIN SYNDROME.

It has also been used to treat a variety of problems related to poor blood flow to the brain, including Ménière's disease, VERTIGO, sleep problems, mood changes, DEPRESSION, hearing problems, high blood pressure, and so on. However, there has been very little research on the drug and its cognitive enhancement in normal subjects.

See also VINPOCETINE.

vinpocetine   This derivative of VINCAMINE, a periwinkle extract, has fewer adverse effects and more benefits in memory enhancement. Marketed in Europe as Cavinton, the drug improves brain metabolism by improving blood flow and enhancing the use of GLUCOSE and oxygen.

It is often used to treat memory problems and other cerebral circulation disorders, such as STROKE, APHASIA, APRAXIA and HEADACHE.

In one Hungarian study involving 882 patients with a range of neurological disorders, significant improvements, including memorization of word lists, were noted in 62 percent of the patients.

In addition, at least one double-blind study of normal subjects indicated that the drug seemed to show significant short-term memory improvement within one hour after taking the drug.

vision   The visual system is an extremely complex unit in both organization and function. While vision occurs almost effortlessly for most people, it is far from a simple process.

The ability to see involves two main structures: the eye and the brain. When light reaches the eye, it passes into the retina, a thin web of nerve cells at the back of the eye. These cells respond to a wide range of information (such as color) in addition to filtering incoming information and sending it on to the optic nerves. At the back of the eyes, these optic nerves cross at the optic chiasma. This means that the left optic tract carries information about objects in the right-hand field of vision, and vice versa.

Visual information is transmitted to a pair of nuclei on each side of the brain (the lateral geniculate nuclei) in an ordered pattern so that each half of the other visual field is precisely mapped onto the lateral geniculate on the opposite side of the brain. Scientists understand this map so well that in cases of STROKE or TUMOR, for example, they can pinpoint the exact location of BRAIN DAMAGE based on the type of visual deficit a person has. The lateral geniculate nuclei relay visual information to the primary VISUAL CORTEX, where it is again mapped in an extremely orderly fashion. From the visual cortex, the information is then transmitted to many other cortical areas involved in the higher aspects of visual processing, which is necessary in order to carry out activities associated with vision such as reading, writing, or recognizing objects. There are many regions of the cortex known to be involved in visual processing, each serving a specific function and linked by many separate pathways. This division of labor could explain some of the more unusual aspects of some brain problems, such as why a stroke patient can recognize some types of objects (like a book or chair) but not recognize a spouse's face. Because these different objects have different features, damage to one area of the cortex may affect the perception of one type of feature but not others.

The brain must conduct extensive processing of visual information, allowing for pattern recognition and interpretation. These processes are based on work by the NEURONS, which are contained within an intricate pathway involving billions of individual NERVE CELLS. Scientists have discovered that many neurons are only involved with specific features of objects, such as orientation, color, directional movement, or complex shapes. The retina also sends visual information to nuclei involved in controlling eye muscles responsible for turning the eyes to track objects and to coordinate movement of both eyes.

Proper functioning of the visual system depends on how well the neurons communicate in a coordinated fashion, using electrical and chemical signals generated by NEUROTRANSMITTERS, messengers, and other molecules.

The basic mechanism for vision is built into the brain at birth. Experiments with newborns reveal that they are already trying to find and fixate on objects around them. While babies cannot see as well as adults, the basic reflexes important to vision are in place at birth, although the retinas are not well developed and the nerves from the eyes through the brain have not yet been covered with MYELIN. By two weeks of age, some babies' eye-brain development has progressed to the point where they can recognize patterns. Scientists reach this conclusion because babies who have reached this point spend more time looking at a pattern resembling a face than at patterns with random elements.

At birth, babies' eyes do not move as a unit and they find it difficult to look at an object. As the brain begins to improve its ability to control eye muscles, the ability to gaze at an object improves. By six weeks of age, infants can move their eyes to follow a ball through a 90-degree arc, and both eyes can focus on an object. Depth of field likewise develops during an infant's first months of life; experts estimate a six-month-old baby has visual acuity at about 20/120 (that is, objects can be clearly seen at 20 feet that a person with normal vision could see at 120 feet). By one year of age, an infant's vision (if developing normally) is 20/20.

Infant animal experiments have revealed that there appears to be a sensitive time for visual development. A two-month-old kitten deprived of visual stimuli for just four days may be permanently blind because the brain cells that register signals from the eyes stop working. Infants, too, reach a critical stage when use of their eyes is essential for the development of the ability to see.

visual-evoked responses (VERs)   Changes in brain functioning following presentation of visual stimuli. For example, neurologists may measure changes in brain activity following flashing lights, using EEG readings or brain-imaging data such as a PET SCAN. VERs are useful in diagnosing neurological disorders including MULTIPLE SCLEROSIS. Increasingly, improved imaging abilities are replacing the use of VERs in diagnosing disorders.

visual fields   The total area a person can see while looking straight ahead. Normally, the visual fields extend to about 90 degrees on either side of the middle of the face, but the field is narrower above and below (especially among people with deep-set eyes). Because the visual fields overlap in the middle ("binocular vision"), a defect in the field of one eye may not be apparent if both eyes are open.

While the total visual field is wide, visual acuity (sharpness) is not the same in all parts of the field. Objects on the periphery of the point at which a person focuses are far less sharp.

Similarly, partial loss of visual field is less noticeable than loss of central vision; even those who have had extensive damage to their visual field (such as from glaucoma or STROKE) may not be aware of it if their central visual acuity remains sharp.

visual memory   The ability to take in, store, and retrieve information presented visually. Short-term visual memory is the ability to hold visual information in short-term memory in order to process it, either moving it into long-term memory or shifting focus.

Visual working memory (or nonverbal working memory) involves the ability to hold visual information in mind while considering it, reflecting on it, or in some other fashion processing it.

Long-term memory also involves visual forms, in which images are stored on a long-term basis and are available for recall.

visual occipital cortex   The area at the back of each cerebral HEMISPHERE, this is the part of the brain where humans "see"—that is, where a person registers electrochemical impulses that arrive from the eyes. In the primary visual cortex,

different columns of BRAIN CELLS register signals from different parts of the retina. From here, the signals are passed on to nearby visual areas for more refinement. In each visual area in the visual cortex, special cells react only to signals produced by special visual stimuli, such as movements in certain directions. Working together, these visual areas of the brain help understand size, shape, and position of objects that a person sees. (See also VISION.)

visual perception   The ability to recognize and interpret visual information provided to the brain. Difficulties in visual perception are unrelated to impairment in the visual system that may diminish visual acuity or result in visual impairment or blindness. Visual perception involves the determination and discrimination of spatial information, as well as performance on such tasks as the discrimination of letters and words, geometric designs, and pictures.

vitamins   Lack of sufficient vitamins can have an impact on brain function.

- **Vitamin A**—Vision problems such as night blindness and decreased sense of taste.
- **Vitamin B$_1$ (thiamine)**—Beriberi, loss of motor coordination, paralysis, pain in arms and legs, headache, loss of myelin sheath, attacks on motor and sensory axons of the brain cell
- **Vitamin B$_2$ (riboflavin)**—Sensitivity to light, burning sensations around mouth, peripheral nerve damage
- **Vitamin B$_3$ (niacin)**—Pellagra, mental problems of disorientation, confusion, depression, memory loss, mania, paranoia
- **Vitamin B$_5$ (pantothenic acid)**—Burning sensations on hands and feet, headaches
- **Vitamin B$_6$ (pyridoxine)**—Abnormal touch sensations, mania, convulsions
- **Vitamin B$_9$ (folic acid)**—Peripheral nerve problems, memory disorders, convulsions, neural tube defects such as spina bifida and anencephaly

- **Vitamin B$_{12}$ (cobalamin)**—Memory problems, pain, abnormal touch sensations, movement problems, weakness, degeneration of white matter in cerebral hemispheres, optic nerves, and spinal cord
- **Vitamin E (tocopherol)**—Affects peripheral nerves and the nerve supply to muscle; walking and balance problems, eye movement problems

All communication in the brain depends on the function of NEUROTRANSMITTERS—chemicals that relay signals through the brain. To manufacture these important neurotransmitters, the brain needs adequate supplies of at least three B vitamins: FOLIC ACID, B$_6$ and B$_{12}$.

While the link between vitamins and cognition and memory is controversial, some studies have shown that better nutrition can lead to improved learning, IQ, and behavior, and several studies suggest that getting too little of these vitamins—especially folic acid and B$_{12}$—may interfere with mental or emotional well-being. Studies suggest that some people who are depressed or who show evidence of senile DEMENTIA may in fact have deficiencies of folic acid or B$_{12}$; correcting these deficiencies improved the DEPRESSION or the memory problems. More important, studies suggest that even a slight lack of these B vitamins may slow down the thinking in otherwise healthy people. In a study, 250 apparently healthy older people revealed that those with the lowest blood levels of B$_{12}$ and folic acid also scored lowest on memory and reasoning tests.

See also VITAMINS, B-COMPLEX.

vitamins, B-complex   The most important vitamins for nervous system function. Vitamins B$_1$ (thiamine), B$_6$, and niacin must be obtained from the diet (especially organ meats, beans, and fresh vegetables) because they are not made by the body.

A lack of vitamin B$_{12}$ may affect the healthy development of the NERVOUS SYSTEM (especially NERVE CELLS) because it synthesizes protein and fat. Without B$_{12}$, the MYELIN sheath (outer covering of the nerve cell) cannot develop properly. Vegetarians are at high risk for B$_{12}$ deficiency unless they consume alternate sources (including lentils, beans, sunflower seeds, peanuts, brown rice, asparagus, leafy greens, and broccoli).

A lack of vitamin B$_1$ causes peripheral nerve dysfunction and numbness in the hands and feet. Severe lack of this vitamin is often linked to alcoholism (because of poor diet) and can lead to the neurological disorder KORSAKOFF SYNDROME.

Excesses of these vitamins may also cause problems with the nervous system. Too much vitamin B$_6$ (doses exceeding 2 grams per day) can cause a severe neuropathy and impair senses of pain, touch, and temperature.

Wechsler Adult Intelligence Scale–Fourth Edition

(WAIS-IV) One of the most widely used IQ TESTS in the United States, this test is designed for older teenagers and adults (from ages 16 through 74 years, 11 months). Written by David Wechsler, it was first introduced in 1939 and has been updated to reduce bias in testing and scoring. This version is a harder edition of the WECHSLER INTELLIGENCE SCALE FOR CHILDREN-IV (WISC-IV). Although the WAIS-IV will result in scores about four points higher than those resulting from the WISC-IV, the test of choice for 16-year-olds is still the WISC-IV because it offers a larger number of valid subtest items to which the teenager can respond, and is therefore more likely to yield reliable and valid findings.

The WISC-IV and the STANFORD-BINET intelligence test are the two most commonly used IQ tests in U.S. schools. Many other tests are also used to assess overall intelligence, academic achievement, and specific LEARNING DISABILITY.

Wechsler Intelligence Scale for Children-IV

(WISC-IV) The IQ TEST of choice for most situations; appropriate for children between the ages of 6 and 16 years, 11 months. This test does a good job of measuring the ability to process visual and verbal information, allowing the child to demonstrate strengths and weaknesses in several areas. These include

- interpretation and problem solving with words or visual images
- speed of information processing
- planning and organization
- attention

- short-term and long-term memory

As with all other intelligence tests in the Wechsler series, the WISC-IV yields three IQ scores

- verbal IQ, reflecting a child's ability to reason using verbal language
- performance IQ, reflecting a child's ability to reason nonverbally
- full-scale IQ, reflecting overall intelligence

Wechsler Preschool and Primary Scale of Intelligence–Third Edition (WPPSI-III)

The WPPSI-III is the version of the Wechsler tests that assesses intellectual abilities from ages two years, six months through seven years, three months. Dr. David Wechsler developed the first edition of the WPPSI-III in 1967. The measure consists of 14 subtests and yields a Verbal Intelligence Quotient, a Performance (i.e., nonverbal) Intelligence Quotient, a Full-Scale Intelligence Quotient that is a composite of the Verbal and Performance IQs, and a Processing Speed Quotient.

As with other intelligence measures in the Wechsler series, the WPPSI-III scores have a mean of 100 and a standard deviation of 15. The subtest scores have a mean of 10 and a standard deviation of 3.

weight of the brain See BRAIN WEIGHT.

Wernicke, Carl (1848–1905) A 19th-century German neurologist who related nerve diseases to specific areas of the brain and also investigated

Subtest	Description	Scale
Block Design	The child copies designs using one- and two-color sides of blocks.	Performance
Information	The child responds to pictures or verbal questions regarding a broad range of general knowledge topics.	Verbal
Matrix Reasoning	The child looks at an incomplete matrix and chooses the missing element from four or five choices.	Performance
Vocabulary	The child names pictures or gives definitions for words.	Verbal
Picture Concepts	The child is presented two or three rows of pictures and chooses one picture from each row that forms a group with common characteristics.	Performance
Symbol Search	The child scans a search group and states whether a target symbol matches any of the symbols in the search group.	Processing Speed
Word Reasoning	The child names the common concept described in a series of clues.	Verbal
Coding	The child uses a "key" for pairing symbols with their corresponding shapes to fill in missing shapes when presented with their symbols.	Processing Speed
Comprehension	The child answers questions based on his/her understanding of general principles and social situations.	Supplemental
Picture Completion	The child names an important missing part for a picture.	Supplemental
Similarities	The examiner reads the child an incomplete sentence containing two concepts that share a common characteristic and asks the child to complete the sentence with a response that is consistent with the shared characteristic.	Supplemental
Receptive Vocabulary	The examiner presents plates with four pictures on each and asks the child to select the picture that best describes the cue the examiner presents.	Optional
Object Assembly	The examiner presents puzzle pieces scrambled in a specified order and asks the child to put together the puzzle.	Supplemental
Picture Naming	The child names pictures from a stimulus book.	Optional

the localization of MEMORY. He is best known for his descriptions of the APHASIAS (disorders interfering with the ability to communicate in speech or writing).

Wernicke studied at the University of Breslau before entering practice in Berlin, later joining the faculty at Breslau, where he remained until the year before his death.

In his book *Der aphasische Symptomenkomples,* published in 1874, he tried to relate the various aphasias to impaired psychic processes in different parts of the brain and included the first accurate description of a sensory aphasia in the TEMPORAL LOBE. He showed that auditory word images appear to be located in a memory bank separate from that containing the images of the articulated words. Wernicke also noted a second language center farther back in the brain known today as WERNICKE'S AREA, which contains the records of individual words.

Wernicke went on to elaborate on different clinical syndromes in terms of damage to either the Wernicke area or the area of the brain discovered by PIERRE-PAUL BROCA.

He published *Textbook of Brain Disorders (Lehrbuch der Gehirnkrankheiten)* in 1891, trying to illustrate cerebral localization for all brain disease. Among the disorders he described in the book was WERNICKE'S ENCEPHALOPATHY, which is caused by a thiamine deficiency.

See also WERNICKE'S APHASIA; WERNICKE-KORSAKOFF SYNDROME.

Wernicke-Korsakoff syndrome This acute neurological condition is an uncommon brain disorder almost always due to the malnutrition that occurs in chronic alcohol dependence, although it can also appear in other conditions such as cancer. The disease consists of two stages: WERNICKE'S ENCEPHALOPATHY followed by Korsakoff's psychosis, each characterized by separate symptoms.

The disease is caused by a deficiency of thiamine (vitamin B_1), which affects the brain and NERVOUS SYSTEM. This deficiency is probably caused by poor eating habits or an inherited defect in thiamine metabolism.

Symptoms and Diagnostic Path

In the first stage (Wernicke's encephalopathy), the patient usually develops symptoms suddenly, including abnormal eye movements, problems in coordinating body movements, slowness, and confusion. There are also signs of NEUROPATHY, such as loss of sensation, pins and needles, or impaired reflexes. The level of consciousness progressively

falls, and without treatment, this syndrome may lead to COMA and death.

The second stage (Korsakoff psychosis, or KORSAKOFF SYNDROME) may follow if treatment is not instituted soon enough. In this stage, sufferers experience severe AMNESIA, apathy, and disorientation. Recent memories are affected more than distant memory; often, patients cannot remember what they did even a few moments ago, and they may make up stories to cover for their loss of memory.

Treatment Options and Outlook

Wernicke's encephalopathy is a medical emergency requiring large doses of intravenous thiamine if the diagnosis is even suspected. Often, this treatment can reverse symptoms within a few hours.

In the absence of treatment, however, the disease will progress to Korsakoff psychosis and at that stage is usually irreversible. The patient will experience permanent impairment of memory and is in need of constant supervision.

See also WERNICKE, CARL; WERNICKE'S APHASIA.

Wernicke's aphasia A disturbance of language characterized by poor comprehension but fluent production, albeit with many word and sound substitutions. It is caused by damage to WERNICKE'S AREA in the brain, a particular area in the dominant cerebral hemisphere.

Symptoms and Diagnostic Path

Despite fluent speech, "internal speech" is impaired because of impaired comprehension, and speech content includes many errors in word selection and grammar. Writing is also impaired, and spoken or written commands are not understood. Wernicke's aphasia is associated with difficulty in accessing the meaning of words such as nouns.

Patients suffering from damage to Wernicke's area have difficulty understanding language in any form. They can speak fluently, forming long and complex sentences, but their strings of words often lack coherent meaning. They frequently use vague terms and roundabout descriptions that never coalesce into complete thoughts. From the prolific speech production of patients, it is easy to see that this is not a difficulty with speech production, but with language production.

See also WERNICKE, CARL; WERNICKE-KORSAKOFF SYNDROME.

Wernicke's area A part of the brain located in the TEMPORAL LOBE near the primary AUDITORY CORTEX that is critical to language comprehension, especially at the level of the meaning of individual words (rather than syntax, which is regulated by BROCA'S AREA). Damage to this part of the brain results in WERNICKE'S APHASIA, which makes individuals unable to understand words while listening, and unable to produce meaningful sentences.

See also WERNICKE, CARL; WERNICKE-KORSAKOFF SYNDROME.

Wernicke's encephalopathy See WERNICKE-KORSAKOFF SYNDROME.

white matter Another term for white nerve fibers (as opposed to cell bodies, which appear as gray) in the brain. The white appearance comes from MYELIN, a fatty substance that surrounds axons, acting as an insulator to enhance electrical conduction of action potentials.

Willis, Thomas (1621–1675) Oxford physician who studied cranial nerves, tracing blood flow to the brain. He believed that thought occurred in the CEREBRUM. He coauthored a book in 1664 in which he described the arterial system at the base of the brain (the Circle of Willis).

Wisconsin Card-Sorting Test A common way to assess FRONTAL LOBE damage. The subject is given a deck of cards marked by a pattern with various symbol shapes, numbers, and colors. A card might have three blue stars or one red star or two green triangles.

The subject begins to sort cards and is given hints as to how they should be sorted by the tester's comments (such as placing all the cards with green triangles in one pile). A normal person quickly learns the proper sorting method; once the subject has learned to sort by the rule, the rule is changed and the subject must figure out what the new sorting rule is. Patients with frontal lobe damage or KORSAKOFF SYNDROME tend to make a perseveration error at this point, continuing to sort the cards by the first rule. They have not lost the ability to understand that the rules have changed, but their understanding does not improve their behavior. They continue to sort by color, although each error brings the news that the action was wrong. Their mistake is not one of imagination or reasoning or any other type of intelligence but is an inflexibility in voluntary motor behavior.

xanthinol nicotinate This form of niacin passes into cells much more easily than niacin itself; therein, it increases the rate of GLUCOSE metabolism and improves blood flow to the brain.

In recent studies, it was found to improve performance of healthy elderly subjects in a variety of short- and long-term memory tasks. Like niacin, however, excess doses can cause flushing and a variety of other mild symptoms.

X-rays Invisible electromagnetic waves of very short wave length, some of which are absorbed and others of which pass through tissues; the shadow that is cast is projected onto a fluorescent screen or a film. X-rays are used to produce images of the brain and skull, in addition to other bones, organs, and internal tissues.

Discovered in 1895 by Wilhelm Conrad Roentgen, X-rays can be used to penetrate all substances, but they have been used most often in medicine to diagnose and treat disease. While X-ray images of bone are quite distinct, pictures of soft tissues are less clear and are therefore of minimal benefit today in visualizing the brain. Still, they are used to evaluate skull fractures, cancer, and general alterations in the appearance of the skull (such as changes seen in PAGET'S DISEASE).

Since the 1920s, radiologists have used substances opaque to radiation as part of the X-ray technique. In ANGIOGRAPHY, contrast dye is injected into an artery or vein to provide images of blood vessels. Since the 1970s, many X-ray techniques have been surpassed by newer procedures that are both easier and safer to perform.

Instead, computer-aided X-rays can show sections of the brain or scan its chemical activity. For example, in COMPUTERIZED AXIAL TOMOGRAPHY (CAT SCAN), an X-ray tube rotates around a patient's head, bombarding it with narrow X-ray beams. With computer help, the technique produces a brain cross-section projected on a TV screen that can be used to pinpoint blood clots, TUMORS, birth defects, or other damage.

Z

zatosetron   A drug that increases the release of ACE-TYLCHOLINE, a neurotransmitter linked to improved learning and memory and deficient in many types of memory impairment. By selectively blocking serotonin (a brain substance that inhibits the release of acetylcholine), zatosetron increases acetylcholine release and enhances memory and performance, accordng to some research. Initial research suggests that zatosetron, like its cousin ondansetron, may improve memory in some healthy older adults with AGE-ASSOCIATED MEMORY IMPAIRMENT.

Scientists at the Memory Assessment Clinics in Bethesda, Maryland, and Scottsdale, Arizona, are testing zatosetron in preliminary double-blind studies of 200 subjects over age 50 with age-associated memory impairment.

APPENDIXES

I. Self-Help Organizations

II. Professional Organizations

III. Governmental Organizations

IV. Helpful Web Sites

V. Read More about It

VI. Research Periodicals

APPENDIX I
SELF-HELP ORGANIZATIONS

Acoustic Neuroma

Acoustic Neuroma Association
600 Peachtree Parkway, Suite 108
Cumming, GA 30041
(770) 205-8211
http://www.anausa.org

Alcoholism

Al-Anon and Ala-Teen
Al-Anon Family Group Headquarters, Inc.
1600 Corporate Landing Parkway
Virginia Beach, VA 23454-5617
(888) 4AL-ANON
http://www.al-anon.alateen.org/

Alcoholics Anonymous
A.A. World Services, Inc.
P.O. Box 459
New York, NY 10163
(212) 870-3400
http://www.alcoholics-anonymous.org

Alzheimer's Disease

Alzheimer's Association
919 N. Michigan Avenue, Suite 1100
Chicago, IL 60611
(312) 335-8700; (800) 272-3900
http://www.alz.org

Alzheimer's Disease Education and Referral Center

National Institute on Aging
PO Box 8250
Silver Spring, MD 20907

(800) 438-4380
http://www.alzheimers.org

Amyotrophic Lateral Sclerosis

Amyotrophic Lateral Sclerosis Association
27001 Agoura Road, Suite 150
Calabasas Hills, CA 91301
(818) 880-9007; (800) 782-4747
http://www.alsa.org

ALS Research Foundation
Pacific Medical Center
PO Box 7999
San Francisco, CA 94120
(415) 923-3604

Aphasia

National Aphasia Association
156 Fifth Avenue, Suite 707
New York, NY 10010
(800) 922-4622
http://www.aphasia.org

Anxiety Disorders

Anxiety Disorders of America
11900 Parklawn Drive, Suite. 100
Rockville, MD 20852
(301) 231-9350
http://www.adaa.org

Freedom from Fear
308 Seaview Avenue
Staten Island, NY 10305
(718) 351-1717
http://www.freedomfromfear.org

National Anxiety Foundation
3135 Custer Drive
Lexington, KY 40517
http://www.lexington-on-line.com/naf.html

Arnold-Chiari Malformation

World Arnold-Chiari Malformation
31 Newtown Woods Road
Newtown Square, PA 19073
http://www.pressenter.com/~WACMA/

Ataxia

National Ataxia Foundation
2600 Fernbrook Lane, Suite 119
Minneapolis, MN 55447-2751
(763) 553-0020
http://www.ataxia.org

Friedreich's Ataxia Group in America
PO Box 116
Oakland, CA 94611
(415) 655-0833

Attention Deficit Disorder/ Hyperactivity

(see also LEARNING DISABILITIES)

Center for Hyperactive Child Information
PO Box 66272
Washington, DC 20035
(703) 920-7495

Children and Adults with Attention Deficit Disorder (CHADD)
8181 Professional Place, Suite 201
Landover, MD 20785
http://chadd.org

Coalition for the Education and Support of Attention Deficit Disorder
PO Box 242
Osseo, MI 55369
(612) 425-0423

Council for Learning Disabilities
PO Box 40303
Overland Park, KS 66204
(913) 492-8755

Learning Disabilities Association of America
4516 Library Road
Pittsburgh, PA 15234
(412) 341-1515

National Attention Deficit Disorder Association
PO Box 488
West Newbury, MA 01985
(508) 462-0495; (800) 487-2282

National Center for Learning Disabilities
381 Park Avenue South, Suite 1420
New York, NY 10016
(212) 545-7510

National Networker
PO Box 32611
Phoenix, AZ 85064
(602) 941-5112

Time Out to Enjoy (TOTE)
c/o CDR
208 S. La Salle, No. 1330
Chicago, IL 60604
(312) 444-9484

Autism

Autism Network International
PO Box 35448
Syracuse, NY 13235
http://www.autistics.org

Autism Services Center
605 9th Street
PO Box 507
Huntington, WV 25710
(304) 525-8014

Autism Society of America
7910 Woodmont Avenue, Suite 300
Bethesda, MD 20814
(301) 657-0881; (800) 3-AUTISM
http://www.autism-society.org

Autism Genetic Resource Exchange
5225 Wilshire Boulevard, Suite 226
Los Angeles, CA 90036
(888) 288-4762
http://www.agre.org

Cure Autism Now Foundation
5455 Wilshire Boulevard, Suite 715
Los Angeles, CA 90036
(323) 549-0500
http://www.cureautismnow.org

National Alliance for Autism Research
414 Will Street
Princeton, NJ 08540
(888) 777-6227
http://www.naar.org

Autoimmune Diseases

**American Autoimmune Related Diseases
   Association**
22100 Gratiot Avenue
East Detroit, MI 48021
(810) 776-3900
http://www.aarda.org

Batten Disease

**Batten Disease Support and Research
   Association**
120 Humphries Drive, Suite 2
Reynoldsburg, OH 43068
(800) 448-4570
http://www.bdsra.org

Behcet's Disease

American Behcet's Disease Association
PO Box 280240
Memphis, TN 38168
(800) 723-4238
http://www.pweb.netcom.com/~mharting

Birth Defects

Birth Defect Research for Children
930 Woodcock Road, Suite 225
Orlando, FL 32803
(407) 245-7035
http://www.birthdefects.org

March of Dimes Birth Defects Foundation
1275 Mamaroneck Avenue

White Plains, NY 10605
(888) 663-4637
http://www.modimes.org

Blindness/Vision Problems

**Helen Keller National Center for Deaf/Blind
   Youth and Adults**
111 Middle Neck Road
Sands Point, NY 11050
(516) 944-8900
http://www.helenkeller.org

Lighthouse International
111 E. 59th Street
New York, NY 10022
(212) 821-9200
http://www.lighthouse.org

Prevent Blindness America
500 E. Remington Road
Schaumburg, IL 60173
(800) 331-2020
http://www.preventblindness.org

Brain Damage

**The Family Survival Project for Brain-
   Damaged Adults**
1736 Divisadero Street
San Francisco, CA 94115
(415) 921-5400

Brain Injury Association, Inc.
105 N. Alfred Street
Alexandria, VA 22314
(703) 236-6000
http://www.biausa.org

Brain Injury Services
10340 Democracy Lane, Suite 305
Fairfax, VA 22030
(703) 352-1656
http://www.braininjurysvcs.org

Think First Foundation
5550 Meadowbrook Drive, Suite 110
Rolling Meadows, IL 60008
(800) 844-6556
http://www.thinkfirst.org

Brain Research

Division of Basic Brain and Behavioral Sciences
National Institute of Mental Health
National Institute of Neurological Disorders and Stroke
9000 Rockville Pike
Building 31, Room 8A06
Bethesda, MD 20892
(800) 352-9424

National Foundation for Brain Research
1250 24th Street NW, Suite 300
Washington, DC 20037
(202) 293-5453
http://www.brainnet.org

Brain Tumors

Acoustic Neuroma Association
600 Peachtree Parkway, Suite 108
Cumming, GA 30041
(770) 205-8211
http://www.anausa.org

American Brain Tumor Association
2720 River Road, Suite 146
Des Plaines, IL 60018
(800) 886-2282; (847) 827-9910
http://www.abta.org

Brain Tumor Foundation for Children
1835 Savoy Drive, Suite 316
Atlanta, GA 30341
(770) 458-5554
http://www.btfcgainc.org

Brain Tumor Society
124 Watertown Street, Suite 3-H
Watertown, MA 02472
(617) 924-9997
http://www.tbts.org

Children's Brain Tumor Foundation
274 Madison Avenue, Suite 1301
New York, NY 10016
(212) 448-9494
http://www.cbtf.org

National Brain Tumor Foundation
414 13th Street, Suite 700
Oakland, CA 94612
(800) 934-CURE
http://www.braintumor.org

Cancer

National Cancer Institute
(800) 4-CANCER

Caregivers

Family Caregiver Alliance
690 Market Street
Suite 600
San Francisco, CA 94104
http://www.caregiver.org
e-mail: info@caregiver.org
(415) 434-3388; (800) 445-8106 (CA)
Fax: (415) 434-3508

Cerebral Palsy

United Cerebral Palsy Association
1660 L Street NW, Suite 700
Washington, DC 20036
(800) 872-5827

Charcot-Marie-Tooth Disease

Charcot-Marie-Tooth Association
Crozer Mills Enterprise Center
601 Upland Avenue
Upland, PA 19015
(800) 606-CMTA; (610) 499-7486

Chronic Fatigue

The CFIDS Association of America, Inc.
PO Box 220398
Charlotte, NC 28222-0398
(800) 442-3437; (704) 365-2343
http://www.cfids.org

Coma

Coma Recovery Association
100 E. Old Country Road, Suite 9
Mineola, NY 11501

(516) 997-1826
http://www.comarecovery.org

Craniosynostosis

Society for Children with Craniosynostosis
PO Box 1522
Denver, CO 80201
(303) 722-9992

Creutzfeldt-Jakob Disease

Creutzfeldt-Jakob Disease Foundation
PO Box 611625
Miami, FL 33261-1626
http://www.cjdfoundation.org
e-mail: crjakob@aol.com.
Fax: (954) 436-7591

Cri Du Chat Syndrome

5p– Society
7108 Katella Avenue, #502
Stanton, CA 90680
(888) 970-0777
http://www.fivepminus.org

Deafness/Hearing Loss

Self Help for Hard of Hearing People
7910 Woodmont Avenue, Suite 1200
Bethesda, MD 20814
(301) 657-2248
http://www.shhh.org

Alexander Graham Bell Association for the Deaf and Hard of Hearing
3417 Volta Place
Washington, DC 20007
(202) 337-5220; TDD: (202) 337-5220
http://www.agbell.org

American Society for Deaf Children
PO Box 3355
Gettysburg, PA 17325
(800) 942-2732; TDD: (717) 334-7922
http://www.deafchildren.org

Better Hearing Institute
515 King Street, Suite 420
Alexandria, VA 22314
(800) 327-9355
http://www.betterhearing.org

Developmental Disabilities

(see DOWN SYNDROME; MENTAL RETARDATION)

Down Syndrome

Association for Children with Down Syndrome
4 Fern Place
Plainview, NY 11803
(516) 933-4700
http://www.acds.org

National Association for Down Syndrome
PO Box 4542
Oakbrook, IL 60521
(312) 325-9112
http://www.nads.org

National Down Syndrome Adoption Exchange
(914) 428-1236

National Down Syndrome Congress
7000 Peachtree-Dunwoody Road NE
Suite 100
(800) 232-6372; (770) 604-9500
http://www.ndsccenter.org

National Down Syndrome Society
666 Broadway, Suite 810
New York, NY 10012
(212) 460-9330; (800) 221-4602 (except New York); (800) 460-9330 in New York
http://www.ndss.org

Dysautonomia

Dysautonomia Foundation
633 Third Avenue, 12th Floor
New York, NY 10017
(212) 949-6644
http://www.med.nyu.edu/fd/fdcenter.html

National Dysautonomia Research Foundation
421 W. Fourth Street, Suite 9
Red Wing, MN 55066
(651) 267-0525
http://www.ndrf.org

Epilepsy

Epilepsy Concern Service Group
1282 Wynnewood Drive
West Palm Beach, FL 33417
(407) 683-0044

Epilepsy Foundation of America
4351 Garden City Drive, Suite 406
Landover, MD 20785
(301) 459-3700; (800) EFA-1000
http://www.efa.org

Fetal Alcohol Syndrome

**National Organization on Fetal Alcohol
   Syndrome**
216 G Street NE
Washington, DC 20002
(800) 666-6327
http://www.nofas.org

Gaucher's Disease

National Gaucher Foundation
11140 Rockville Pike, Suite 350
Rockville, MD 20852
(800) 925-8885
http://www.gaucherdisease.org

Guillain-Barré Syndrome

**Guillain-Barré Syndrome Foundation
   International**
PO Box 262
Wynnewood, PA 19096
(610) 667-0131
http://peabody.webmast.com/gbs/

Headache

National Headache Foundation
5252 N. Western Avenue

Chicago, IL 60625
(800) 843-2256; (800) 523-8858 in IL
http://www.headache.org

**American Council for Headache Education
   (ACHE)**
19 Mantua Road
Mt. Royal, NJ 08061
(800) 255-ACHE; (856) 423-0258
http://www.achenet.org

**Association for Applied Psychophysiology
   and Biofeedback**
10200 W. 44th Avenue, Suite 304
Wheat Ridge, CO 80033
(800) 477-8892
http://www.aapb.org

Head Injury

National Head Injury Foundation
1776 Massachuestts Avenue NW, Suite 100
Washington, DC 20036
(202) 296-6443; (800) 444-6443

Brain Trauma Foundation
523 E. 72nd Street, 8th Floor
New York, NY 10021
(212) 772-0608
http://www.braintrauma.org

Head Injury Hotline
212 Pioneer Bldg.
Seattle, WA 98104
(206) 621-8558
http://www.headinjury.com

Brain Injury Association
105 N. Alfred Street
Alexandria, VA 22314
(800) 444-6443
http://www.biausa.org

**Rehabilitation Research Center for
   Traumatic Brain and Spinal Cord Injury**
950 S. Bascon Avenue, Suite 2011
San Jose, CA 95128
(800) 352-1956
http://www.tbi-sci.org

Huntington's Disease

Hereditary Disease Foundation
11400 W. Olympic Boulevard, Suite 855
Los Angeles, CA 90064
(310) 575-9656
http://www.hdfoundation.org

Huntington Disease Society of America
158 W. 29th Street, 7th Floor
New York, NY 10001
(800) 345-4372; (212) 242-1968 in NY
http://www.hdsa.org

Huntington Society of Canada
151 Frederick Street, Suite 400
Kitchener, Ontario
CANADA N2H 2M2
(519) 749-7063
(800) 998-7398 (in Canada only)
http://www.hsc-ca.org

Hydrocephalus

**Guardians of Hydrocephalus Research
  Foundation**
2618 Avenue Z
Brooklyn, NY 11235
(718) 743-GHRF; (800) 458-8655

National Hydrocephalus Foundation
12413 Centralia
Lakewood, CA 90715
(562) 402-3523
http://www.NHFonline.org

Hydrocephalus Association
875 Market Street, Suite 705
San Francisco, CA 94102
(415) 732-7040
http://www.hydroassoc.org

Infectious Diseases

**CDC National Prevention Information
  Network**
(800) 458-5231

Joseph Disease

International Joseph Disease Foundation
PO Box 2550
Livermore, CA 94551
(510) 443-4600

Learning Disorders

AVKO Dyslexia Research Foundation
3084 W. Willard Road
Clio, MI 48415
(810) 686-9283
http://www.AVKO.org

Council for Learning Disabilities
9013 West Brooke Drive
Overland Park, KS 66212
(913) 492-3840

Learning Disabilities Association
4156 Library Road
Pittsburgh, PA 15234
(412) 341-1515
http://www.ldanatl.org

National Center for Learning Disabilities
381 Park Avenue South, Suite 1401
New York, NY 10016
(212) 545-7510; (888) 575-7373
http://www.ld.org

International Dyslexia Society, The
8600 La Salle Road
Baltimore, MD 21286
(800) ABCD-123; (410) 296-0232
http://www.interdys.org

Leukodystrophy

United Leukodystrophy Foundation
2304 Highland Drive
Sycamore, IL 60178
(800) 728-5483
http://www.ulf.org

Mental Health/Mental Illness

National Alliance for the Mentally Ill
Colonial Place Three

2107 Wilson Boulevard, Suite 300
Arlington, VA 22201
(703) 524-7600; (800) 950-6264
http://www.nami.org

Mental Retardation

(See also DOWN SYNDROME)

**American Network of Community Options
and Resources**
4200 Evergreen Lane, Suite 315
Annandale, VA 22003
(703) 642-6614
http://www.ancor.org

Association for Retarded Citizens
1010 Wayne Avenue, Suite 650
Silver Spring, MD 20910
(301) 565-3842
http://www.thearc.org

**Association for Children with Retarded
Mental Development**
162 5th Avenue, 11th Floor
New York, NY 10010
(212) 741-0100; (800) WOW-ACRM

Fragile X Foundation
PO Box 190488
San Francisco, CA 94119
(800) 688-8765; (510) 763-6030
http://www.fxf.org

FRAXA Research Foundation
45 Pleasant Street
Newburyport, MA 01950
(978) 462-1866
http://www.fraxa.org

Pilot Parents
1941 S. 42 Street, Suite 122
Omaha, NE 68105
(402) 346-5220

Migraine

(see HEADACHE)

Multiple Sclerosis

National Multiple Sclerosis Society
733 Third Avenue
New York, NY 10017
(800) 624-8236
http://www.nmss.org

Multiple Sclerosis Foundation
6350 N. Andrews Avenue
Fort Lauderdale, FL 33309
(305) 776-6805; (800) 441-7055
http://www.msfacts.org

Multiple Sclerosis Association of America
706 Haddonfield Road
Cherry Hill, NJ 08002
(800) 532-7667
http://www.msaa.com

Muscular Dystrophy

MD Association
3300 E. Sunrise Drive
Tucson, AZ 85718
(800) 572-1717
http://www.mdausa.org

Myasthenia Gravis

Myasthenia Gravis Foundation of America
123 W. Madison Street, Suite 800
Chicago, IL 60602
(800) 541-5454
http://www.myasthenia.org

Narcolepsy

(see SLEEP DISORDERS)

Neurofibromatosis

National Neurofibromatosis Foundation
95 Pine Street, 16th Floor
New York, NY 10005
(212) 344-6633
http://www.nf.org

Neurofibromatosis, Inc.
8855 Annapolis Road, Suite 110
Lanham, MD 20706
(800) 942-6825
http://www.nfinc.org

Pain

American Chronic Pain Association
PO Box 850
Rocklin, CA 95677
(916) 632-0922
http://www.theacpa.org

National Chronic Pain Outreach Association
PO Box 274
Millboro, VA 24460
(540) 862-9437
http://www.chronicpain.org

Parkinson's Disease

American Parkinson Disease Association, Inc.
1250 Hylan Boulevard, Suite 4B
Staten Island, NY 10305
(718) 981-8001; (800) 223-APDA
http://www.apdaparkinson.org

Michael J. Fox Foundation for Parkinson's Research
840 Third Street
Santa Rosa, CA 95404
(800) 850-4726
http://www.michaeljfox.org

The Parkinson's Institute
1170 Morse Avenue
Sunnyvale, CA 94089
(800) 786-2958
http://www.parkinsonsinstitute.org

National Parkinson Foundation
1501 NW Ninth Avenue
Miami, FL 33136
(800) 327-4545; (800) 433-7022 in FL;
    (305) 547-6666 in Miami
http://www.parkinson.org

Parkinson's Disease Foundation
Wm. Black Medical Building
Columbia-Presbyterian Medical Center

710 West 168th Street
New York, NY 10032
(212) 923-4700; (800) 457-6676
http://www.pdf.org

Parkinson's Educational Program
1800 Park Newport #302
Newport Beach, CA 92660
(800) 344-7872; (714) 640-0218 in CA

United Parkinson Foundation
833 W. Washington Boulevard
Chicago, IL 60607
(312) 733-1893

Pick's Disease

National Niemann-Pick Disease Foundation, Inc.
N1590 Fairview Lane
Ft. Atkinson, WI 53538
http://www.nnpdf.org
(877)-CURE-NPC

Progressive Supranuclear Palsy

Society for Progressive Supranuclear Palsy
1838 Greene Tree Road, Suite 515
Baltimore, MD 21208
(800) 457-4777
http://www.psp.org

Prader-Willi Syndrome Association
Suite 220
2510 S. Brentwood Boulevard
St. Louis, MO 63144
(800) 926-4797; (314) 962-7644
http://www.pwsausa.org

Rett Syndrome

International Rett Syndrome Association
9121 Piscataway Road
Clinton, MD 20735
(301) 856-3334; (800) 818-RETT
http://www.rettsyndrome.org

Rett Syndrome Research Foundation
4600 Devitt Drive
Cincinnati, OH 45246

(513) 874-3020
http://www.rsrf.org

Reye's Syndrome

National Reye's Syndrome Foundation
426 North Lewis
Byran, OH 43506
(419) 636-2679; (800) 233-7393; (800) 231-7393
   in OH
http://www.bright.net/~reyesyn

Shy-Drager Syndrome

Shy-Drager Syndrome
1607 Silver, SE
Albuquerque, NM 87106
(800) 737-4999

Sleep Disorders/Narcolepsy

American Academy of Sleep Medicine
6301 Bandel Road #101
Rochester, MN 55901
(507) 287-6006
http://www.aasmnet.org

American Sleep Apnea Association
1424 K Street NW, Suite 302
Washington, DC 20005
(202) 293-3650
http://www.sleepapnea.org

Narcolepsy and Cataplexy Foundation
   of America
445 E. 68th Street
New York, NY 10021
(212) 570-5506

National Sleep Foundation
1522 K Street NW, Suite 500
Washington, DC 20005
http://www.sleepfoundation.org

Spasmodic Dysphonia

National Spasmodic Dysphonia Association
One E. Wacker Drive, Suite 2430
Chicago, IL 60601
(800) 795-6732
http://www.dystonia-foundation.org/NSDA

Spasmodic Torticollis

National Spasmodic Torticollis Association
9920 Talbert Avenue
Fountain Valley, CA 92708
(800) 487-8385
http://www.torticollis.org

Spina Bifida

Spina Bifida Association of America
4590 MacArthur Boulevard NW, Suite 250
Washington, DC 20007
(800) 621-3141
http://www.sbaa.org

Spina Bifida Adoption Referral Program
1955 Florida Drive
Xenia, OH 45385
(513) 372-2040

Spinal Injuries

American Paralysis Association
500 Morris Avenue
Springfield, NJ 07081
(800) 225-0292; (201) 379-2690 in NJ

Christopher Reeve Paralysis Foundation
500 Morris Avenue
Springfield, NJ 07081
(800) 225-0292
http://www.apacure.com

National Spinal Cord Injury Hotline
2200 Keman Drive
Baltimore, MD 21207
(800) 526-3456
http://www.scihotline.org

National Spinal Cord Injury Association
8701 Georgia Avenue, Suite 500
Silver Spring, MD 20851
(301) 588-6959; (800) 962-9629
http://www.spinalcord.org

Paralyzed Veterans of America
801 18th Street NW
Washington, DC 20006
(202) 872-1300

Spinal Cord Society
Wendell Road
Fergus Falls, MN 56537
(218) 739-5252

Stroke

American Stroke Association
7272 Greenville Avenue
Dallas, TX 75231
(800) 553-6321; (214) 750-5231

National Stroke Association
9707 E. Easter Lane
Englewood, CO 80112
(303) 771-1700
http://www.stroke.org

National Institute of Neurological Disorders and Stroke
PO Box 5801
Bethesda, MD 20824
(800) 352-9424

Stroke Clubs International
805 12th Street
Galveston, TX 77550
(409) 762-1022

Sturge-weber Syndrome

Sturge-Weber Foundation
PO Box 418
Mount Freedom, NJ 07970
(800) 627-5482; (973) 895-4445
http://www.sturge-weber.com

Tardive Dyskinesia/Dystonia

Tardive Dyskinesia/Tardive Dystonia National Association
PO Box 45732
Seattle, WA 98145
(206) 522-3166

Tay-Sachs

National Tay-Sachs and Allied Diseases Association, Inc.
2001 Beacon Street, Suite 204
Brookline, MA 02146

(617) 277-4463; (800) 906-8723
http://www.ntsad.org

Late Onset Tay-Sachs Foundation
1303 Paper Mill Road
Erdenheim, PA 19038
(800) 672-2022
http://www.lotsf.org

Tourette Syndrome

Tourette Syndrome Association
42-40 Bell Boulevard
Bayside, NY 11361
(718) 224-2999; (800) 237-0717
http://www.tsa-usa.org

Tourette Syndrome Foundation of Canada
173 Owen Boulevard
Willowdale, Ontario
CANADA M2P 1GB

Tremor

International Tremor Foundation
7046 105th Street
Overland Park, KS 66212
(913) 341-3880

Trigeminal Neuralgia Association

PO Box 340
Barnegat Light, NJ 08006
(904) 779-0333
http://www.tna-support.org

Tuberous Sclerosis

Tuberous Sclerosis Alliance
801 Roeder Road, Suite 750
Silver Spring, MD 20910
(800) 225-6872; (301) 562-9890
http://www.tsalliance.org

Vestibular Disorders

Vestibular Disorders Association
PO Box 4467
Portland, OR 97208
(503) 229-7705
http://www.vestibular.org

APPENDIX II
PROFESSIONAL ORGANIZATIONS

Academy of Aphasia
150 Muir Road
Martinez, CA 94553
(925) 372-2670
http://www.academyofaphasia.org

American Academy of Cerebral Palsy and
    Developmental Medicine
6300 River Road, Suite 727
Rosemont, IL 60018
(847) 698-1635
http://www.aacpdm.org

American Academy of Neurological and
    Orthopaedic Surgeons
2320 S. Rancho Drive, Suite 202
Las Vegas, NV 89102
(702) 388-7390
http://www.aanos.org

American Board of Neurological Surgery
6550 Fannin Street, Suite 2139
Houston, TX 77030
(713) 790-6015
http://www.abns.org

American Academy of Somnology
PO Box 27077
Las Vegas, NV 89126
(800) 513-2757
http://www.hopperinstitute.com

American Association of Neurological Surgeons
5550 Meadowbrook Drive
Rolling Meadows, IL 60088
(888) 566-2267
http://www.aans.org

American Board of Orthopaedic
    Microneurosurgery
2300 Rancho Drive, Suite 202

Las Vegas, NV 89102
(702) 388-7390

American Epilepsy Society
342 Main Street
West Hartford, CT 06117
(860) 586-7505
http://www.aesnet.org

American Neurological Association
5841 Cedar Lake Road, Suite 204
Minneapolis, MN 55416
(952) 545-6284
http://www.aneuroa.org

American Pain Society
4700 W. Lake Avenue
Glenview, IL 60025
(847) 375-4515
http://www.ampainsoc.org

American Society for Stereotactic and Functional
    Neurosurgery
Houston Stereotactic Center
6550 Fannin Street, No. 2139
Houston, TX 77030
http://www.assfn.org

AVKO Education Research Foundation
3084 West Willard Road, Suite W
Clio, MI 48420
(810) 686-9283
http://www.AVKO.org

Cajal Club
c/o Dr. David Whitlock
Univ. of Colorado Health Sciences Center
Dept. of Cellular & Structural Biology, B-111
4200 E. 9th Avenue
Denver, CO 80262
(303) 270-8201

Child Neurology Society
100 West County Road E, Suite 126
St. Paul, MN 55126
(651) 486-9447

Congress of Neurological Surgeons
10 N. Martingale Road, Suite 190
Schaumburg, IL 60173
(877) 517-1267
http://www.neurosurgery.org/cns/

Council for Learning Disabilities
PO Box 40303
Overland Park, KS 66212
(913) 492-8755

International Association for the Study of Pain
909 NE 43rd Street, Suite 306
Seattle, WA 98105
(206) 547-6409
http://www.iasp-pain.org

International Federation of Clinical
    Neurophysiology
6550 Fannin Street, No. 2139
Houston, TX 77030
(713) 790-6015

International Neural Network Society
19 Mantua Road

Mt. Royal, NJ 08061
(856) 423-0162
http://www.inns.org

National Coalition for Research in Neurological
    Disorders
1250 24th Street NW, Suite 300
Washington, DC 20037
(202) 293-5453

Neuro-Developmental Treatment Association
1550 S. Coast Highway, Suite 201
Laguna Beach, CA 92651
(800) 869-9295
http://www.NDTA.org

Society of Neurological Surgeons
750 Washington Street
Box 178
Boston, MA 02111
(617) 956-5858

Society of Neurosurgical Anesthesia and Critical
    Care (SNACC)
1910 Byrd. Avenue, Suite 100
PO Box 11086
Richmond, VA 23230
(804) 673-9037
http://www.snacc.org

APPENDIX III
GOVERNMENTAL ORGANIZATIONS

Autism Network International (ANI)
PO Box 35448
Syracuse, NY 13235-5448
jisincla@mailbox.syr.edu
http://ani.autistics.org

MAAP Services for Autism, Asperger's, and PDD
PO Box 524
Crown Point, IN 46308
info@maapservices.org
http://www.maapservices.org
(219) 662-1311
Fax: 219-662-0638

National Cancer Institute/Cancer Information Service
31 Center Drive, Building 31, MSC 2580
Bethesda, MD 20892
(800) 422-6237
http://www.nci.nih.gov

National Dissemination Center for Children with Disabilities
U.S. Dept. of Education, Office of Special Education Programs
P.O. Box 1492
Washington, DC 20013-1492
nichcy@aed.org
http://www.nichcy.org
(800) 695-0285
Fax: 202-884-8441

National Eye Institute
2020 Vision Place
Bethesda, MD 20892
(301) 496-5248
http://www.nei.nih.gov

National Institute of Child Health and Human Information Resource Center
PO Box 3006
Rockville, MD 20847
NICHDInformationResourceCenter@mail.nih.gov
http://www.nichd.nih.gov
(800) 370-2943; (888) 320-6942 (TTY)
Fax: 301-984-1473

National Institute of Mental Health
6001 Executive Boulevard, Room 8184, MSC 9663
Bethesda, MD 20892
(301) 443-4513
http://www.nimh.nih.gov

National Institute of Neurological Disorders and Stroke
National Institutes of Health
9000 Rockville Pike
Building 31, Room 8A-16
Bethesda, MD 20205
(301) 496-5751
(800) 352-9424
http://www.ninds.nih.gov

National Institute on Aging
9000 Rockville Pike
Bethesda, MD 20205
(301) 496-9265

National Institute on Alcohol Abuse and Alcoholism
6000 Executive Boulevard, Willco Building
Bethesda, MD 20892
(301) 443-3860
http://www.niaaa.nih.gov

National Institute on Deafness and Other Communication Disorders Information Clearinghouse
1 Communication Avenue
Bethesda, MD 20892-3456
nidcdinfo@nidcd.nih.gov
http://www.nidcd.nih.gov
(800) 241-1044; (800) 241-1055 (TTD/TTY)

National Organization for Rare Disorders (NORD)
55 Kenosia Avenue
PO Box 1968
Danbury, CT 06813-1968
(203) 744-0100
Toll free: (800) 999-6673 (voicemail only)
TDD Number: (203) 797-9590
FAX: (203) 798-2291
E-mail: orphan@rarediseases.org

APPENDIX IV
HELPFUL WEB SITES

General Information

http://www.nih.gov/nia/health/agepages/
    forget.htm

Forgetfulness: It's Not Always What You Think.
A National Institute on Health informational page
    with link to the Alzheimer's Disease Education
    and Referral Center (ADEAR).

http://www.mayohealth.org/mayo/common/
    htm/alzheimers.htm

Memory Loss: Not Always Permanent
Informative site that is part of the Mayo Clinic
    Health Oasis. The Alzheimer's Center link leads
    to information for caregivers and quizzes to test
    your knowledge of the disease.

http://www.brain.nwu.edu/core/define.htm

Definitions for the medical terms you might hear
    while seeking treatment for memory loss.

http://www.brain.nwu.edu/core/caregive.
    htm

Information for caregivers of those with Alzheimer's
    and memory disorders.

http://www.alz.uci.edu/CausesofDementia.
    html

A list of the possible causes of dementia.

http://alzheimers.about.com/health/
    alzheimers/msubmemory.htm

A useful site with links to the many aspects of the
    impact of memory loss.

AIDS Dementia Complex

http://alzheimers.about.com/health/alzheimers/
    library/blaidsrelateddementia.htm

A definition of AIDS Dementia Complex.

http://www.natip.org/memory.html

Memory, thinking, and behavior problems associated
    with AIDS.

http://www.cdc.govlhivlpubslfaq/faq5.htm

How can I tell if I'm infected with HIV? What are
    the symptoms?

Alzheimer's Disease

http://www.ahcpr.gov:80/clinic/alzcons.htm

A patient and family guide to early Alzheimer's,
    published by the Agency for Healthcare Re-
    search and Quality.

http://www.alzheimers.com/

Practical information that supports prevention and
    treatment of Alzheimer's disease and the efforts
    of caregivers who deal with those who are
    affected by it.

http://www.ohioalzcenter.org/warn.html

Ten warning signs of Alzheimer's disease.

http://www.brain.nwu.edu/core/dementia.
    htm

A clear definition of dementia, covering Alzheimer's
    and its 10 warning signs.

http://www.drkoop.com/dyncon/article.
    asp?at=&id=1223

A definition of Alzheimer's from a site under the
    name of the former surgeon general of the
    United States, C. Everett Koop.

http://www.drkoop.com/dyncon/article.
    asp?at=&id=6149

Wellness and prevention of Alzheimer's disease.

http://www.drkoop.com/dyncon/article.
    asp?at=&id=4037
How a diagnosis of Alzheimer's disease is reached.

http://www.drkoop.com/dyncon/article.
    asp?at=&'id=5906
Treatment and management of Alzheimer's disease.

http://home.mira.net/~dhs/ad3.html
The Alzheimer's Web. A site devoted to Alzheimer's research. This site is for patients and physicians but takes a more academic approach.

http://www.alzheimer.ca/
The site for the Alzheimer Society of Canada.

http://www.ahaf.org/alzdis/about/adsymp.
    htm
The symptoms of Alzheimer's disease from the American Health Assistance Foundation.

http://www.ahaf.org/aFlzdis/about/adcare.
    htm
Practical information on creating a safe environment and solving day-to-day problems for caregivers of those with Alzheimer's.

http://www.alzhelmers.org/pubs/adcdir.html
A list of national Alzheimer's disease centers.

http://alzheimers.about.com/health/
    alzheimers/ library/weekly/aa051300a.
    htm?terms= MEMORY+LOSS
Coping with memory loss and links to other information.

Behcet's Disease

http://www.ninds.nih.gov/health and
    medical/disorders/behcet doc.htm
A fact sheet from the National Institute of Neurological Disorders and Stroke.

Chronic Fatigue Syndrome and Fibromyalgia

http://familydoctor.org/handouts/031.html
How Do I Know If I Have Chronic Fatigue Syndrome. A series of questions with links to informational sites about the syndrome.

http://www.cdc.gov/ncidod/diseases/cfs/
    cfshome.htm
Chronic Fatigue Syndrome information and links to support groups from the Centers for Disease Control.

http://chronicfatigue.about.com/health/chronic
    fatigue/library/weekly/aa051999.htm
Information, support, and links.

http://chronicfatigue.about.com/
    health/ chronicfatigue/msubfmdef.
    htm?terms=fibromyalgia
Links to definitions of fibromyalgia, information, and how to tell if you might have the condition.

Creutzfeldt-Jakob Disease

http://www.ninds.nih.gov/health_and_
    medical/pubs/creutzfeldt-jakob_disease
    _fact_sheet.htm
A fact sheet containing information about Creutzkldt-Jakob disease from the National Institute of Neurologic Disorders and Stroke.

http://members.aol.com/larmstr853/cjdvoice/
    facts.htm
A fact sheet on Creutzfeldt-Jakob disease from the CJD-Voice, an e-mail based support and discussion group.

Dementia With Lewy Bodies

http://www.ninds.nih.gov/
    health_and_medical/disorders/
    dementiawithlewybodies doc.htm
A page defining Dementia with Lewy Bodies, a dementia with elements of both Alzheimer's and Parkinson's.

Depression

http://onhealth.com/conditions/resource/
    conditions/item,291.asp
A definition of the condition and description of symptoms.

http://onhealth.com/conditions/in-depth/
item/item,14931_1_1.asp
Depression checklist.

http://www.nimh.nih.gov/publicat/
depressionmenu.cfm
Information on depression from the National
Institute of Mental Health.

Electroconvulsive Therapy

http://www.ect.org/effects.shtml
The effects of electroconvulsive therapy.

Huntington's Disease

http://alzheimers.about.com/health/
alzheimers/msubhuntingtons.htm
Links to information and support.

http://www.noah.cuny.edu/neuro/hunting.html
Ask NOAH (New York Online Access to Health)
about Huntington's. Useful information and
links.

Lewy Body Dementia
Lewy-Net

http://www.ccc.nottingham.ac.uk/~mpzjlowe/
lewy/lewyhome.html

Lyme Disease

http://library.LymeNet.org/domino/file.nsf
Links to information about the effects and treatment
of Lyme Disease.

http://www/geocities.com/HotSprings/Oasis/
6455/lyme-links.html
Lots of links to exhaustive information about Lyme
disease.

Memory Quizzes and Memory Improvement Information

http://www.nymemory.org/devig/
memoryquiz.html
Memory Quiz from the New York Memory and
Healthy Aging Services.

http://www.alzheimers.com/health library/
risk/risk_04_sharp.html
How to Stay Mentally Sharp for Life, Part 1.

http://www.alzheimers.com/health library/
risk/risk.05_sharp2.html
How to Stay Mentally Sharp for Life, Part II.

http://www.alzheimers.com/health library/
risk/risk_06_quiz.html
Memory Quiz: How Sharp Are You?

http://www.brain.nwu.edu/core/memory.
htm
A memory test offered by the Cognitive Neurology
and Alzheimer's Disease Center of Northwestern
University.

Menopause

http://www.nymemory.org/devig/index.
html
A site for women addressing memory loss in
menopause, the effect of estrogen therapy and
Alzheimer's.

http://www.alzheimers.com/health library/
treatment/treatment_02_estro.html
Estrogen therapy in women and its apparent effect
on Alzheimer's.

http://pharmacology.about.com/health/
pharmacology/library/weekly/aa980815
.htm
Definition of and treatment for menopause.

Mild Cognitive Impairment

http://www.mayohealth.org/mayo/9903/htm/
memoryto.htm
Definition of Mild Cognitive Impairment. A
state of memory loss somewhere between
that associated with normal aging and that of
Alzheimer's disease.

Multiple Sclerosis

http://www.htlnet.com/msen.html
The online Multiple Sclerosis Education Network.

http://www.ninds.nih.gov/health_and_
    medical/disorders/multiple_sclerosis.htm
Information on multiple sclerosis from the
National Institute of Neurological Disorders
and Stroke.

Niemann-Pick Disease

http://easyweb.easynet.co.uk/vob/alzheimers/
    information/picks_disease.htm
What is Pick's Disease?

http://www.ninds.nih.gov/health_and_
    medical/disorders/niemann.doc.htm
Information on Niemann-Pick disease from the
National Institute of Neurological Disorders and
Stroke.

Nutritional Deficiency Dementia

http://www.alzheimers.com/health library/
    diagnosis/diagnosis_12_nutri.html
A short overview of the condition.

Parkinson's Disease

http://www.ninds.nih.gov/health_and_
    medical/pubs/parkinson_diseasehtr.htm
A thorough look at Parkinson's Disease from the
National Institute of Neurologic Disorders and
Stroke.

http://www.ninds.nih.gov/health_and_
    medical/pubs/parkinson_disease..htr.ht
    m#early symptoms
The early symptoms of Parkinson's Disease.

http://alzheimers.about.com/health/
    alzheimers/msubparkinsons.htm
Links to information and support.

Primary Progressive Aphasia

http://www.brain.nwu.edu/core/PPA.HTM
A site defining Primary Progressive Aphasia.

http://www.cdc.gov/hiv/pubs/faq/faq5.htm
What is Primary Progressive Aphasia?

Pseudodementia of Depression

http://midwestneuro.com/deg/dd
    pseudodemen.htm
The difference between dementia and pseudodementia.

http://midwestneuro.com/deg/dd_
    pseudodemen.htm
A test for pseudodementia.

Stroke/Multi-Infarct Dementia

http://www.ninds.nih.gov/healthandmedical/
    pubs/stroke_hope_through_research.htm
An exhaustive brochure on stroke—types, causes
and therapies.

http://www.alzheimers.com/healthlibrary/
    diagnosis/diagnosis 08 mid.html
Information on multi-infarct dementia.

http://www.ninds.nih.gov/health_and_
    medical/disorders/multi-infarctdementia
    _doc.htm
A mini fact sheet on multi-infarct dementia from
the National Institute of Neurological Disorders
and Stroke.

Wernicke-Korsakoff Syndrome
(Alcohol-related Dementia)

http://www.caregiver.org/factsheets/wks.html
A definition of alcohol-related dementia plus
information on treatment and recommendations
for caregivers.

http://my.webmd.com/content/asset/Miller_
    keane_35782
Definition and information about symptoms.

http://netwellness.org/mhc/top/000771.htm
Causes, incidence, and risk factors.

Wilson's Disease

http://www.ninds.nih.gov/health_and_
    medical/disorders/wilsons_doc.htm
An information sheet on Wilson's Disease from the
National Institute of Neurological Disorders and
Stroke.

APPENDIX V
READ MORE ABOUT IT

AIDS/HIV

Ford, Michael Thomas. *100 Questions & Answers About AIDS: What You Need to Know Now.* New York: William Morrow, 1993.

Stine, Gerald J. *AIDS Update 2000.* Upper Saddle River, N.J.: Prentice Hall, 1999.

Ward, Darrell E. *The Amfar AIDS Handbook: The Complete Guide to Understanding HIV and AIDS.* New York: W. W. Norton, 1998.

ALZHEIMER'S DISEASE

Bellenir, Karen, ed. *Alzheimer's Disease Sourcebook: Basic Consumer Health Information About Alzheimer's Disease, Related Disorders, and Other Dementias.* Detroit, Mich.: Omnigraphics, Inc., 1999.

Cohen, Elwood. *Alzheimer's Disease: Prevention, Intervention, and Treatment.* New Canaan, Conn.: Keats Publishing, 1999.

Davies, Helen D., Jensen, Michael P. *Alzheimer's: The Answers You Need.* Forest Knolls, Calif.: Elder Books, 1998.

Gray-Davidson, Frena. *Alzheimer's Disease Frequently Asked Questions: Making Sense of the Journey.* Lowell, Mass.: Lowell House, 1999.

Hay, Jennifer. *Alzheimer's & Dementia: Questions You Have . . . Answers You Need.* Allentown, Pa.: Peoples Medical Society, 1996.

Kuhn, Daniel, Bennett, David A. *Alzheimer's Early Stages: First Steps in Caring and Treatment.* Alameda, Calif.: Hunter House, 1999.

Lindemann, Nelson, James Lindemann, and Nelson Hilde. *Alzheimer's: Answers to Hard Questions for Families.* New York: Main Street Books, 1997.

Molloy, William, and Paul Caldwell. *Alzheimer's Disease.* Willowdale, Ont., Canada: Firefly Books, 1998.

Rogers, Joseph. *Candle and Darkness: Current Research in Alzheimer's Disease.* Chicago: Bonus Books, 1998.

Snyder, Lisa, LCSW. *Speaking Our Minds: Personal Reflections from Individuals With Alzheimer's.* New York: W. H. Freeman, 1999.

CAREGIVERS' BOOKS

Dowling, James R., and Nancy L. Mace. *Keeping Busy: A Handbook of Activities for Persons With Dementia.* Baltimore: Johns Hopkins University Press, 1995.

Driskoll, Eileen. *Alzheimer: A Handbook for the Caretaker.* Boston:Branden Publishing, 1994.

Edwards, Allen Jack. *When Memory Fails: Helping the Alzheimer's and Dementia Patient.* Cambridge, Mass.: Perseus Press, 1994.

Gray-Davidson, Frena. *The Alzheimer's Sourcebook for Caregivers: A Practical Guide for Getting Through the Day.* Los Angeles: Lowell House, 1996.

Gruetzner, Howard. *Alzheimer's: A Caregiver's Guide and Sourcebook.* New York: John Wiley & Sons, 1992.

Haisman, Pam. *Alzheimer's Disease: Caregivers Speak Out.* Fort Myers, Fla.: Chippendale House Publishers, 1998.

Hamdy, R. C., James M. Turnbull, Joellyn Edwards, and James M. Turnball, eds. *Alzheimer's Disease: A Handbook for Caregivers.* St. Louis: Mosby, 1997.

Hodgson, Harriet. *Alzheimer's: Finding the Words: A Comunication Guide for Those Who Care.* New York: John Wiley & Sons, 1995.

Mace, Nancy L., Peter V. Rabins, M.D., and Paul R. McHugh. *The 36-Hour Day: A Family Guide to Caring for Persons with Alzheimer Disease, Related Dementing Illnesses, and Memory Loss in Later Life.* Baltimore: Johns Hopkins University Press, 1999.

Sheridan, Carmel B. *Failure-Free Activities for the Alzheimer Patient: A Guidebook for Caregivers.* Forest Knolls, Calif.: Elder Books 1987.

CHRONIC FATIGUE

Bell, David S. *The Doctor's Guide to Chronic Fatigue Syndrome.* Cambridge, Mass.: Perseus Press, 1995.

DEMENTIA

Rabens, Peter, et al. *Practical Dementia Care.* Oxford: Oxford University Press, 1999.

DEPRESSION

Mondimore, Francis Mark. *Depression: The Mood Disease (Johns Hopkins Health Book)* Baltimore: Johns Hopkins University Press, 1995.

Perry, Angela R., ed. *Essential Guide to Depression: American Medical Association.* New York: Pocket Books, 1998.

LYME DISEASE

Lang, Denise. *Coping With Lyme Disease: A Practical Guide to Dealing With Diagnosis and Treatment.* New York: Henry Holt, 1997.

MEMORY IMPROVEMENT

Crook, Thomas H., and Brenda D. Adderly. *The Memory Cure.* New York: Pocket Books, 1999.

Green, Cynthia R. *Total Memory Workout: 8 Steps to Maximum Memory Fitness.* New York: Bantam Doubleday Dell, 1999.

Lorayne, Harry, and Jerry Lucas. *The Memory Book.* New York: Ballantine Books, 1996.

Mark, Vernon H., M.D., and Jeffrey P. Mark. *Reversing Memory Loss: Proven Methods for Regaining, Strengthening, and Preserving Your Memory.* Boston: Houghton Mifflin, 2000.

Turkington, Carol A. *12 Steps to a Better Memory.* New York: Plume, 1996.

Yutsis, Pavel, and Lynda Toth. *Why Can't I Remember?: Reversing Normal Memory Loss.* East Rutherford, N.J.: Avery Publishing Group, 1999.

MENOPAUSE

Warga, Claire L. *Menopause and the Mind: The Complete Guide to Coping with Memory Loss, Foggy Thinking, Verbal Confusion, and Other Cognitive Effects of Perimenopause and Menopause.* New York: Simon & Schuster, 1999.

MULTIPLE SCLEROSIS

Barnes, David, and Ian McDonald. *Multiple Sclerosis: Questions and Answers.* Coral Springs, Fla.: Merit Publishing International 2000.

PARKINSON'S DISEASE

Cram, David L. *Understanding Parkinson's Disease: A Self-Help Guide.* Omaha, Neb.: Addicus Books, 1999.

Hutton, J. Thomas, Raye Lynne Dippel, and Nathan Slewett, eds. *Caring for the Parkinson Patient: A Practical Guide.* Amherst, N.Y.: Prometheus Books, 1999.

STROKE

Caplan, Louis R., Dyken, Mark L., Easton, J. Donald. *American Heart Association Family Guide to Stroke Treatment, Recovery, and Prevention.* New York: Times Books, 1996.

Tanner, Dennis C. *The Family Guide to Surviving Stroke and Communication Disorders.* Needham Heights, Mass.: Allyn & Bacon, 1998.

APPENDIX VI
RESEARCH PERIODICALS

American Journal of Clinical Hypnosis
American Society of Clinical Hypnosis 130 East
    Elm Court
Suite 201 Roselle, IL 60172-2000
630-980-4740
Fax: 630-351-8490
e-mail: info@asch.net www.asch.net/journal. him

American Journal of Psychiatry
American Psychiatric Association
1400 K Street NW
Washington, DC 20005
(202) 682-6020
Fax: 202-682-6850
e-mail: apa@psych.org www.ajp.psychiatryonline.
    org
    Presents clinical research and discussion on
current psychiatric issues.

American Journal of Psychology
University of Illinois Press
1325 South Oak Street
Champaign, IL 6 1820-6903
217-333-0950
Fax: 217-244-8082
e-mail: uipress@illinois.edu
www.press.uillinois.edu/journals/ajp.html

American Journal of Physiology
American Physiological Society
9650 Rockville Pike
Bethesda, MD 20814
301-530-7071
http://ajpcon.physiology.org

APA Monitor
American Psychological Association
750 First Street NE
Washington, DC 20002-4242
202-336-5500
800-374-2721
www.apa.org/monitor

American Psychologist
American Psychological Association
750 First Street NE
Washington, DC 20002
202-336-5500
800-374-2721
http://www.apa.org/journals/amp.html

Annals of the New York Academy of Science
New York Academy of Science
2 E. 63rd Street
New York, NY 10021
212-838-0230
e-mail: nyas@nyas.org www.nyas.org

Annual Review of Neuroscience
Annual Reviews, Inc.
4139 El Camino Way
Box 10139
Palo Alto, CA 94303-0139
800-523-8635
650-493-4400
Fax: 650-424-0910 or 650-855-9815
    Presents original reviews of critical literature
and current developments in neuroscience

Annual Review of Psychology
Annual Reviews, Inc.
4139 El Camino Way
Box 10139
Palo Alto, CA 94303
650-493-4400
Fax: 650-424-0910 or 650-855-9815

Apasiology
Taylor and Francis, LTD
Rankine Road
Basingstoke. Hants
England RG24 8PR
+44(0)1256 813000
Fax: +44 (0) 1256 479438
e-mail: Enquiry@taudfco.uk
www.taylorandfrancis.com/jnls/aph.htm
   Presents information on all aspects of brain damage-related language problems.

Journal of Comparative Psychology
American Psychological Association
750 First Street NE
Washington, DC 20002-4242
202-336-5500
800-374-2721
   Presents laboratory and field studies of behavioral patterns of various species as they relate to development, evolution, etc.

Journal of Experimental Child Psychology
Academic Press
Journals Division
525 B Street
Suite 1900
San Diego, CA 92101-4495
619-231-0926
800-321-5068
http://www.academicpress.com/jecp
   Covers all aspects of behavior in children.

Journal of Experimental Psychology
American Psychological Association
750 First Street NW
Washington, DC 20002-4242
202-336-5500
800-374-2721
http://www.apa.org/journals/xge.html

*Journal of Experimental Psychology: Learning,
   Memory & Cognition*
American Psychological Association
750 First Street NE
Washington, DC 20002-4242
202-336-5500

800-374-2721
http://www.apa.org/journals/xlm.html
   Presents experimental studies of fundamentals of encoding, transfer, memory and cognition processes in human behavior.

Journal of General Psychology
Heldref Publications
1319 18th Street NW
Washington, DC
20036-1802
202-296-6267
800-365-9753
Fax: 202-296-5149
e-mail: tkelly@heldref.org
www.heldref.org

Journal of Geriatric Psychiatry
International Universities Press
Journals Dept.
59 Boston Post Road
P.O. Box 1524
Madison, CT 06443-1524
203-245-4000
   Presents research in the field of geriatric psychiatry, Auheimer's disease.

Journal of Gerontology
Gerontological Society of America
1030 15th Street NW
Suite 250
Washington, DC 20005-1503
202-842-1275
Fax: 202-842-1150
www.geron.org/journals/gsapub.html

Journal of Mind and Behavior
Institute of Mind and Behavior
Box 522
Village Station, NY 10014
212-595-4853
   Presents articles on the theory of consciousness, mind and body epistemology, etc.

Journal of Nervous and Mental Disease
Lippincott Williams and Wilkins
2107 Insurance Way

Hagerstown, MD 21740
www.jonmd.com.custserv/ww.com
   Presents studies in social behavior and neurological science.

Journal of Neurology, Neurosurgery and Psychiatry
BMJ Publishing Group
BMA House
Tavistock Square
London, England WC1H 9JR
+44 (0) 171 387 4499
http://jnnp.bmjjournals.com
   Presents reports on clinical neurology, neurosurgery, neuropsychology, neuropsychiatry

Journal of Neuroscience
Society for Neuroscience
11 Dupont Circle NW
Suite 500
Washington, DC 20036
202-462-6688
Fax: 202-462-1547
e-mail: Jn@sfn.org
www.jneurosci.org

Allschwilerstr. 10
P.O. Box CH4009
Basel Switzerland
061-3061111
   Presents information on the neural bases of cognitive dysfunction (such as in Parkinson's disease, Alzheimer's disease, Huntington's disease).

Developmental Psychbiology
John Wiley & Sons
Journals
605 3rd Avenue
New York, NY 10158-0012
212-850-6000

Developmental Psychology
American Psychological Association
750 First Street NE
Washington, DC 20002-4242
202-336-5500
800-374-2721
http://www.apa.org/journals/dev.html

Experimental Neurology
Academic Press
525 B Street
Suite 1900
San Diego, CA 92101
619-231-0926
800-321-5068
http://www.academicpress/com/en
   Presents original research in neuroscience.

International Journal of Neuroscience
Gordon & Breach, Science Publishers
P.O. Box 32160
Newark, NJ 07102
800-545-8398

Journal of Abnormal Psychology
American Psychological Association
750 First Street
Washington, DC 20002-4242
202-336-5500
800-374-2721
http://www.apa.org/journals.abn.html
   Artides on basic research and theory in abnormal behavior.

Journal of Applied Developmental Psychology
Ablex Publishing Co.
355 Chestnut Street
Norwood, NJ 07648
201-767-8450

Journal of Applied Psychology
American Psychological Association
750 First Street NE
Washington, DC 20002-4242
202-336-5500
800-374-2721
http://www.apa.org/journals/apa.html
   Presents research on applications of psychology in work settings.

Journal of Child Psychology and Psychiatry and Allied Disciplines
Pergamon Press
Journals Division
660 White Plains Road
Tarrytown, NY 10591-5153

Primarily concerned with child and adolescent psychiatry and psychology.

Journal of Clinical Psychiatry
Physician's Postgraduate Press
P.O. Box 752870
Memphis TN 38175
901-751-3800
Fax: 901-751-3444
   Presents original material on psychiatric behavior and neurological science.

Journal of Clinical Psychology
Clinical Psychology Publishing Co.
4 Conant Square
Branden, VT 05733
802-247-6871

Journal of Cognitive Neuroscience
MIT Press
5 Cambridge Center
Cambridge, MA 02142-1493
617-253-5646
Fax: 617-258-6779
   Presents research on the brain and behavior.

Archives of Child Neuropsychology
Pergamon Press
Journals Division
660 White Plains Road
Tarrytown, NY 19591-5153

Archives of General Psychiatry
American Medical Association
515 N. State Street
Chicago, IL 60610
312-464-0183
http://archneur.ama-assn.org

Behavioral Brain Research
Elsevier Science Publishing Co.
655 Avenue of the Americas
New York, NY 10010-5107
212-633-3730
Fax: 212-633-3680
e-mail: Usinfo-f@elsevier.com

Behavioral Neuroscience
American Psychological Association
750 First Street NE
Washington, DC 20002-4242

202-336-5500
800-374-2721
http://www.apa.org/journals/bne.html

Biological Psychiatry
Elsevier Science Publishing Co.
655 Avenue of the Americas
New York, NY 10010-5107
212-633-3730
Fax: 212-633-3680
e-mail: Usinfo-f@elsevier.com
   Covers the whole range of psychiatric research.

Brain Research
Elsevier Science Publishing Co.
655 Avenue of the Americas
New York, NY 10010-5107
212-633-3730
Fax: 212-633-3680
e-mail: Usinfo-f@elsevier.com
   Presents information on behavioral science and neurology.

Brain Research Bulletin
Pergamon Press
Journals Division
660 White Plains Road
Tarrytown, NY 10591-5153
   Presents a broad spectrum of articles in neuroscience.

Clinical Neurology and Neurosurgery
Elsevier Science Publishing Co.
655 Avenue of the Americas
New York, NY 10010-5107
212-633-3680
Fax: 212-633-3680
e-mail: Usinfo-f@elsevier.com

Cognition
Elsevier Science Publishing Co.
655 Avenue of the Americas
New York, NY 10010-5107
212-633-3680
Fax: 212-633-3680
e-mail: Usinfo-f@elsevier.com

Cognitive Development
Ablex Publishing Co.
355 Chestnut Street
Norwood, NJ 07648

Cognitive Psychology
Academic Press
Journals Division
525 B Street
Suite 1900
San Diego, CA 92101-4495
619-231-0926
800-321-5068
http://www.academic.press.com/cogpsych

Cognitive Science
Ablex Publishing Co.
355 Chestnut Street
Norwood, NJ 07648

Journal of Neuroscience Research
John Wiley & Sons
Journals
605 Third Avenue
New York, NY 10158-0012
212-850-6000
  Presents basic research in molecular cellular aspects of neuroscience.

Journal of Psychology: Interdisciplinary and
  Applied
Heidref Publications
1319 18th Street NW
Washington, DC 20036-1802
202-296-6267
800-365-9753
Fax: 202-296-5149
e-mail: Tkelly@heldref.org
www.heldref.org

The Lancet
655 Avenue of the Americas
New York, NY 10010
800-462-6198
212-633-3850
e-mail: custserv@lancet.com
www.thelancet.com

Neurobiology of Aging
Pergamon Press
Journals Division
660 White Plains Road
Tarrytown, NY 10591-5153

Neuropsychology
American Psychological Association
750 First Street NE
Washington, DC 20002-4242
202-336-550
800-374-2721
http://www.apa.org/journals/neuro.html
  Presents information in clinical neuropsychology, especially neuropsychological measurement techniques and psychosocial adjustment of patients.

New England Journal of Medicine
Massachusetts Medical Society
860 Winter Street
Waltham Woods Corporate Center
Waltham, MA 02451-1411
781-893-3800
www.nejm.org

Proceedings of the National Academy of Science
National Academy of Science
2102 Constitution Avenue
Washington, DC 20418
202-334-2672
Fax: 202-334-2739

Psychiatry Research
Elsevier Science Publishing Co.
655 Avenue of the Americas
New York, NY 10010-5107
212-633-3730
e-mail: Usinfo-f@elsevier.com

Psychological Bulletin
American Psychological Association
750 First Street NW
Washington, DC 20002-4242
202-336-5500
800-374-2721
http://www.apa.org/journals/bul.html

Psychology and Aging
American Psychological Association
750 First Street NE
Washington, DC 20002-4242
http://www.apa.org/journals/pag.html

Surgical Neurology
Elsevier Science Publishing Company
655 Avenue of the Americas
New York, NY 10010-5107

212-633-3730
Fax: 212-633-3680
e-mail: Usinfo-f@elsevier.com

Trends in Neuroscience
Elsevier Science Publishing Co.

655 Avenue of the Americas
New York, NY 10010-5107
212-633-3730
Fax: 212-633-3730
e-mail: Usinfo-f@elsevier.com

GLOSSARY

absolute refractory period The period after an impulse has been triggered during which a nerve fiber cannot carry a second impulse.

acetylcholine A neurotransmitter that appears to be involved in learning and memory. Acetylcholine is severely diminished in the brains of people with Alzheimer's disease.

acetylcholinesterase (AchE) Enzyme that stops the action of acetylcholine.

action potential The electrical "all-or-none" impulse that transmits information within the nervous system.

activities of daily living (ADLs) Personal care activities necessary for everyday living, such as eating, bathing, grooming, dressing, and toileting. People with dementia may not be able to perform necessary functions without assistance. Professionals often assess a person's ADLs to determine what type of care is needed.

adrenergic Term that means "associated with catecholamines."

agonist Chemical that increases the effect of a neurotransmitter.

allele One of two or more alternative forms of a gene. For example, one allele of the gene for eye color may code for blue eyes, while another allele may code for brown eyes.

amino acids The basic building blocks of proteins. Genes contain the code for the production of the 20 amino acids necessary for human growth and function.

amyloid A protein deposit associated with tissue degeneration; amyloid is found in the brains of individuals with Alzheimer's.

amyloid plaque Abnormal cluster of dead and dying nerve cells, other brain cells, and amyloid protein fragments. These plaques are one of the characteristic abnormalities found in the brains of people with Alzheimer's disease. The presence of amyloid plaques and neurofibrillary tangles on autopsy positively diagnose Alzheimer's disease.

amyloid precursor protein (APP) A normal protein found in the brain, heart, kidneys, lungs, spleen, and intestines from which beta amyloid protein is formed. In Alzheimer's disease, APP is cut and releases beta amyloid protein, which then forms clumps called amyloid plaques.

antagonist Chemical that blocks the action of a neurotransmitter.

anterior A directional term meaning "toward the front."

apolipoprotein E (ApoE) A protein that ferries cholesterol through the bloodstream. The ApoE gene has three variants, E2, E3, and E4. Each person inherits one variant from each parent. ApoE4 is the form of the gene that occurs more often in people with Alzheimer's disease than in the general population. E2 and E3 may protect against the disease.

astrocyte (astroglia) A glial cell that supports nerve cells.

axon A long wirelike nerve fiber extending from the cell body of a neuron that sends nerve impulses (messages) to other neurons. In large nerves, the axon is covered with a sheath made of myelin.

beta-amyloid protein A specific type of protein normally found in humans and animals. In Alzheimer's disease, it is found in the core of plaques in the brain.

blood-brain barrier The selective barrier membrane that controls the entry of substances from the blood into the brain.

caudal A directional term that means "toward the tail end."

cell The smallest unit of a living organism that is capable of functioning independently.

cell body Also called the soma, this is the part of the cell that contains the nucleus.

central nervous system (CNS) One of the two major divisions of the nervous system. Composed of the brain and spinal cord, the CNS is the control network for the entire body.

cerebral cortex The outer layer of the brain, consisting of nerve cells and the pathways that connect them. The cerebral cortex is the part of the brain in which thought processes (including learning, language and reasoning) take place.

cerebrospinal fluid (CSF) The fluid that fills the areas surrounding the brain and spinal cord.

choline A natural substance required by the body that is obtained from various foods, such as eggs; an essential component of acetylcholine.

choline acetyltransferase (CAT) An enzyme that controls the production of acetylcholine.

cholinergic system The system of nerve cells that uses acetylcholine as its neurotransmitter.

cholinesterase Members of a class of enzymes that break down choline esters, such as acetylcholine.

chromosome An H-shaped structure inside the cell nucleus made up of tightly coiled strands of genes. Each chromosome is numbered (in humans, 1–46), and contains DNA, sequences of which make up genes.

cognitive abilities Mental abilities such as judgment, memory, learning, comprehension, and reasoning.

cortisol The major natural glucocortocoid (GC) in humans. It is the primary stress hormone.

cytoplasm Cell material (including membranes, organelles, and fluid), not including the nucleus.

dendrites Branched extensions of the nerve cell body that receive signals from other nerve cells. Each nerve cell usually has many dendrites.

differentiation Process of change during the development of a cell.

DNA The abbreviation for deoxyribonucleic acid, the genetic material of the cell located in the nucleus.

enzyme A protein produced by living organisms that promotes or otherwise influences chemical reactions.

excitability The general capacity of cells to respond to irritation; this is highly enhanced in neurons and receptors.

extracellular spaces Fluid-filled areas between neighboring cells.

fibril A very tiny fiber or hairlike structure at the end of the axon.

free radicals Also called oxygen free radicals, these are oxygen molecules with an unpaired electron that is highly reactive, combining easily with other molecules and sometimes damaging other cells. Antioxidants deactivate free radicals.

ganglia Small groups of neurons in which nerve signals are processed.

gene The biological unit of heredity. Each gene is located at a specific spot on a particular chromosome, and is made up of a string of chemicals arranged in a certain sequence along the DNA molecule.

glia A cell type that makes up the supportive tissue of the central nervous system. The brain is made up of glial cells and the much larger nerve cells.

habituate Gradual adaptation to an irritation (in nerve cells) that causes a decrease or halt to the generation of nerve impulses.

hippocampus An area buried deep in the forebrain that helps regulate emotion and is important for learning and memory.

homeostasis The general capacity of a living organism to adjust to a chemical or physical stress so as to preserve a stable activity.

hormones Chemicals used by the endocrine system to transmit messages.

hyperpolarization An increase in the resting electrical potential across a nerve cell membrane.

infarct A small area of dead brain tissue.

ions Charged particles generated from atoms or molecules by the loss or acquisition of electrons; this is important in neurons as a source of electrical potential.

lesions Tissue damage that may be caused by trauma or disease.

membrane Thin covering of a cell or tissue. Neurons are covered by a very thin membrane through which transmitter chemicals pass.

mitochondria   Organelles found in all animal cells that are concerned with energy transformation.

motor end plate   A flat disk at the end of a nerve. Motor end plates connect the nerve to the muscle.

myelin   The fatty substance that surrounds axons and insulates the nerve.

myelin sheath   A protein-based membrane surrounding the body of the nerve cell that acts as insulation. The growth of the myelin sheath is associated with increased efficiency in the neuron's ability to carry nerve impulses. Brain damage frequently takes the form of destruction of the myelin sheath, causing death of the neuron.

nerve   Bundle of axons through which signals pass to and from the brain.

nerve cell (neuron)   The basic working unit of the nervous system. The nerve cell is typically composed of a cell body containing the nucleus, several short branches (dendrites), and one long arm (the axon) with short branches along its length and at its end.

nerve fiber   Structures of a neuron, aside from the cell body; nerve fibers include such things as dendrites and axons.

nerve growth factor   A substance that occurs naturally in the body and enhances the growth and survival of cholinergic nerves.

nerve tracts   Concentrations of parallel nerve axons running through the body.

neuroglial cells   Special cells that are packed around and between the neurons that help support the delicate nervous tissue.

neuromuscular junction   The synapse where motor nerves contact a muscle.

neuron   The cellular unit of the central and peripheral nervous systems.

neurotransmitter   A chemical the nervous system uses to carry messages from one neuron to another.

paresis   Muscular weakness caused by disease of the nervous system that is usually considered to be a lesser degree of weakness than full paralysis, although the two words may be used interchangeably.

peptide   Short chain of amino acids.

permeability   A measure of how porous a membrane is to molecules.

polarization   The net difference in electrical charge generated across a membrane.

protein   A molecule made up of amino acids arranged in a certain order. Proteins include neurotransmitters, enzymes, and many other substances.

receptor   A site on a nerve cell that receives a specific neurotransmitter; the message receiver.

reflex   An automatic response of the body that, at first, does not involve the brain, such as jerking away a hand from a flame.

refractory period   The period of time necessary for the nerve-cell membrane to repolarize so that another impulse can pass.

resting membrane potential   The electrical imbalance that exists across a normal, living cell membrane.

rods   Light-sensitive cells in the retina in the shape of rods.

semipermeable membrane   A type of membrane that only certain small molecules can penetrate.

skull   The part of the skeleton that makes up the head, protecting the brain, eyes, and ears.

synapse   The tiny gap between two nerve cells; messages are transmitted across this gap from one nerve cell to another, usually by a neurotransmitter.

synaptic vesicle   A capsule that contains sacs of neurotransmitters behind the presynaptic membrane.

threshold   The level at which a depolarization is just enough to cause an action potential in an axon.

transmitter   See *neurotransmitter.*

vesicle   A small saclike structure that forms the brain during fetal development.

REFERENCES

Aartson, M. J., M. Martin, and D. Zimprich. "Gender Differences in Level and Change of Cognitive Functioning: Results from the Longitudinal Aging Study in Amsterdam." *Gerontology* 50 (2003): 35–38.

Abel, E. L. "Fetal Alcohol Syndrome: A Cautionary Note." *Current Pharmacy Design* 12 (2006): 1,521–1,529.

Accornero, V. H., et al. "Prenatal Cocaine Exposure: An Examination of Childhood Externalizing and Internalizing Behavior Problems at Age 7 Years." *Epidemiology, Psychiatry, and Society* 15 (2006): 20–29.

Achenbach, T. M. "What Is Normal? What Is Abnormal: Developmental Perspectives on Behavioral and Emotional Problems." In *Developmental Psychopathology: Perspectives on Adjustment, Risk, and Disorder,* edited by S. S. Luthar et al., 93–114. New York: Cambridge University Press, 1997.

Adolph, K. E., and A. S. Joh. "Multiple Learning Mechanisms in the Development of Action." In *Learning and the Infant Mind,* edited by A. Needham and A. Woodward. New York: Oxford University Press, 2008.

Aggarwal, N. T., et al. "The Apolipoprotein E Epsilon4 Allele and Incident Alzheimer's Disease in Persons with Mild Cognitive Impairment." *Neurocase* 11(2005): 3–7.

Aimone, J. B., J. Wiles, and F. H. Gage. "Potential Role for Adult Neurogenesis in the Encoding of Time in New Memories." *Nature Neuroscience* 9 (June 1, 2006): 723–727.

Alessi, C. A. "Sleep." In *Encyclopedia of Gerontology,* edited by J. E. Birren. San Diego, Calif.: Academic Press, 2007.

Allen, P. A., E. Ruthru, and M. C. Lien. "Attention." In *Encyclopedia of Gerontology,* edited by J. E. Birren. San Diego, Calif.: Academic Press, 2007.

Alvik, A, et al. "Alcohol Consumption before and during Pregnancy Comparing Concurrent and Retrospective Reports." *Alcohol: Clinical and Experimental Reports* 30 (2006): 510–515.

American Chronicle. "Christmas Cheer—Leaded or Unleaded?" Available online. URL: http://www.americanchronicle.com/articles/viewArticle.asp?articlelD=45463. Accessed January 3, 2008.

American Psychological Association. "Getting in Touch with Your Inner Brainwaves through Biofeedback." Available online. URL: http://www.psychologymatters.org/biofeedback.html. Downloaded February 14, 2008.

Amos, D., and S. P. Johnson. "Learning by Selection: Visual Search and Object Perception in Young Infants." *Developmental Psychology* 42 (2006): 1,236–1,245.

Anderson, C. A. "Video Games and Aggressive Behavior." In *Kids Stuff: Marketing Sex and Violence to America's Children.* Baltimore, Md.: Johns Hopkins University Press, 2003.

Anderson, C. A., D. A. Gentile, and K. E. Buckley. *Violent Video Game Effects on Children and Adolescents.* New York: Oxford University Press, 2007.

Anstey, K. J., et al. "Smoking as a Risk Factor for Dementia and Cognitive Decline: A Meta–Analysis of Prospective Studies." *American Journal of Epidemiology* 166 (2007).

Anthony, A. C. "Role of Folic Acid in Nutrient Delivery and Fetal Development." *American Journal of Clinical Nutrition* 85 (2007): 5,985–6,035.

Arendt, R. E., et al. "Children Prenatally Exposed to Cocaine: Developmental Outcomes and Environmental Risks at Seven Years of Age." *Journal of Developmental and Behavioral Pediatrics* 25 (2004): 83–90.

Arkowitz, Hal, and Scott O. Lilienfeld. "Can Antidepressants Cause Suicide?" *Scientific American Mind* 18 (September 1, 2007): 80–83.

———. "Facts and Fictions in Mental Health." *Scientific American Mind* 18 (March 1, 2007): 80–81.

Arvanitakas, Z., et al. "Diabetes and Function in Different Cognitive Systems in Older Adults Without Dementia." *Diabetes Care* 29 (2006): 560–565.

Aslin, R. N., and A. L. Lathrop. "Visual Perception." In *Handbook of Infant and Early Childhood Development,* edited by M. Haith and J. Benson. London: Elsevier, 2008.

Associated Press. "Mattel Issues New Massive China Toy Recall." Available online. URL: http://www.msnbc.msn.com/id/20254745/. Accessed January 3, 2008.

Avgil, M., and A. Ornoy. "Herpes Simplex Virus and Epstein-Bar Virus Infections in Pregnancy: Consequences of Neonatal or Intrauterine Infection.' *Reproductive Toxicology* 21 (2006): 436–445.

Babcock, Hilary M., with National Institutes of Health. *"Acute Cytomegalovirus (CMV) Infection."* Available online. URL: http://www.nlm.nih.gov/medlineplus/ency/article/000568.htm.

Beaver, John D., et aI. "Individual Differences in Reward Drive Predict Neural Responses to Images of Food." *Journal of Neuroscience* 26, no. 19 (2006): 5,160–5,166.

Binns, Corey. "The Hidden Power of Culture." *Scientific American Mind* 18 (September 1, 2007): 9.

———. "Social Rhythm." *Scientific American Mind* 18 (September 1, 2007): 10.

Blakeslee, Sandra, and Matthew Blakeslee. *The Body Has a Mind of Its Own: How Body Maps in Your Brain Help You Do (Almost) Everything Better.* New York: Random House, 2007.

———. "Where Mind and Body Meet." *Scientific American Mind* 18 (September 1, 2007): 44–49.

Bouvier, S. E., and S. A. Engel. "Behavioral Deficits and Cortical Damage Loci in Cerebral Achromatopsia." *Cerebral Cortex* 16, no. 2 (February 1, 2005): 183–191.

Canadian Pediatric Society. Infectious Diseases and Immunization Committee. "Autistic Spectrum Disorder: No Causal Relationship with Vaccines." Available online. URL: http://www.cps.ca/ENGLISH/statements/ID/PlDnoteJun07.htm. Accessed January 14, 2008.

Centers for Disease Control and Prevention. *Fact Sheet:* "Toxoplasmosis." Available online. URL: http://www.cdc.gov/toxoplasmosis/. Accessed February 15, 2008.

Choisser, Bill. "Face Blind!" Available online. URL: http://www.choisser.com/faceblind/. Accessed January 1, 2007.

Citizencain. "Slouching Toward Truth: Autism and Mercury." Available online. URL: http://citizencain.blogspot.com/2005/11/slouching–toward–truth–autism–and–30.html. Accessed February 15, 2008.

Diamond, Marian C., and Arnold B. Scheibel. *The Human Brain Coloring Book.* New York: Collins, 1986.

Doja, A., and W. Roberts. "Immunizations and Autism: A Review of the Literature." *Canadian Journal of Neurological Sciences* 33, no. 4 (2006): 341–346.

Dweck, Carol S. "The Secret to Raising Smart Kids." *Scientific American Mind* 18 (January 1, 2007): 37–41.

Ebbinghaus, Hermann. *Memory: A Contribution to Experimental Psychology.* New York: Dover Publications, 1964.

Education.Com. "Toy Recall Update: Mattel Recalls 9 Million Toys." Available online. URL: http://www.education.com/magazine/article/Mattel/education.com. Accessed January 3, 2008.

Egner, T., and J. H. Gruzelier. "Ecological Validity of Neurofeedback: Modulation of Slow Wave EEG Enhances Musical Pertormance." *NeuroReport* 14 (2003): 1,221–1,224.

Fields, R. Douglas. "New Brain Cells Go to Work." *Scientific American Mind* 18 (September 1, 2007): 30–35.

———. "Sex and the Secret Nerve." *Scientific American Mind* 18 (March 1, 2007): 20–27.

Frenkel, Karen A. "Continuing Effects of 9/11." *Scientific American Mind* 18 (September 1, 2007): 9.

———. "How Do Neurons Communicate?" *Scientific American Mind* 17 (January 1, 2007): 12–13.

Freud, Sigmund. *The Psychopathology of Everyday Life.* New York: W. W. Norton, 1960.

Frith, Chris. *Making up the Mind: How the Brain Creates Our Mental World.* Hoboken, N.J.: Wiley–Blackwell, 2007.

Frost, Randy O., Gail Steketee, and Kamala A. I. Greene. "Cognitive and Behavioral Treatment of Compulsive Hoarding." *Brief Treatment and Crisis Intervention* 3 (2003): 323–338.

Fuchs, T., et al. "Neurofeedback Treatment for Attention–Deficit/Hyperactivity Disorder in Children: A Comparison with Methylphenidate." *Applied Psychopathology & Biofeedback* 28 (2003): 1–12.

Gardner, Howard. "Mind Explorers Merge Their Maps." Books of the Times. *New York Times* (February 8, 1991). Available online. URL: nytimes.com. Accessed May 28, 2008.

Geier, D. A., and M. R. Geier. "An Assessment of Downward Trends in Neurodevelopmental Disorders in the United States Following Removal of Thimerosal from Childhood Vaccines." *Medical Science Monitor* 12, no. 6 (May 29, 2006): CR231–239.

Goldacre, B. "Opinions from the Medical Fringe Should Come with a Health Warning." Available online. URL: http://www.guardian.co.uk/science/2007/feb/24/badscience.uknews. Accessed January 14, 2008.

Grimm, Oliver. "Addicted to Food?" *Scientific American Mind* 18 (May 1, 2007): 36–39.

Grueter, Thomas. "Forgetting Faces." *Scientific American Mind* 18 (September 1, 2007): 68–73.

Grueter, Thomas, and Martina Grueter. "Prosopagnosia in Biographies and Autobiographies." *Perception* 36, no. 2 (2007): 299–301.

Halpern, Diane F., et al. "Sex, Math, and Scientific Achievement." *Scientific American Mind* 18 (January 1, 2007): 44–49.

Hammad, T. A., T. Laughren, and J. Racoosin. "Suicidality in Pediatric Patients Treated with Antidepressant Drugs." *Archives of General Psychiatry* 63, no. 3 (March 1. 2006): 332–339.

Healy, D. *Let Them Eat Prozac: The Unhealthy Relationship Between the Parmaceutical Industry and Depression.* New York: New York University Press, 2004.

Hervey, A. S., J. N. Epstein, and J. F. Curry. "Neuropsychology of Adults with Attention-Deficit/Hyperactivity Disorder: A Meta-Analytic Review." *Neuropsychology* 18, no. 3 (July 1, 2004): 485–503.

Hodges, J. R., et al. "The Differentiation of Semantic Dementia and Frontal Lobe Dementia (Temporal and Frontal Variants of Frontotemporal Dementia) from Early Alzheimer's Disease: A Comprehensive Neuropsychological Study." *Neuropsychology* 13, no. 1 (January 1, 1999): 31–40.

Inman, Mason. "White Matter Listens In." *Scientific American Mind* 18 (September 1, 2007): 8.

Institute of Medicine. "Immunization Safety Review: Measles-Mumps-Rubella Vaccine and Autism." 2001. Available online. URL: http://www.iom.edu/Object.File/Master/4/132/ISR-MMR-4Pager.pdf. Accessed January 14, 2007

Janet, Pierre-Marie-Félix. *La Medicine Psychologique.* Paris: E. Flammarion, 1923.

———. *The Mental State of Hystericals: A Study of Mental Stigmata and Mental Accidents.* New York: G. P. Putnam's Sons, 1901.

Kaufman, Alan S., and Elizabeth O. Lichtenberger. *Assessing Adolescent and Adult Intelligence,* 3rd ed. New Haven, Conn.: Worth Publishers, 2005.

Kee, N., et al. "Preferential Incorporation of Adult-Generated Granule Cells into Spatial Memory Networks in the Dentate Gyrus." *Nature Neuroscience* 10 (March 1, 2007): 355–362.

Kennerknecht, Ingo, et al. "First Report of Prevalence of Non-Syndromic Hereditary Prosopagnosia (HPA)." *American Journal of Medical Genetics* 140, no. 15 (2006): 1,617–1,622.

KidsHealth for Parents. "Infections: Cytomegalovirus" Available online. URL: http://www.kidshealth.org/parent/infections/bacterial_viral/cytomegalovirus.html. Accessed November 1, 2007.

———. "Pervasive Developmental Disorders." Available online. URL: http://kidshealth.org/parent/medical/learning/pervasive_develop_disorders.html. Accessed November 1, 2007.

Kolb, Brian, and Ian O. Whishaw. *Fundamentals of Human Neuropsychology.* New Haven, Conn.: Worth Publishers, 2008.

Lezak, M. *Neuropsychological Assessment.* New York: Oxford University Press, 2004.

Lorayne, Harry, and Jerry Lucas. *The Memory Book.* New York: Dorset Press, 1974.

Luria, A. R. *The Mind of a Mnemonist.* New York: Basic Books, 1968.

Lynchburg News & Advance. "Protecting Virginia's Toy Shelves." Available online. URL: http://www.newsadvance.com/servlet/Satellite?pagename=LNA%2FGMArticle%2FLNA_BasicArticle&c=MGArticle&cid=1173354074839&path=!news!opinion. January 3, 2008.

Monastra, V. J., D. M. Monastra, and S. George. "The Effects of Stimulant Therapy, EEG Biofeedback, and Parenting Style on the Symptoms of Attention-Deficit/Hyperactivity Disorder." *Applied Psychopathology & Biofeedback* 27 (2002): 231–249.

"Most Americans Can't Spot Stroke Warning Signs." Available online. URL: http://ori.msnbc.msn.com/id/24527358/wid/11915829/. Accessed June 23, 2008.

National Institute of Neurological Disorders and Stroke. "NINDS Pervasive Developmental Disorders Information Page." Available online. URL: http://www.ninds.nih.gov/disorders/pdd/pdd.htm. Accessed November 1, 2007.

National Institutes of Health. "Acute Cytomegalovirus (CMV) Infection. MedlinePlus." Available online. URL: http://www.nlm.nih.gov/medlineplus/ency/article/000568.htm. Accessed February 15, 2008.

National Stroke Association. "Act F.A.S.T. If Someone Might Be Having a Stroke." Available online. URL: http://www.stroke.org. Accessed June 20, 2008.

NewsInferno.Com. "Worst Toy Recall List Includes Aqua Dots, Fisher-Price Power Wheels." Available online. URL: http://www.newsinferno.com/archives/2293. Accessed January 3, 2008.

Novella, Stella. "The Anti-Vaccination Movement." *Skeptical Inquirer* 31 (November 1, 2007): 26–31.

O'Toole, M. E. *The School Shooter: A Threat Assessment Perspective.* Washington, D.C.: Federal Bureau of Investigation, 1999.

Ramachandran, Vilayanur S., and Diane Rogers Ramachandran. "Touching Illusions." *Scientific American Mind* 17 (January 1, 2007): 14–16.

Robertz, Frank J. "Deadly Dreams." *Scientific American Mind* 18 (September 1, 2007): 52–59.

Sachan, Dinsa. "Behave Yourself!" *Scientific American Mind* 18 (September 1, 2007): 11.

Sanfey, A. G., et al. "The Neural Basis of Economic Decision–Making in the Ultimatum Game." *Science* 300 (June 13, 2003): 1,755–1,758.

School Violence Resource Center. "Fact Sheet: Youth Risk Factors. 2001." Available online. URL: http://www.svrc.net/Files/RiskFactors.pdf. Accessed December 1, 2007.

Schrock, Karen. "Freeing a Locked-in Mind." *Scientific American Mind* 18 (May 1, 2007): 40–45.

Snyder, Peter J., Paul D. Nussbaum, and Diana L. Robins, eds. *Clinical Neuropsychology: A Pocket Handbook for Assessment.* Washington, D.C.: American Psychological Association, 2005.

Strauss, Esther, Elisabeth M. S. Sherman, and Otfried Spreen. *A Compendium of Neuropsychological Tests: Administration, Norms, and Commentary,* 3rd ed. Oxford: Oxford University Press, 2006.

Volkow, Nora D., and Roy A. Wise. "How Can Drug Addiction Help Us Understand Obesity?" *Nature Neuroscience* 8, no. 5 (2005): 555–560.

whonamedit.com. "Pierre Marie Felix Janet." Available online. URL: http://www.whonamedit.com/doctor.cfm/2467.html. Accessed February 15, 2008.

WRAL-TV. "Toy Recalls Due to Lead Are 'a Real Concern.'" Available online. URL: http://www.wral.com/5onyourside/story/1994322/. Accessed January 3, 2008.

INDEX

Note: Page numbers in **boldface** indicate the major discussion of a topic.

A

AAMI (age-associated memory impairment). *See* mild cognitive impairment

AAP. *See* American Academy of Pediatrics

abacavir 12

abaissement du niveau mental **1**, 176

abducens nerve (sixth cranial nerve) **1**, 63, 75. *See also* cranial nerves

abortive poliomyelitis 299

ABR test. *See* auditory brain stem response (ABR) test

abscess, brain **1–2**

absence seizure. *See* petit mal seizure

abstract memory **2**

academic skills disorders 191, 194–195

acalculia **2–3**, 68–69

ACE (angiotensin-converting enzyme) inhibitors 41

acetaminophen 101, 159, 233, 234, 321

acetylcholine **3**

    Alzheimer's disease and 3, 6, 9, 18, 19, 20, 58, 93–94, 121, 135, 149, 316, 348

    blockers 30, 319

    drop in, with age 6, 9

    functions 63, 65, 93

    levels of, increasing 92, 93–94, 120, 269, 375

    and memory 293

    myasthenia gravis and 246

    nicotine and 268

    nucleus basalis of Meynert and 273

    parasympathetic nervous system and 282

    production of 55, 93, 364

acetylcholinesterase 3, 149, 316

acetylcholinesterase inhibitors 20, 149

acetyl-L-carnitine (ALC) **3**

achievement tests 70, 79, 175

acoustic nerve (auditory nerve; cochlear nerve) **3**, 4, 162, 366

acoustic neuroma **3–4**, 70

acoustic reflex **4**

acquired immunodeficiency syndrome. *See* AIDS

acquisition **4–5**

ACTH. *See* adrenocorticotropic hormone

ACTH-secreting pituitary tumors 296

action potential 118

activities of daily living (ADLs) 68

Actonel (risedronate sodium) 281

acupuncture 134, 234

acute idiopathic polyneuritis. *See* Guillain-Barré syndrome

acute (reversible) organic brain syndrome 322

acyclovir 57, 131

Adam. *See* Ecstasy

adaptive skill areas, assessment of 227

ADC. *See* AIDS dementia complex

ADD. *See* attention deficit disorder (ADD) with or without hyperactivity

Adderall (amphetamine) 46

addiction **5–6**

    alcohol 5, 13, 360. *See also* alcoholism

    amphetamines 5, 26

    barbiturates 5, 54

    brain systems underlying 344

    cocaine 5, 97, 344

    defined 5

    endorphins and 134

    and hallucinogens 158

    nicotine 5, 268–269

    opiates 164, 277

    Ritalin exposure and 46

adenosine receptors, caffeine and 82

adenosine triphosphate (ATP) 152, 171

Ader, Robert 171

ADH (antidiuretic hormone). *See* vasopressin

ADLs. *See* activities of daily living

adolescents, antidepressants and 32

adrenal gland 6, 116, 137, 272

adrenaline **6**. *See also* epinephrine

adrenocorticotropic hormone (ACTH) **6**, 104, 143, 296

advertising, subliminal 344

AFP. *See* alpha-fetoprotein

African Americans, stroke risk 342

age-associated memory impairment (AAMI). *See* mild cognitive impairment

age spots 87

aging and memory **6–9**, 297, 310

aging and the brain **9–10**. *See also* elderly; senility

    brain plasticity 297–298

    brain weight 79

    cognitive changes, normal, *vs.* dementia 114

    context processing **102–103**

    dementia risk 114

    dopamine levels 102

    melatonin levels 212

    mental decline

        causes of 6–7, 9–10, 16

        diagnosis and treatment 3, 7, 8–9, 10, 16

        types of 7–8, 9

    and stroke risk 341, 342

agnosia **10–11**. *See also* anosognosia; auditory agnosia; prosopagnosia

agraphia **11**, 34, 36–37, 68–69, 275. *See also* apraxia; dysphasia

AIDS and the brain **11**. *See also* TORCH disorders

    in children 12, 229

    complications 11–12, 70, 109, 116

    neurological manifestations **259–260**

    treatment and outlook 260

AIDS dementia complex (ADC) **11–12**, 70

Albert, Marilyn 61

ALC. *See* acetyl-L-carnitine

Alcmaeon de Croton 62

alcohol and the brain **12–15**. *See also* alcoholism; fetal alcohol effects; fetal alcohol syndrome

    action and effects 5, 12–15, 14, 71, 86, 88, 112, 287, 365

    addiction 5, 13, 360

    bootleg whiskey, and lead poisoning 185–186

    drug interactions 36, 54, 58

    and drug-related dementia 116

    fetal damage 14, 71, 119–120, 189, 227

    memory 7, 14, 23, 25, 60–61, 123, 217, 292

Alcoholics Anonymous 113

alcohol idiosyncratic intoxication **15**. *See also* Korsakoff syndrome

alcoholism

    amnesia in 15, 23, 25, 217, 292

    genetic predisposition toward 14

    imaginary smells in 333

    and neurological damage 13

treatment 113, 308
vitamin deficiency in 14, 208, 369
and Wernicke-Korsakoff syndrome 178–179, 372
alendronate sodium (Fosamax) 281
alertness, and ultradian rhythms 363
Alexandria, library at 164
alexia **15**, 34, 68–69, 275. *See also* agraphia; aphasia; apraxia; dyslexia; dysphasia
Alhazen 63
Alpers' disease **15**, 304
alpha antagonists, uses 349
alphabetical searching **15**
alpha-fetoprotein (AFP) 27, 247, 253
alpha receptor blockers 33
alpha waves **15–16**, 78, 129, 210
alprazolam (Xanax) 20
ALS. *See* amyotrophic lateral sclerosis
altered states of consciousness **16**, 176. *See also abaissement du niveau mental;* dissociation; sleep
aluminum, and Alzheimer's disease 17
Alzheimer, Alois 16, **16**, 58, 273
Alzheimer's disease **16–22**. *See also* Lewy body dementia
    acetylcholine dysfunction in 3, 6, 9, 18, 19, 20, 58, 93–94, 121, 135, 149, 316, 348
    amnesia in 23, 217
    basal forebrain and 55
    beta-amyloid plaques and 16, 17, 18, 21, 22, 26, **58**, 256, 349–350
    causes 35, 72, 93, 333
    cholinergic hypothesis of **93**
    dopamine deficiency in 3
    early onset 16–17, **22**
    incidence 16
    and neurofibrillary tangles 16, 58, **256**, 349–350
    and nucleus basalis of Meynert 93
    prevention 111
    protein kinase C levels 306
    research on 16–18
    risk factors and prevention 16–17, 21–22, 35
    sundowning effect 20
    symptoms and diagnosis 16, 18–19, 20, 114, 116, 235–236
    tau protein and 58, 256, 349–350
    treatment and outlook 3, 17, 19, 58, 93–94, 100, 118, 121, 137, 149, 152, 167, 171, 198, 212, 251, 269, 293, 316, 364, 366
Amanita muscaria mushrooms 157, 158
amantadine 86, 349
ambenonium chloride (Mytelase) 246
amblyopia **22–23**
American Academy of Pediatrics (AAP) 45, 52, 290, 299
American Bar Association 67
American Board of Neurological Surgery 265

American Board of Psychiatry and Neurology (ABPN) 260, 264
American Medical Association 67
American Neurological Association 67
American Psychological Association 92
amino acids **23**
aminoglutethimide 86
amitriptyline (Elavil) 32–33, 46, 235, 305, 320, 360
amnesia **23–25**
    alcohol and 15, 23, 25, 217, 292
    anterograde 23, 217, 352, 358
    basal forebrain and 55
    causes 23–24, 30, 66, 93, 144, 161, 210
    combat **100**
    continuous 25, **103**
    defined 23
    hysterical 24–25, **170**
    infantile 52, **171–172**
    medial temporal lobectomy and 136
    mixed types 24
    organic 24, 217, **279**
    postencephalitic 217
    posthypnotic 24, 229
    posttraumatic 23, 100, 300, 358
    psychogenic 24–25, 103
    research on 178
    retrograde 23, 61, 179, 217, **313–314**, 352, 357, 358
    shrinking retrograde **329**
    source 7, **334**
    transient global **357**, 358
    treatment 24, 220, 364
    types 23–25
amnesia and crime **25**
amnesic drugs 30–31
amnesic syndrome **25**
amniocentesis 27, 247
amobarbital 54
amoxapine (Asendin) 32, 360, 361
amphetamines **25–26**
    action and effects 5, 25–26, 86, 158, 273, 298, 339–340, 364–365
    addiction 5, 26
    chemical similarity to noradrenaline 340
    circadian rhythm and 96
    uses 36, 46
Amphotericin B 109
ampicillin 225
amputated limbs, phantom pain in 297
amusia 26, 68–69
amygdala 6, 9, **26**, 55, 64, 136, 210, 213
amyloid. *See* beta-amyloid protein
amyloid precursor protein (APP) 17, **26**, 58
amyotrophic lateral sclerosis (ALS; Lou Gehrig's disease) 17, **26–27**, 72, 240, 252
Anafranil. *See* clomipramine
analgesics, uses 282
anandamide 210

anaphylactic shock, treatment of 137
anaplastic astrocytoma 40
anencephaly **27**, 72, 252, 336
anesthetics 86, 98, 282
aneurysm, brain 27, **27–28**, 30
angiography **28**, 128, 374
angioma 342, 343
angiotensin-converting enzyme (ACE) inhibitors 41
animal(s), limbic system in 130
animal magnetism 229, 230
animal memory **28–29**
aniracetam (Draganon; Sarpul; RO 13-5057) **29**, 272, 308
Anna O **29–30**, 79, 121
anoetic consciousness 101–102
anomia **30**, 35
anosmia 333
anosognosia 11, **30**
anoxia **30**, 60, 165
anterior commissure **30**, 327
anterior communicating artery **30**, 343
anterior pituitary 104
anterograde amnesia 23, 217, 352, 358
antianxiety drugs 20, 34, 57–58, 357
antibiotics 123, 333
anticholinergics 3, **30–31**, 53, 112, 116, 241
anticholinergic syndrome 31
anticholinesterase drugs 31, 246
anticoagulant drugs 31, 41, 333, 342, 358
anticonvulsant drugs 31, 60, 86, 131, 132, 136, 149, 342, 361
antidementia drugs 260
antidepressant drugs **31–33**. *See also* cyclics; monoamine oxidase (MAO) inhibitors; selective serotonin reuptake inhibitors; tricyclic antidepressants
    action and effects 86, 119, 268
    side effects 32–33, 123
    tryptophan and 361
    uses 20, 40, 46, 160, 235, 250, 287, 305, 320
antidiuretic hormone (ADH). *See* vasopressin
anti-dyskinetics 86
antiemetic drugs **33**, 131, 234
antifungal drugs 178
antihistamines 31, 46, 86, 123, 333, 365
antihypertensives 123, 333
anti-inflammatory drugs 20, 171. *See also* nonsteroidal anti-inflammatory drugs
antioxidant(s) 20, 21, **33**, 152
antiplatelet drugs 41, 358
antipsychotic drugs 20, 31, **33–34**, 71–72, 128, 258–259, 357. *See also* lithium; neuroleptics
anti-Rh immune globulin 228
antiseizure medications 253, 287, 320
antispasmodic drugs 319
ants, behavioral stimuli 28–29
anvil (incus) 162

anxiety **34**
   antianxiety drugs 20, 34, 57–58, 357
   causes 34, 340
   defense mechanisms **111**
   and déjà vu 112
   GABA and 149
   hallucinogens and 158
   physiological changes in 143
   Tourette syndrome and 355
   treatment of 57, 307, 357
aphasia 11, **34–35**, 79, 371–372. See also
   anomia; Broca's aphasia; conduction
   aphasia; optical aphasia; Wernicke's
   aphasia
Der aphasische Symptomenkomples
   (Wernicke) 372
apnea **35**. See also sleep apnea
apoE. See apolipoprotein E
apolipoprotein E (ApoE) 16–17, **35**
apomorphine 86
apoplexy **35–36**
APP. See amyloid precursor protein
appestat **36**
appetite **36**, 166. See also appestat
appetite stimulants **36**
appetite suppressants **36**, 86
apraxia **36–37**, 315
aprosodia **37**, 180
arachnoid 293
arachnoiditis **37**
arachnoid mater 222
arachnoid membrane **37**
archetype theory (Jung) 98–99
archicortex **37**. See also hippocampus
arcuate fasciculus 180
arecoline 94
Aredia (pamidromate disodium) 281
Aretaeus of Cappadocia **37**
Aricept. See donepezil
Aristotle 63, 74
arithmetic, developmental disorders 195
Arnold-Chiari malformation **37–38**
Aropax. See paroxetine
arteriogram **38**. See also angiography
arteriography, cerebral **38**
arteriosclerosis 38, 116
artery. See anterior communicating artery;
   arteriogram; arteriography, cerebral;
   carotid artery; endarterectomy
articulation, developmental disorders
   194
artificial somnambulism 229
ascending paralysis. See Guillain-Barré
   syndrome
ascending reticular activating system **38**
ASDs. See autism spectrum disorders
Asendin. See amoxapine
Ashkenazi Jews 350
Asians, alcohol and 14
asparate 17
Asperger, Hans 38
Asperger's syndrome **38–40**
aspirin 101, 159, 233, 316, 342, 358

assistive technology, for learning
   disabilities 196
association 40
association areas **40**, 113
Association for Brain Tumor Research
   154
astrocytes 152
astrocytoma **40**, 294
asymmetry in the brain **40–41**, 43
ataxia **41**, 88, 146. See also Friedreich's
   ataxia; Machado-Joseph disease
ataxic gate 211
atenolol (Tenormin) 235
atherosclerosis 35, **41–42**, 133, 174, 212,
   342
athetosis **42**, 124. See also tardive
   dyskinesia
athetotic symptoms, of cerebral palsy 89
ATP. See adenosine triphosphate
atropine 31, 86, 123, 158
attention and the brain **42**, 143
attention deficit disorder (ADD) with or
   without hyperactivity **42**, 193
attention deficit hyperactivity disorder
   (ADHD) **42–48**. See also attention
   disorders; hyperactivity
   brain areas involved in 43
   causes 42–43, 230, 290
   classification of 237
   incidence 42
   and memory 217
   symptoms and diagnosis 39, 43–45,
      191, 193
   Tourette syndrome and 355
   treatment and outlook 45–48, 197,
      230–231
attention disorders 195
attention span, and development of adult
   intelligence 59
auditory agnosia **48**
auditory and visual processing disabilities
   188
auditory brain stem response (ABR) test
   48
auditory cortex **48–49**, 89, 180, 181
auditory-evoked potentials (AEP) **49**,
   261. See also auditory brain stem
   response (ABR) test
auditory hallucinations 353
auditory memory **49**. See also echoic
   memory
auditory nerve. See acoustic nerve
auditory nerve tumor. See acoustic
   neuroma
auditory perception **49**
autism. See autistic disorder
autism, early onset **49–50**
autism spectrum disorders (ASDs) **50–51**,
   51, 72. See also Asperger's syndrome;
   autistic disorder
autistic disorder (autism) 39, 49, **51–52**,
   72, 152, 193, 328. See also Asperger's
   syndrome; autism, early onset

autistic savants **52**, 216
autobiographical memory **52**
autoimmune disorders 245–246, 249,
   345–346. See also multiple sclerosis
automatic gestures **52**
automatic processing **52**
L'Automatisme Psychologique (Psychological
   automatism; Janet) 120, 176
automatism plea 25
autonomic nervous system **52–53**. See also
   dysautonomia; parasympathetic nervous
   system
   damage to 263
   functions 137, 143, 171, 311
   hypothalamus and 200
   neurotransmitters 272
autonomous consciousness 101
Aventyl. See nortriptyline
averaged evoked response **53**
Avonex 245
AX-Continuous Performance Test 102–
   103
axon(s) **53**
   damage to 262
   formation and growth 137, 254
   functions 63, 65, 134, 212–213, 261
   long-term potentiation 162
Ayres, A. Jean 324
AZT. See zidovudine
Aztecs, and hallucinogenic mushrooms
   157

B

Babinski reflex 259
baclofen 86, 205, 304, 334, 349, 361
balance **54**, 87, 143, 366. See also vertigo
balloon angioplasty 28, 41–42
band of Broca 93
Barbital 54
barbiturates 5, **54**, 58, 86, 100, 153. See
   also central nervous system depressants
Bardet-Biedl syndrome 183
Bartlett, Sir Frederic C. **54–55**
basal forebrain 6, 9, **55**. See also
   cholinergic basal forebrain
basal ganglia 43, **55–56**, 64, 85, 89, 163,
   178, 240–241, 284. See also striatum;
   substantia nigra
basic fibroblast-growth factor 252
basilar membrane **56**
Batten disease **56**
B-complex vitamins. See vitamin(s), B-
   complex
behavior, factors affecting 151, 369
behavioral disabilities, classification of
   237
behavioral treatments of memory
   disorders **57**
Bell's palsy **57**, 73
Bender, Lauretta 57
Bender-Gestalt test **57**
benign intracranial hypertension. See
   pseudotumor cerebri

benzodiazepines **57–58**, 120
    action and effects 5, 86, 149
        side effects 58, 123
        uses 34, 54, 338, 357
Berger, Hans 260
besipirdine **58**
beta-amyloid protein 16, 17, 18, 21, 22, 26, **58**, 256, 349–350
beta blockers 40, 41, 123, 235, 357
beta-endorphins. *See* endorphin(s)
beta-interferon, uses 317
Betaseron 245
beta waves **58**, 78, 129, 210
Bias, Len 97
bilateral acoustic NF (BAN). *See* neurofibromatosis
bilirubin 178
Binet, Alfred **58–59**
Binswanger's disease **59**
biofeedback **59–60**, 234
biological clock. *See* circadian rhythm; jet lag; melatonin; seasonal affective disorder
bipolar disorder (manic depression) 32, 33, 48, 60, 201, 212, 319, 356, 357
birds, memory in 29
birth defects 33, 165–166, 262, 266, 354. *See also* anencephaly; Arnold-Chiari malformation; fetal hydantoin syndrome; hydrocephalus; meningocele; microcephaly; myelomeningocele; Prader-Willi syndrome; spina bifida
birth injury to the brain **60**
bisphosphonates 281
blackouts, alcoholic **60–61**
blepharospasm 241
blindsight 275
blood alcohol level 13
blood-brain barrier **61**, 78, 252, 266–267
blood circulation, discovery of 159
blood clots. *See* clot, blood
blood pressure 41, 96–97, 238, 272, 362
blood salts and protein levels, regulation of 280
blood supply to the brain. *See* circulation and the brain
blood transfusion, and West Nile encephalitis 131
blood vessels. *See* angiography; anterior communicating artery; arteriogram; arteriography, cerebral; atherosclerosis; carotid artery; circulation and the brain; endarterectomy
bodily/kinesthetic intelligence 243
body position, sensing of 323
Boe, Franz de la. *See* Sylvius, Franciscus
bone marrow transplantation 255–256
Book of Optics (Alhazen) 63
Boston remote memory battery **61**, 314
Botox 241
Botulinum toxin 205
botulism **61–62**
bovine spongiform encephalopathy. *See* mad cow disease

Boxer's encephalopathy 132
brachytherapy (interstitial radiation; seeding) 154
brain **62–65**. *See also* abscess, brain; aging and the brain; brain in history
        energy source for 138, 155, 169, 173, 208
        structure and function 62, 63–65
brain cancer. *See* cancer, brain
brain cells **65**. *See also* glial cells; neuron(s)
        alcohol's effect on 13
        in brain development 119
        energy source for 138, 155, 169, 173, 208
        number of 67
        research on 209
brain damage **65–66**. *See also* head injury; traumatic brain injury
        effects of 42, 71, 116–117, 163, 168, 188, 324
        exogenous *vs.* endogenous 57
        glutamate and 155
        localized 66
        punch drunk syndrome **307**
        recovery, gender differences 151–152
        transorbital lobotomy and 198
        treatment of 76
brain death **66–67**, 129, 311
brain-derived neurotrophic factor 252
brain development in children **67–68**, 174, 189–190, 208, 267. *See also* development of the brain; fetal brain development; lead poisoning and the brain
brain disorders **68–73**, 82, 217, 264
brain food **73**, 92–93, 198. *See also* malnutrition; nutrition and the brain
brain function tests. *See* electroencephalography; PET scan
brain in history 62–63, **73–74**, 260–261. *See also* Smith, Edwin, surgical papyrus of
brain injury. *See* brain damage
brain mapping. *See* brain scans
brain scans **74–75**
brain size 8, 14–15, 150–151
brain stem **75–76**. *See also* diencephalon; midbrain (mesencephalon); pons
        ascending reticular activating system **38**
        and brain development 67, 119
        coma and 99
        and consciousness 101, 363
        cranial nerves and 104
        functions 62, 64, 75, 162, 163, 311, 323
        locus coeruleus **203**
        osmoreceptors in 280
        research on 143
brain stem encephalitis, rabies and 309
brain syndrome, organic **279**, 366
brain tissue transplants 76

brain tumors **76–78**. *See also* acoustic neuroma; astrocytoma; craniopharyngioma; ependymoma; glioblastoma; hemangioblastoma; medulloblastoma; meningioma; oligodendroglioma
        amnesia in 24
        brain disorders from 70
        cell phones and 77, **85–86**
        in children 77, 78, 255
        and dementia 116–117
        diagnosis 28, 153
        and memory 217–281
        primary v. secondary 70, 76
        staging 255, 276
        symptoms and diagnosis 74, 77
        treatment and outlook 77–78, 339
        types of 70, 76–77
brain waves **78–79**, 190, 210. *See also* alpha waves; beta waves; delta waves; electroencephalography; theta waves
brain weight **79**, 120
BRAT battery **79**
breast cancer, risk factors 138
Breasted, James Henry 334
breathing, control of 79
breathing center **79**
Breuer, Josef 29, **79**, 120–121
British Medical Journal 360
Broca, Pierre-Paul 63, **79–80**, 80, 150, 182–183, 292. *See also* speech
Broca's aphasia 34–35, **80**, 180
Broca's area 34, 63, 65, **80**, 180, 181, 243, 373
bromocriptine (Parlodel) 285, 296
bronchodilators 86
Brown-Peterson task **80–81**
Brown-Sequard, Charles Edouard **81**
buclizine 86
bulbar polio 299
bupropion HCl (Wellbutrin; Zyban) 32
Bush, George H. W. 76
Bush, George W. 76
Buspar. *See* buspirone
buspirone (Buspar) 20, 112
butalbital 234
Butler, Robert 8
Butters, Nelson 141
bypass surgery 42

C

cacosmia 333
CADASIL (cerebral autosomal dominant arteriopathy with subcortical infarcts and leukoencephalopathy) 242
Cade, John 201
cadmium, and brain development in children 189
Cafergot (ergotamine tartrate) 234
caffeine 36, **82**, 86, 339–340
calcium **82–83**, 216
calcium channel blockers 41, 235, 269
calpain 83, **83**, 216

cancer
  AIDS-related 259
  nervous system 254–256
  spinal cord tumors **337**
cancer, brain. *See* acoustic
  neuroma; astrocytoma; brain
  tumors; craniopharyngioma;
  ependymoma; glioblastoma; glioma;
  hemangioblastoma; medulloblastoma;
  meningioma; neuroblastoma;
  neuroectodermal tumors;
  oligodendroglioma; pituitary adenoma;
  pituitary tumors; retinoblastoma
cannabinoid receptors 209–210
cannabinols 158
canned food, botulism and 61–62
Capgras, Jean Marie Joseph 83, **83**
Capgras syndrome **83**
carbamazepine (Tegretol) 31, 40, 60, 86,
  320, 361
carbidopa-L-dopa (Sinemet) 199, 284,
  349
carbon disulfide 356
carbon monoxide poisoning **83–84**
carboplatin 255
carboxylic acid. *See* pyroglutamate
cardiovascular system. *See* circulation and
  the brain
carotid angiography 28
carotid artery **84**, 133
carotid endarterectomy 42, 133
cataplexy **84–85**, 249–250
Catapres. *See* clonidine
catecholamine(s) **85**. *See also* dopamine;
  norepinephrine
CAT scan (computed axial tomography;
  CT scan) 74, **85**, 161, 207, 236, 374
caudate nucleus 43, 55, 64, **85**, 166, 242.
  See also striatum
Cavinton. *See* vinpocetine
CDC. *See* Centers for Disease Control
Celexa. *See* citalopram
cell(s), brain. *See* brain cells; glial cells;
  neuron(s)
cell body **85**
cell phones and brain tumors 77, **85–86**
cellular rhythms. *See* circadian rhythm
Centers for Disease Control (CDC) 12, 62,
  95, 110, 184, 185, 253, 299, 341, 357
central hearing loss 162
Central Linguistic Auditory Milestones
  Scale (CLAMS) 173, 175
central nervous system (CNS) 61–62, **86**,
  138, 197, 340
central nervous system depressants **86**,
  99, 112, 150
central nervous system stimulants **86**
central sleep apnea 331
central sulcus **86**, 88
centrophenoxine (Lucidril) **87**
cephalosporin 225
cerebellar astrocytoma. *See* astrocytoma
cerebellar ataxia 41

cerebellum **87–88**. *See also* cerebellum,
  diseases of the; medulloblastoma
  in brain development 119
  and cerebral palsy 89
  damage to 87–88
  functions 54, 62, 64, 76, 87, 143, 163
  location of 76
  and memory 222
  neurons in 261
cerebellum, diseases of the **88**
cerebral angiography 28
cerebral blood-flow studies **88**. *See also*
  PET scan; SPECT
cerebral commissures **88**. *See also* anterior
  commissure; corpus callosum
cerebral cortex 64–65, 88, **88**, 91. *See also*
  motor cortex; occipital lobe; parietal
  cortex; parietal lobes
  alcohol and 13–14
  archicortex **37**
  and cerebral palsy 89
  development of 68
  functions 2, 64–65, 88, 130, 323, 340
  interneurons in 174
  limbic system and 200
  neurons in 261
cerebral embolism 341
cerebral hemispheres 62, 63–64, **88–89**,
  90. *See also* anterior commissure; corpus
  callosum; left brain; left brain-right
  brain; right brain
  asymmetry in 40–41
  complementarity **100**
  dominant hemisphere **121**
  ependymoma **135**
  functions 143
  gender differences 151
  and handedness 158–159
  hemispherectomy **163**
  hemisphericity **163**
  and language 180, 183, 338
  lateralization **182–183**
  nondominant hemisphere **269**
  specialization with age 151
cerebral hemorrhage **89**, 341. *See also*
  hemorrhage, brain
cerebral palsy (CP) 70, 73, **89–90**, 170,
  290, 328
cerebral thrombosis **90**, 341
cerebral toxoplasmosis 259–260
cerebrospinal fluid (CSF) **90**, 104, 247, 365.
  See also hydrocephalus; lumbar puncture
cerebrovascular accident (CVA). *See* stroke
cerebrovascular disease 38, **90**
cerebrum 1, 15, 62, **90–91**, 101, 153. *See
  also* cerebral hemispheres; intracerebral
  hemorrhage
cerebrum, diseases of the **91**
CFIDS. *See* chronic fatigue and immune
  dysfunction syndrome
CFS (chronic fatigue syndrome). *See*
  chronic fatigue and immune dysfunction
  syndrome

chaining **91**
Chamorro natives (Guam) 17
ChAT. *See* choline acetyltransferase
chelation therapy, for lead poisoning 185
chemical brain stimulation **91**
chemoreceptors **91**, 333, 349
chemotherapy
  blood-brain barrier and 61, 78
  side effects 190, 211, 333
  uses 78, 135, 153–154, 211, 255, 277,
    295, 313, 337
Cheung Shu-hung 184
chicken pox 132, 315–316
child abuse, memory of **91–92**
childhood absence seizures. *See* petit mal
  seizure
childhood diseases, and mental retardation
  227
childhood memories, repression of 91–92,
  146
children. *See also* brain development in
  children
  acalculia in 2–3
  AIDS in 12, 229
  appetite loss in 36
  brain tumors in 77, 78, 255
  brain weight 120
  coma in 100
  ependymomas in 135
  febrile seizures **320–321**
  hemispherectomy in 163
  language delay in 181–182
  language processing disabilities 182
  lead poisoning 183–187
  medulloblastoma in 77, 211
  petit mal epilepsy in 289
  retinoblastoma in 312–313
  speech development in 335
  traumatic brain injury in 358–359
  visual processing deficits in 2
Child Study Team 190
chloral hydrate 86
chloramphenicol 225
chlordiazepoxide/amitriptyline (Limbitrol)
  32
chlorpromazine (Thorazine) 33, 71, **92**,
  121, 167, 202, 318, 357
chlorzoxazone 86
cholesterol medication 41
choline **92–93**, 198
choline acetyltransferase (ChAT) 3, 18,
  93, 135
cholinergic 3, **93**
cholinergic basal forebrain **93**
cholinergic hypothesis of Alzheimer's
  disease **93**
cholinergic system 210, 268. *See also*
  anticholinergics
cholinesterase inhibitors 19, **93–94**, 121
cholinomimetic agents **94**
chorea **94**. *See also* Sydenham chorea
choreoathetosis 42, 124
choroid plexus 365

chromosome 11 60
chromosome 14 16
chromosome 16 56
chromosome 19 16–17
chromosome 21 16, 17
chronic fatigue and immune dysfunction syndrome (CFIDS) 73, **94–96**
chronic fatigue syndrome (CFS). *See* chronic fatigue and immune dysfunction syndrome
chronic organic brain syndrome 322
chronic wasting disease (CWD) 304
chunking 364
cigarettes and the brain. *See* nicotine
ciliary-neurotrophic factor 252
cimetidine, and delirium 112
cingulate gyrus 64
Cipralex. *see* escitalopram oxalate
Cipramil. *See* citalopram
circadian rhythm 96, 151, 176, 211–212, 294, 319–320, 330. *See also* infradian rhythm; ultradian rhythms
circle of Willis 84
circulation and the brain 35, 84, **96–97**, 116, 174, 366, 374. *See also* angiography; atherosclerosis; cerebral blood-flow studies; cerebrovascular disease; embolism, cerebral; stroke; transient ischemic attack; vertebrobasilar insufficiency
cisplatin 255
13-cis-retinoic acid 256
citalopram (Celexa; Cipramil; Emocal; Sepram; Seropram) 32, 112, 321
CJD. *See* Creutzfeldt-Jakob disease
CLAMS. *See* Central Linguistic Auditory Milestones Scale
clang associations 353
Clinton, William J. "Bill" 76
clioquinol 123
clomipramine (Anafranil) 32, 40, 250, 360
clonazepam (Klonopin) 31, 112, 289, 334, 338, 355, 361
clonidine (Catapres) 40, 46, **97**, 349, 355
clophedianol 86
Clostridium botulinum 61
clot, blood
  anticoagulant drugs **31**, 41, 333, 342, 358
  antiplatelet medications 41, 358
  cerebral thrombosis 90, 341
  high blood pressure and 116
  thrombolytic therapy 42
clozapine 112
club moss 20
cluster headaches 160
CMV. *See* cytomegalovirus
CNS. *See* central nervous system
cobalamin. *See* vitamin B$_{12}$
cocaine **97–98**
  action and effects 86, 97, 273, 339
  addiction 5, 97, 344

and fetal damage 189
and vasopressin levels 364–365
cocaine psychosis 97
cochlea 162
cochlear nerve. *See* acoustic nerve
codeine 234
coexistence hypothesis 218
Cognex. *See* tacrine
cognition 98, 363
cognitive-behavioral therapy 47
cognitive development 98
Cognitive Failures Questionnaire 98
cognitive map **98**
cognitive triage 98
coil embolization 28
collective unconscious **98–99**
colliculus **99**
color agnosia 11
coma **99–100**. *See also* brain death; Glasgow Coma Score
combat amnesia **100**
combat fatigue. *See* combat amnesia
commissures, cerebral. *See* cerebral commissures
commissurotomy **100**. *See also* split-brain research
Compazine (prochlorperazine) 234
complementarity **100**
complex seizure 136
computed axial tomography. *See* CAT scan
computer use and memory **100**
COMT inhibitor 285
concentration. *See* attention
concussion **100–101**. *See also* postconcussion syndrome
conditioned reflexes 311
conduction aphasia 180
confabulation 11, 83, **101**
congenital brain defects 101
congenital hypothyroidism, and mental retardation 228
consciousness **101–102**, 312. *See also* altered states of consciousness; dissociation
consolidation, of memory **102**, 215
consumer Product Safety Commission 184
context processing **102–103**
continuous amnesia 25, **103**
continuous positive airway pressure (CPAP) 331
contraceptives, oral, and stroke risk 342
contrecoup effects 71, **103**, 161, 300
Controlled Substances Act 25
conversion **103**
Copaxone 245
copper, metabolizing of 242
cornea transplants, and Creutzfeldt-Jakob disease 106, 107
corona radiata 144
corpus callosum 62, **103**
  anterior commissure and 30
  changes with age 151
  commissurotomy **100**

functions 88, 271
  gender differences 151
  and split-brain research 338
corpus striatum. *See* striatum
cortex. *See* cerebral cortex
cortex, limbic. *See* limbic system
cortical deafness 11
cortical lobes **103**
corticobasal degeneration **103–104**
corticospinal tract 240
corticosteroids 6, 77–78, 131, 132, 153, 154, 316, 317
corticotropin. *See* adrenocorticotropic hormone
corticotropin-releasing factor **104**
cortisol 6, 9, 68, 72, 104
Cotugno, Domenico **104**
Coumadin (warfarin) 41
CP. *See* cerebral palsy
CPAP. *See* continuous positive airway pressure
crack 5, 97, 189
cranial nerves 63, 75, 76, **104–105**, 149, 211. *See also* specific nerves
craniopharyngioma **105**
craniosynostosis **105**
craniotomy 28, **106**, 138, 344, 360
cranium **106**
creatine phosphokinase 258–259
Creutzfeldt-Jakob disease (CJD) **106–108**
  causes 18, 70, 106–107, 166, 206–207, 304, 333
  classic 166, 205–206
  dementia in 115
  new variant (nvCJD) 107, 166, 205–207, 304
  types 304
cri du chat syndrome **108–109**
criminals, amnesia in **25**, 60–61
cry of the cat syndrome. *See* cri du chat syndrome
cryptococcosis 70, **109**, 116
Cryptococcus neoformans 70, 109
CSF. *See* cerebrospinal fluid
CT scan. *See* CAT scan
cue-dependent forgetting 68–69, **109**
Cushing's syndrome 6, 296
CVA (cerebrovascular accident). *See* stroke
CWD. *See* chronic wasting disease
cyclics, action and effects 32
cyclophosphamide 255
Cylert. *See* pemoline
Cymbalta (duloxetine) 32
cysticercosis **110**
cytomegalovirus (CMV) **109–110**, 232. *See also* TORCH disorders

D

D4T 12
d-amino-d-arginine vasopressin (DDAVP) 216
dapoxetine 321
Daraprim (pyrimethamine) 357

date-rape drugs 150
DDAVP. *See* d-amino-d-arginine
   vasopressin
death, definition of 67
decay **111**
decerebrate **111**
declarative memory **111**
deep brain stimulation 285
defense mechanism **111**. *See also*
   dissociation
deferoxamine 256
degenerative diseases and the brain **111**,
   117. *See also* Alpers' disease; Alzheimer's
   disease; amyotrophic lateral sclerosis;
   Batten disease; Binswanger's disease;
   corticobasal degeneration; Creutzfeldt-
   Jakob disease; encephalopathy; Lewy
   body dementia; Machado-Joseph
   disease; mad cow disease; motor neuron
   disease; multiple sclerosis; Parkinson's
   disease; Pick's disease; primary lateral
   sclerosis; progressive supranuclear palsy;
   Rett syndrome; Shy-Drager syndrome;
   Tay-Sachs disease; tuberous sclerosis
dehydroepiandrosterone (DHEA) **111**
déjà vu **111–112**
delirium **112**, 117
delirium tremens (DTs) 5, 13, 71, **113**
delta-9 tetrahydrocannabinol (THC) 209
delta waves 78, **113**, 129, 210, 330
demand characteristics hypothesis 218
dementia **113–117**. *See also* Alzheimer's
   disease; Creutzfeldt-Jakob disease; Pick's
   disease; pseudodementia
   acute (reversible) organic brain
      syndrome 322
   AIDS dementia complex **11–12**, 70
   amnesia in 23
   Binswanger's disease **59**
   causes 369
   chronic organic brain syndrome 322
   defined 72, 113
   diseases capable of causing 115–117
   drug-related 2, 115–116
   Lewy body 115, **199–200**
   lifestyle factors in 72
   multi-infarct 115, 116, **242–243**, 308
   presenile 322
   risk factors 273–274
   senile **322**
   treatment and outlook 115, 167, 357,
      364
dementia praecox 16, **117**, 318
dementon 288
demyelinating disorders **117–118**, 146,
   244, 317
demyelination 246, 251
dendrite(s) **118**
   formation and growth 8, 137, 254
   functions 63, 65, 134, 261, 346
   and memory 213
Denver II intelligence test 173, 175
Depakote. *See* valproate

deprenyl (Eldepryl; Jumex; selegiline;
   Emsam) **118**, 238, 285, 301
depression **118–119**. *See also*
   antidepressant drugs
   amnesia in 25
   and dementia 117
   in elderly 2
   exercise and 138
   imaginary smells in 333
   and IQ score 175
   melatonin levels and 212
   nutrition and 274
   thought disorder in 353
   treatment and outlook 119, 201, 307,
      321, 360–361
   tryptophan and 361
Deroxat. *See* paroxetine
Descartes, René **119**, 294
desegregation 120, 176
desipramine (Norpramin)
   side effects 32, 360
   uses 32, 40, 46, 85, 235, 250, 320
despiramine 360
Desyrel. *See* trazodone
developmental aphasia 35
developmental arithmetic disorders 195
developmental articulation disorder 194,
   196
developmental disability, as term 228
developmental disorders 191, 194–197,
   324. *See also* pervasive developmental
   disorders; schizencephaly
developmental expressive language
   disorder 194
developmental reading disorder 194. *See
   also* dyslexia
developmental receptive language disorder
   194, 237
developmental speech and language
   disorders 191, 194, 196, 197
developmental writing disorder 195
development of the brain **119–120**, 262,
   297, 326. *See also* brain development in
   children; fetal brain development
Dexedrine. *See* dextroamphetamine
dextroamphetamine (Dexedrine;
   Dextrostat) 40, 46, 340
Dextrostat. *See* dextroamphetamine
DHA, and brain function 273–274
DHE. *See* dihydroergotamine
DHEA. *See* dehydroepiandrosterone
diabetes insipidus, causes 296
diabetes mellitus
   associated health risks 35, 41, 169,
      253, 342
   history of research on 37
   treatment of 364
   tricyclics and 360
*Diagnostic and Statistical Manual, III-Revised
   (DSM-III-R)* 42
*Diagnostic and Statistical Manual, Fourth
   Edition—Text Revision (DSM-IV-TR)* 38,
   42, 44, 193–194

diagnostic tests. *See* achievement
   tests; auditory brain stem response
   (ABR) test; AX-Continuous
   Performance Test; Bender-Gestalt
   test; Boston remote memory
   battery; cerebral blood-flow studies;
   Cognitive Failures Questionnaire;
   Early Language Milestone Scale;
   electroencephalography; imaging
   techniques; intelligence tests; Iowa Test
   of Basic Skills; Iowa Test of Educational
   Development; Jordan Left-Right
   Reversal Test; lumbar puncture; memory
   tests; mental status examination; mini-
   mental state examination; Multiple
   Sleep Latency Test; nerve conduction
   velocity study; neurological exam;
   neuropsychological assessment; New
   Adult Reading Test; Peabody Picture
   Vocabulary Test-Fourth Edition;
   Wisconsin Card-Sorting Test
diazepam (Valium) 20, 31, 57–58, 112,
   113, **120**, 289, 334, 338, 346, 349
dichioraiphenazone 234
Didronel (etidronate disodium) 281
diencephalon (interbrain) 25, **120**, 163.
   See also telencephalon; thalamus
dietary supplements, side effects 333
diethylpropion 36
dihydroergotamine (DHE; Migranal) 234
Dilantin. *See* phenytoin
dimercaprol 185
dimethylaminoethanol (DMAE) 87, **120**
diphenoxylate 86
diplegia, in cerebral palsy 89
discrepancy, in learning disabilities 197
dissociation 1, 29–30, 92, **120–121**, 176
dissociative disorders 120
disulfiram 86
disulfotan 288
DMAE. *See* dimethylaminoethanol
dominant hemisphere **121**
domipramine 40
donepezil (Aricept) 19, 20, 93, 94, **121**,
   236
dopamine **121**
   ADHD and 43, 230
   aging and 102
   Alzheimer's disease and 3
   blocking reuptake of, side effects 321
   breakdown of 238
   as catecholamine 85
   and depression 118
   drug effects on 25, 32, 97, 127, 143,
      210, 268, 344, 357
   fetal brain cell transplants and 76
   functions 102, 103, 121, 130, 344–
      345
   Lewy body dementia and 121
   in nucleus accumbens 273
   and Parkinson's disease/Parkinsonism
      55, 198–199, 284
   and personality 287

pleasure centers and 298
and psychoses 33
and schizophrenia 318
substantia nigra and 121, 199
synthesis of 344
and tic disorders 241, 356
dopamine blockers 32, 33
dopamine hypothesis **121**
dopaminergic, defined **121**
dopaminergic receptor blockers 92
Down, J. Langdon 52
Down syndrome 17, 70–71, **121–122**, 227
doxapram 86, 340
doxepin (Sinequan) 32, 320, 360
doxorubicin 255
Draganon. *See* aniracetam
dreams 99, **122–123**, 330–331
dronabinol, as central nervous system
depressant 86
Drug Enforcement Agency, U.S. 150, 231
drug-related dementia 2, 115–116
drugs. *See also* addiction; prescription
medication; substance abuse; *specific
drugs*
dementia caused by 2, 115–116
and fetal damage 189, 227
and hearing 162
overdose, treatment 99
drugs and memory **123**
DSI. *See* sensory integration dysfunction
*DSM-III-R. See Diagnostic and Statistical
Manual, III-Revised*
*DSM-IV-TR. See Diagnostic and Statistical
Manual, Fourth Edition—Text Revision*
DTs. *See* delirium tremens
duloxetine (Cymbalta) 32
dura mater **123**, 222
dynorphin 263
dysarthria 88, **123–124**
dysautonomia **124**
dyscalculia 188
dysgraphia 188
dyskinesia **124**
dyslexia **124–125**, 152, 158, 188, 194, 197, 310
dysmyelination disease 117–118, **125**
dysosmia 333
dysphasia 34, **125**. *See also* agraphia;
alexia; aphasia; apraxia
dysplasia, septo-optic (SOD) **325–326**
dyspraxia 324
dystonia **125**, 241

E

E. *See* Ecstasy
ear, structure of 56, 162. *See also* hearing
eardrum 162
Early Language Milestone Scale (ELMS)
126, 173, 175
early onset autism **49–50**
Ebbinghaus, Hermann 54–55, 145–146
Eccles, Sir John Carew **126**
echoencephalography **126–127**

echoic memory **127**. *See also* auditory
memory
Ecstasy (MDMA) 6, **127**
ECT (electroconvulsive therapy) 358
edetate calcium disodium 185
EDS. *See* excessive daytime sleepiness
Edwin Smith surgical papyrus. *See* Smith,
Edwin, surgical papyrus of
EEG. *See* electroencephalogram;
electroencephalography
Effexor (venlafaxine HCl) 32
effortful processing **127**
Egas Moniz, António Caetano de Abreu
Freire **127–128**, 145
Egyptians, on brain 62, 73
eidetic memory **128**, 214
eight cranial nerve. *See* vestibulocochlear
nerve
eighth-nerve tumor. *See* acoustic neuroma
elaborative encoding 132
Elavil. *See* amitriptyline
Eldepryl. *See* deprenyl
elderly. *See also* aging and memory; aging
and the brain; Alzheimer's disease; mild
cognitive impairment
acalculia in 2
and context processing 102–103
depression in 2
fluid imbalance in 143
folic acid deficiency in 144
loss of taste 333
memory in 100, 215
organic brain syndrome in **279**
prescription medications, dementia
from 2, 116
sleeping problems 212, 331
electrical stimulation of the brain **128–129**, 209, 285–286, 351
electroconvulsive therapy (ECT) 358
electroencephalogram (EEG) 66, **129**
electroencephalography (EEG) 75, 78,
129, 138, 260
electrolytes, and brain function 143
electromagnetic fields (EMFs) 77, 85–86, 208
eleventh cranial nerve. *See* spinal
accessory nerve
ELMS. *See* Early Language Milestone
Scale
embolism, cerebral **129**
embolization, coil 28
EMFs. *See* electromagnetic fields
EMG. *See* single fiber electromyography
Emocal. *See* citalopram
emotional development, brain
development and 68
emotions and the brain **129–130**. *See also*
limbic system
amygdala 26
chemical basis of emotions 129–130
defense mechanisms **111**
endorphins and 133–134
and memory 26, 203, 213

nutrition and 369
regulation of 64, 65
Emsam. *See* deprenyl
en bloc blackouts 61
encephalitis 12, 23, 89, 116, **130–131**,
217, 259. *See also* Rasmussen's
encephalitis
encephalitis lethargica **131–132**
encephalitis periaxialis diffusa. *See*
Schilder's disease
encephalocele 72
encephalograph 129
encephalomyelitis 116, **132**
encephalon **132**
encephalopathy **132**. *See also* toxic
encephalopathy; transmissible
spongiform encephalopathies (TSEs);
Wernicke's encephalopathy
encoding 7, 31, 127, **132**, 134
endarterectomy 42, **133**
endbrain. *See* telencephalon
endocrine system 169, 211, 295
endogenous *vs.* exogenous brain damage
57
endorphin(s) 63–65, **133–134**, 239, 263,
268, 277, 295
endovascular therapy, for brain aneurysm
28
engram (memory trace) **134**, 213, 286, 347
enkephalin 63–65, **134**, 239, 263
enteroviruses 130
environmental factors
in brain development 67–68, 120
in learning disabilities 189
in multiple sclerosis 244
Environmental Protection Agency (EPA)
77, 184, 266
environmental toxins. *See* toxins
enzyme(s) **134–135**
EPA. *See* Environmental Protection Agency
ependymoma 135
epilepsy **135–137**
causes 2, 135, 299, 342
childhood absence (petit mal) 289
idiopathic, causes 165
imaginary smells in 333
meningitis and 70
risk factors 321
seizures
first aid for 136–137
types 135–136
status epilepticus **339**
symptoms and diagnosis 135–136
temporal lobe 112, 136, 307
treatment and outlook 136, 163, 210,
291, 307, 338, 353
epilepsy medications, and neural tube
defects 72
epinephrine (adrenaline) 32, 63, 82, 85,
137, 143, 346, 359
epirubicin 255
episodic memory 7, 10, 203
equilibrium. *See* balance

equine encephalitis 130
Erasistratus of Chios **137**
ergoloid mesylates. *See* Hydergine
ergotamine 160
ergotamine tartrate (Cafergot) 234
ERT. *See* estrogen replacement therapy
Escherichia coli 225
escitalopram oxalate (Lexapro, Cipralex,
    Esertia) 32, 321
Esertia. *see* escitalopram oxalate
essential tremor 359
estrogen and the brain 111, **137–138**
estrogen replacement therapy (ERT)
    21–22
ethanol. *See* alcohol
ethchlorvynol, as central nervous system
    depressant 86
ethinamate 86
ethmoid bone 106
ethosuximide 31, 289
etidronate disodium (Didronel) 281
etomidate 86
etoposide 255
Etrafon (perphenazine/amitriptyline) 32
Etudes cliniques (Morel) 117
EUE. *See* exotic ungulate encephalopathy
event-related potentials (ERPs) 75
evoked potentials (EPs) 161, 236. *See also*
    auditory-evoked potentials
evoked response **138**
evolution of brain, and brain development
    119
excessive daytime sleepiness (EDS)
    249–250
excitotoxins 17
exclusion, in learning disability diagnosis
    197
executive function 7, 69, 148
Exelon. *See* rivastigmine
exercise and the brain 7–8, 10, 138, **138**,
    221
exogenous *vs.* endogenous brain damage
    57
exotic ungulate encephalopathy (EUE)
    304
experimental neuropsychology 264–265
*Experimental Studies on the Properties and
    Functions of the Nervous System in Vertebrate
    Animals* (Flourens) 143
*Experimental Surgery in the Treatment of
    Certain Psychoses* (Egas Moniz) 128
expressive language disorders 36–37, 80
external locus of control. *See* field
    dependence
extradural hemorrhage **138–139**
extrapyramidal system 139, **139**
eye 1, 366–367. *See also* vision

F

faces, memory for **219**
facial agnosia. *See* prosopagnosia
facial nerve (seventh cranial nerve) 63,
    75, 76, 105, **140**. *See also* cranial nerves

fainting **140**
Fallopio, Gabriel **140**
false memory 91–92, 101, 112, 134, 214,
    218. *See also* memory distortions
false recollection. *See* Freudian slip
falx cerebri 123
familial dysautonomia (FD) 124
familial insomnia 166
Famous Faces Test **140–141**
Faria, Abbe 230
FAS. *See* fetal alcohol syndrome
fatal familial insomnia (FFI) 106, **141**,
    166, 304
Faverin. *See* fluvoxamine
FD. *See* familial dysautonomia
FDA. *See* Food and Drug Administration,
    U.S.
Federal Communications Commission 86
feline encephalopathy 106, 304
fenfluramine 36, 86
fetal alcohol effects (FAE) 141
fetal alcohol syndrome (FAS) 14, 71,
    141–142, 189
fetal brain cells, in brain damage
    treatment 76
fetal brain development 142, 189, 208,
    266–267, 318. *See also* development of
    the brain
fetal hydantoin syndrome 72, **142**
fetus
    nervous system, development of 144
    TORCH disorders **354**
    viral infection in, and schizophrenia
        318
FFI. *See* fatal familial insomnia
fibrates, for atherosclerosis 41
field dependence **142**
field independence **142–143**
field sensitivity. *See* field dependence
fifth cranial nerve. *See* trigeminal nerve
fight-or-flight response 52, 63, 65, 143,
    169, 272, 346, 360
fipexide **143**
first cranial nerve. *See* olfactory nerve
Fissure of Sylvius (sylvian fissure) **143**,
    346
fissures, cerebral. *See* sulci
flashbacks, temporal lobe epilepsy and
    136
flavoxate 86
Fleischl-Marxow, Ernst von 98
Flourens, Marie-Jean-Pierre **143**
flucytosine 109
fluent aphasia. *See* Wernicke's aphasia
fluid imbalances and the brain **143**, 292,
    352, 364. *See also* thirst
fluoxetine (Prozac, Fontex, Seromex,
    Seronil, Sarafem)
    action and effects 321
    side effects 32, 33, 360
    uses 32, 40, 46, 112, 160, 235, 250,
        305, 326
fluphenazine 33, 357

fluvoxamine (Luvox, Faverin) 20, 32,
    40, 321
fly agaric. *See Amanita muscaria*
    mushrooms
fMRI. *See* functional magnetic resonance
    imaging
folate. *See* vitamin B_9 (folic acid)
folic acid. *See* vitamin B_9
fontanelles, craniosynostosis and 105
Fontex. *See* fluoxetine
food, for brain function **73**, 92–93, 198
Food and Drug Administration, U.S.
    (FDA) 62, 144, 150, 167, 198, 206, 269,
    285, 342, 348, 360, 362
food poisoning, botulism **61–62**
forebrain 30, 119, 142, **144**, 167
fornix **144**
Fosamax (alendronate sodium) 281
fourth cranial nerve. *See* trochlear nerve
Fowler, L. N. 292
Fowlers 292
fractionated stereotactic radiosurgery
    (FSR) 4
fragile X syndrome 39, 71, **144–145**, 227
Franklin, Benjamin 229
freebasing 97
Freeman, Walter 128, **145**, 198, 201–203
free radicals 9, 20, 21, 33, **145**, 167
free radical scavengers 305
Freud, Sigmund **145–146**
    on agnosia 11
    Anno O (patient) and 29–30
    Breuer (Josef) and 79
    on cocaine 97–98
    on déjà vu 112
    on dissociation 29–30, 120–121
    on dreams 123
    hypnosis studies 24
    on hysterical amnesia 24–25, 170
    on infantile amnesia 52, 171
    on memory 55, 145–146
    on repression 170, 171
Freudian slip 146
Friedreich, Nicholas 146
Friedreich's ataxia 41, **146–147**
frontal aphasia. *See* Broca's aphasia
frontal bone 106
frontal lobe **147–148**. *See also* premotor
    cortex; supplementary motor area
    abscesses 1
    and ADHD 43
    damage, assessment of 373
    functions 7, 64, 88, 91, 130
    location 64
    Pick's disease and 293
frontal lobotomy. *See* leucotomy;
    lobotomy
FSH-secreting pituitary tumors 296
FSR. *See* fractionated stereotactic
    radiosurgery
functional magnetic resonance imaging
    (fMRI) 74–75, **148**
fundal cells 148

fundus **148**
fusiform gyrus **148**, 310

G

GABA (gamma-aminobutyric acid) 149, **149**
GABAergic systems 149, 184, 210
GABA neurotransmitter system, muscimol and 158
gabapentin 361
Gage, Phineas A. 287
galanin 166
galantamine hydrobromide (Razadyne) 19, 93, 94, **149**
galantine, side effects 94
Galen 74, 104, **149**
Gall, Franz Joseph **149–150**, 291–292
gamma-aminobutyric acid. *See* GABA
gamma hydroxybutyrate (sodium oxybate; GHB; Xyrem) **150**, 250
gamma knife. *See* stereotactic radiosurgery
ganciclovir 131
ganglia **150**
ganglioneuroblastoma 254
ganglioneuroma 254
gangliosides 350
Gardner, Howard 243–244
gastrostomy 305
gender differences **150–152**
    in ADHD incidence 44, 168
    anterior commissure and 30
    and autistic savants 52
    in corpus callosum 103
    in learning disorder incidence 39
    in medulloblastoma incidence 211
    in MS incidence 244
    in myasthenia gravis incidence 245
generalized amnesia 25
gene therapy 42, 337
genetic disorders of the brain 70–71, **152**.
    See also anencephaly; Batten disease;
    birth defects; Creutzfeldt-Jakob disease;
    cri du chat syndrome; Down syndrome;
    fragile X syndrome; Friedreich's ataxia;
    Huntington's disease; hydrocephalus;
    infantile neuroaxonal dystrophy; Lewy
    body dementia; Machado-Joseph
    disease; microcephaly; narcolepsy;
    neurofibromatosis; phenylketonuria;
    Prader-Willi syndrome; Sandhoff
    disease; Tay-Sachs disease; Wilson's
    disease
    and mental retardation 227
    prion diseases as 304
    sex-linked 71
    Tourette syndrome as 356
genital herpes, and neonatal microcephaly 232
gerinoma 294
Gerstmann's syndrome 282
Gerstmann-Sträussler-Scheinker disease (GSS) 18, 106, 166, 304
GHB. *See* gamma hydroxybutyrate

gigantism 296
Ginger Jake syndrome 286–287
ginkgo biloba **152**
Glasgow Coma Score 359
glaucoma, treatment 293
glia cells. *See* glial cells
glial cells 65, 142, **152–153**, 338. *See also* glioma
glial-growth factor 252
glial-maturation factor 252
glioblastoma **153–154**
glioblastoma multiforme 40, 153
glioma 77, **154**. *See also* astrocytoma;
    ependymoma; glioblastoma;
    oligodendroglioma
glioma of the optic nerve **154–155**
global amnesia. *See* organic amnesia
global aphasia 34
globus pallidus 43, 55, 64, 285
glossopharyngeal nerve (ninth cranial nerve) 63, 75, **155**. *See also* cranial nerves
glucocorticoids 104
glucose **155**. *See also* hypoglycemia
    blood level 166, 169
    as brain energy source 138, 155, 169, 173, 208
    metabolism 138, 152, 173, 374
    storage 155
glucose utilization scan. *See* PET scan
glutamate 12, 17, 19–20, 26, **155**, 167, 268, 269
glutethimide 86
glycine 267
glycogen 155
glycopyrrolate 31
Goldstein, Avram 263
Golgi, Camillo 63
grand mal seizures 135–136, **155**, 320
grasp reflex 311
gray matter 64, 88, 150, **155**, 207, 336–337. *See also* cerebral cortex
growth hormone **155**, 251–252
growth hormone-secreting pituitary tumors 296
GSS. *See* Gerstmann-Straussler-Scheinker disease
guanabenz 86
guanfacine (Tenex) 86, 355
Guillain-Barré syndrome **155–156**, 204, 251
Guillotin, J. I. 229
Guthrie, Robert 290

H

habituation **157**
Hagsberg, Bengt 315
hair cells 366
Haldol. *See* haloperidol
Hales, Stephen 260
Haller, Albrecht von **157**
hallucinations 18, 29, 136, **157**, 199, 353
hallucinogenic mushrooms **157–158**

hallucinogens 5, 6, **158**. *See also* LSD;
    marijuana
haloperidol (Haldol) 20, 33, 40, 86, 112, 283, 318, 355, 357
hammer (malleus) 162
handedness **158–159**, 182, 183
happiness, smell-related memories and 221
harmatine 158
Harvey, William **159**
hashish 5, 6, 209–210
HD. *See* Huntington's disease
headaches **159–160**
head injury **160–162**. *See also* brain
    damage; concussion; postconcussion
    syndrome
    and agnosia 10
    and cerebral palsy 89
    contrecoup effects 71, **103**, 161, 300
    mild **236–237**
    and nonverbal learning disabilities 271
    REM sleep in 123
    seeing stars **338–339**
    and subdural hemorrhage 344
health, and memory 216
hearing **162**, 366. *See also entries under*
    acoustic *and* auditory
heart disease 35, 138, 147
Hebb, Donald 102, 162, **162**, 163
Hebb's rule **162**
Hebb synapse **163**
hemangioblastoma **163**
hematoma 116, 138, **163**
hemiballismus **163**
hemiplegia 89
hemispatial neglect **163**
hemispherectomy **163**
hemispheres, brain. *See* cerebral
    hemispheres
hemisphericity **163**
Hemophilus influenzae type B (Hib) 224, 228–229
hemorrhage, brain **164**. *See also*
    extradural hemorrhage; intracerebral
    hemorrhage
    cerebral **89**, 341
    diagnosis of 74
    extradural **138–139**
    intracerebral hemorrhage **174**
    subarachnoid 24, **343**
    subdural **343–344**
heparin 41
hereditary degenerative diseases, of
    cerebellum 88
heroin and the brain 5, **164**, 239, 298
Herophilus of Chalcedon 74, **164**
herpes simplex 217. *See also* TORCH
    disorders
Herpes simplex encephalitis (HSE) 130
herpes virus 6 (HHV-6) 95
herpes virus family, cytomegalovirus **109–110**

heterocyclic antidepressants, as
  anticholinergic 31
hexosaminidase 317, 350
HHV-6 (herpes virus 6) 95
Hib. *See Hemophilus influenzae* type B
high blood pressure 97, 116, 174, 342
high-density lipoprotein (HDL) 41
hindbrain (rhombencephalon) **164**
hippocampus (archicortex) **164–165**
    cell loss, with age 6, 9
    evolution of 64
    functions 64, 164–165
    glutamate and 155
    marijuana use and 210
    and memory 6, 9, 64, 66, 111, 136,
      164–165, 172, 210, 213–214, 215,
      351–352
Hippocrates 37, 62–63, 73–74, **165**
Hispanics, stroke risk 342
histamine Hl blockers 32, 33
histamine receptors, tricyclics and 360
HIV (human immunodeficiency virus)
  11–12. *See also* AIDS and the brain
H.M. (lobectomy patient) 136, 203, 210,
  213
hologramic brain **165**
homosexual men, brain structure in 327
hormone(s) **165**. *See also* norepinephrine;
  steroid hormones
    and adult sexual difference 326
    and chronic fatigue and immune
      dysfunction syndrome 95
    control of 65
    epinephrine (adrenaline) 32, 63, 82,
      85, **137**, 143, 346, 359
    functions 165
    and hunger regulation 166
    nerve-growth factor (NGF) 21, 137,
      251–252
    neurohormones **258**
    pituitary gland and 295
    secreting pituitary tumors **295–296**
    steroid 111, 279, 303, 337
    stress 6, 9, 68, 72, 143
hot tubs, pregnancy and **165–166**
HSE. *See* Herpes simplex encephalitis
Hughes, John 263
human immunodeficiency virus. *See* HIV
human prion diseases **166**
humors 37, 164, 165
hunger 36, **166**
Huntington, George 166
Huntington's disease (HD) 85, 115, **166–
167**, 217, 242
hydantoin 142
Hydergine (ergoloid mesylates) 20, **167**
hydrocephalus 90, **167–168**. *See also*
  normal-pressure hydrocephalus
    causes 38, 70, 90, 294, 299, 336
    and nonverbal learning disabilities 271
    normal-pressure 117
    obstructive 117
hydrocodone 234

hydrocortisone, and ACTH production 6
hydrophobia. *See* rabies
hydroxyzine. 86
hyperactive-impulsive subtype of ADHD
  44, 45
hyperactivity 142, 152, **168–169**,
  193, 195. *See also* attention deficit
  hyperactivity disorder
hyperbilirubinemia. *See* kernicterus
hyperglycemia 155
hyperkinesis. *See* hyperactivity
hyperkinetic syndrome. *See* attention
  deficit hyperactivity disorder;
  hyperactivity
hyperlipidemia 342
hypertensive headaches 160
hyperthermia therapy, for spinal cord
  tumors 337
hyperthyroidism, and Tourette syndrome
  355
hyperzine A 20
hypnagogic hallucinations 250
hypnosis 24, 29–30, **169**, 170, 176, 203,
  214. *See also* mesmerism
hypnotic drugs 31
hypocretin-1 249
hypocretin-2 249
hypoglossal nerve (twelfth cranial nerve)
  63, 75, **169**. *See also* cranial nerves
hypoglycemia 155, **169**, 292
hypothalamus **169–170**. *See also* appestat;
  suprachiasmatic nucleus
    damage to 169–170
    and depression 118
    functions 6, 36, 130, 143, 166, 169,
      200, 311, 326, 350–351, 352, 364
    gender differences 151
    GHB and 150
    in homosexual men 327
    and immune system 171
    and Laurence-Moon-Biedl syndrome
      183
    limbic system and 200
    and memory 66, 213
    osmoreceptors in 280
    pleasure center in **298**
    radiation therapy and 211
    secretions 104, 121
hypothyroidism 39, **170**, 228
hypoxia **170**
hysteria, dissociation in 176
hysterical amnesia 24–25, **170**

I

ibogaine 158
ibotenic acid 158
ibuprofen 20, 159, 233, 234
ice-pick lobotomy. *See* transorbital
  lobotomy
ICP. *See* intracranial pressure
idebenone **171**
IDEIA. *See* Individuals with Disabilities
  Education Improvement Act

ideomotor apraxia 36–37
idiopathic epilepsy 165
IEP. *See* individualized educational
  program
ifosfamide 255
IGF-1. *See* insulin-like growth factor
l'illusion des sosies 83
imaging techniques **171**. *See also* brain
  scans; CAT scan; echoencephalography;
  magnetic resonance imaging (MRI); PET
  scan; pneumoencephalography; SPECT;
  SQUID; tomography; ultrasound scan;
  ventriculography
    advances in 69
    and brain research 296
    and language areas of brain 181
    optical imaging 353
imipramine (Tofranil)
    side effects 32, 360
    uses 40, 46, 85, 112, 250, 305, 320,
      360
imipramine pamoate (Tofranil-PM) 32
Imitrex. *See* sumatriptan
immune system 51, 156, **171**, 245
immunotherapy 154, 246, 256, 317
INAD. *See* infantile neuroaxonal
  dystrophy
inattentive subtype of ADHD 44
incus (anvil) 162
Inderal. *See* propranolol
individualized educational program (IEP)
  2–3, 196
Individuals with Disabilities Education
  Improvement Act (IDEIA) 190, 197
indole alkaloid derivatives 158
indomethacin **171**, 233
infant(s)
    habituation in 157
    hormonal activity in 326
    kernicterus 178
    neonatal meningitis **225–226**
    neonatal microcephaly 232
    Ohtahara syndrome **276**
    prematurity, and sensory integration
      dysfunction 324
    reflexes in 311
    REM sleep in 123
    shaken baby syndrome **327–328**
    speech in 335
    traumatic brain injury in 358–359
    vision in 367
infant botulism 62
infantile amnesia 52, **171–172**
infantile neuroaxonal dystrophy (INAD)
  172
infantile paralysis. *See* poliomyelitis
infantile progressive spinal muscular
  atrophy (Werdnig-Hoffmann paralysis)
  240
infection 70, 116, **173**, 204. *See also*
  virus(es)
inflammation of the brain. *See*
  encephalitis; infection; meningitis

influenza 120, 315–316
infradian rhythm **173**
Innocent XII (pope) 209
insect-borne diseases 130–131
insecticide, acetylcholinesterase disrupters 3
insomnia 332, 356
instinctive behavior 312
Institute of Medicine (IOM) 52, 92
insulin 123, 169
insulin-coma shock therapy 202
insulin-like growth factor (IGF-1) 302
intelligence 79, 173, **173–174**
intelligences, multiple **243–244**
intelligence tests 59, 69, 173, 243. *See also* BRAT battery; Denver II; IQ tests; Kohs Block Design Test; Stanford-Binet Intelligence Scale; Wechsler Adult Intelligence Scale; Wechsler Intelligence Scale for Children; Wechsler Preschool and Primary Scale of Intelligence
interbrain. *See* diencephalon
interference, aging and 9
interferon 86, 123, 154
interleukin-2 154, 256
interneuron **174**
interpersonal intelligence 244
interstitial radiation. *See* brachytherapy
intracerebral hemorrhage **174**
intracranial pressure (ICP) **174–175**
intrapersonal intelligence 244
invasive Hib (*Hemophilus influenzae* type B) disease 224, 228–229
involuntary functions, autonomic nervous system and 52
IOM. *See* Institute of Medicine
Iowa Test of Basic Skills **175**
Iowa Test of Educational Development 175
iproplatin 255
IPV (inactivated polio vaccine) 299
IQ 216, 268, 369
IQ tests **175**. *See also* intelligence tests
irreversible coma. *See* brain death
ischemia, *vs.* anoxia 30
ischemic attacks, transient. *See* transient ischemic attack
isocarboxazid (Marplan) 32
isometheptene (Midrin) 234

J

Jacksonian epilepsy 136
James, William 8–9
Janet, Pierre 1, 120, **176**
Jansky-Bielschowsky disease 56
JC virus 305
jet lag **176–177**, 212, 332
Jordan Left-Right Reversal Test **177**
Joseph disease. *See* Machado-Joseph disease
jugular vein **177**
Jumex. *See* deprenyl
Jung, Carl 1, 98–99, 176

K

K252 compounds 252
Kennedy, Rosemary 203
kernicterus **178**
ketoconazole (Nizoral) **178**
Klonopin. *See* clonazepam
knee-jerk reflex 311
Kohs Block Design Test **178**
Korsakoff, Sergey Sergeyevich **178**
Korsakoff psychosis. *See* Korsakoff syndrome
Korsakoff's dementia 116
Korsakoff syndrome 14, 71, **178–179**, 217, 364, 372
Kosterlitz, Hans 263
Kraepelin, Emil 16, 117, 318
Kufs' disease 56
kuru 18, 106, **179**, 304, 333

L

LaCrosse encephalitis 131
Lamotrigine 123
language **180**. *See also* agraphia; alexia; aphasia; apraxia; auditory agnosia; developmental speech and language disorders; dyslexia; dysphasia; language processing disabilities; learning disability; reading; speech
    and autobiographical memory 52
    developmental receptive language disorder 194, 237
    development of 68
    mixed receptive-expressive language disorder **237–238**
    neurological mechanisms 183
    optical aphasia **278**
    Pervasive Developmental Disorders and 288
    receptive **310**
    stroke and 341
language areas of the brain 34, **180–181**, 338, 351, 373
language delay 68–69, **181–182**
language processing disabilities **182**
languages, memory for **219**
Lashley, Karl **182**
late-onset autism 49
lateral geniculate bodies **182**
lateralization **182–183**. *See also* lateral preference
lateral preference **183**
lateral sulcus 88
Laurence-Moon-Biedl syndrome 169–170, **183**
Lavoisier, A. L. 229
lazy eye. *See* amblyopia
LD. *See* learning disability
L-dopa. *See* levodopa
lead poisoning and the brain **183–187**, 189–190, 229, 265–266, 356
learning 120, 164, **187–188**, 306, 369. *See also* nootropics

learning disability (LD) 68–69, **188–198**. *See also* acalculia; aphasia; auditory and visual processing disabilities; dyscalculia; dysgraphia; dyslexia; pervasive developmental disorders
    causes 73, 144, 170, 188–190, 211, 256–257, 290, 302, 325, 327, 355
    classification of 237
    definition of 188, 196–197
    gender and 39
    language processing disabilities **182**
    lead poisoning and 266
    and memory 217
    and sensory integration dysfunction 324
    symptoms and diagnosis 43, 190–195, 193, 197, 227
    treatment and outlook 195–198
    types 188, 194–195
learning problem, v. learning disability 193
Leber's optic neuropathy 278
lecithin 92–93, **198**
left brain (left hemisphere) 63–64, 88, 91, 180, 183, 198, 338
left brain-right brain **198**
Lehrbuch der Gehirnkrankheiten (*Textbook of Brain Disorders*; Wernicke) 372
Lejeune, Jerome 122
Leksell, Lars 339
Leonardo da Vinci 74, **198**
leptomeningitis 116
leucotomy 127, 145, **198**. *See also* lobotomy
leu-enkephalin 263
levamisole, for glioblastoma 154
LeVay, Simon 327
levodopa 55, 131, **198–199**, 205, 283, 284, 305, 345
Levy, Jerre 152
Lewy body 115, 199
Lewy body dementia 115, **199–200**
Lexapro. *See* escitalopram oxalate
Librium 57–58
lidocaine 112
lidocaine hydrochloride 96
lifestyle, brain disorders from 71–72
limbic system **200–201**. *See also* amygdala; cingulate gyrus; hippocampus; nucleus accumbens
    in animals 130
    components of 120, 200, 302–303
    damage to 200–201
    development of 68
    drugs and 13, 97, 277
    functions of 64, 130, 200, 221, 326, 340
    mammillary bodies and 209
    and memory 64, 203, 213–214, 221
    neuropeptides in 263
    pleasure centers and 298
Limbitrol (chlordiazepoxide/amitriptyline) 32

Lindau's tumor. *See* hemangioblastoma
lipofuscin 3, 87
lithium 32, 33, 40, 60, 123, **201**, 357
liver disease, and encephalopathy 132
lobectomy 201
lobotomy 145, 198, **201–203**, 202,
    307. *See also* leucotomy; transorbital
    lobotomy
localized amnesia 25
locus coeruleus **203**, 272
lodestone. *See* magnetite
Loftus, Elizabeth 203, 214, 218
logic, brain development and 68
logical/mathematic intelligence 243
longitudinal cerebral fissure 88
long-term memory **203**, 215
    aging and 7, 10
    characteristics *vs.* short-term memory
        203
    disorders of 217
    recall 213, 217, **310**
    storage in brain 102, 112, 134, 137,
        164, 203, 212–214, 261, 286, 296–
        297, 328–329, 347
    transfer of short-term memory into
        328–329
    visual 368
long-term potentiation (LTP) 162
Lou Gehrig's disease. *See* amyotrophic
    lateral sclerosis
Louis XVI (king of France) 229
low blood sugar. *See* hypoglycemia
low-density lipoprotein (LDL) 41
low-grade astrocytoma 40
loxapine 86
LP. *See* lumbar puncture
LSD (lysergic acid diethylamide) 5, 6,
    158, **204**, 364–365
LSH-secreting pituitary tumors 296
LTP. *See* long-term potentiation
L-tryptophan **204**
lucid dreaming **204**
Lucidril (centrophenoxine) **87**
lucid sleep 230
Ludiomil (maprotiline) 32
lumbar puncture (LP) 90, **204**
lung cancer, marijuana use and 210
Lustral. *See* sertraline
Luvox. *See* fluvoxamine
lysergic acid diethylamide. *See* LSD

M

M1-Mouth Area 181
Machado-Joseph disease (MJD) **204**
mad cow disease (bovine spongiform
    encephalopathy) 70, 106, 107, **205–
    207**, 304
magnesium sulfate, as central nervous
    system depressant 86
magnetic resonance imaging (MRI) 74,
    161, 207, **207**, 236
magnetite **207–208**
magnetoencephalography (MEG) 75

maidenhair tree 152
maintenance encoding 132
malathion 288
malleus (hammer) 162
malnutrition 120, 178–179, **208–209**,
    227, 292–293, 372. *See also* brain food
Malpighi, Marcello **209**
mammalian brain. *See* limbic system
mammillary bodies **209**
manganese, as neurotoxin 265–266
mania, treatment ,92
manic-depressive disorder. *See* bipolar
    disorder
mannitol 316
MAO. *See* monoamine oxidase
mapping the brain **209**. *See also* imaging
    techniques; motor homunculus
maprotiline (Ludiomil) 32
marijuana 5, 6, 158, **209–210**, 365
Marplan (isocarboxazid) 32
maternal serum alpha-fetoprotein blood
    test 253
mathematical ability 68, 243
matprotiline 86
Maxalt (rizatriptan) 234
Mayo Clinic 20
mazindol 36
MBD. *See* minimal brain dysfunction
MDMA. *See* Ecstasy (MDMA)
measles 132
measles-mumps-rubella (MMR) vaccine
    51–52
meclizine 86
medial septum 93
medial temporal lobe 25, 136, **210**
meditation and the brain 134, **210**
medulla 13, 64, 75, 76, 143, **210–211**
medulla oblongata. *See* medulla
medulloblastoma 70, 77, **211**
MEG. *See* magnetoencephalography
melanin, Rett syndrome and 315
melatonin 176, **211–212**, 294, 319–320,
    330
memantine (Namenda) 19, 94, **212**
memory **212–216**. *See also* acquisition;
    aging and memory; cue-dependent
    forgetting; encoding; engram; long-term
    memory; recall; retrieval; short-term
    memory
    aging and **6–9**, 297, 310
    alcohol and 7, 14, 23, 25, 60–61, 123,
        217, 292
    alteration of 134
    in animals **28–29**
    anoxia and 165
    auditory **49**
    autistic savants 52
    autobiographical **52**
    automatic gestures and 52
    automatic processing and **52**
    biochemical basis of 216
    brain areas used in 26, 40, 91, 213–
        214. *See also specific areas*

brain damage and 65–66
centrophenoxine and 87
of child abuse **91–92**
consolidation of **102**, 215
decay 111
declarative **111**
DMAE and 120
eidetic **128**, 214
emotions and 26, 203, 213
episodic 7, 10, 203
estrogen and 137–138
false 91–92, 101, 112, 134, 214, 218.
    See also memory distortions
formation process 215, 216
Freud on 55, 145–146
limbic system and 64, 203, 213–214,
    221
mammillary bodies and 209
marijuana use and 210
mnesic syndromes **238**
motor association **239**
multi-infarct dementia and 242
nonverbal **272**
nonverbal learning disabilities and
    271
nutrition and 273–274, 292–293,
    369
passive storage 102
photographic **128**, 214
physostigmine and 319
pregnancy and **303**
procedural 111, 203
protein kinase C and 306
racial. *See* collective unconscious
recall 213, 217, **310**
recovered **91–92**
registration of 215
research on 54–55, 59, 162, 182, 216,
    285–286
scopolamine and 319
semantic 7, 9, 203, **322**
sensory 215
stimulus-response **340**
storage in brain 102, 112, 134, 137,
    164, 203, 212–214, 261, 286, 296–
    297, 328–329, 347
types of 66, 214–216
verbal **365**
voluntary and involuntary 215
memory, active working **216–217**
memory, disorders of **217–218**, 292–293.
    See also agnosia; Alzheimer's disease;
    amnesia; Korsakoff syndrome;
    mild cognitive impairment; mnesic
    syndromes; prosopagnosia
    associated cognitive disorders 113
    causes 72, 82, 114, 116, 161, 217–
        218, 322
    confabulation in 101
    cue-dependent forgetting 68–69, **109**
    drugs and **123**
    evaluation of 70
    in hypothyroidism 170

medial temporal lobectomy and 136,
   351–352
   transient **358**
   treatment of 57, 92–93, 93–94, 100,
   293, 303, 308, 364, 366, 375
memory aids 8–9, 216
   alphabetical searching **15**
   association **40**
   behavioral treatments **57**
   for brain damage victims 66
   chaining **91**
   choline 92–93
   computer use **100**
   face-name association method 220
   first-letter cueing 220
   Hydergine 20, **167**
   lecithin 198
   for names 220
   nootropics 3, 29, 83, 216, **272**, 308
   for numbers 220
   visual imagery method 220
Memory Assessment Clinics 375
memory distortions 7, 55, 134, 218, **218**.
   See also false memory
memory for crime. *See* amnesia and crime
memory for events **218–219**
memory for faces **219**
memory for languages **219**
memory for music **219**
memory for names 7, 219, **219–220**
memory for numbers **220–221**
memory for objects 219, **221**
memory for odors **221**
memory for places **221–222**
memory for rote movements **222**
memory for stories **222**
memory for taste **222**
memory for voices **222**
memory quotient (MQ) 25
memory tests 80–81, 98, 140–141
memory trace. *See* engram
Menactra. *See* meningococcal conjugate
   vaccine
meninges **37**, **222**, 233, 337. *See also*
   meningioma; meningitis
meningioma **222–223**, 294, 333
meningitis 37, 70, 89, 109, **223–224**, 232,
   259, 337
meningitis, hemophilus **224–225**
meningitis, meningococcal **225**
meningitis, neonatal **225–226**
meningitis, pneumococcal **226**
meningocele **226**, 247, 253, 336
meningococcal conjugate vaccine
   (Menactra) 224, 225, 226
meningococcal polysaccharide vaccine
   (Menomune) 224, 225, 226
meningococcal vaccines 224, 225, 226
meningomyelocele 253
Menomune (meningococcal
   polysaccharide vaccine) 224, 225, 226
"mental aura" 286
mental disorders, organic **279–280**

mental illness 226, **226**
mental retardation **227–229**. *See also*
   autistic savants
   causes 14, 89, 108, 122, 141, 144,
      185, 208, 227, 228–229, 290, 299,
      302, 326, 327, 342, 362
   degrees of severity 228
   incidence 227
   treatment 308
   v. dementia 113
   v. learning disability 193, 227
mental status examination 19, **229**
mental stimulation, and mental function
   7–8, 10, 22
meperidine 5
meprobamate 86
mercury 265–266, 356
mescaline 5, 6, 158
mesencephalon. *See* midbrain
Mesmer, Franz Anton **229**. *See also*
   mesmerism
mesmerism **229–230**. *See also* Mesmer,
   Franz Anton
message transmission in brain, research
   on 126
Mestinon (pyridostigmine bromide) 246
metabolic diseases, and dementia 116
metachromatic leukodystrophy 116, 118,
   125
metacognition **230**
metencephalon 164
met-enkephalin 263
methamphetamine 40
methyldopa 86, 123
3,4 methylenedioxymethamphetamine
   (MDMA). *See* Ecstasy
methylphenidate hydrochloride
   (Ritalin) 40, 43, 46, 86, **230–231**,
   340, 364–365
methyl-phenyl tetrahydropyridine
   (MPTP) 283
methyprylon 86
methysegide 160
metoclopramide 86, 283
metyrosine 86
MG. *See* myasthenia gravis
microcephaly 142, **231–232**
microglia 152
microscope, invention of 63
microsleeps 249
midbrain (mesencephalon) 64, 75, 168,
   232, 239. *See also* colliculus; tectum,
   midbrain
Midrin (isometheptene) 234
mifepristone (RU-486) 223
migraine 73, 159–160, **232–235**, 339,
   342, 345
Migranal. *See* dihydroergotamine
mild cognitive impairment 19, 72, **235–
   236**, 375
mild head injury **236–237**
Miller, Irene Frances 126
minerals and the brain 73, 208

minimal brain dysfunction (MBD) 42,
   237
mini-mental state examination (MMSE)
   19, 69, **237**
mink encephalopathy 106, 304
Mirapex. *See* pramipexole
mirtazapine (Remeron) 32
misidentification syndromes 83
mitotane 86
mixed nonfluent aphasia 34
mixed receptive-expressive language
   disorder **237–238**. *See also* language
   processing disabilities
MMR (measles-mumps-rubella) vaccine
   51–52
MMSE. *See* mini-mental state examination
mnemonics 328
mnesic syndromes **238**. *See also* agnosia;
   agraphia; alexia; Alzheimer's disease;
   anosognosia; aphasia; apraxia; Broca's
   aphasia; dissociative disorders;
   dysphasia; hysterical amnesia; organic
   amnesia; retrograde amnesia; selective
   amnesia; transient global amnesia
modafinil 250
molecular neurobiology **238**
molindone, as central nervous system
   depressant 86
Mongolism. *See* Down syndrome
monoamine neurotransmitters 32, 238
monoamine oxidase (MAO) 238, **238**
monoamine oxidase (MAO) inhibitors 32,
   33, 118, 238, 321, 340
monoclonal antibodies 256
mononucleosis, infectious 132
mood 138, 144. *See also* emotions and the
   brain; limbic system
mood disorders, Tourette syndrome and
   355
mood stabilizers 40
Moreau de Tours, Jacques Joseph 120,
   210
Morel, Benedict Augustin 117
Moro's reflex 311
morphine 5, **239**, 282, 298
mosquito-borne diseases, encephalitis
   130–131
motor aphasia. *See* Broca's aphasia
motor area. *See* motor cortex
motor association **239**
motor behavior, frontal lobe damage and
   373
motor cortex 87, 180, **239–240**. *See also*
   motor homunculus
motor homunculus **240**
motor nerves 74, **240**, 286, 334, 337
motor neuron disease **240**. *See also*
   primary lateral sclerosis
motor neurons 26, **240**, 311, 330–331, 336
motor symptoms of brain disorders 69
motor system, striatum and 340
motor system disease. *See* motor neuron
   disease

motor tics 241
movement, control of 87, 345
movement disorders **240–242**. *See
also* dystonia; Huntington's disease;
Parkinson's disease; Tourette syndrome;
tremor
MPTP (methyl-phenyl tetrahydropyridine)
283
MQ. *See* memory quotient
MRI. *See* magnetic resonance imaging
MS. *See* multiple sclerosis
MSLT. *See* Multiple Sleep Latency Test
multi-infarct dementia 115, 116, **242–
243**, 308
multiple area IQ scores (S.A.S's) 338
multiple intelligences **243–244**
multiple personality disorder, dissociation
in 176
multiple sclerosis (MS) 117, 138, 204,
244–245, 278, 333, 361. *See also*
Schilder's disease
Multiple Sleep Latency Test (MSLT) 250
muscarine 94
muscarinic blockers 32, 33
muscimol 158
muscle(s), cataplexy **84–85**
mushrooms, hallucinogenic **157–158**
music, memory for **219**
musical/rhythmic intelligence 243
myalgic encephalomyelitis. *See* chronic
fatigue and immune dysfunction
syndrome
myasthenia gravis (MG) 73, **245–246**
myelencephalon 164
myelin 152, **246**, 266, 301, 373. *See also*
demyelinating disorders; dysmyelination
disease
myelination 120, 262, 318, 367
myelin sheath 63, 156, 245, **246**, 305,
369
myelogram **246**
myelography 37, **246–247**
myelomeningocele 247–248, **247–248**,
336
myoclonus 124
mysoline (Primidone) 31, 241
Mytelase (ambenonium chloride) 246

N

N.A. (thalamic damage patient) 213, 352
nadolol 40
Najab ud-din Muhammad 63
naloxone **249**
Namenda (memantine) 19, 94, **212**
names, memory for 7, 219, **219–220**
naproxen 123, 233
narcolepsy 73, 85, 150, **249–250**, 332,
340
narcotics and the brain 134, **250–251**,
283, 298. *See also* morphine; opiates
Nardil (phenelzine) 32
NART. *See* New Adult Reading Test
National Center of Health Statistics 216

National Conference of Commissioners on
Uniform State Laws 67
National Council on Alcoholism and Drug
Dependence, Inc. 13
National Institute of Aging 9, 235–236, 293
National Institute of Child Health and
Human Development (NICHD) 52
National Institute of Mental Health 43
National Institute of Neurological
Disorders and Stroke 133
National Institute of Occupational Safety
and Health (NIOSH) 267
National Institute on Aging (NIA) 22, 121
National Institutes of Health 39, 109,
190, 342
National Joint Committee on Learning
Disabilities 196
Native Americans, alcohol and 14
naturalistic intelligence 244
natural opiates. *See* endorphin; limbic
system
nausea, antiemetic drugs **33**, 234
nefazodone (Serzone) 20, 32
neglect 42
Neisser, Ulric 172
Neisseria meningitidis 225
neocortex 64, 166, **251**. *See also*
association areas
neostigmine bromide (Prostigmin) 246
neostriatum. *See* caudate nucleus
neotic consciousness 101
nerve cells. *See* neuron(s)
nerve conduction velocity study **251**
nerve-growth factor (NGF) 21, 137,
251–252
nerve impulse **252**
nerves, spinal 337
nerve signal. *See* nerve impulse
nervous coordination 143
nervous exhaustion. *See* neurasthenia
nervous system 12, 144, **252**. *See also*
autonomic nervous system; central
nervous system; peripheral nervous
system
neural graft **252**
neural plate **252**
neural tube, development 119
neural tube defects **252–254**. *See also*
anencephaly; hydrocephalus; spina bifida
Arnold-Chiari malformation and 38
causes of 72, 144
folic acid deficiency and 27, 72, 229,
247, 248, 253–254
neurapraxia **254**
neurasthenia **254**
neurinoma. *See* acoustic neuroma
neurite 251, **254**
neuritis. *See* neuropathy
neuroanatomy **254**
neurobiology **254**
neuroblastic tumors 254
neuroblastoma **254–256**
neurochemistry **256**

neurocranium **256**
neurocysticercosis 110
neurodevelopmental treatment **256**
neuroectodermal tumors 144
neuroendocrine functions, melatonin
cycle and 212
neurofibrillary tangles 16, 58, **256**,
349–350
neurofibromatosis 4, 39, **256–258**
neuroglial cells **258**
neurohormone **258**
neurolemmoma. *See* acoustic neuroma
neuroleptic malignant syndrome (NMS)
71–72, **258–259**, 360
neuroleptics 40, 123, 307, 348
neurolinguistics **259**
neurological exam 69, **259**, 311
neurological manifestations of AIDS
259–260
neurological structure, gender differences
151–152
neurologist 260, 264
neurology 69, 209, **260–261**
neuroma 70, **261**. *See also* acoustic
neuroma
neurometrics **261**
neuron(s) **261–262**. *See also* axon(s);
motor neurons; receptor(s); synapse(s)
beta-amyloid and 58
in cerebellum 87
free radical damage to 33
functions 65, 134, 212–213, 261, 346
fundal cells 148
growth of 119, 142
history of research on 63
inability to reproduce 261, 297
learning-induced changes in 187–188
loss of, with aging 297
neurotoxins and 266
number of 296, 346
and pain 281
plasticity of **296–298**
research on 126
structure 65, 261, 281, 306
and visual processing 367
neuronal ceroid lipofuscinoses. *See* Batten
disease
neuronal migration disorders (NMDs) 262
neuronal storage diseases 116
neuron doctrine 63
neuropathology 262
neuropathy **262–263**. *See also* optic
neuritis
neuropeptides 166, **263**. *See also* substance
P
neuropeptide Y 166
neuropharmacology. *See*
psychopharmacology
neuropsychiatry 69, **263–264**
neuropsychological assessment 69, 161,
236, **264**
neuropsychologist 264
neuropsychology 69, **264–265**

neurosis 226
neurosonography. *See* ultrasound scan
neurosurgeon **265**
neurosurgery **265**
neurosyphilis **265**, 347
neurotensin **265**
neurotoxic drugs **265**
neurotoxin(s) 12–13, 67, 184, **265–267**,
   286. *See also* lead poisoning and the
   brain; pesticides and the brain; toxic
   encephalopathy; toxic mood disorders;
   toxins, environmental
neurotransmitter(s) **267–268**. *See also*
   acetylcholine; catecholamine(s);
   dopamine; endorphin; enkephalin;
   epinephrine; GABA (gamma-
   aminobutyric acid); glutamate; glycine;
   norepinephrine; receptor(s); serotonin;
   substance P; vasopressin
      and Alzheimer's disease 17
      amino acids and 23
      amphetamines and 25
      antidepressants and 31–32
      balance of 268
      bipolar disorder and 60
      blocking of, side effects 321
      chemical brain stimulation 91
      decreased production, with age 6
      depression and 118–119
      engrams and 134
      enzymes and 135
      functions 63, 134, 212–213, 261, 346
      lithium and 201
      neurohormones **258**
      neurotensin **265**
      neurotoxins and 266
      nicotine and 268
      and personality 287
      research on 126
      synthesis of, and nutrition 369
neurotrophin-3 252
neurotrophin-4/5 252
nevirapine 12
New Adult Reading Test (NART) **268**
New Idea in Medicine (Sylvius) 346
new variant Creutzfeldt-Jakob disease
   (nvCJD) 107, 166, 205–207, 304
NGF. *See* nerve-growth factor
niacin. *See* vitamin B₃
NICHD. *See* National Institute of Child
   Health and Human Development
nicotine 5, 94, **268–269**, 339
nikethamide 340
nimodipine (Nimotop) **269**
ninth cranial nerve. *See* glossopharyngeal
   nerve
NIOSH. *See* National Institute of
   Occupational Safety and Health
Nissl, Franz 16
Nizoral (ketoconazole) **178**
NLD. *See* nonverbal learning disabilities
NMDA (N-methyl-D-aspartate) 12, 269
NMDA receptor 12, 167, **269**

NMDA receptor antagonists 19–20, 212
NMDs. *See* neuronal migration disorders
N-methyl-D-aspartate. *See* NMDA
NMR (nuclear magnetic resonance). *See*
   magnetic resonance imaging
NMS. *See* neuroleptic malignant syndrome
Nobel Prize 126, 127, 128
No Child Left Behind (NCLB) 190
nominal aphasia 34
nondominant hemisphere **269**
nonparalytic poliomyelitis 299
non-REM (NREM) sleep 309, 331
nonsecreting pituitary tumors 295–296
nonsomniacs 330
nonsteroidal anti-inflammatory drugs
   (NSAIDs) 20, 233
nonverbal learning disabilities (NLD)
   269–272
nonverbal memory **272**
nootropics 3, 29, 83, 216, **272**, 308
noradrenaline. *See* norepinephrine
norepinephrine (noradrenaline) **272–273**
      ADHD and 230
      breakdown of 238
      and depression 118
      drug effects on 5, 25, 32, 97, 210,
         339–340, 357
      functions 63, 85, 130, 143, 216, 360
      pleasure centers and 298
      regulation of 65
      REM sleep and 330
      sympathetic nervous system and 346
      synthesis of 203, 290
norepinephrine blockers, side effects
   32–33, 321
normal-pressure hydrocephalus (NPH)
   117, **273**
Norpramin. *See* desipramine
nortriptyline (Aventyl; Pamelor) 32, 40,
   235, 360
Norvasc 235
NPH. *See* normal-pressure hydrocephalus
NREM (non-REM) sleep 309, 331
NSAIDS. *See* nonsteroidal anti-
   inflammatory drugs
nuclear magnetic resonance (NMR). *See*
   magnetic resonance imaging
nucleus accumbens 97, **273**
nucleus basalis of Meynert 93, **273**
nutritional disorders, and dementia 116
nutrition and the brain **273–274**. *See also*
   brain food; malnutrition; vitamin(s)
      brain development 142, 208–209
      memory 273–274, 292–293, 369
      and neurotransmitters 268
      variation in individual needs 208
nystagmus, aberrant 88

O

obesity, genetic causes 302
objects
      memory for 219, **221**
      misplacing 221

Observationes anatomicae (Fallopio) 140
*Observations and Experiments Investigating the
   Physiology of Senses* (Purkinje) 308
obsessive-compulsive disorder (OCD)
   280, 307, 353, 355
obstructive hydrocephalus 117
obstructive sleep apnea 331
occipital bone 106
occipital cortex. *See* visual cortex
occipital lobe 64, 88, 89, 91, 181, 275,
   275
occipital neuralgia **275**
OCD. *See* obsessive-compulsive disorder
ocular dominance columns **275**
oculomotor nerve (third cranial nerve)
   63, 75, 105, **275**. *See also* cranial nerves
odors, memory for **221**
Ohtahara syndrome **276**
olanzapine 112
olanzapine/fluoxetine (Symbyax) 32
olfactory bulbs **276**
olfactory fatigue **276**
olfactory nerve (first cranial nerve) 63,
   105, **276**, 333. *See also* cranial nerves
oligodendrocytes 152
oligodendroglioma **276–277**
olivopontocerebellar atrophy (OPCA)
   329
Omega-3 fat, and brain function 273–
   274
ondansetron 375
OPCA. *See* olivopontocerebellar atrophy
operant conditioning 311
opiate receptors 239, 263, 277, 298
opiates **277–278**. *See also* heroin;
   morphine; opium
      action and effects 5, 164, 239, 277
      addiction 5
      endogenous 134, 164, 277–278. *See
         also* endorphin
      manufacture of 239
      and memory impairment 123
      uses 86, 234, 277
opium and opium derivatives 239, 282
optical aphasia **278**
optical imaging 353
optic chiasm **278**, 367
optic nerve (second cranial nerve) 63,
   105, **278**. *See also* cranial nerves
optic neuritis **278–279**
optic tectum **279**
OPV (oral poliovirus vaccine) 299
oral contraceptives, and stroke risk 342
Orap. *See* pimozide
organ donation 67
organic amnesia (global amnesia) 24,
   217, **279**
organic brain syndrome **279**, 366
organic mental disorders **279–280**
The Organization of Behavior (Hebb) 162
organ of Corti 56, 162
organology 292
organophosphates 288

organ transplants, and West Nile
  encephalitis 131
osmoreceptors **280**
osteogenic sarcoma 281
osteoporosis, risk reduction 138
oval window 162
oxidative stress 20
oxiracetam 272, 308
2-oxo-pyrrolidone. *See* pyroglutamate
oxybutynin 86
oxycodone 234
oxytocin **280**

P

Paget's disease **281**
pain **281–282**, 323
pain control, endorphins and 133
painkillers 112, 123, **282**
paleocortex **282**
pallidotomy 285
Pamelor. *See* nortriptyline
pamidromate disodium (Aredia) 281
P-amyloid 18
panic disorders, Tourette syndrome and
  355
pantothenic acid. *See* vitamin B₅
Pappenheim, Bertha. *See* Anna O
Paracelsus 229
paradoxical sleep **282**. *See also* rapid eye
  movement (REM) sleep
paraldehyde 86
paralytic poliomyelitis 299
paranoid delusions, in Alzheimer's disease
  18
parasympathetic nervous system (PNS)
  52–53, 64, 65, **282**
parathyroid disease, and dementia 116
paregoric 86
pargyline 86
parietal bones 106
parietal cortex **282**
parietal lobes 2, 10–11, 64, 65, 88, 91,
  181, 223, **282**
Parkinson, James 284
parkinsonism 17, 34, 55, 69, 131,
  283–284
Parkinson's disease **284–285**
  basal ganglia and 55
  causes of 76, 121, 345
  dementia in 115
  incidence 284
  and memory 217
  symptoms and diagnosis 69, 284
  treatment and outlook 55, 76, 100,
    118, 198–199, 252, 284–285, 297
Parlodel. *See* bromocriptine
Parnate (tranylcypromine sulfate) 32
Paroxat. *See* paroxetine
paroxetine (Paxil, Seroxat, Aropax,
  Deroxat, Paroxat) 20, 32, 33, 235, 321,
  326
paroxetine mesylate (Pexeva) 32

partial seizures 136
Paxil. *See* paroxetine
PCA. *See* pyroglutamate
PCR analysis. *See* polymerase chain
  reaction (PCR) analysis
PDD. *See* Pervasive Developmental
  Disorders
Peabody Picture Vocabulary Test-Fourth
  Edition (PPVT-IV) 310
pediatric AIDS 229
pemoline (Cylert) 40, 86, 364–365
Penfield, Wilder 209, **285–286**
penicillamine 185
penicillin 225–226, 346, 347
pentamidine 12
pentobarbital 54
peptides **286**
perception **286**
  field dependence 142
  field independence 142–143
perceptual disorder **286**
pergolide (Permax) 285
peripheral nervous system (PNS) **286**
  components of 252
  defined 86
  functions 86
  neuropathy 262–263, **286–287**
  nutrition and 369
peripheral neuropathy **286–287**
peripheral NF. *See* neurofibromatosis
Permax (pergolide) 285
perphenazine 357
perphenazine/amitriptyline (Etrafon;
  Triavil) 32
personality 15–16, **287**
Pert, Candace 171, 263
Pervasive Developmental Disorders
  (PDDs) 38, 39, 50, **288**. *See also*
  Asperger's syndrome; autistic disorder;
  Rett syndrome
pesticides and the brain **288**, 356
petit mal seizure 135–136, **288–289**
PET scan (positron emission tomography)
  75, 161, 173, 209, 236, **289–290**
PETT (positron emission transaxial
  tomography). *See* PET scan
Pexeva (paroxetine mesylate) 32
phase sequences 163
phenelzine (Nardil) 32
phenmetrazine 36
phenobarbital 31, 54, 320
phenothiazines 33, 86, 283, 318, 357
phentermine 36
phenylalanine 71, **290**, 290–291
phenylethyamine 118
phenylketonuria (PKU) 71, 227, 228,
  290–291
phenylpropanolamine 36
phenytoin (Dilantin) 31, 72, **291**, 320
pheromones 326
phosphatidyl choline 93
photographic memory 128, 214

phototherapy 319
phrenology 74, 149–150, **291–292**
physiological causes of memory loss
  292–293
Physiological Elements of the Human Body
  (Haller) 157
physostigmine **293**, 319
pia-arachnoid 293
Piaget, Jean 214
pia mater 222, **293**
Pick, Arnold 293
Pick's disease 115, **293–294**
pimozide (Orap) 86, 355
pineal gland 211–212, **294**, 319, 330
pineal gland tumors **294–295**
pineoblastomas 294
pineocytomas 294
piperidine derivatives 158
piracetam 29, 272, 308
pituitary adenoma **295**
pituitary gland **295**
  endorphins and 133, 134
  functions 143, 352
  hormones 6, 155, 280, 364
  hypothalamus and 169, 200
pituitary gland disease 116
pituitary tumors 6, 105, **295–296**
PKC. *See* protein kinase C
PKU. *See* phenylketonuria
placebo effect, in nutrition 208–209
places, memory for **221–222**
plantar reflex 311
planum temporale 40, **296**
plaques, neuritic
  in Alzheimer's disease 16, 17, 18, 21,
    22, 26, **58**, 256, 349–350
  in fatal familial insomnia 141
plasma, as term 308
plasticity **296–298**
play therapy, for ADHD 48
pleasure centers 130, **298**
PLS. *See* primary lateral sclerosis
PML. *See* progressive multifocal
  leukoencephalopathy
PMS (premenstrual syndrome) 212
pneumatic school of medicine 37
pneumococcal vaccine 226
pneumoencephalography **298**
PNS. *See* parasympathetic nervous system;
  peripheral nervous system
poisoning, carbon monoxide **83–84**
polio. *See* poliomyelitis
polioencephalitis **298**
polioencephalomyelitis **298**
poliomyelitis (polio) 298, **298–299**
polycythemia 342
polymerase chain reaction (PCR) analysis
  145
polypeptides 23
polysomnogram (PSG) 250
pons 64, 75, **299**, 330
Pool, J. Lawrence 354

porencephaly **299–300**, 317
positron emission tomography. *See* PET scan
positron emission transaxial tomography (PETT). *See* PET scan
postcentral gyrus (somatosensory cortex) **300**
postconcussion syndrome 71, 100, 160, **300–301**
postencephalitic amnesia 217
posthypnotic amnesia 24, 229
postpolio syndrome (PPS) **301–302**
posttraumatic amnesia 23, 100, 300, 358
potassium **302**
poverty, and mental retardation 227
powassan encephalitis 130
PPS. *See* postpolio syndrome
PPVT-IV. *See* Peabody Picture Vocabulary Test-Fourth Edition
Prader-Willi syndrome (PWS) **302**
pramipexole (Mirapex) 283, 284–285
pramiracetam 272, 308
praxia **302**
prednisone 57
prefrontal cortex 43, 64, 102, 148, 287, **302–303**
prefrontal lobe 7
prefrontal lobotomy 307
pregnancy. *See also* development of the brain; neural tube defects
    alcohol and 14, 71, 119–120, 189, 227. *See also* fetal alcohol effects; fetal alcohol syndrome
    antiemetic drugs and 33
    drug use and 189, 227
    hot tubs and **165–166**
    labor, initiation of 280
    and mental retardation, problems resulting in 227, 229
    and multiple sclerosis 245
    and neurofibromatosis 257
    and nutrition 208
    phenytoin during 72
    PKU and 290
    screening for Down syndrome 122
    smoking and 119–120, 189, 227
    and stroke risk 342
    and syphilis transmission 347
    temperature, excessive, and 165–166, 253
    TORCH disorders and 354
    and toxoplasmosis 357
pregnancy and memory **303**
pregnenolone **303**
premotor cortex **303**
prescription medication
    brain disorders from 2, 71–72, 116
    caffeine in 82
presenile dementia 322
President's Commission for the Study of Ethical Problems in Medicine 67
primary lateral sclerosis (PLS) **303–304**

primary visual cortex 275, **304**
Primidone. *See* mysoline
primitive brain. *See* reptilian brain
primitive reflexes 311
prion(s) (proteinaceous infectious particle) 70, 106–108, 141, 206–207, **304–305**. *See also* human prion diseases; transmissible spongiform encephalopathies
prion protein molecule (PrP) 304–305
procaine 98
procarbazine 86
procedural memory 111, 203
prochlorperazine (Compazine) 234
progressive bulbar palsy 240
progressive multifocal leukoencephalopathy (PML) 260, **305**
progressive muscular atrophy 240
progressive supranuclear palsy (PSP) 241–242, **305**
prolactin 296
prolactin-secreting pituitary tumors 295–296
promethazine 86
propiomazine 86
propoxyphene 234
propranolol (Inderal) 235, 241
prosopagnosia 72, 275, **306**
Prostigmin (neostigmine bromide) 246
protein(s) and brain function 73. *See also* amino acids
protein kinase C (PKC) **306**
protoplasm, as term 308
protriptyline (Vivactil) 32, 250, 332, 360
Prozac. *See* fluoxetine
PrP. *See* prion protein molecule
Prusiner, Stanley B. 304
pseudodementia **306**
pseudotumor cerebri (benign intracranial hypertension) **306**
psilocybin 158
psilocybin/psilocin mushrooms 157–158
PSP. *See* progressive supranuclear palsy
psychedelic drugs **306**. *See also* hallucinogens
Psychiatrie (Kraepelin) 117
psychiatrists, views on mental illness 202
psychic blindness **306**
psychoactive drugs 30, 298
psychoanalysis, development of 79, 145
psychogenic amnesia 24–25, 103
psychoneuroimmunology 171
The Psychopathology of Everyday Life (Freud) 146
psychopharmacology **307**
psychosis. *See also* antipsychotic drugs
    in Alzheimer's disease 18
    causes 226
    cocaine psychosis 97
    symptoms and diagnosis 226
    thought disorder in 353
    v. dementia 113

psychosurgery **307**. *See also* leucotomy; lobectomy; lobotomy; surgery
Psychosurgery (Freeman and Watts) 145
psychotherapy 47, 98–99, 214
psychotropic drugs 123, 307
5p– syndrome. *See* cri du chat syndrome
Public Health Service, U.S. 254
Public Law 94-142 197
public schools, special education services 190–191
punch drunk syndrome 71, **307**
pure word deafness 11
Purkinje, Jan Evangelista **307–308**
Purkinje cells 308
Purkinje effect 308
Purkinje fibers 308
putamen. *See* striatum
putamen nucleus 55, 64
Puysegur, Marquis de 229
PWS. *See* Prader-Willi syndrome
pyramidal cells **308**
pyridostigmine 301
pyridostigmine bromide (Mestinon) 246
pyridoxine. *See* vitamin B_6
pyrimethamine (Daraprim) 357
pyroglutamate (2-oxo-pyrrolidone; carboxylic acid; PCA) **308**
pyrrolidone derivatives 272, **308**
Pythagoras **308**

Q

qEEG. *See* Quantitative EEG
quadriplegia, in cerebral palsy 89
quantitative EEG (qEEG) 161, 236
quetiapine (Seroquel) 32
quinidine 123
quinolinic acid 167
quinolones 123

R

RA. *See* retrograde amnesia
rabies (hydrophobia) 130, **309**
rabies vaccine 132
racial memory. *See* collective unconscious
radiation therapy
    side effects 190, 211, 271
    uses 4, 78, 105, 135, 153–154, 154–155, 211, 255, 277, 294–295, 296, 313, 337
radionuclides 334–335
Rain Man (film) 52
Ramon y Cajal, Santiago 63
raphe nuclei. 204, 330
rapid eye movement (REM) sleep (paradoxical sleep) 123, 182, 249, **309**, 330–331
Rasmussen's encephalitis, treatment 163
RASY. *See* reticular activating system
rauwolfia, as central nervous system depressant 86
Razadyne. *See* galantamine hydrobromide
reading 148, **309–310**. *See also* developmental reading disorder; dyslexia

Reagan, Ronald W. 76
Rebif 245
Reboul-Lachaux, J. 83
recall 213, 217, **310**
receptive language **310**. *See also*
  developmental receptive language
  disorder; mixed receptive-expressive
  language disorder
receptor(s) **310**. *See also* chemoreceptors
    depression and 118–119
    drug abuse and 189
    functions 134, 212–213, 261, 346
    heat 350
    myasthenia gravis and 245
    substance abuse and 344
Recklinghausen, Friedrich von 256–257
recovered memory 91–92
reduplicative paramnesia. *See* Capgras
  syndrome
reflex(es) 14, **310–311**, 366
reflex arc 311
registration, of memory 215, 217
regressive autism 49
*Remembering: A Study in Experimental and
  Social Psychology* (Bartlett) 55
Remeron (mirtazapine) 32
REM sleep. *See* rapid eye movement
  (REM) sleep
repair of brain tissue, neural plasticity
  and 297
repression, Freud on 146, 171. *See also*
  hysterical amnesia
reproductive cycle 138, 151, 173
reptilian brain (primitive brain) 64, 75,
  312
Requip. *See* ropinirole
research
    on Alzheimer's disease 16–18
    on brain cells 209
    chemical brain stimulation **91**
    electrical brain stimulation **128–129**,
      209, 285–286, 351
    evoked response **138**
    future of 65
    history of 126, 149–150
    on localization of brain function 80
    on message transmission in brain 126
    split-brain research **338**
    on temporal lobe 351
    on thought 353
    visual-evoked responses (VERs)
      367–368
reserpine 349
respiratory stimulants 340
response bias hypothesis 218
reticular activating system (RASY) 43,
  312, 340
reticular core **312**
reticular formation **312**
    alcohol and 13
    cochlear nerve and 4
    and consciousness 101, 363
    damage to 76, 99

functions of 75
    limbic system and 200
    location of 64, 75
retinoblastoma **312–313**
retrieval 313
    aging and 7
    cue-dependent forgetting 68–69, **109**
    effortful processing **127**
    engrams and 134
    head injury and 161
    infantile amnesia 171–172
    in memory process 215
    scopolamine and 319
retrograde amnesia (RA) 23, 61, 179,
  217, **313–314**, 352, 357, 358. *See also*
  shrinking retrograde amnesia
retrovirus, in spinal fluid (spumavirus) 95
Rett, Andreas 314
Rett syndrome 71, **314–315**
Reye's syndrome 73, **315–316**
Rh disease 228
rhombencephalon. *See* hindbrain
riboflavin. *See* vitamin B$_2$
ribonucleic acid. *See* RNA
rifampicin 225
right brain (right hemisphere) **316**. *See
  also* left brain-right brain
    functions of 63–64, 88, 91, 198, 338
    and language 180, 183
right-hemisphere learning disorders. *See*
  nonverbal learning disabilities
riluzole (Rilutek) 26–27
risedronate sodium (Actonel) 281
Risperdal. *See* risperidone
risperidone (Risperdal) 40, 112, 355
Ritalin. *See* methylphenidate
  hydrochloride
rivastigmine (Exelon) 19, 93, 94, 121,
  316
rizatriptan (Maxalt) 234
RNA (ribonucleic acid) 216
RO 13-5057. *See* aniracetam
Roentgen, Wilhelm Conrad 374
Rohypnol 150
rooting reflex 311
ropinirole (Requip) 283, 284–285
RU-486 (mifepristone) 223
rubella 132, 229, 232. *See also* TORCH
  disorders

S

saccule 366
Sacks, Oliver 131
SAD. *See* seasonal affective disorder
St. Louis encephalitis 131
St. Vitus' dance 94, 345
Sandhoff disease **317**
Santavuori-Haltia disease 56
Sarafem. *See* fluoxetine
sarcoma, osteogenic 281
Sarpul. *See* aniracetam
saunas, and pregnancy 165–166
savant, autistic **52**

scala tympani 56
Schaie, K. Warner 8
schema, in memory 55
Schilder's disease 117, **317**
schizencephaly **317–318**
schizophrenia **318–319**
    amnesia in 25
    brain asymmetry and 40–41
    causes and risk factors 55, 97, 120,
      121, 165, 318
    cerebellum and 88
    corpus callosum and 103
    imaginary smells in 333
    and IQ score 175
    Jung (Carl) on 176
    and memory 217
    thought disorders in 353
    treatment 33, 92, 121, 357
Schwann cells 257
schwannoma. *See* acoustic neuroma
scopolamine 31, 86, 293, **319**
scrapie 106, 107, 206, 304
searching technique, aging and 9
seasickness patches, and memory
  impairment 123
seasonal affective disorder (SAD) 212,
  319–320
secobarbital 54
second cranial nerve. *See* optic nerve
secreting pituitary tumors 295–296
sedatives 131, **320**. *See also* barbiturates;
  central nervous system depressants
seeing stars **338–339**
seizure(s) **320**. *See also* anticonvulsant
  drugs; grand mal seizures; petit mal
  seizure
    causes 15, 320
    epileptic 320
      first aid for 136–137
      types of 135–136
    status epilepticus **339**
    and Todd's paralysis **353**
    treatment 163, 210, 291
seizure, febrile **320–321**
seizure disorder 320
selective amnesia 25
selective serotonin reuptake inhibitors
  (SSRIs) **321–332**
    side effects 32–33, 321
    uses 60, 160, 235, 250, 320, 326
selegiline. *See* deprenyl
self, sense of 351. *See also*
  autobiographical memory
self-hypnosis. *See* hypnosis
semantic memory 7, 9, 203, **322**
semicircular canals 365
senile dementia **322**
senility 111, 113, 167, 308, **322**. *See also*
  aging and memory; dementia praecox
sense of direction 221
senses and the brain **322–323**, 352. *See
  also entries under* sensory
sensory agnosia 11

sensory area **323**
sensory ataxia 41
sensory cortex **323**
sensory defensiveness 325
sensory deprivation **323**
sensory integration **323–324**
sensory integration dysfunction (DSI) **324–325**
sensory memory 215
sensory nerves 74, 286, 323, 334, 337
Sepram. *See* citalopram
septo-optic dysplasia (SOD) **325–326**
septum 64
Serlain. *See* sertraline
Seromex. *See* fluoxetine
Seronil. *See* fluoxetine
Seropram. *See* citalopram
Seroquel (quetiapine) 32
serotonin **326**. *See also* selective serotonin reuptake inhibitors
    breakdown of 238
    cyclics and 32
    and depression 118
    functions 63, 130, 360
    hallucinogenic drugs and 5, 127, 157–158, 204
    migraine and 160, 233
    precursors 204
    seasonal affective disorder and 320
    synthesis of 345
    and Tourette syndrome 356
    tryptophan and 361
serotonin receptor medications 234
serotonin receptors 322
serotonin system 235, 321
Seroxat. *See* paroxetine
sertraline (Zoloft, Lustral, Serlain) 32, 33, 40, 235, 250, 321, 326
Serzone. *See* nefazodone
seventh cranial nerve. *See* facial nerve
sex differences in the brain. *See* gender differences
sex-linked genetic disorders 71
sexual abuse, delayed memory of 91–92
sexual function, antidepressant drugs and 32–33
sexuality and the brain **326**
sexual orientation and the brain **326–327**
shaken baby syndrome 71, **327–328**
Sherrington, Sir Charles 126
short-term memory **328–329**
    aging and 7, 9, 10
    alcohol abuse and 14
    characteristics v. long-term memory 203
    drugs to improve 143, 366
    head injury and 161
    protein kinase C and 306
    transfer into long-term memory 328–329
    visual 368
shrinking retrograde amnesia **329**
shunt, brain **329**

Shy-Drager syndrome 73, **329–330**
SIDS. *See* sudden infant death syndrome
sight. *See* vision
Simon, Theodore 59
simple seizures 136
Sinemet. *See* carbidopa-L-dopa
Sinequan. *See* doxepin
single fiber electromyography (EMG) 246
single-photon emission computerized tomography. *See* SPECT
sixth cranial nerve. *See* abducens nerve
skeletal muscle relaxants 86
Skelid (tiludronate disodium) 281
skull bones. *See* craniosynostosis; fontanelles
sleep and the brain 211–212, 230, **330–331**. *See also* rapid eye movement (REM) sleep
sleep apnea **331–332**, 332
sleep cycle 96, 332, 352, 363
sleep disorders 95, 176, **332**. *See also* apnea; familial insomnia; fatal familial insomnia
sleeping sickness **332**
sleep paralysis 250
slow viruses of the brain **332–333**
smell, sense of 200, **333**, 349. *See also* entries under olfactory
Smith, Edwin, surgical papyrus of 62, 160, 300, **333–334**
smoking 7, 84, 119–120, 189, 227, 333. *See also* nicotine
snoring 331
SNS. *See* sympathetic nervous system
Snyder, Solomon 263
social functioning. *See* nonverbal learning disabilities
social skills training, for ADHD 47
social stress, impact of 340
socioeconomic status, as predictor of mental decline 8
SOD. *See* septo-optic dysplasia
sodium amytal therapy 202
sodium oxybate (gamma hydroxybutyrate; GHB; Xyrem) 250
sodium pentothal 100, 361
somatic nervous system **334**
somatosensory agnosia 11
somatosensory cortex. *See* postcentral gyrus
somnambulism, artificial 229
source amnesia 7, **334**
southern blot analysis 145
spasmodic torticollis 241
spasticity **334**
spastic symptoms, of cerebral palsy 89
spatial information, types of 221–222
spatial memory 221–222
spatial visualization skills, aging and 7, 10
special education services 2–3, 190–191, 195–196

SPECT (single-photon emission computerized tomography) 161–162, 236, **334–335**
speech 68, 180, 181, **335**
speech disorders 327, 335. *See also* developmental speech and language disorders; dysarthria
speech-language pathologist **335**
speech therapist. *See* speech-language pathologist
speech therapy, for aphasia 35
Speigel, David 214
Sperry, Roger 198
sphenoid bone 106
Spielmeyer-Vogt disease 56
spina bifida 27, 72, 165–166, 167, 247, 252, **335–336**. *See also* meningocele; myelomeningocele
spina bifida occulta 247, 336
spinal accessory nerve (eleventh cranial nerve) 63, 75, **336**. *See also* cranial nerves
spinal cord 81, 152, 252, 261, **336–337**. *See also* neurosyphilis
spinal cord tumors 163, **337**
spinal nerves 337
spinal tap. *See* lumbar puncture
spino-cerebellar ataxia, type 3 (SCA/3). *See* Machado-Joseph disease
spiroplasmas 70
spleen, neural connections 171
split-brain research **338**
spongiform encephalopathies 70, 106, 206–207, **338**. *See also* Creutzfeldt-Jakob disease; fatal familial insomnia; kuru; mad cow disease; prion(s); scrapie
spumavirus 95
SQUID (superconducting quantum interference device) **338**
SSRIs. *See* selective serotonin reuptake inhibitors
Stanford-Binet Intelligence Scale: Fifth Edition (SB 5) 173, 175, **338**
stapes (stirrup) 162
stars, seeing **338–339**
state of mind, and immune system function 171
statins 41
status epilepticus **339**
stem cell transplantation 255–256
stent, arterial 42
stereogram **339**
stereotactic radiosurgery (gamma knife) 78, **339**
stereotaxic surgery 307
steroid hormones 111, 279, 303, 337
stimulants and the brain 45–46, 168, 203, **339–340**
stimulus 312, **340**
stimulus-response memory **340**
stirrup (stapes) 162
Stokes-Adams syndrome 140, **340**
strabismus 1

Streptococcus 225, 226, 345, 355
stress and the brain 57, 68, 104, 171, 214, **340**
stress hormones 6, 9, 68, 72, 143
stress management, for parents of ADHD children 48
striate cortex. *See* visual cortex
striatonigral degeneration 329
striatum **340–341**
stroke **340–342**. *See also* apoplexy
    and agnosia 10
    and amnesia 24
    brain damage following 269
    brain-wave evaluations following 78
    causes and risk factors 38, 41, 84, 90, 129, 133, 174, 341, 342, 343
    cerebellum and 88
    and memory 213
    and multi-infarct dementia 242
    symptoms and diagnosis 74, 341–342
    treatment and outlook 2, 133, 252, 269, 342
    warning signs of 24, 341
Student Assistance Team 190
Studien über Hysterie (*Studies on Hysteria*; Freud and Breuer) 29, 79, 120–121
Sturge-Weber syndrome **342–343**
stuttering 152, 158
subacute sclerosing panencephalitis 333
subarachnoid hemorrhage 24, **343**
subarachnoid space 204, 298, **343**
subclavian artery 84
subconscious activity 102
subdural hematoma 116
subdural hemorrhage **343–344**
subliminal learning **344**
substance abuse **344**. *See also* addiction; alcoholism
    effects of 71, 112, 116, 189, 197, 227, 232
    Ritalin exposure and 46
substance P 267, **344**
substantia gelatinosa **344**
substantia nigra **344–345**
    and basal ganglia 55, 64
    damage to 76
    deprenyl and 118
    dopamine and 121, 199, 284
    GHB and 150
    in Lewy body dementia 199
    opiate receptors in 239
    and Parkinson's disease 121
substitution hypothesis 218
sudden infant death syndrome (SIDS) 331
sugar, and memory 273–274
suicide
    antidepressants and 32, 360
    bipolar disorder and 60
sulci **345**. *See also* central sulcus; lateral sulcus
sulfadiazine 357
sumatriptan (Imitrex) 234, **345**

superconducting quantum interference device. *See* SQUID
superior colliculus **345**
supplementary motor area **345**
suprachiasmatic nucleus 151, **345**
surgery. *See also* hemispherectomy; leucotomy; lobectomy; lobotomy
    brain tissue transplants **76**
    and Creutzfeldt-Jakob disease 106, 107
    for epilepsy 136
    pallidotomy 285
    psychosurgery **307**
    stereotactic radiosurgery 78, **339**
    thalamotomy 285
    topectomy **354**
    trephining **360**
    ventriculoatriostomy **365**
    ventriculostomy **365**
Surmontil. *See* trimipramine
Sydenham chorea **345**
sylvian fissure (Fissure of Sylvius) **143**, **346**
Sylvius, Franciscus **346**
Symbyax (olanzapine/fluoxetine) 32
sympathetic nervous system (SNS) 52–53, 64, 65, 81, 158, 169, **346**. *See also* parasympathetic nervous system
sympathomimetics 86
synapse(s) **346–347**
    development of 67
    functions 212–213
    learning-induced changes in 187–188
    number of 346
    plasticity of **296–298**
    pruning of 262
    reproductive cycle and 138
    research on 126
synaptic change and memory **347**. *See also* memory, storage in brain
synaptic gap, functions 134
synaptic vesicles 3
syncope. *See* fainting
syphilis 116, **347**

T

Taborikova, Helena 126
tacrine (Cognex) 19, 20, 93, 94, 121, 293, 348, **348**
Taenia solium 110
tangles, neurofibrillary. *See* neurofibrillary tangles
tapeworms, and cysticercosis 110
tardive dyskinesia 33–34, 71, 92, **348–349**, 361
Tasmar (tolcapone) 284–285
taste 222, 349, **349**
taste buds 349
tau protein 58, 256, **349–350**
Tay-Sachs disease **350**. *See also* Sandhoff disease
tectum, midbrain **350**
tegmentum **350**

Tegretol. *See* carbamazepine
telencephalon (endbrain) 144, **350**. *See also* prefrontal cortex
temperature, sensation of 323
temperature regulation **350–351**
temporal artery **351**
temporal bones 106
temporal cortex. *See* temporal lobe
temporal lobe(s) **351**. *See also* leucotomy; Wernicke's area
    abscesses 1
    and déjà vu 112
    electrical stimulation of 128–129, 285–286, 351
    functions 48–49, 65, 88, 89, 91, 162, 351
    location 64, 65
    and memory 66, 128–129, 213, 285–286, 351
    tumors of 223
temporal lobectomy 136, **351–352**
Tenex. *See* guanfacine
teniposide 255
Tenormin (atenolol) 235
tension headaches 159
TENS units. *See* transcutaneous nerve stimulator (TNS) unit
tenth cranial nerve. *See* vagus nerve
tentorium 123
teratogenic effects, of marijuana and hashish 6
teratomas 294
terpenes 152
testosterone 111
tetrabenazine 349
tetracyclics 32
tetrahydroaminoacridine (THA). *See* tacrine
Textbook of Brain Disorders (*Lehrbuch der Gehirnkrankheiten*; Wernicke) 372
THA (tetrahydroaminoacridine). *See* tacrine
thalamotomy 285
thalamus **352**. *See also* superior colliculus
    and fatal familial insomnia 141
    functions 87
    GHB and 150
    limbic system and 64
    and memory 66, 213–214
    opiate receptors in 239
    and schizophrenia 318
    and senses 322–323, 352
    thalamotomy 285
THC (delta-9 tetrahydrocannabinol) 209
theta waves 78, 129, 210, 352
thiamine. *See* vitamin B_1
thimerosal 51–52
thiopental 54
thioridazine 357
thiothixene 33
thioxanthenes 86
third cranial nerve. *See* oculomotor nerve
thirst **352**. *See also* fluid imbalances and the brain

Thorazine. *See* chlorpromazine
thought 352–353
thought disorders **353**, 358
thrombolytic therapy 42
thymosine 154
thymus 171, 246
thyroid gland 116, 170
thyroid stimulating hormone (TSH;
    thyrotropin) **353**, 355
thyrotropin. *See* thyroid stimulating
    hormone
thyroxine 170
TIA. *See* transient ischemic attack
tic disorders 124, 241. *See also* Tourette
    syndrome
tic douloureux. *See* trigeminal neuralgia
Ticlid 342
tiludronate disodium (Skelid) 281
time out (behavior modification tool) 48
tizanidine 304
TNS unit. *See* transcutaneous nerve
    stimulator (TNS) unit
tocopherol. *See* vitamin E
Todd's paralysis **353**
Tofranil. *See* imipramine
Tofranil-PM (imipramine pamoate) 32
tolcapone (Tasmar) 284–285
tomogram **353**
tomography **353**
tonic neck reflex 311
topectomy **354**
TORCH disorders **354**
torticollis, spasmodic 241
touch, sensation of 323
Tourette syndrome 46, 241, **354–356**
toxic encephalopathy 72, 132, **356**
toxic headaches 160
toxic mood disorders **356**
toxins, environmental. *See also* lead
    poisoning and the brain; neurotoxin
    and brain disorders 72
    and brain tumors 77
    and dementia 116
    and fetal damage 120, 227
    and glioblastoma risk 153
    and neural tube defects 254
    toxic headaches 160
    and transient global amnesia 357
Toxoplasma gondii 356
toxoplasmosis 232, 259–260, **356–357**.
    See also TORCH disorders
tramadol (Ultram) 234
tranquilizers 5, 283, **357**. *See also*
    antianxiety drugs; antipsychotic drugs;
    barbiturates; benzodiazepines
transcutaneous nerve stimulator (TNS)
    unit 234, 287
transient global amnesia 24, **357**, 358
transient ischemic attack (TIA) 341,
    358
    Broca's aphasia in 80
    causes of 41, 84
    diagnosis of 28

and stroke risk 342
    treatment of 31, 133
transient memory disorders 358
transmissible mink encephalopathy (TME)
    106, 304
transmissible spongiform encephalopathies
    (TSEs) 70, 106, 206–207, 338. *See also*
    Creutzfeldt-Jakob disease; fatal familial
    insomnia; kuru; mad cow disease;
    prion(s); scrapie
transorbital lobotomy 198, 202
transsphenoidal operation 295
tranylcypromine 32
tranylcypromine sulfate (Parnate) 32
trauma-induced headache 160
traumatic amnesia. *See* posttraumatic
    amnesia
traumatic brain injury **358–359**
trazodone (Desyrel) 32, 86, 112, 320
tremor 124, 241, **359–360**
trephining **360**
Treponema pallidum 347
Triavil (perphenazine/amitriptyline) 32
tricyclic antidepressants 32–33, 40, 235,
    250, 320, 321, **360–361**
trifluoperazine 357
trigeminal nerve (fifth cranial nerve)
    63, 75, 105, 233, **361**. *See also* cranial
    nerves
trigeminal neuralgia **361**
trimeprazine, as central nervous system
    depressant 86
trimethobenzamide, as central nervous
    system depressant 86
trimipramine (Surmontil) 32
triptans 234
trisomy 21. *See* Down syndrome
trochlear nerve (fourth cranial nerve) 63,
    75, **361**. *See also* cranial nerves
truth drugs **361**
Trypanosoma brucei 332
tryptophan 23, 273, **361–362**
TSEs. *See* transmissible spongiform
    encephalopathies
tsetse fly 332
TSH. *See* thyroid stimulating hormone
TSH-secreting pituitary tumors 296
tuberous sclerosis 39, **362**
Tulving, Endel 101
tumors. *See also* brain tumors
    nerve 256–258, 261
    parietal lobe 10–11
    pineal gland **294–295**
    pituitary 6, 105, **295–296**
    retina 312–313
    spinal cord 163, **337**
    sympathetic nervous system **254–256**
Turgenev, Ivan 79
Twelfth cranial nerve. *See* hypoglossal
    nerve
Type M person 16
Type P person 16
Type R person 15

tyramine 36, 238
tyrosine 23, 71, 290, **362**

U

Über Coca (Freud) 97–98
ultradian rhythms **363**
Ultram (tramadol) 234
ultrasound scan **363**
unconscious mind 103, **111**, 146. *See also*
    collective unconscious
unconsciousness 100–101, 102, **363**
Uniform Determination of Death Act 67
Usher, JoNell Adair 172
utricle 366

V

vacant slot hypothesis 218
vaccine(s)
    for Alzheimer's disease 21
    and autistic disorder 51–52, 72
    meningococcal 224, 225, 226
    and mental retardation prevention
        228–229
    pneumococcal 226
    polio 298–299
    rabies 132, 309
    swine flu 156
vagus nerve (tenth cranial nerve) 63, 75,
    105, 140, **364**. *See also* cranial nerves
Vagus Nerve Stimulator 136
Valium. *See* diazepam
valproate (Depakote) 15, 40, 60, 235
valproic acid 31, 289, 320, 349, 361
Varolio, Constanzo **364**
vascular headaches 159–160
vascular surgery 342
vasculitis, and dementia 116
vasopressin (antidiuretic hormone) 352,
    364, **364–365**, 365
vegetarians, malnutrition in 292, 369
venlafaxine HCl (Effexor) 32
ventricles 90, 164, 165, 298, **365**
ventriculitis **365**
ventriculoatriostomy **365**
ventriculography **365**
ventriculoscopy **365**
ventriculostomy **365**
verapamil 160, 235
verbal/linguistic intelligence 243–244
verbal memory **365**
VERs. *See* visual-evoked responses
vertebrobasilar insufficiency 140, **365**
vertigo **365**
Vesalius, Andreas 74, 364
vestibular nerve **366**
vestibular system **366**
vestibulocochlear nerve (eight cranial
    nerve) 3, 63, 75, 257, 258, **366**. *See also*
    cranial nerves
vestibulo-ocular reflex **366**
Vigabatrin 123
vincamine **366**. *See also* vinpocetine
vincristine 255

vinpocetine (Cavinton) **366**
virinos, and mad cow disease 206
virus(es). *See also* poliomyelitis; rabies
   and Alzheimer's disease 17, 18
   and Bell's palsy 57
   and dementia 18
   and encephalitis 130
   and Guillain-Barré syndrome 156
   and mad cow disease 206
   in pregnancy, and schizophrenia
     318
   slow viruses of the brain **332–333**
vision **366–367**. *See also* eye;
  stereogram; superior colliculus;
  suprachiasmatic nucleus; *entries under*
  optical
   amblyopia **22–23**
   blindsight 275
   brain development and 67–68
   brain pathways 275
   in infants 367
   primary visual cortex **304**
   processing of visual information
     367, 368
   psychic blindness **306**
   seeing stars **338–339**
   vestibulo-ocular reflex **366**
visual agnosia 11
visual association areas, and language
  function 180
visual cortex (striate cortex) 89, 180,
  181, 367
visual-evoked responses (VERs) **367–368**
visual fields **368**
visual memory **368**
visual-motor integration tests, BRAT
  battery **79**
visual occipital cortex **368**
visual perception **368**
visual processing deficits, in children 2
visual/spatial intelligence 244
vitamin(s) 14, 73, 208, **368–369**. *See*
  also vitamin deficiency
vitamin(s), B-complex 116, 292–293,
  369
vitamin A 56, 333, 368
vitamin B_1 (thiamine)
  deficiency 14, 23, 116, 132, 178–
    179, 217, 368, 369, 372
  for delirium 112
  and memory 292
  sources of 369
vitamin B_2 (riboflavin) 368
vitamin B_3 (niacin) 116, 292, 368, 369
vitamin B_5 (pantothenic acid) 254, 368
vitamin B_6 (pyridoxine) 72, 368, 369

vitamin B_9 (folic acid) **143–144**
  deficiency
   effects of 27, 72, 116, 229, 247,
    248, 253–254, 368
   in elderly 144
  functions 143–144, 369
  sources of 144
vitamin B_{12} (cobalamin)
  deficiency 116, 253, 254, 292–293, 369
  functions 333, 369
vitamin C 20, 33, 56
vitamin D 333
vitamin deficiency. *See also specific*
  vitamins
  in alcoholism 14, 208, 369
  causes of 208
  and fetal damage 120
vitamin E (tocopherol) 20, 21, 33, 56,
  236, 369
Vivactil. *See* protriptyline
vocabulary, brain development and 68
vocal tics 241, 354–355
voices, memory for **222**
von Hippel-Lindau disease 163
von Recklinghausen's disease. *See*
  neurofibromatosis

W

WAIS-IV. *See* Wechsler Adult Intelligence
  Scale–Fourth Edition
walking or stepping reflex 311
warfarin (Coumadin) 41
water on the brain. *See* hydrocephalus
Watts, James 128, 145, 198, 201–202
Wechsler, David 370
Wechsler Adult Intelligence Scale–
  Fourth Edition (WAIS-IV) 25, 173,
  175, 338, **370**
Wechsler Intelligence Scale for Children–
  Fourth Edition (WISC-IV) 173, 175,
  370, **370**
Wechsler Preschool and Primary Scale of
  Intelligence–Third Edition (WPPSI-III)
  370, 371
weight of the brain. *See* brain weight
Wellbutrin. *See* bupropion HCl
Werdnig-Hoffmann paralysis (infantile
  progressive spinal muscular atrophy)
  240
Wernicke, Carl 63, 183, 292, **370–372**
Wernicke-Korsakoff syndrome 71, 116,
  178–179, **372**
Wernicke's aphasia 180, **372–373**
Wernicke's area 34, 63, 65, 80, 180,
  181, 372, 373, **373**
Wernicke's encephalopathy 14, 71, 132,
  372

West Nile encephalitis 131
Whipple's disease 116
white blood cells, communication by
  171
white matter 88, **373**
  color, reason for 152, 246
  damage to 161, 236, 301
  imaging of 207
  metachromatic leukodystrophy and
   125
  research on 150
  in spinal cord 336–337
Why Survive? Being Old in America
  (Butler) 8
Whytt, Robert 260
Willis, Thomas **373**
Wilson's disease 116, 242
WISC-IV. *See* Wechsler Intelligence Scale
  for Children–Fourth Edition
Wisconsin Card-Sorting Test **373**
witnesses to crime, questioning of 98
women, alcohol and 14
women's intuition 152
word recognition, fusiform gyrus and
  148
working memory, visual 368
WPPSI-III. *See* Wechsler Preschool and
  Primary Scale of Intelligence–Third
  Edition
writing. *See* agraphia; developmental
  writing disorder

X

Xanax (alprazolam) 20
xanthinol nicotinate **374**
X chromosome linked microcephaly
  232
X-rays 171, **374**. *See also*
  angiography; myelography;
  pneumoencephalography; tomography;
  ventriculography
XTC. *See* Ecstasy
Xyrem (sodium oxybate; gamma
  hydroxybutyrate; GHB) 250

Y

young adults, antidepressants and 32

Z

zatosetron **375**
zidovudine (AZT) 12, 229
zinc, and sense of smell 333
Zoghbi, Huda 315
zolmitriptan (Zomig) 234
Zoloft. *See* sertraline
Zomig (zolmitriptan) 234
Zyban. *See* bupropion HCl